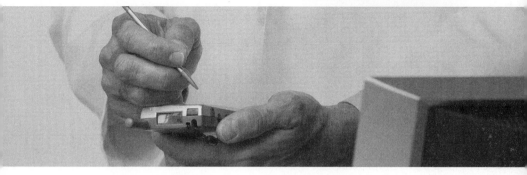

Handbook of Informatics for Nurses & Healthcare Professionals

Fourth Edition

Toni Hebda, RN, MNEd, PhD, MSIS
Professor of Nursing Programs
Chatham University, Pittsburgh, PA

Patricia Czar, RN
Information Systems Consultant
Pittsburgh, PA

PEARSON
Prentice
Hall

Upper Saddle River, New Jersey 07458

Library of Congress Cataloging-in-Publication Data
Hebda, Toni.
   Handbook of informatics for nurses & healthcare professionals / Toni Hebda, Patricia
Czar.—4th ed.
     p. ; cm.
   Includes bibliographical references and index.
   ISBN-13: 978-0-13-504394-3
   ISBN-10: 0-13-504394-8
1. Nursing informatics—Handbooks, manuals, etc. 2. Medical informatics—Handbooks,
manuals, etc. I. Czar, Patricia. II. Title.
   [DNLM: 1. Medical Informatics. 2. Nursing. 3. Allied Health Personnel.
WY 26.5 H443h 2008]

RT50.5.H43 2009
610.73'0285—dc22   2008016034

Publisher: Julie Levin Alexander
Publisher's Assistant: Regina Bruno
Editor-in-Chief: Maura Connor
Assistant to Editor-in-Chief: Marion Gottlieb
Executive Editor: Pamela Lappies
Editorial Assistant: Sarah Wrocklage
Director of Marketing: Karen Allman
Marketing Manager: Francisco Del Castillo
Marketing Specialist: Michael Sirinides
Managing Editor: Patrick Walsh
Production Liaison: Anne Garcia
Operations Manager: Ilene Sanford

Development Editor: Michael Giacobbe
Creative Director: Christy Mahon
Senior Art Director: Maria Guglielmo-Walsh
Interior Design: Elm Street Publishing Services
Cover Design: Cheryl Asherman
Cover Illustration/Photo: Getty Images
Composition: Integra Software Services Pvt. Ltd.
Full-Service Project Management: Elm Street
Publishing Services
Cover Printer: Phoenix Color Corporation,
Hagerstown, MD
Printer/Binder: Bind-Right Graphics

Pearson Prentice Hall™ is a trademark of Pearson Education, Inc.
Pearson® is a registered trademark of Pearson plc
Prentice Hall® is a registered trademark of Pearson Education, Inc.

Pearson Education Ltd., London
Pearson Education Singapore, Pte. Ltd
Pearson Education, Canada, Inc. Toronto
Pearson Education–Japan
Pearson Education Australia PTY, Limited

Pearson Education North Asia Ltd., Hong Kong
Pearson Educación de Mexico, S.A. de C.V.
Pearson Education Malaysia, Pte. Ltd.
Pearson Education, Inc., Upper Saddle River, New Jersey

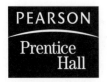

10 9 8 7 6 5 4 3 2 1
ISBN-13: 978-0-13-504394-3
ISBN-10: 0-13-504394-8

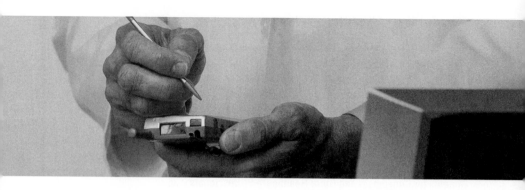

Contents

CHAPTER 2   Hardware, Software, and the Roles of Support Personnel   49

CHAPTER 3   Ensuring the Quality of Information   78

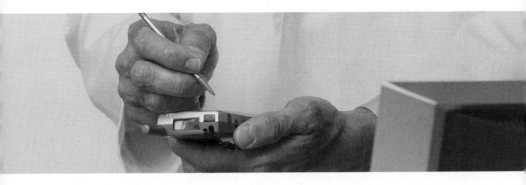

Preface

The original idea for this book came from the realization that there were few comprehensive sources available with practical information about computer applications and information systems in healthcare. From its inception this book was envisioned as a guide for nurses and other healthcare professionals who need to learn how to adapt and use computer applications in the workplace. As the outline developed, it became apparent that this book could also serve as an informatics text for students in the healthcare professions.

This fourth edition contains updates and revisions to reflect changes that have occurred in the rapidly evolving technology of health. The authors endeavor to provide an understanding of the concepts, skills, and tasks that are needed for healthcare professionals today and to achieve the national information technology goals set forth by President Bush in 2004 as a means to help transform our healthcare delivery system. Both of the primary authors have a long-standing interest and involvement in nursing informatics, having worked in the field, been active in informatics groups, and presented nationally and internationally.

Previous editions were accompanied by the *Internet Resource Guide for Nurses & Health Care Professionals*. For this edition we have integrated that material into the body of this text. The extensive listing of Web sites now resides on the Companion Website, along with many additional resources and activities.

ORGANIZATION

The book is divided into three sections: General Computer Information, Healthcare Information Systems, and Specialty Applications. The major themes of privacy, confidentiality, and information security are woven throughout the book.

The first section, General Computer Information, reviews information common to all information systems. It assumes no prior knowledge or experience with computers. Chapter 1 introduces informatics as an area of specialty, addresses major issues in healthcare that are driving the adoption of information technology, and talks about nurses as knowledge workers and the Technology Informatics Guiding Education Reform (TIGER) initiative as a means to transform the profession by establishing informatics competencies for all nurses. Chapter 1 has been revised to reflect the growing move toward transparency in healthcare and technology as a tool to improve healthcare delivery, improve retention of nurses, and support the journey to magnet status. Chapter 2 reviews basic information and terminology related to computer hardware and software and includes an updated section on computer and information services support positions that reflects new and changing roles. There is a section on mobile and handheld devices. Chapter 3 emphasizes the significance of good data integrity and management. It also addresses the burgeoning area of data mining and its applications within the healthcare delivery system. Chapter 4 addresses basic Internet use to support healthcare including basic search strategies and criteria for evaluating the quality of online information. Additional information on Internet use and resources is found in the appendices at the end of the book.

The second section, Healthcare Information Systems, covers information and issues related to the use of computers and information systems in healthcare. This section bridges the gap between the theory and practice of nursing informatics. Chapter 5 covers basic information on healthcare information systems, including computerized provider order entry (sometimes referred to as computerized physician or provider order entry), decision support, and expert systems. It has been updated to include physician practice management systems and longterm and homecare systems. Chapters 6 through 15 discuss all aspects of selecting, implementing, and operating these systems. Chapters 6 through 8 discuss the processes of overall and system strategic planning, system selection, and implementation. Content was added to Chapter 6 to reflect the growing recognition of the need to integrate information technology into the strategic plan of the organization. Chapter 7 provides practical advice on the selection of an information system while Chapter 8 discusses implementation and routine maintenance. The new Chapter 9 offers a fresh perspective on information systems training from a nurse working in the training venue at a large medical center. Chapter 10 discusses information security and confidentiality; it includes practical information on ways to protect information housed on mobile devices. Chapter 11, System Integration and Interoperability, addresses issues that impact the exchange of data from one information system to another as well as their significance for healthcare professionals. Chapter 12, The Electronic Health Record, discusses the components of the electronic record and introduces the concept of the personal health record. Chapter 13 is a new chapter on Regional Health Information Organizations (RHIOs), which have been identified as a key step in the process of developing a birth-to-death electronic record for every individual with information that is accessible to providers dealing with an increasingly mobile population. Chapter 14, Regulatory and Accreditation Issues, discusses key legislation for healthcare information systems such as the Health Insurance Portability and Accountability Act (HIPAA) and the Patriot Act and identity theft issues as well as recent developments that impact reimbursement. Chapter 15, Continuity Planning and Disaster Recovery, discusses the relationship between strategic planning for the organization and the significance of maintaining uninterrupted operations for patient care as well as legal requirements to maintain and restore information. Much of Chapter 15 is geared to the professional working in information services or preparing to work in this area.

The third section covers three specialty applications of computers in healthcare. Chapter 16 discusses ways that computers can support healthcare education. It contains content on Web-based education as well as the use of wireless and handheld computers in education. Chapter 17, Telehealth, discusses the applications and issues associated with this area of practice with a special section on telenursing. Chapter 18 looks at ways that informatics can support evidence-based practice and healthcare research.

Three appendices are included at the end of the book. The first two provide detailed information on getting up and running on the Internet and using the Internet to perform a job search. The third appendix provides suggested responses to the case studies that are found at the end of each chapter.

FEATURES

Each chapter contains pedagogical aids that help the readers learn and apply the information discussed.

Learning Objectives: Learning Objectives are listed at the beginning of each chapter to let the readers know what they can expect to learn from their study of it.

Future Directions: As the last heading in each chapter, Future Directions forecasts how the topic covered in the chapter might evolve in the upcoming decades.

Case Study Exercises: Case studies at the end of each chapter discuss common, real-life applications that review and reinforce the concepts presented in the chapter.

MediaLink: At the end of each chapter, the MediaLink box encourages students to use the Companion Website (www.prenhall.com/hebda) to apply what they have learned in multiple-choice review questions, discussion questions, case studies, and other interactive exercises, as well as additional resources. The purpose of the MediaLink feature is to further enhance the student experience, build on knowledge gained from the textbook, and foster critical thinking.

Summary: To assist in the review of the chapter, the Summary at the end of each chapter highlights the key concepts and information from the chapter.

References: Resources used in the chapter are listed at the end.

Glossary: The Glossary at the back of the book serves to familiarize readers with the vocabulary used in this book and in healthcare informatics.

We recognize that healthcare professionals have varying degrees of computer and informatics knowledge. This book does not assume that the reader has prior knowledge of computers. All computer terms are defined in the chapter, in the Glossary at the end of the book, and on the Companion Website.

HOW TO USE THIS BOOK

This book may be used in the following different ways:

- It may be read from cover to cover for a comprehensive view of nursing informatics.
- Specific chapters may be read according to reader interest or need.
- It may serve as a reference for nurses and other clinicians involved in system design, selection and implementation, and ongoing maintenance.
- It may be useful for the educator or researcher who wants to make better use of information technology.
- It can serve as a review for the American Nurses Association's Informatics Credentialing examination.

RESOURCES

Companion Website (www.prenhall.com/hebda): The Companion Website offers additional case studies, review questions, discussion questions, and other interactive exercises, as well as links to other Websites and other related items of interest for each chapter. Toni Hebda wrote and compiled all material for the Companion Website.

TestGen Test Bank: Twenty-five questions for instructors to use for assessment are provided for each chapter. They are available for download at the Prentice Hall Website, in the Instructor's Resource Center (www.prenhall.com).

PowerPoint Lecture Slides: Author-written PowerPoint slides accompany each chapter for use in classroom presentations and for student review.

Course Management Systems: Educators using this book to introduce students to the world of informatics will find materials available for course management systems that include instructor and student online course materials. For more information about adopting an online course management solution to accompany *Handbook of Informatics for Nurses &*

Healthcare Professionals, Fourth Edition, please contact your Pearson Education Sales Representative or go online to the appropriate Website below and select "Course," then "Nursing," and search for the book cover and select "Adopt Now" or "Preview."

WebCT: *http://cms.prenhall.com/webct/index.html*

BlackBoard: *http://cms.prenhall.com/blackboard/index.html*

Toni Hebda

Patricia Czar

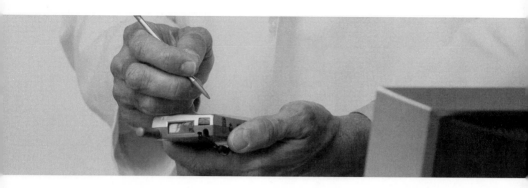

Acknowledgments

We acknowledge our gratitude first and foremost to our families, especially our mothers, for their support as we wrote and revised this book. We are excited to have work from our contributors in this edition. We are grateful to our co-workers and professional colleagues who provided encouragement and support throughout the process of conceiving and writing this book. We appreciate the many helpful comments offered by our reviewers. Finally, we thank Pamela Lappies, Executive Acquisitions Editor; Michael Giacobbe, Development Editor; Sarah Wrocklage, Editorial Assistant; and Anne Garcia, Production Liaison; and the staff at Pearson Health Science for their encouragement, suggestions, and support as we developed this fourth edition. Many thanks to Amanda Grant, Project Editor at Elm Street, for her part in production.

When we first started to write together, we knew each other only on a professional basis. As we worked on this book, we found that different professional backgrounds, experiences, and personalities complemented each other well and added to the quality of the final product. The best part of this project, however, has been the friendship that we have developed as we have worked together.

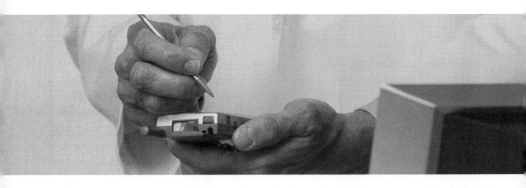

Contributors

This edition brings in work from contributors for a fresh look at informatics applications in education, as a support for evidence-based practice and research and information system training.

Terri L. Calderone, EdD, RN
Chapter 9: Information Systems Training
Dr. Calderone has a background in information technology, nursing informatics, and corporate training and development. Her professional experience includes clinical information systems design for hospital and outpatient applications and the development of a corporate university for a large business organization. She currently serves as Manager of Nursing Informatics, Excela Health, Greensburg, Pennsylvania. Her interests include instructional technology, strategic planning, and designing e-learning for nursing education. She earned a baccalaureate nursing degree and graduate degree in education from Pennsylvania State University. She earned a doctoral degree in Instructional Technology and Distance Education from Nova Southeastern University.

Dr. Margaret Hansen, EdD, MSN, RN
Chapter 16: Using the Computer to Support Healthcare and Patient Education
Dr. Hansen has written and presented extensively on informatics applications in education and has developed several multimedia educational programs. Dr. Hansen is an Associate Professor at the University of San Francisco. She earned her undergraduate nursing degree from Seton Hall University, a Master's in Nursing Science degree from San Jose State University, and her Doctorate in Education from the University of San Francisco. Dr. Hansen holds post-Master's certificates in Nursing Informatics from Duquesne University and Distance Education from the University of Wisconsin-Madison. She is currently Visiting Associate Professor at the University of Technology, Sydney.

Dr. Dee McGonigle, MSN, PhD
Chapter 16: Using the Computer to Support Healthcare and Patient Education—section on personal digital assistants (PDAs)
Dr. McGonigle presently serves as Editor-in-Chief of the *Online Journal of Nursing Informatics* (OJNI). She is an Associate Professor of Nursing and Information Sciences and Technology at Pennsylvania State University and a valued colleague from shared time together in a local user's group called Tri-State Nursing Computer Network. Dr. McGonigle earned her baccalaureate nursing degree at Pennsylvania State University, her MSN from Indiana University of Pennsylvania, and her PhD in Education from the University of Pittsburgh. She has authored numerous publications on informatics.

Dr. Carol Patton, MSN, PhD
Chapter 18: Evidence-Based Practice and Research
Dr. Patton is a Professor and the Director of Nursing Programs at Chatham University in Pittsburgh, Pennsylvania. Her expertise is varied, including teaching nursing skills, primary prevention, and outcome assessment and research. She has also managed faculty development, and designed, promoted, and developed research and nursing scholarship in a variety of higher education settings. Dr. Patton also does consulting focusing on feasibility and accreditation studies for nursing and health science programs. She received her Doctorate of Public Health from the University of Pittsburgh, Master's of Science in Nursing, West Virginia University, and Bachelor's of Science in Nursing, Pennsylvania State University. She is a National League for Nursing Certified Nurse Educator (CNE) as well as ANCC Family Nurse Practitioner. Dr. Patton has conducted international research focusing on primary prevention in Nicaragua. Dr. Patton designed and implemented the RN – BSN, the Master of Science in Nursing, and the Doctor of Nursing Practice programs at Chatham.

MEDIA CONTRIBUTOR

TestGen Test Bank Questions
Mary Ruth Hassett, PhD, RN-BC
Division Chair and Professor
Nursing and Health Sciences
Lewis-Clark State College
Lewiston, Idaho

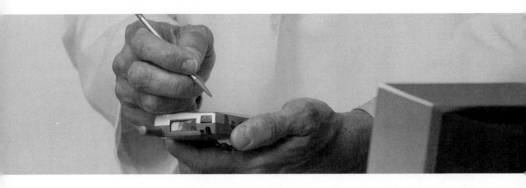

Reviewers

Mary T. Boylston, RN, MSN, EdD
Chair and Professor
Eastern University
St. Davids, Pennsylvania

Mary Ruth Hassett, PhD, RN-BC
Division Chair and Professor
Nursing & Health Sciences
Lewis-Clark State College
Lewiston, Idaho

Carol Kilmon, PhD, RN
Associate Professor
The University of Texas at Tyler
Tyler, Texas

Helen Lerner, RN, EdD, CPNP
Associate Professor and Coordinator
Lehman College
Bronx, New York

Sharon Loury, BSN, MSN, PhD, RN
Assistant Professor
East Carolina University
Greenville, North Carolina

Darlene Mathis, DNP, CRNP
Nurse Practitioner
Sylacauga Pediatrics
Sylacauga, Alabama

Rhonda Reed, RN, MSN, CRRN
Instructor, Technology Coordinator,
Staff Nurse
Indiana State University
Terre Haute, Indiana

Leanne M. Waterman, MS, RN, FNP
Assistant Professor
Onondaga Community College
Syracuse, New York

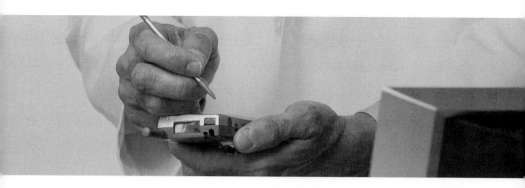

About the Authors

Toni Hebda, RN, MN Ed, PhD, MSIS, is the Professor of Nursing Programs at Chatham University, Pittsburgh, PA. She has worked as a system analyst for a major healthcare delivery system and previously taught a nursing informatics certificate program at Duquesne University School of Nursing. Her interest in informatics provided a focus for her dissertation and subsequently led her to help establish a regional nursing informatics support group and obtain a graduate degree in information science and ANCC certification as informatics nurse. She is a reviewer for the *Online Journal of Nursing Informatics.*

Patricia Czar, RN, is an Information Systems Consultant. She has been active in informatics for more than 25 years, serving as manager of clinical systems at a major medical center where she was responsible for planning, design, implementation, and ongoing support for all of the clinical information systems. She has been an active member of several informatics groups and has presented nationally and internationally. Ms. Czar has served as mentor for nursing and health informatics students and has a Microcomputer Specialist certificate.

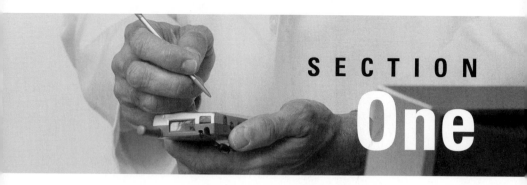

SECTION
One

General Computer Information

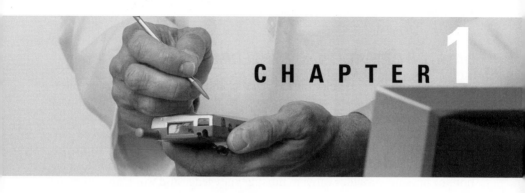

Informatics in the Healthcare Professions

After completing this chapter, you should be able to:

1 Define the terms *data*, *information*, *knowledge*, and *wisdom*.

2 Describe the role of the nurse as knowledge worker.

3 Discuss the significance of good information and knowledge management for healthcare delivery, the healthcare disciplines, and healthcare consumers.

4 Distinguish between *medical informatics, nursing informatics*, and *consumer informatics*.

5 Differentiate between *computer* and *information literacy*.

6 Discuss the TIGER Initiative and contrast the different informatics competencies needed for nurses entering into practice, experienced nurses, and informatics nurses and nurse specialists.

7 Discuss the relationship between major issues in healthcare and the deployment of information technology.

8 Identify characteristics that define nursing informatics as a specialty area of practice.

9 Provide specific examples of how nursing informatics impacts the healthcare consumer as well as professional practice, administration, education, and research.

10 Forecast the roles that nursing informatics and health information technology will play in the healthcare delivery system 5 years from now.

11 Compare the types of educational opportunities available in nursing informatics.

DATA, INFORMATION, KNOWLEDGE, AND WISDOM

During the course of any day, nurses handle large amounts of data and information and apply knowledge. This is true for all nurses, whether they provide direct care or serve as administrators, educators, researchers, or in some other capacity. Informatics provides tools to help process, manage, and analyze data and information collected for the purposes of documenting and improving patient care, as well as to support knowledge that adds to the scientific foundation for nursing, provides value to nursing knowledge and work, and improves the public image for nursing by building a knowledge-based identity for nurses (ANA 2007).

Data are a collection of numbers, characters, or facts that are gathered according to some perceived need for analysis and possibly action at a later point in time (Anderson 1992). Examples of data include a client's vital signs. Other examples of data are the length of hospital stay for each client; the client's race, marital, or employment status; and next of kin. Sometimes this type of data may be given a numeric or alphabetic code, as shown in Table 1–1.

A single piece of datum has little meaning. However, a collection of data can be examined for patterns and structure that can be interpreted (Saba and McCormick 1996; Warman 1993). **Information** is data that have been interpreted. For example, individual temperature readings are data. When they are plotted onto a graph, the client's change in temperature over time and comparison with normal values become evident, thus becoming information. Table 1–2 provides examples of data and information. Although it is possible to determine whether individual values (data) fall within the normal range, the collection of several values over time creates a pattern, which in this case demonstrates the presence of a low-grade fever (information).

TABLE 1–1	Example of Coded Data: Employment Status Codes	
Code	**Status**	**Explanation**
1	Employed full-time	Individual states that he or she is employed full-time.
2	Employed part-time	Individual states that he or she is employed part-time.
3	Not employed	Individual states that he or she is not employed full-time or part-time.
4	Self-employed	Self-explanatory
5	Retired	Self-explanatory
6	On active military duty	Self-explanatory
7	Unknown	Individual's employment status is unknown.

TABLE 1–2   Examples of Data and Information

Time	Temperature	Pulse	Respirations
7 AM	37.8° C	88	24
12 NOON	38.9° C	96	24
4 PM	38° C	84	22
8 PM	37.2° C	83	20

(The values in the table above represent data: a client's vital signs over the course of a day. Each individual value is limited in meaning. The pattern of the values represents information, which is more useful to the healthcare provider.)

Data and information are collected when nurses record the following activities:

- Initial client history and allergies
- Initial and ongoing physical assessment
- Vital signs such as blood pressure and temperature
- Response to treatment
- Client response and comprehension of educational activities

Knowledge is a more complex concept. **Knowledge** is the synthesis of information derived from several sources to produce a single concept or idea. It is based on a logical process of analysis and provides order to thoughts and ideas and decreases uncertainty (Ayer 1966; Engelhardt 1980). It is dynamic and derives meaning from its context (Steyn 2004). Validation of information provides knowledge that can be used again. Historically, nursing has acquired knowledge through tradition, authority, borrowed theory, trial and error, personal experience, role modeling, reasoning, and research. Current demands for safer, cost-effective, quality care require evidence of the best practices supported by research. Computers and information technology provide tools that aid data collection and the analysis associated with research to support the overall work of nurses. **Information technology** (IT) is a general term used to refer to the management and processing of information with the assistance of computers.

An example of knowledge can be seen in the determination of the most effective nursing interventions for the prevention of skin breakdown. If a research study produces data related to the prevention of skin breakdown achieved through specific interventions, these data can be collected and analyzed. The trends or patterns depicted by the data provide information regarding which treatment is more effective than others in preventing skin breakdown. The validation of this information through repeated studies provides knowledge that nurses can use to prevent skin breakdown in their clients.

Wisdom occurs when knowledge is used appropriately to manage and solve problems (Ackoff 1989; ANA 2007). It results from understanding and requires human effort. The trip from data to wisdom is neither automatic nor smooth (Murray 2000). Wisdom comes from cumulative experiences, as the result of learning skills and ways of thinking that can be viewed as predecessors to wisdom, and via the creation of conditions that help participants to use their accumulated knowledge effectively (Gluck & Baltes 2006). It represents the human part of the equation in the move along the continuum from data to information to knowledge to wisdom.

Large-scale use of data, information, and knowledge requires that they be accessible. Traditionally, client data and information have been handwritten in an unstructured format on paper and placed in multiple versions of the patient record at hospitals, clinics, physician offices, and long-term and home health agencies. This process makes the location, abstraction, and comparison of information slow and difficult, limiting the creation of knowledge. Increasingly demands for improvements in healthcare delivery call for the use of information for quality measurement and improvement, research, and education through information technology as a means to automate and share information. Technology exists to move from paper-based to computer-based records. It is essential that nurses collaborate with technical personnel to plan what information to include, the source of the information, and how it will be used. Nurses must be active participants in the design of automated documentation to ensure that information is recorded appropriately and in a format that can be accessed and useful to all healthcare providers. Nurses also have a responsibility to safeguard the security and privacy of client information via education, policy, and technical means.

In 1994, Harsanyi, Lehmkuhl, Hott, Myers, and McGeehan argued that understanding current and evolving technology for the management and processing of nursing information helps the nursing profession assume a leadership position in health reform. That argument remains true now. If nurses understand the power of informatics, they can play an active role in evaluating and improving the quality of care, cost containment, and other consumer benefits. For example, nurses who are able to understand and use an information system that analyzes trends in client outcomes and cost can initiate appropriate changes in care. Nurses empowered by IT may also design computer applications that enhance client education, such as individualized discharge instructions, medication instructions and information, and information about diagnostic procedures. In these and other ways, nurses can integrate IT into nursing practice and administration as a means to manage client care, document observations, and monitor client outcomes for ongoing improvement of quality.

Nurses also handle information in the roles of educator and researcher. For example, educators must track information about students' classroom and clinical performance. Computers facilitate this process and allow educators to compare individuals with group norms. Nursing education must also prepare students to handle data. This is accomplished in several steps: teaching basic computer and information literacy, using nursing information systems, realizing the significance of automated data collection for quality assurance purposes, and recognizing the benefits of using computers to manage clinical data for research.

Researchers use computers to expedite the collection and analysis of data. One possible project, for example, uses data obtained from nursing documentation systems to study the relationship between frequent turning and positioning and the client's skin integrity. Nursing information systems are rich in data to support this type of research, and the growing prevalence of information systems increases research opportunities. As a result, nurses can expand the scientific base of their profession.

THE NURSE AS KNOWLEDGE WORKER

Healthcare professionals need to know more today to perform their daily jobs than at any previous point in history. Healthcare delivery systems are knowledge-intensive settings with nurses as the largest group of knowledge workers within those systems. Advancements in knowledge, skills, interventions, and drugs are growing at an exponential rate. This makes it impossible for any one individual to keep up with all the knowledge needed to practice nursing or any of the other healthcare disciplines without making use of available resources and continuing education. Unfortunately there is a failure on the part of the present healthcare delivery system to consistently translate new knowledge into practice and apply new technologies safely, appropriately, and expediently (IOM 2007). Several years typically elapse before new knowledge and advancements make it into the clinical setting. At the same time, the acuity level of clients continues to rise, changing the actual work that healthcare workers do and how they do it. One constant in this scenario is the ongoing need for knowledge and evidence. Information technology (IT) can bridge the gap as healthcare delivery continues its evolution from a task-based to a knowledge-based industry. Nurses need to be adept at using patient-centered IT tools to access information to expand their knowledge in a just-in-time, evidence-based fashion. There must be a shift from critical thinking to critical synthesis. In short nurses must optimize their value as intellectual capital (Haase-Herrick & Herrin 2007; Simpson 2007). Work must also be done to develop workload measurements for knowledge workers. Pesut (2006) notes that a change has occurred in the nursing process and how nurses represent clinical thinking. The development of standardized nursing languages, electronic record systems, and sophisticated analyses all serve to facilitate this transformation to knowledge work.

The nurse assumes several roles during the course of client care (Snyder-Halpern et al. 2001). Each role requires a different level of decision making and a different type of decision support. These roles include:

- *Data gatherer.* In this role the nurse collects clinical data such as vital signs.
- *Information user.* The nurse interprets and structures clinical data, such as a client's report of experienced pain, into information that can then be used to aid clinical decision making and patient monitoring over time. Quality assurance and infection control activities exemplify other ways in which nurses use information to detect patterns.

- *Knowledge user.* This role is seen when individual patient data are compared with existing nursing knowledge.
- *Knowledge builder.* Nurses display this role when they aggregate clinical data and show patterns across patients that serve to create new knowledge or can be interpreted within the context of existing nursing knowledge.

IT can support the nurse in each of these roles. Computerized assessment and documentation forms facilitate data collection by including prompts to help nurses to remember questions that they should ask and facts that should be recorded. These same tools strengthen the quality of clinical databases. The data gatherer role is also facilitated when input from monitoring devices is fed directly into clinical documentation systems. The information user role is supported when computer capability quickly discerns patterns that help translate data into information. This saves time and labor for the nurse and provides useful information in a timely fashion. Applications to support the knowledge user in clinical settings at the point of care are becoming more prevalent. These might include clinical practice guidelines, expert systems to support decision making, or research that supports evidence-based care and/or online drug databases. Although clinical information systems have the capability to aggregate data, this capability is not available at the bedside in all facilities. Knowledge builders examine aggregate data for relationships among variables and interventions. According to Davenport, Thomas, and Cantrell (2002), managers of knowledge workers have the responsibility to optimize the work process through improvements in design of the workplace as well as the application of technology. The unfortunate reality is that resource allocation for health information technology has lagged behind other industries and the current healthcare environment has yet to fully realize its potential. IT can streamline paperwork, transform data into information and knowledge, and eliminate redundancy. A recent survey of American hospitals found that almost one third of the best facilities also had the most advanced information technology (Fischman 2006; Sensmeier 2006).

As healthcare delivery systems continue to evolve additional changes in the ways that nurses and other healthcare professionals work are expected. The next expected metamorphosis is from knowledge worker to self-directed innovator. The innovator uses a holistic view, works across settings, and is enabled by access to information. This information is derived from multiple sources and formats but ideally may be accessed from a single platform (Hulford, Gough, & Krieger 2007).

THE SIGNIFICANCE OF GOOD INFORMATION AND KNOWLEDGE MANAGEMENT

Good information management ensures access to the right information at the right time to the people who need it. Vast amounts of information are produced daily. This information may or may not be readily available when it is needed. Its volume exceeds the processing capacity of any single human being. Part of good information management ensures that care providers have the resources that they need to provide safe, efficient, quality care. Some examples of these resources include clinical guidelines, standards of practice, policy and procedure manuals, research findings, drug databases, and information on community resources. IT can help to ensure access to the most recent versions of these types of resources via tools such as intranets, electronic communities, or blogs (Watson 2007). This solution eliminates the uncertainties of whether reference books are available in all clinical areas of any given facility and whether all areas have the most recent version. Good information management also eliminates redundant data collection. Redundant data collection wastes time and irritates clients (HIMSS 2002).

Although the terms information management and knowledge management are sometimes used interchangeably, **knowledge management** refers to the creation of systems that enable organizations to tap into the knowledge, experiences, and creativity of their staff to improve their performance (Davidson & Voss 2002). It is a structured process for the generation, storage, distribution, and application of both tacit knowledge (personal experience) and explicit knowledge (evidence) in organizations (Sandars & Heller 2006).

THE DEFINITION AND EVOLUTION OF INFORMATICS

Informatics is the science and art of turning data into information. The term can be traced to a Russian document published in 1968 (Bemmel & Musen 1997). It is an adaptation of the French term *informatique,* which refers to "the computer milieu" (Saba 2001). Broadly, informatics has been defined as "the study of the application of computer and statistical techniques to the management of information" (Academic Medical Publishing & CancerWEB 1997). The term has been applied to various disciplines. **Medical informatics** refers to the application of informatics to all of the healthcare disciplines as well as to the practice of medicine. Some sources distinguish medical informatics from health informatics in the following manner. Medical informatics focuses primarily upon information technologies that involve patient care and medical decision making while health informatics refers to the use of educational technology for healthcare clients or the general public. Informatics has subsequently emerged as an area of specialization within the various healthcare disciplines and is one of the fastest growing career fields in healthcare. Overlap occurs among medical, dental, and nursing informatics primarily in the areas of information retrieval, ethics, patient care, decision support, human-to computer interactions, information systems, imaging, computer security, and computerized health records (Guenther & Caruth 2006). Table 1–3 displays some informatics terms and definitions; many are similar, but not all can be used interchangeably.

Nursing informatics may be broadly defined as the use of information and computer technology to support all aspects of nursing practice, including direct delivery of care, administration, education, and research. The definition of nursing informatics is evolving as advances occur in nursing practice and technology; there have been many different definitions throughout the years as the discipline has evolved. According to the American Nurses Association (ANA)

TABLE 1–3   Informatics Definitions

Informatics. The science and art of turning data into information.

Medical informatics. May be used to refer to the application of information science and technology to acquire, process, organize, interpret, store, use, and communicate medical data in all of its forms in medical education, practice and research, patient care, and health management; the term may also refer more broadly to the application of informatics to all of the healthcare disciplines as well as the practice of medicine.

Nursing informatics. Specialty "that integrates nursing science, computer science, and information science to manage and communicate data, information, knowledge and wisdom into nursing practice. Nursing informatics facilitates the integration of data, information, knowledge and wisdom to support patients, nurses, and other providers in their decision-making in all roles and settings. This support is accomplished through the use of information structures, information processes, and information technology" (American Nurses Association [ANA] 2007, p. 1).

Health informatics. The application of computer and information science in all basic and applied biomedical sciences to facilitate the acquisition, processing, interpretation, optimal use, and communication of health related data. The focus is the patient and the process of care, and the goal is to enhance the quality and efficiency of care provided.

Bioinformatics. The application of computer and information technology to the management of biological information including the development of databases and algorithms to facilitate research.

Consumer health informatics. Branch of medical informatics that studies the use of electronic information and communication to improve medical outcomes and the healthcare decision-making process from the patient/consumer perspective (AMIA May 3, 2007).

Dental informatics. Computer and information sciences to improve dental practice, research, education, and management.

Clinical health informatics. Multidisciplinary field that focuses on the enhancement of clinical information management at the point of healthcare through improvement of information processes, implementation of clinical information systems, and the use and evaluation of clinical decision support (CDS) tools as a means to improve the effectiveness, quality, and value of the services rendered.

Public health informatics. Application of information and computer science and technology to public health practice, research, and learning.

Sources: American Medical Informatics Association (AMIA) (May 3, 2007). Working Groups Consumer Health Informatics (CHI-WG). Retrieved May 31, 2007 from http://www.amia.org/mbrcenter/wg/chi/. Used by permission of AMIA.

(2001) and Staggers and Thompson (2002), these may be broken down into the following categories: 1) definitions with an information technology focus, 2) conceptually oriented definitions, and 3) definitions that focus on roles. Early definitions emphasized the role of technology. This may be seen in the statement by Scholes and Barber (1980) that nursing informatics is the "application of computer technology to all fields of nursing." Ball and Hannah (1984) later used a definition of medical informatics to define nursing informatics as the "collected informational technologies which concern themselves with the client care decision-making process performed by healthcare practitioners" (p. 3).

In 1985 Hannah added the role of the nurse within nursing informatics to the definition that she and Ball developed. It retained its technical focus. The emphasis on technology remained evident in several later definitions as well. Critics note that many definitions emphasize technology and downplay the role of the informatics nurse in processing information that can be done without the aid of a computer. Staggers and Thompson (2002) also note that when clients are mentioned, it is usually in the role of passive recipients of care rather than as active participants in the care process.

The conceptually driven definitions started to appear in the mid-1980s as models and relationships were added to definitions (ANA 2001; Staggers & Thompson 2002). Schwirian (1986) used Hannah's 1985 definition but added a model that depicted users, information, goals, and computer hardware and software connected by bidirectional arrows. Schwirian called for a solid foundation of nursing informatics knowledge built on research that was model driven and proactive rather than problem driven. Graves and Corcoran (1989, p. 227) built on Hannah's definition to include "a combination of computer science, information science and nursing science designed to assist in the management and processing of nursing data, information and knowledge to support the practice of nursing and the delivery of nursing care." This definition addressed the purpose of technology and provided a link between information and knowledge. It built on an earlier model developed by Graves and Corcoran. In 1996 Turley introduced his model, which shows nursing informatics using theory from cognitive science, computer science, and information science on a base of nursing science with information present at the point that all areas overlap.

Role-oriented definitions began to appear at the same time that nursing informatics gained acceptance as an area of specialty practice. In 1992 the ANA's Council on Computer Applications in Nursing incorporated the role of the informatics nurse specialist into a definition derived from work by Graves and Corcoran. According to this definition, the purpose of nursing informatics was "to analyze information requirements; design, implement and evaluate information systems and data structures that support nursing; and identify and apply computer technologies for nursing." The ANA revised its definition again in 1994 to "legitimize the specialty and to guide efforts to create a certification examination" (ANA 2001, p. 16). The 1994 definition follows.

> Nursing informatics is the specialty that integrates nursing science, computer science, and information science in identifying, collecting, processing, and managing data and information to support nursing practice, administration, education, research, and expansion of nursing knowledge. Nursing informatics supports the practice of all nursing specialties in all sites and settings whether at the basic or advanced level. The practice includes the development of applications, tools, processes, and structures that assist nurses with the management of data in taking care of patients or in supporting their practice of nursing. (p. 3)

The ANA revised its definition of nursing informatics again in 2001, noting the need to address the core elements of "nurse, patient, health environment, decision making and nursing data, information knowledge, information structures, and information technology" (p. 17). The ANA prepared its definition for North America. This definition attempted to recognize the more active role of the patient in his or her own care and to more clearly articulate the role of the informatics nurse in the healthcare environment. This definition follows:

> Nursing informatics is a specialty that integrates nursing science, computer science, and information science to manage and communicate data, information, and knowledge in nursing practice. Nursing informatics facilitates the integration of data, information and knowledge to support patients, nurses, and other providers in their decision making in all roles and settings. This support is accomplished through the use of information structures, information processes, and information technology. (ANA, 2001, p. 17)

Groups and individuals in other parts of the world continued their work on definitions as well. The Nursing Informatics Special Interest Group of the International Medical Informatics Association (2003) amended their definition of *nursing informatics* in 1998 to read that nursing informatics "is the integration of nursing, its information, and information management with information processing and communication technology, to support the health of people worldwide." At approximately the same time, a National Steering Committee in Canada solicited feedback via the National Nursing Informatics Project (Hebert 1999) from nursing organizations, educational institutions, and employers to arrive at the following definition for Canada.

> Nursing Informatics (NI) is the application of computer science and information science to nursing. NI promotes the generation, management and processing of relevant data in order to use information and develop knowledge that supports nursing in all practice domains. (p. 5)

Despite national differences, there was a consensus on the need for a definition to shape the specialty, obtain funding for studies, design educational programs, and help other disciplines define informatics practice within their own areas and to set expectations for employers (Hebert 1999; Staggers & Thompson 2002). There was also agreement that the goal of nursing informatics was to ensure that data collected and housed within automated record systems would be available as information that can be used by healthcare professionals at the bedside as well as by those in administrative and research positions (Newbold 2002).

In subsequent years the practice of nursing informatics has continued to evolve, leading to a review and revision of both the definition and scope of practice statements by the American Nurses Association (ANA 2007). This most recent definition incorporates the concept of wisdom to read as below:

> Nursing informatics is a specialty that integrates nursing science, computer science, and information science to manage and communicate data, information, knowledge and wisdom into nursing practice. Nursing informatics facilitates the integration of data, information, knowledge and wisdom to support patients, nurses, and other providers in their decision making in all roles and settings. This

support is accomplished through the use of information structures, information processes, and information technology. (ANA 2007, p. 1)

Medical Informatics, Nursing Informatics, and Consumer Informatics

Medical informatics is generally used as a broad term to include all the disciplines in the field with specific health-related areas beneath it, including nursing informatics and consumer informatics. Consumer informatics is driven by several factors including technological advances, an increasingly Internet-savvy population, a need for increased accountability in the selection of healthcare services, an acceptance of online and telephone transactions in lieu of face-to-face interactions, concerns for safety, the advent of health savings accounts, and a change in the revenue model that calls for individuals to assume greater responsibility for payment for services (Singh, Hummel, & Walton 2005).

COMPUTER AND INFORMATION LITERACY

The terms *computer literacy* and *information literacy* are not synonymous. **Computer literacy** is a popular term used to refer to a familiarity with the use of personal computers, including the use of software tools such as word processing, spreadsheets, databases, presentation graphics, and e-mail. The majority of students admitted to nursing schools now enter with some level of computer literacy.

Information literacy has a broader meaning. Information literacy is defined as the ability to recognize when information is needed as well as the skills to find, evaluate, and use needed information effectively (Association of College and Research Libraries [ACRL] 2002). Information literacy is particularly important in today's environment of rapid technological change and knowledge growth, with information available from many sources and in different formats, including text, graphics, and audio. Information literacy is important to all disciplines because it forms the basis for ongoing learning. In its related, definition of information and communication literacy, the Educational Testing Service (ETS) (2007) focuses on the ability to use digital technology, communication tools, and networks as tools to problem solve and communicate, and to maintain a fundamental understanding of ethical and legal issues. In healthcare the definition of information literacy must also include an awareness of the conceptual differences between various classifications and standardized languages, critical thinking skills, the ability to use the tools offered by technology to solve information problems, as well as an understanding of the ethical and legal issues surrounding the access and use of information (Kisilowska 2006; Skiba 2005).

The significance of information literacy for nursing is that it represents an important step in promoting evidence-based nursing practice because the information literate nurse can weigh the quality and significance of research findings for application (DiCecco 2005). Despite the recognition of information literacy as a bridge to evidence-based practice the connection is not automatic. Problems include a lack of awareness of the importance of evidence-based practice, inconsistent role modeling by RNs, a lack of comfort in using database searches, and a lack of exposure to evidence-based clinical practice (Courey, Benson-Soros, Deemer, & Zeller 2006; Pravikoff, Tanner, & Pierce 2005).

In a survey of U.S. nurses to determine perceptions of access to tools to obtain evidence and assess skill levels with these tools, Pravikoff, Tanner, and Pierce (2005) found that the majority of respondents recognized the need for information to support practice but the most frequently consulted resources included peers and general searches of the Internet. There was limited use of established bibliographic databases or crucial evaluation of research findings for application in practice. The majority of the respondents had never conducted a database search and claimed that they had never received instruction in the use of electronic resources. While the researchers noted that the majority of participants had graduated prior to the mid 1980s, these findings raise questions about the true levels of information literacy among practicing nurses and have led many nursing leaders to call for an evaluation of nursing curricula for the incorporation of information literacy and evidence-based practice. In another study of undergraduate nursing programs McNeil et al. (2005) found that approximately one-half of undergraduate nursing programs were teaching information literacy skills and required students to enter with proficiency in word processing and e-mail. However the inclusion of content on data standards and unified language systems was less obvious. Another study that relied upon self-reports by baccalaureate students found a significant improvement in skills over an 8-year period ending in 2005 but concluded that nursing education may not be providing entry level nurses with all the skills needed in today's technology rich environment, noting low reported levels of experience with databases, spreadsheets, and statistical packages (McDowell & Ma 2007).

This situation has ramifications for both nursing education and current practice. Ornes and Gassert (2007) found nursing faculty to be the greatest block to incorporating technology into curricula. Faculty need to examine their own knowledge and skills in information literacy, attitudes, the incorporation of information literacy throughout the curriculum, and assessment measures for information literacy. An important part of this evaluation includes consideration of how these foundation level skills are used and whether students and graduates progress to the critical review of research and its application into practice (Booth 2006; Skiba 2005). Institutions also need to put mechanisms into place to help develop information literacy among staff and to encourage evidence-based practice (McBride 2006).

INFORMATICS COMPETENCIES FOR NURSES

In past years there was little agreement on the skills required for informatics competencies and the level of competencies required for each level of practice. This situation made it difficult for educators and employers to ensure that all nurses possessed appropriate skills. Arnold (1996) noted the need for familiarity with presentation graphics, data analysis, and decision support for administrators and educators. In 1998 the American Association of Colleges of Nursing (AACN) identified information management as a skill needed by baccalaureate nursing graduates. More specifically, the AACN wanted graduates to be able to use existing and evolving methods of discovering, retrieving, and using information in their practice. This requirement was partially addressed through the requirement for courses in basic computer skills as a gateway to information literacy and information management skills. Hobbs' (2002) review of previous studies of informatics competencies found conceptual, methodology, and measurement problems that made it difficult to make generalizations across the research, although there was agreement that nurses should have skills in basic word processing and the ability to use databases, spreadsheets, document care, and e-mail. Yee (2002) found that employers wanted graduates to have these skills as well as Internet search skills and the ability to use statistical software, clinical information systems, and scheduling systems. Heller, Oros, and Durney-Crowley (2003) saw a need for nurses to be adept at accessing patient information in electronic records and the use of telehealth applications. Garde, Harrison, and Hovenga (2005) called for the development of a comprehensive health informatics education framework for nurses as well as other health professionals. An increasing number of nursing leaders have called for greater attention to the development of informatics competencies, including information literacy, as a necessary stepping stone to evidence-based practice (Barton 2005; Desjardins, Cook, Jenkins, & Bakken 2005; Dreher & Miller 2006; Skiba 2005). McDowell and Ma (2007) emphasized the need for competence in e-mail, Web surfing, database searches, spreadsheets, and statistical analysis.

Other compelling reasons for the development of informatics competencies include the fact that the way that health information is accessed is changing as a result of the Internet and the migration toward electronic records. The federal mandate that all Americans have an electronic medical record by 2014 makes informatics competencies necessary for all healthcare professionals (Ornes & Gassert 2007). Nurses also need familiarity with spreadsheets and statistics software and analysis for use in quality improvement activities, the creation and monitoring of budgets, and a better understanding of research findings (McDowell & Ma 2007). The tools and technology that nurses need to perform their work efficiently are also changing.

Work on the identification of informatics competencies is ongoing and there is a growing consensus upon required skills. Several parties—including individual researchers, academics, employers, and various professional organizations such as the American Nurses Association, the American Medical Informatics Association, the Nursing Informatics Working Group of the Healthcare Information Management System Society (HIMSS), the National League for Nursing Task Group on Informatics Competencies, the Healthcare Leadership Alliance (HLA), and the Alliance for Nursing Informatics (ANI)—have turned their attention to this issue. Informatics competencies are deemed essential as a means to facilitate the delivery of safer, more efficient care, to add to the knowledge base for the profession, and to transition toward evidence-based practice (Smedley 2005). The *Scope and Standards of Nursing Informatics Practice* (ANA 2007) includes an updated matrix of competencies that expands upon earlier work by Staggers, Gasser, and Curran. The ANA document categorizes competencies into one of three areas—computer literacy, information literacy, and professional development/leadership—considering the knowledge and skills needed at each level of practice.

Weiner and Trangenstein (2006) noted that public health nursing leaders need informatics skills particularly since many of them graduated in an era when informatics was not recognized as a necessary part of their curriculum. With informatics skills, they will have the ability to work more efficiently, provide greater influence on public policy, and better respond to public health threats including bioterrorism.

The Technology Informatics Guiding Education Reform (TIGER) Initiative

The TIGER Initiative emerged from a national gathering of leaders from nursing administration, practice, education, informatics, technology, and government, as well as other key stakeholders, who realized that nursing must transform itself as a profession to realize the benefits that electronic patient records can provide (HIMSS Nursing Task Force 2007; Sensmeier 2007; TIGER 2007). Its purpose was to create a vision for the future of nursing to provide safer, higher quality patient care through the use of information technology. It requires informatics competencies for every nurse and active involvement in advancing health information technology. The group identified leadership, education, technology-enabled processes that facilitate teamwork and relationships throughout the care continuum, systems that support education and practice, and a supportive culture and policies as key factors to attain this vision. It was funded by federal funds and grants from the Robert Wood Johnson Foundation. The TIGER Initiative called for the redesign of nursing education to keep up with rapid changes in technology, active participation by nurses in the design of informatics tools, and increased visibility by nurses in the national health IT agenda. It organized teams to work toward the common goals, obtained additional funding, developed workplans and outcomes for each team, and identified informatics competencies for all levels of nursing personnel, including nursing assistants. Achievement of the TIGER initiative is particularly important as healthcare providers move toward adoption of all-electronic records by 2014.

Entry-Level Core Competencies

The beginning nurse focuses primarily on developing and using skills that rely upon the ability to retrieve and enter data in an electronic format that is relevant to patient care, the analysis and interpretation of information as part of planning care, the use of informatics applications designed for nursing practice, and the implementation of policies relevant to information. The *Scope and*

Standards of Nursing Informatics Practice (ANA 2007) calls for the following competencies for the beginning nurse:

- Basic computer literacy, including the ability to use basic desktop applications and electronic communication.
- The ability to use information technology to support clinical and administrative processes, which presumes information literacy to support evidence-based practice.
- The ability to access data and perform documentation via computerized patient records.
- The ability to support patient safety initiatives via the use of information technology.
- Recognition of the role of informatics in nursing.

The Experienced Nurse

The experienced nurse builds upon the competencies required for entry-level practitioners using basic computer skills to information regarding the patient. This practitioner has the expertise to serve as a content expert in system design; to see relationships among data elements; to execute judgments based on observed data patterns; to safeguard access to quality of information; and to participate in efforts to improve information management and communication. The ANA (2007) has identified competencies to include:

- Proficiency in his or her area of specialization and the use of IT and computers to support that area of practice including quality improvement and other related activities (ANA 2007).
- Knowledge representation methodologies for evidence-based practice.
- The ability to use information systems and work with informatics specialists to enact system improvements.
- Proficiency in using evidence-based databases.
- The promotion of innovative applications of technology in healthcare.

The Informatics Nurse

This individual has advanced preparation in information management and possesses the following skills (ANA 2007):

- Proficiency with informatics applications to support all areas of nursing practice including quality improvement activities, research, project management, system design, development, analysis, implementation, support, maintenance, and evaluation.
- Fiscal management.
- Integration of multidisciplinary language/standards of practice.
- Skills in critical thinking, data management and processing, decision making, and system development and computer skills.
- The identification and provision of data for decision making.

The Informatics Nurse Specialist (INS)

The INS possesses a sophisticated level of understanding and skills in information management and computer technology, demonstrating most of the competencies seen at the previous three levels. The INS is the innovator who sees the broad vision of what is possible and how it may be attained. The *Scope and Standards of Practice* (ANA 2007) calls for educational preparation for the INS that enables him or her to conduct informatics research and generate informatics theory. This preparation and expertise makes the INS well suited to work in a variety of areas and functional roles including project management and administration.

THE PUSH FOR PATIENT SAFETY

Patient safety is a priority for health systems, professionals, and consumers around the world. In 2004 the World Health Organization (Joint Commission International Center for Patient Safety 2007; WHO 2007) launched the World Alliance for Patient Safety in response to a World Health Assembly Resolution urging WHO and Member States to consider the problem of patient safety. The Alliance addressed 10 major action issues, which included a focus on new technologies as a means to improve patient safety. In 2005 WHO designated the Joint Commission and Joint Commission International (JCI) as a WHO Collaborating Centre on Patient Safety Solutions. The Collaborating Centre established an international network of experts and organizations with expertise in patient safety to identify, evaluate, adapt, and disseminate patient safety solutions across the globe. WHO defines patient safety solutions as "any system design or intervention that has demonstrated the ability to prevent or mitigate patient harm stemming from the processes of healthcare." The Centre plans to identify problems and present evidence-based solutions along with supporting documentation. In 2007 the International Steering Committee of the Centre approved solutions for the following:

- look-alike, sound-alike medication names
- patient identification
- communication during patient hand-over
- correct procedure and body site
- electrolyte solution concentration control
- medication accuracy
- catheter and tubing misconnections
- needle reuse and injection device safety
- hand hygiene

The Centre then began work on the second round of patient safety solutions. The latter group of patient safety issues include follow-up on critical test results, falls, hospital acquired central line infections, pressure ulcers, care of the rapidly deteriorating patient, patient and family involvement in care, provider apology and disclosure, and medications with names that look or sound similar. The Centre coordinates the High 5s Project, which is developing standard operating procedures to address widespread patient safety problems across the globe (Monegaom 2007).

The Institute for Healthcare Improvement (IHI) (2007) is another group dedicated to the improvement of global healthcare. IHI challenged U.S. hospitals to join in a campaign to save 100,000 lives during an 18-month period that commenced in 2005. The 3,100 participating hospitals managed to save an estimated 122,000 lives during that period through the implementation of specific evidence-based and life-saving protocols that included:

- Special Rapid Response Teams that were called at the first sign of patient decline.
- Evidence-based care for acute myocardial infarction.
- Medication reconciliation as a means to prevent adverse drug events (ADEs).
- Steps to prevent central line infections.
- Prophylactic use of perioperative antibiotics to prevent surgical site infections.
- Preventive measures against the development of ventilator-associated pneumonia.

In 2006 IHI kicked off the 5 Million Lives Campaign with the goal of sparing 5 million lives from medical harm during a 2-year period based upon estimates that nearly 15 million instances of medical harm occur in the United States each year. Four thousand U.S. hospitals participated in the adoption of 12 interventions designed to save lives and reduce injuries. Earlier standards were retained with new standards added to:

- Reduce the incidence of surgical complications.
- Reduce methicillin-resistant staphylococcus aureus (MRSA) infection.
- Prevent pressure ulcers.
- Prevent harm from high-alert medications starting with anticoagulants, sedatives, narcotics, and insulin.
- Decrease readmissions for the treatment of congestive heart failure.
- Obtain cooperation from hospital boards of directors to accelerate organizational progress toward safe care.

These and many other concurrent efforts are the outgrowth of the landmark reports published by the Institute of Medicine (IOM), *To Err Is Human: Building a Safer Health System* and *Crossing the Quality Chasm: A New Health System for the 21st Century,* which served to heighten awareness of safety issues in the healthcare delivery system. The IOM is a division of the National Academy of Sciences, which was created by the United States government to advise in scientific and technical matters. Its Committee on the Quality of Health Care in America was formed in 1998 with the charge to develop a strategy that would substantially improve the quality of healthcare over a 10-year period. According to the IOM (1999), at least 44,000 to 98,000 deaths per year in U.S. hospitals are due to medication errors. The IOM included recommendations for the use of IT to prevent adverse drug interactions, inappropriate doses, potential side effects, and other types of mistakes.

The Joint Commission, formally known as the Joint Commission on Accreditation of Healthcare Organizations, (2007) is an independent, nonprofit organization dedicated to improving the safety and quality of health care. The Joint Commission provides accreditation of healthcare organizations and related services to ensure that safety and quality standards are met. National Patient Safety Goals are identified annually to address problem areas. Accredited facilities must demonstrate compliance. Medication reconciliation became an accreditation requirement because it was noted that medication errors often occurred when patients were transferred from unit to unit, from one level of care to another, and at the time of discharge (Rogers 2006; Thompson 2005). Medication reconciliation entails getting a list of all pre-admission meds, which is then used when medications are ordered as a basis for comparison at the time of admission, transfer, and discharge to note discrepancies.

Many other organizations and groups have an interest in patient safety as well. A partial list includes:

- American Nurses Association
- American Medical Association
- Healthcare Information and Management System Society (HIMMS)
- Agency for Healthcare Research and Quality (AHRQ)
- American Hospital Association (AHA)
- Centers for Medicare and Medicaid Services
- Leapfrog Group
- National Advisory Council on Nurse Education and Practice (NACNEP)
- Council on Graduate Medical Education (COGME)
- National Committee for Quality Assurance (NCQA)
- National Patient Safety Agency (United Kingdom)
  - National Patient Safety Foundation
  - Patient Safety Institute
- Patient Safety Task Force of the U.S. Department of Health and Human Services
- Institute for Healthcare Improvement
- Institute for Safe Medication Practice
- Centers for Disease Control (CDC)
- U.S. Food and Drug Administration (FDA)
- Partnership for Patient Safety

Interest in patient safety spawned legislation. *The Patient Safety and Quality Improvement Act of 2005* sought to improve patient safety by encouraging voluntary and confidential reporting of events that adversely affect patients. It created Patient Safety Organizations (PSOs) to collect, aggregate, and analyze confidential information reported by healthcare providers. The bulk of other federal legislative efforts focus on incentives to the adoption of information technology as a means to promote efficiency and improve safety. The Patient Safety Act represents an important move in the correct direction where information is shared about adverse events for learning purposes for the benefit of all. Approximately one-half of the states have passed their own medical error reporting laws with a few establishing patient safety centers. Pennsylvania's *Medical Care Availability and Reduction of Error (MCARE) Act* requires the submission of reports of both adverse events and near misses (Rabinowitz et al. 2006). The National Reporting and Learning System in England and Wales coordinates the national reporting of patient safety incidents and determines solutions (Cousins & Baker 2004). This type of reporting allows institutions to compare their error rates with the statewide rate and produces safety alerts that help organizations to act proactively (Simpson 2005a). Prior to this time institutions neither shared this type of data nor was there widespread learning from incidents and failures.

The IOM reports heightened public awareness of the threat of medical errors. Burroughs et al. (2007) found that inpatients defined medical errors more broadly to include falls, communication problems, and responsiveness. Many of the problems that threaten patient safety result from failed process or communication particularly when patients are transferred or shifts change. For this reason some experts call for a review of practices used by other fields, including the aviation industry and military, for guidance in creating a safer environment (Bauer 2006; Doucette 2006; Hohenhaus, Powell, & Hohenhaus 2006). The Federal Aviation Authority (FAA) requires the development and use of practices designed to improve the recognition and utilization of all available resources to acheive safe operations. These practices include cross monitoring and situational awareness in a cooperative, nonpunitive environment to create a culture of safety. Cross-monitoring is a process for double-checking high risk work and verification of inaccurate or ambiguous information. This process may be manual or built into information systems. Situational awareness is awareness of what's going on. Unfortunately awareness may be decreased with poor communication, group think/mindset, and task overload/underload. SBAR (situation, background, assessment, recommendations) represents an adaptation of aviation procedures by the U.S. Navy for the express purpose of improved communication of critical information. SBAR has since been used with success in healthcare. Its reliance upon redundancy establishes an expected pattern of communication, making deviations from the pattern and errors obvious. Situation and background are used to communicate objective information while assessment and recommendation allow the sharing of opinion and requests. Variations of the technique to standardize report information have also been successful (Shendell-Falik, Feinson, & Mohr 2007). Prompts can be built into information systems to facilitate this process and improve care (Sidlow & Katz-Sidlow 2006). Some examples of information that nurses identify as important to care but are sometimes not communicated include attending physician, code and allergy status, reason for admission, identification of anticipated status changes, and daily plan of care inclusive of discharge plans.

The creation of a culture of safety requires a nonpunitive environment in which errors, near misses, and potential problems can be reported without fear of reprisal. Nurses are committed to patient safety initiatives because they are involved in care at all levels (Manno, Hogan, Heberlein, Nyakiti, & Mee 2006).

The Joint Commission announced plans to provide a data management system to accredited hospitals in 2007 to help identify and prioritize areas for improvement using current data, past survey findings, complaints, and reports of sentinel events. Resulting information could be used to drive quality and safety improvement efforts through comparative performance information, benchmark reports, and quality risk profiles. Aggregate data could be used to identify trends or common areas for improvement. The Minnesota Alliance for Patient Safety (MAPS) is a collaborative effort that encourages statewide sharing of key safety information through electronic databases (Apoid, Daniels, & Sanneborn 2006).

Patient Identification

Errors in the patient identification process threaten patient safety. For this reason, the Joint Commission now requires organizations to investigate and plan for technology that can assist with the process of positive patient identification when it designated improving the accuracy of patient identification as a potential National Patient Safety Goal for 2008. There have also been national initiatives to reduce identification errors for procedures and during medication administration, laboratory testing, bedside glucose checks and blood transfusion, and the administration of intravenous fluids (Wickham 2006). Barcodes and radio frequency identification (RFID) are the dominant technologies for this area.

Barcodes have been used in sales and various businesses for many years. Sometimes known as UPC codes, they can be found on most products including medications and intravenous fluids. Barcodes come in simple linear format or two-dimensional forms. Linear codes can include a medical record number while two-dimensional forms can include more information such as name, age, provider, and gender (Halamba 2006). Barcode technology is inexpensive. Barcode technology does require line-of-sight scanning, which requires awakening or repositioning the patient. It may not read well on objects that have been bent, wrinkled, wet, or torn.

RFID tags are used in merchandise tags. RFID technology is durable, can contain more information, does not require direct visualization, and may be reprogrammable (Halamka 2006; Roark & Miguel 2006). It is available in passive and active forms. The passive form contains a chip and antenna, is generally small, and may be flat. It broadcasts data when stimulated by radio frequency energy. Active RFID uses batteries and transmitters to constantly provide location information, making it ideal for tracking equipment, patient, and even staff. RFID tends to be more expensive, although research developments may soon make it more cost effective. Consequently there is no single technology solution for ensuring patient identification at present.

IT Safeguards

Hospitals and healthcare providers have been slow to adopt IT that is commonly found in the business sector. IT advocates claim that it can support the work of healthcare professionals and benefit consumers by improving efficiency, quality, and safety. The desire to reduce or eliminate medication errors focuses attention on computerized physician order entry (CPOE), barcode medication administration, and e-prescribing. When properly used, technologies such as automated drug dispensing systems, smart IV pumps, electronic medical records, computerized documentation at the beside, barcoding, and computerized prescriber order entry reduce adverse events through the introduction of additional checks and balances to existing systems (Manno, Hogan, Heberlein, Nyakiti, & Mee 2006). There are also IT applications for evidence-based medical error reporting, risk management, clinical alerts, electronic medication administration, and clinical decision support that provides information that allows clinicians to be proactive. Evidence-based error identification and reporting applications collect data from external sources such as extant databases and applications to determine where errors occur to help focus resources (Simpson 2005a).

Computerized Physician (or Provider/Prescriber) Order Entry (CPOE)

Computerized Physician (or Provider/Prescriber) Order Entry (CPOE) is the process by which the physician or another healthcare provider, such as a nurse practitioner, physician's assistant, or physical or occupational therapist, directly enters orders for client care into a hospital information system. Its benefits include a reduction in transcription errors, a decrease in elapsed time from order to implementation, standardization and more completeness of orders, fewer medication errors, and the ability to incorporate clinical decision support, alerts for critical lab values, and prompts for when certain tests are due. Information is drawn from separate systems such as the hospital information, pharmacy, and laboratory systems with drug databases to warn prescribers of potential problems with dosages, potential drug interactions, allergies, and contraindications such as pregnancy or other health conditions (Alliance for Health Reform 2006; Simpson 2005a).

Despite its purported benefits, it is essential to recognize that CPOE is a tool, not a guarantee, of safety (Simpson 2005a). There have been a few reports that CPOE has contributed to errors, particularly since not all CPOE are created equal. Its low adoption rate to date, rated ease of use, lack of standardization of systems, poor integration with clinical information systems, and poor design and inadequate training must be factored when looking at actual efficiencies. Basic CPOE includes entry of orders with simple checking for allergies and drug interactions. At the intermediate level CPOE allows some flexibility in displaying results. Advanced clinical order management (ACOM) is a subset of CPOE. ACOM incorporates guided ordering or mentored ordering with formulary management. At its most advanced level ACOM makes use of artificial intelligence and collective knowledge from national standards of care, order sets, alerts, and best practices in workflow efficiencies (McCoy 2006).

Widespread adoption of CPOE has been hampered by the perception that it requires additional time with no benefits to the provider (Bauer 2006; McCoy 2006). Physicians associate data entry as a clerical task and resist any tasks that require additional time. There is also the belief by physicians that they already provide high-quality care and do not need to have their decisions made for them. Systems need to be responsive to the user or risk not being used.

E-prescribing

E-prescribing refers to the electronic transmission of drug prescriptions from a hospital-based inpatient ordering system (CPOE) or handheld device (Blair 2006; Gooch 2006; Wojcik 2007). It may be done from a location at, or near, the patient. Associated advantages include fewer errors, improved communication, greater efficiency, improved compliance with recommended treatment guidelines, lower costs, and less time to fill prescriptions. Errors are reduced because problems with illegible handwriting are eliminated, and the system incorporates lists of patient allergies and other medications. Information may also be available that suggests the best drug for a particular problem, dosing recommendations, drug interactions, contraindications, off-label uses, allowable formulary drugs for a particular individual, and insurance co-payments. As is the case with CPOE e-prescribing systems vary in the features offered.

Adoption has been slow as physicians have cited the need for more reliable, secure systems that are easy to use, do not impede their workflow, and are affordable or subsidized. The National E-Prescribing Patient Safety Initiative (NEPSI) recently announced a program to offer free e-prescribing to physicians across the United States. Some third-party payers have programs that underwrite a portion of an e-prescribing system for physicians (Krizner 2006). Many states have legislation that supports e-prescribing.

Successful e-prescribing requires commitment to training and technical support, access to accurate and current information, incentives from insurance companies and employers, and the ability of prescribers to change their workflow. A growing number of employers and insurance companies support e-prescribing as a means to curtail costs. E-prescribing does require more time than writing a paper prescription, but it permits the creation of a more comprehensive record than the many disparate pieces of paper still found in many physician offices and patient records. The IOM report *Preventing Medication Errors* (2006) estimates 1.5 million persons incur harm annually from medication errors. The same report calls for all providers to have plans in place by 2008 for electronic prescriptions with implementation by 2010.

Barcode and RFID Medication Administration

The FDA issued a rule in 2004 requiring barcodes on most prescription and some over-the-counter medications as a means to decrease medication errors. Barcode scanning technology for medication administration automates the storage, dispensing, returning, restocking, and crediting of barcoded medications, improving safety by ensuring that the right medication is dispensed to the right patient particularly when used with barcoded patient ID bands. It is frequently referred to as barcode medication administration (BCMA). Several varieties of barcode software and multiple barcode formats exist. Matching organizational needs to the appropriate hardware and software requires interdisciplinary collaboration between clinical, information systems (IS), financial, and supply management teams. According to the U.S. Food and Drug Administration (2004) barcode implementation will reduce medication errors by 50 percent. Barcode technology is also available for IV infusion pumps for integration into the medication administration system, point-of-care glucose meters, and blood products. RFID technology can be used in lieu of barcode technology for medication administration purposes. It offers several advantages but comes with a higher cost and is not as widely used at present.

Decision-Support Software

Decision-support software (DSS) is a type of computer application that analyzes data and presents it in a fashion that facilitates decision making. It can incorporate lab values, standards of care, and other patient specific information. It also contains alerts that help to promote safety. The underlying premise of DSS is that the amount of knowledge today exceeds the retention abilities of any one person. DSS is a tool that extends human capabilities. It may be an integral part of CPOE and e-prescribing programs. It can be found in other settings as well. An example that is relevant to nurses is when DSS guides the triage nurse through a series of observations, questions, and interventions when a patient presents with a specific complaint. There are also tools related to drugs and clinical pathways. The value of DSS is contingent upon both the quality of the individual tools and the willingness of users to use them. The selection of a tool has the potential to directly and indirectly impact patient care and outcomes (Clauson, Marsh, Polen, Seamon, & Ortiz 2007).

OTHER MAJOR ISSUES IN HEALTHCARE WITH INFORMATICS IMPLICATIONS

The Nursing Shortage

There are numerous projections of a severe global nursing shortage. The nursing shortage has the attention of the public and healthcare providers because numerous studies have shown a relationship between the number of patients assigned to a nurse and clinical outcome. This shortage comes at a time when the overall population is aging, placing greater demands on the healthcare system. Unfilled positions force hospitals to close units and curtail services. The ramifications of the shortage extend beyond vacant positions. There is also an issue of lost knowledge as nurses retire or opt to leave the profession, which can seriously impact an organization's performance (Hatcher et al. 2006; Trossman 2006a).

The causes of the nursing shortage are numerous. They include dissatisfaction, a decreased interest in the field, and decreased enrollment. The situation necessitates redesign of care delivery models and the way that nurses are educated. There must be an increased emphasis upon the development of problem solving and analytical skills in an increasingly complex, rapidly changing environment where there is an exponential growth of knowledge that exceeds any individual's ability to keep up-to-date (Donley 2005). Technology cannot solve problems that result from staffing shortages, but it can help prevent errors by giving busy nurses a system of double checks.

Work Flow Changes

The way that nurses and other healthcare providers work is changing for many reasons. There is a shift away from tasks to knowledge work and the demand for best practices. This change in clinical thinking is likely to continue its evolution. It is enabled through nursing informatics, standardized nursing knowledge and language systems, electronic records, and more sophisticated data analysis techniques (Pesut 2006). Hospitalized patients are more acutely ill. More treatment is rendered in outpatient settings. Rising costs demand greater efficiencies, forcing individual nurses and administrators to look for innovative, better methods to utilize all resources.

Information Technology as a Means to Retain Aging Nurses

The Robert Wood Johnson Foundation report *Wisdom at Work* examines retention of the older nurse to retirement age and beyond as a means to deal with the "nursing shortage," noting that aging baby boomers represent the largest untapped labor market and the value of the accumulated wisdom found within this group (Hatcher 2006). It emphasizes the need to use well-designed technology to enable the work of the nurse, not complicate it. This is in concert with the ANA view that technology has a crucial role in healthcare with the potential to benefit nurses and patients if it is well used (Trossman 2005). Technology enhanced environments make it easier to direct care. Electronic records eliminate the need for a centralized nurses' station; automated alerts facilitate safety and remind staff when medications and treatments are due, and when tasks need to be done. Smart technology tracks devices eliminating wasted steps and time. Cell phone communication serves to decrease steps, quickly relay call light messages, and provide a means to record or listen to shift report.

Hart (2007) notes the need to plan for an aging workforce. From a technology perspective this includes improved ergonomics both in high tech equipment as well as low tech applications that allow the older worker to effect patient transfers safely without risk of injury to either the patient or themselves. Additional modifications include better product design for the older nurse such as the use of white letters on a dark background, efforts to reduce glare, lowering monitor placement to accommodate for bifocal wearers, and better lighting. All nurses, including older nurses, need to be active participants in technology design and testing.

Evidence-Based Practice

Nursing leaders have long emphasized the need to establish a set of knowledge that is uniquely nursing. Evidence provides the means necessary to provide consistent, quality care. Current practice leaves little time or opportunity to conduct literature searches, evaluate research, and make clinical decisions based upon research. Even fewer nurses have actually conducted research. The current work environment does not support these efforts. The widespread adoption of electronic patient records, CPOE, and other point of care technologies that support nursing workflow will help remove barriers to information and evidence-based practice (Simpson 2006). Nurses also need increased exposure to evidence-based nursing in the preliminary and continuing education (Simpson 2005b).

Genomics

The delivery of quality care increasingly calls for an understanding of the genetic contribution to diseases and human response to illness and interventions. For this reason an interdependent group of nurse leaders drafted *Essential Nursing Competencies and Curricula Guidelines for Genetics and Genomics* in 2005 to establish the minimum requirements to prepare nurses to deliver competent genetic- and genomic-focused care (ANA 2006). Information literacy and informatics skills are essential to the attainment of these competencies, which call for all registered nurses to:

- Demonstrate a knowledge of the relationship of genetics and genomics to health, prevention, screening and monitoring.
- Identify clients who may benefit from genetic information and services and provide appropriate, accurate information.
- Make referrals as needed.
- Provide appropriate services.
- Evaluate the effectiveness of current technology and interventions.

Pressures to Implement Information Technology

There is widespread acknowledgment that the current healthcare system cannot be sustained and must be transformed as costs continue to rise, the budget deficit grows, threats to national well-being mount, and demands for care increase as the population ages. Information technology is seen as a necessary tool for reform (Weiner & Trangenstein 2006). The Bush administration set 2014 as the timeframe for widespread adoption of electronic medical records. Bush and many others identified the need for healthcare consumers to have the information and tools they needed to make the healthcare choices right for them by making it easier to compare quality and cost of care. Gingrich (2006) called for the following changes: the establishment of a National Health Information Network as a part of national security preparedness; increased reimbursement from Medicare and Medicaid to reward quality outcomes and drive the adoption of technology; and legislative changes that would allow hospitals and other entities to provide community physicians with technology for up-to-date systems that would save lives, improve quality of care, and save money. Some third party payers have determined that they will reimburse physicians for teleconsults while some employers and vendors participate in programs to provide physician offices with financial bonuses for the use of information technology to improve the quality of care (Lang 2006). The Center for Health Transformation, founded by Newt Gingrich, represents a collabora-tion of public and private sector leaders dedicated to creation of a 21st Century Intelligent Health System (Alliance for Health Reform 2006). One organization that advocates patient safety through technology is the Leapfrog Group. The Leapfrog Group is a coalition of large corporations that have mobilized their purchasing power to promote changes, including the adoption of technology and CPOE, in the healthcare delivery system by channeling patients to facilities that meet specified safety standards (Alliance for Health Reform 2006). The Institute for Safe Medication Practices has called for healthcare delivery systems to enact changes to provide safer, more effective care. One initiative of this group is the compilation of a list of error-prone abbreviations, symbols, and dose designations that should never be used in any communication because they have frequently been misinterpreted in the past.

Despite these factors the adoption of information technology in healthcare in the United States lags behind that of other countries. It is plagued by insuffi-cient funding, a lack of interoperability that hinders the ability to exchange information with other systems, and issues surrounding data storage, security, and privacy. The Office of the National Coordinator of Health Information Technology (ONC formerly ONCHIT) is the federal body responsible for promoting health IT in the United States.

The Move Toward Magnet Hospital Status

Magnet designation is one of the healthcare industry's most celebrated indicators of quality patient care. Magnet recognition was developed by the American Nurses Credential Center (ANCC) as a measure to recognize organizations that provide the very best nursing care. Magnet facilities use technology to promote, support, and improve patient and staff safety, integrate research and evidence-based prac-tice into clinical processes, and support communication among the disciplines. Healthcare information technology provides a means to reduce errors, improve efficiency, patient safety, and knowledge. It facilitates the incorporation of evi-dence-based guidelines into documentation and helps to compensate for the nursing shortage while improving care (Sensmeier 2006; Winter 2006). The infor-matics nurse plays a key role to obtaining and maintaining magnet hospital status.

Consumer Demands for Quality and Cost-effective Care

As consumers become more sophisticated and knowledgeable about medical and information technologies they hold providers to higher standards (Consumer Influence 2006). They are not content to wait for care but increasingly expect to have a voice in determining what services are delivered and how. This has been particularly clear with the Veterans Health Administration where customer desires and needs have driven changes (Wertenberger, Yerardi, Drake, & Parlier 2006). It has implications for investment in technology as well so that providers can maintain a competitive edge. Another expectation is 24-hour availability to health information via interactive services that allow consumers to schedule appointments, e-mail their physicians, look up beneficial information, and learn about their conditions (Baldwin 2006). Marketing and delivery of promised services is extremely important in this situation (Burgess 2004). Consumers expect quality and often have already reviewed information about the quality of services provided.

Online Report Cards

The concept of healthcare quality report cards has existed for several years. These documents contain evaluated care data of individual physicians, facilities, health plans, and other care providers, serving as a tool to help healthcare consumers by allowing them to compare the quality and other characteristics of providers and health plans. The Agency for Healthcare Research and Quality (AHRQ) supports The Healthcare Report Card Compendium web page, a searchable directory of over 200 sources of comparative information.

Consumer Transparency

Consumer transparency actually refers to consumer's ability to compare the quality and cost of care to make a value-driven decision (Kyle & Ridley 2007). Prices are transparent when the buyer knows his price and the prices paid by others in advance. President Bush, WHO, and many scholars have called for greater transparency. Traditionally healthcare institutions have not advertised prices. In theory price transparency may help to establish more uniform prices but some fear that it will increase prices paid by the poor, reduce competition, or be used in a misleading fashion.

Remote Clinical Monitoring

An aging population, a shortage of healthcare professionals, and a move to keep the ill and elderly in their homes as long as possible—all while trying to contain costs—has led to a spate of programs that use technology to remind people to check their blood sugar or blood pressure, take their medications, and otherwise monitor them in their own homes. Measures range from monitoring glucose levels, weight, general well-being, and cardiac rhythms, to checking pace maker function, to determining whether the refrigerator was opened. This type of monitoring helps individuals to better manage their own health, minimize travel, and forestall moving to a facility for care (Nugent, Wallace, Kernohan, McCreight, Mulvenna, & Martin 2007).

Disease Management

Successful disease management requires two-way communication between providers and consumers with active participation and involvement in treatment decisions. Consumers may not have the skills to accomplish these tasks or have difficulty understanding healthcare information and instructions due to language and culture differences and difficulty navigating the healthcare system (Nath 2007). Health literacy is needed. Health literacy connotes that an individual possesses the problem-solving and decision-making skills needed to comprehend and use new information and to navigate the healthcare system. Nurses need to be sensitive to the health literacy levels of their clients particularly as it impacts their outcomes, and assist them to develop a greater understanding of their health issues.

Research

The move to evidence-based practice as a means to meet demands for quality and cost-effective care now lies within the grasp of virtually every healthcare professional with the implementation of the electronic record. Electronic records and the systems that house them make it easier and faster to collect information. Data stripped of individual patient identifiers can then be downloaded into other applications for the identification of patterns and further analysis. Much of this process can be performed automatically so that the timeframe from data collection to interpretation is shortened and findings can be disseminated and applied more quickly.

Payment for Performance

In years past healthcare institutions, nurses, and consumers were affected by managed care. This system imposed limits upon what providers could charge, and payers provided a set reimbursement by diagnosis. Downsizing, acquisitions, and mergers occurred in an attempt to increase efficiency along with automation and cross-training of personnel. One legacy of this era was that fewer people were left to do the work. Another result was that remaining providers had the ability to extend their reach by offering a more comprehensive set of services and encouraging consumers to stay within their healthcare network. These types of alliances foster the sharing of information as merged entities gravitate to computer systems that can exchange information and as administrators turn to information technology as a means to maximize efficiencies. While the emphasis remains on the "bottom line" the healthcare delivery system is moving toward a model where providers are paid for performance (Donley 2005). A recent report by the IOM (2006) notes problems with the healthcare delivery system, including incentives for a high volume of services rather than quality services and better outcomes. This same report calls for better coordination of care among providers and across episodes of illness and identifies design principles for payment for performance and its implementation. An earlier report provides a set of starter measures. The IOM notes that public reporting of outcomes would motivate improved provider behavior and provide consumers with information that they could use to make treatment decisions.

NURSING INFORMATICS AS A SPECIALTY AREA OF PRACTICE

Nursing informatics was first recognized as a specialty by the ANA in 1992. Informatics nurses are knowledgeable about patient care and technology; for that reason, they provide a valuable communication link between healthcare and technology professionals (Abbott 2002). Informatics nurses work in hospitals and other healthcare settings, in educational facilities, in research, as consultants, with medical device and software vendors or web content providers, and in government agencies focusing on disease management.

The Scope and Standards of Nursing Informatics Practice (ANA 2001) noted that nursing informatics displays 5 of the 12 defining characteristics that must be present for a nursing specialty. These attributes were derived from earlier work by Styles (1989) and later modified by Panniers and Gassert (1996) and include the following:

- *A differentiated practice.* Nursing informatics differs from other specialties within nursing because it focuses on data, information, and knowledge; the structure and use of the same; and efforts to guarantee that nursing information is represented in efforts to automate health information. It shares an interest in the client, the environment, health, and nurses in other areas of specialty practice.
- *Defined research priorities.* Target areas for research were identified and published in the early 1990s. These centered primarily on the development of a standard language for use within nursing, which would allow nurses from different regions of a country or the world to establish that they were describing the same phenomenon and to conduct studies that could be replicated. In more recent years, survey results identified additional areas deemed critical for research, although the development of a standard nursing language remains crucial. The development of databases for clinical information is another priority area.
- *Representation by one or more organization(s).* This criterion is met because nursing informatics interests are represented by work groups within the American Medical Informatics Association (AMIA) and the International Medical Informatics Association, in a number of regional groups within the United States, and in national groups abroad. Table 1–4 displays some of these groups, and Table 1–5 lists official publications for informatics groups as well as other journals and resources.
- *Formal educational programs.* Early leaders in nursing informatics obtained their expertise through experience as well as classes in related areas such as computer science and information science. Grant monies from the Division of Nursing of the Health Resources and Services Administration (National Advisory Council on Nurse Education and Practice 1997) were used to establish the first two graduate programs in nursing informatics at the University of Maryland in 1988 and at the University of Utah in 1990.

TABLE 1–4 A Partial Listing of Nursing Informatics Organizations and Groups

United States

National

Academy of Ambulatory Care Nursing—Informatics Special Interest Group

American Medical Informatics Association (AMIA): Nursing Informatics Working

American Nurses Association

National League for Nursing (NLN): Nursing Education Research, Technology, and Information Management Advisory Council

American Medical Informatics Association (AMIA): Nursing Informatics Working Group Informatics Special Interest Group

Health Information and Management Systems Society (HIMSS): Nursing Informatics Committee

Regional

American Nursing Informatics Association (ANIA)—California

Boston Area Nursing Informatics Consortium (BANIC)—Greater Boston Area

British Columbia Computer Nurse Group

Capitol Area Roundtable on Informatics in Nursing (CARING)—Washington, DC

Connecticut Healthcare Informatics Network (CHIN)

Delaware Valley Nursing Computer Network (DVNCN)

Informatics Nurses from Ohio (INFO)

Michigan Nursing Informatics Network (MNIN)

Minnesota Nursing Informatics Group (MINING)

New Jersey State Nurses Association (NJSNA) Computer Forum on Nursing Informatics

North Carolina State Nurses Association Council on NI (CONI)

Nursing Information Systems Council of New England (NISCNE)

Puget Sound Nursing Informatics Group–Northwest Washington State

South Carolina Informatics Nursing Network (SCINN)

South West Michigan Informatics

Tennessee Nursing Association Nursing Informatics Council

Texas Nursing and Healthcare Informatics Association

Utah Nursing Informatics Network (UNIN)

International

IMIA Nursing Informatics Special Interest Group

Australian Nursing Informatics Council (ANIC)

Brazilian Nursing Association Nursing Informatics Group at Brazilian Nursing Association

Canadian Organisation for Advancement of Computers in Health (COACH)

Health Informatics New Zealand (HINZ) (www.hinz.org.nz)

Spanish Society of Nursing Informatics and Internet (SEEI)

Swiss Special Interest Group Nursing Informatics (SIG-NI)

There are now several graduate programs as well as certificate programs and doctoral education in this area. Some nurses still elect to enter programs in healthcare informatics and medical informatics as a means to pursue their interests.

- *A credentialing process.* The American Nurses Credentialing Center (ANCC 2001) used the foundation provided by the ANA in its 1994 definition of nursing informatics and scope and standards of practice.

TABLE 1–5 Health Care Informatics Journals	
ADVANCE for Health Information Executives Online	Journal of the American Medical Informatics Association (JAHIMA)
Artificial Intelligence in Medicine	Journal of Clinical Monitoring and Computing
Bioinformatics (formerly: Computer Applications in the Biosciences)	Journal of Healthcare Information Management (HIMSS publication)
BioSystems	Journal of Medical Internet Research
British Journal of Healthcare Computing & Information Management	Journal of the Medical Library Association (formerly Bulletin of the Medical Library Association)
Computerized Medical Imaging and Graphics	
Computer Methods and Programs in Biomedicine	Journal of Telemedicine and Telecare
Computers in Biology and Medicine	LinuxMed News
Computers, Informatics, Nursing (formerly Computers in Nursing)	Mathematical and Computer Modeling
	MD Computing
European Journal of Information Systems	Medical and Biological Engineering and Computing
Health Data Management	
Health Informatics Europe	Medical Computing Today
Health Informatics Journal	Medical Decision Making
Health Information & Libraries Journal (formerly Health Libraries Review)	Medical Engineering & Physics
	Medical Informatics and the Internet in Medicine
Healthcare Information Management and Communications Canada	
	Medical Science Monitor
Health Management Technology Online	Methods of Information in Medicine
Healthcare Informatics Online	Micron
Informatics in Primary Care	Neural Networks
Informatics Review	Online Chronicle of Distance Education and Communication
International Journal of Medical Informatics (formerly International Journal of Bio-Medical Computing)	
	Online Journal of Nursing Informatics Corporation (OJNIC)
International Journal of Technology Assessment in Health Care	RN Palm: The Journal of Mobile Informatics
	SCAR News: Society for Computer Applications in Radiology
Journal of Biomedical Informatics (formerly Computers and Biomedical Research)	
	Telemedicine Today Magazine

Applicants for the credentialing examination are required to meet the following criteria:

a) Have a baccalaureate or higher degree in nursing or a baccalaureate in a relevant field

b) Possess a current, active license as a professional nurse in the United States or a legally recognized equivalent in another country

c) The equivalent of two years of full time professional practice as a nurse

d) Thirty contact hours of continuing education applicable to nursing informatics within the past 3 years
e) Have a minimum of 2,000 hours of practice in informatics nursing in the past 3 years, or a minimum of 12 semester hours of graduate credits in nursing informatics courses with at least 1,000 hours of practice in informatics nursing within the previous 3 years, or completion of a graduate program in nursing informatics that includes at least 200 hours of faculty supervised clinical practicum

The certification examination covers content on the theory, information management principles and database management, human factors, and the analysis, design, implementation, evaluation, support, and marketing of information systems as well as trends and issues (ANCC 2007).

Nursing informatics is a specialty practice within a broader field that shares commonalities with other informatics areas (ANA 2007). It is interdisciplinary in nature. It is important to nursing because it represents the nursing perspective, identifies a practice base for nurses, produces unique knowledge, and provides needed standardized nursing language. Informatics nurses have a role in the development of health policy and in assessing the usability of devices for consumers and other healthcare professionals.

THE ROLES OF THE INFORMATICS NURSE AND INFORMATICS NURSE SPECIALIST

The ANA (2007) revised the language in its Scope of Nursing Informatics Practice statement to be consistent with that used to describe other clinical nurse specialists and to move away from job titles to role functions. The result led to a distinction between the **Informatics Nurse (IN)** and **Informatics Nurse Specialist (INS).** The Informatics Nurse refers to the RN who works in the area of informatics. This individual has experience or an interest in the area but no formal informatics preparation. In contrast the INS has advanced, graduate education in nursing informatics or a related field and may hold ANCC certification. Both the IN and INS may work under a variety of different titles and in various settings. The IN employs strategies that transforms data into information and information into knowledge, and ensures that information is disseminated at appropriate times for appropriate uses in the healthcare continuum. The INS needs to play an active role in research and theory development and in the design and testing of information systems and the human-computer interface; he or she also needs to help shape policy and serve as an advocate for the design and use of informatics to serve other healthcare professionals and the public. Other facets of the INS role include responsibilities in administration, telehealth, education and professional development, compliance issues, and discovery in databases and analysis. The INS is prepared to assess work processes and subsequently design, select, implement, and evaluate data structures and suggested technology intended to improve productivity and contribute to the body of nursing knowledge. Both the IN and INS must be aware of uniform language efforts and have a concept of the value of documentation from healthcare information systems.

APPLICATIONS OF NURSING INFORMATICS

Informatics offers many solutions to support the work of healthcare professionals and healthcare consumers as they seek self-help and care (Brennan 2000). Some examples of how informatics and computers support the various areas of nursing and consumer health follow.

Nursing Practice
- Worklists to remind staff of planned nursing interventions
- Computer-generated client documentation including discharge instructions and medication information
- Monitoring devices that record vital signs and other measurements directly into the client record
- Computer-generated nursing care plans and critical pathways
- Automatic billing for supplies or procedures with nursing documentation
- Reminders and prompts that appear during documentation to ensure comprehensive charting
- Quick access to computer-archived patient data from previous encounters
- Online drug information

Nursing Administration
- Automated staff scheduling
- Online bidding for unfilled shifts
- Electronic mail for improved communication
- Cost analysis and finding trends for budget purposes
- Quality assurance and outcomes analysis
- Patient tracking and placement for case management

Nursing Education
- Online completion of mandatory education requirements
- Online course registration and scheduling
- Computerized student tracking, testing, and grade management
- Course delivery and support for Web-based education
- Remote access to library and Internet resources
- Teleconferencing and Webcast capability
- Presentation software for preparing slides and handouts
- Online test administration
- Communication with students

Nursing Research
- Computerized literature searching
- The adoption of standardized language related to nursing terms

- The ability to find trends in aggregate data, which is data derived from large population groups
- Use of the Internet for obtaining data collection tools and conducting research
- Collaboration with other nurse researchers

These examples demonstrate the importance of information sharing. Nursing informatics, through the use of computers, can facilitate and speed information sharing in all practice areas. For this to be most effective, nurses must have a basic understanding of informatics.

Consumers turn to the Internet for health information and services as well. Additional consumer applications may include:

- Communication with healthcare providers via e-mail and instant messaging
- Remote monitoring and other telehealth services
- Support groups
- Online scheduling

BENEFITS FOR CONSUMERS AND OTHER HEALTHCARE PROFESSIONALS

Nursing informatics benefits nurses and other healthcare professionals and consumers, healthcare organizations, education planners, and resource managers (ANA 2007). For example, other providers can use data collected and documented by nurses using automated systems, thereby helping to eliminate silos of information typically amassed by each individual group. In addition, multidisciplinary critical pathways are used by nurses and providers to plan and document care for a client. The aggregate critical pathway data may be analyzed for trends related to overall effectiveness of client care.

Other healthcare disciplines may have information systems that use data collected by nursing systems. For example, pharmacy information systems make use of data collected by nursing information systems, such as current medications, allergies, client demographic information, and diagnosis. This feature eliminates redundant data collection by different professionals, saving them time. Laboratory information systems may also connect to nursing systems. When a laboratory test is ordered and entered into the computer on the hospital unit, the information is transferred to the laboratory computer system. This replaces handwritten paper requisitions, saving time and improving communication. Similarly, other hospital departments may receive requests for consults.

Other uses of automation within healthcare may also improve communication and increase profitability. One example is inventory control. Healthcare product suppliers use technology to decrease administrative costs and to attract customers with improved inventory control. Specifically, suppliers can more quickly fill orders, check hospital inventory, and allow customers to receive prices, place orders, and confirm orders through information systems. Some suppliers provide the inventory system for customer use. Customers get a more accurate inventory, automatic replacement of supplies as they are used, and the ability to maintain a smaller inventory to reduce costs. This process is known as Web-based purchasing or e-procurement. Thus, client care and consumer demands drive the healthcare delivery system toward working smarter, which is often best accomplished through automation.

Many of the benefits of automation in healthcare are seen with the development of the electronic medical record, which is an electronic version of the client data found in the traditional paper record. Some specific benefits of electronic medical records include the following:

- *Improved access to information.* The electronic medical record can be accessed from several different locations simultaneously, as well as by different levels of providers.
- *Error reduction and improved communication.* Automation eliminates problems associated with illegible handwriting and provides a series of checks and balances.
- *Decreased redundancy of data entry.* For example, allergies and vital signs need be entered only once.
- *Convenience.* Diagnostic images are a part of the record and can be viewed from various locations.
- *Decreased time spent in medication administration and documentation.* Automation facilitates efficient medication administration and allows direct entry from monitoring equipment, as well as point-of-care data entry.
- *Increased time for client care.* More time is available for client care because less time is required for documentation and transcription of physician orders.
- *Facilitation of data collection for research.* Electronically stored client records provide quick access to clinical data for a large number of clients.
- *Improved quality of documentation.* Prompts help to ensure that key information is noted.
- *Improved compliance with regulatory requirements.* Automated systems can require information needed for regulatory bodies, ensuring that it is included in documentation.
- *Improved record security.* Access to the health record is limited to individuals with computer access.
- *Improved quality of care and patient satisfaction.* Built-in tools remind nurses to provide interventions appropriate for certain patient problems.
- *Decreased administrative costs for location and maintenance of client records.*
- *Creation of a lifetime clinical record facilitated by information systems.*

Other benefits of automation are related to decision-support software, computer programs that organize information to aid in decision making for client care or administrative issues. Some of the benefits that can be realized with these systems include the following:

- Decision-support tools as well as alerts and reminders notify the clinician of possible concerns or omissions. For example, the client states an allergy to penicillin, and this is documented in the computer system. The physician orders an antibiotic that is a variation of penicillin, and this order is entered into the computer system. An alert informs the clinician that a potential allergic reaction may result and asks for verification of the order.

- With access to reference databases, nurses can easily review information on medications, diseases, and treatments as part of the automated system.
- Effective data management and trend-finding include the ability to provide historical or current data reports.
- Extensive financial information can be collected and analyzed for trends. Information related to cost by diagnosis and treatment can be more easily tracked using computer systems. For example, one can determine the least expensive drug that is effective for a particular diagnosis.
- Data related to treatment such as inpatient length of stay and the lowest level of care provider required could be used to decrease costs.

EDUCATIONAL OPPORTUNITIES FOR NURSING INFORMATICS

Informatics programs have grown since the first recommendations for education of healthcare professionals in the field in the 1970s (Skiba, Carty, & Nelson 2006). The Health and Medical Informatics Education workgroup of the International Medical Informatics Association (IMIA) (2000) developed recommendations for programs by level and discipline with a particular focus on skills for information processing and communication technology as a foundation. This group defined learning outcomes for all health professionals as users of information technology as well as learning outcomes for informatics specialists. The work of this group provided a framework for curriculum development. Informatics was first introduced into schools of nursing in the late 1970s with the State University of New York at Buffalo offering a course on computers and nursing (Tallberg, Saba, & Carr 2006). In subsequent years other groups offered conferences and training for nurses on the use of information technology. The EDUCTRA project of the European Advanced Informatics in Medicine Programme and the IT-EDUCTRA project of the Telematics Applications Programme, Health Sector provided training materials and courses (Hasman 1998). The European Union funded the Nightingale Project during the 1990s (Mantas 1998). Professional groups also played a part in this process.

Graduate, doctoral, and certificate programs are now available in nursing informatics. Projections for the number of informatics nurses needed range from 6,000 to 12,000 (Gugerty 2006). Nursing, healthcare, clinical informatics graduate programs, and biomedical informatics programs collectively lag behind projected needs. This is due, in part, to a lack of sufficient numbers of qualified faculty.

Abundant continuing education opportunities exist to help bridge the gap between undergraduate and graduate programs and help nurses with preparation in the field up-to-date. The Health Information Technology Scholars Program (HITS 2007) is a year-long faculty development program first offered in 2008 as a result of a collaborative effort among the Universities of Kansas, Colorado, and Indiana and the National League for Nursing (NLN). The American Medical Informatics Association (AMIA) has an initiative to provide

10,000 clinicians in 10 years with training in applied health and medical informatics by the year 2010 (AMIA 2007). This initiative has partners in the informatics education community.

FUTURE DIRECTIONS

Nursing informatics has an important role to play in the improvement of health through its contributions to the development of standard languages, design and evaluation of information technology, assisting peers to develop the competencies needed in an increasingly complex environment, facilitating consumer acceptance and use of technology, and by contributing to nursing's scientific body of knowledge (Brennan 2006; Saranto et al. 2006; Strachan, Delaney, & Sensmeier 2006). Informatics Nurse Specialists must serve as leaders to help drive the changes necessary to transform the healthcare delivery system, improve quality of services delivery, and improve safety. The *Scope and Standards for Practice* (ANA 2007) notes that the discipline is changing rapidly. Some of the competencies now associated with informatics nurses and specialists will transition downward to nurses in general practice. There will be a continued blur between nursing informatics and other health informatics with more interdisciplinary projects. New technologies will impact the practice of nursing informatics in ways that cannot be forecast at present. Nanotechnology, genomics, robotics, wearable monitoring devices, and new developments in educational technology represent some of these new technologies. New educational models are needed to incorporate informatics competencies, and new care models must be developed.

Emerging Trends

The drive for patient safety, transparency in healthcare, error reduction, increased efficiency, and additional requirements on the part of regulatory agencies will continue to shape healthcare delivery and informatics practice for many years to come. Consumers will assume a greater responsibility for their healthcare choices as they shoulder a larger portion of the costs.

Role Changes

As the practice of nursing informatics continues to evolve so will the roles of the informatics nurse and informatics nurse specialist. This evolution will occur in response to the ongoing growth of the nursing profession, changes within the healthcare delivery system, and informatics in general. This process will result in additional differentiation between the levels of practice now seen. These changes will require the INS to actively work to keep aware and abreast of these developments.

Interactions with Consumers

Nursing informatics has been virtually invisible to healthcare consumers up to this point in time. This will change as more professionals specialize in this area of informatics practice either to help consumers to better manage their healthcare conditions through the design and testing of monitoring devices and human-computer interfaces or by helping consumers become more discriminating consumers of Web-based information, whether it represents comparable data on providers or details on specific conditions.

Issues

While the development of nursing informatics promises to deliver many benefits, it will not be without a few bumps along the way. There are many different informatics groups within healthcare. Ideally they present a united front and work together. Individuals are confronted with several choices for entry into the field both in area of focus and programs of study.

CASE STUDY EXERCISE

1.1   A client arrives in the emergency department with shortness of breath and complaining of chest pain. Describe how informatics can help nurses and other healthcare providers to more efficiently help the client.

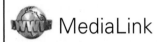 MediaLink

Additional resources for this content can be found on the Companion Website at www.prenhall.com/hebda. Click on "Chapter 1" to select the activities for this chapter.

- Glossary
- Multiple Choice
- Discussion Points
- Case Studies
- MediaLink Application
- MediaLink

SUMMARY

- Data are a collection of numbers, characters, or facts that are gathered according to some perceived need or analysis and possibly action at a later point in time.
- Data have little meaning alone, but a collection of data can be examined for patterns and structure that can be interpreted. At this point, data become information.
- Knowledge is the synthesis of information derived from several sources to produce a single concept or idea.
- Healthcare delivery systems are knowledge-intensive settings with nurses as the largest group of knowledge workers within those systems. Information technology offers several tools to support nurses and other healthcare workers in their knowledge work.
- Good information management ensures access to the right information at the right time to the people who need it. This is particularly important when the volume of information exceeds human processing capacity.

- Informatics is the application of computer and statistical techniques to the management of information.
- Nursing informatics is the use of information and computer technology as a tool to process information to support all areas of nursing, including practice, education, administration, and research. The definition of nursing informatics continues to evolve.
- A formal definition of nursing informatics serves to shape job descriptions and educational preparation for informatics practice.
- Nursing informatics is a necessity, not a luxury, in today's rapidly changing healthcare delivery system. All nurses need basic informatics skills.
- Computer technology facilitates the collection of data for analysis, which can be used to justify the efficacy of particular interventions and improve the quality of care.
- Other healthcare providers also benefit from nursing informatics.
- Nursing informatics allows nurses to have better control over data management.
- According to the American Nurses Association (ANA) the Informatics Nurse Specialist (INS) has advanced graduate education in nursing informatics or a related field and may hold ANCC certification in informatics whereas the Informatics Nurse (IN) is a nurse who works in informatics or has an interest in the area but does not have formal informatics preparation.
- Current educational programs fall short of providing the number of needed informatics nurse specialists.
- New technologies will impact the practice of nursing informatics in ways that cannot be forecast at present.
- Nursing informatics will continue to evolve with changes in the profession, the healthcare delivery system and informatics in general.
- Consumer interactions will become an increasingly important part of nursing informatics practice.

REFERENCES

Abbott, P. A. (2002). Introducing nursing informatics. *Nursing 2002, 32*(1), 14.

Academic Medical Publishing & CancerWEB. (1997). *On-line medical dictionary.* Retrieved December 28, 2002, from http://cancerweb.ncl.ac.uk/cgi-bin/ omd?query=informatics&action=Search+OMD.

Ackoff, R. (1989). From data to wisdom. *Journal of Applied Systems Analysis, Vol. 16,* 3–7.

Agency for Healthcare Research and Quality, (2006). *The Patient Safety and Quality Improvement Act of 2005,* Overview. Retrieved June 13, 2007, from http://www.ahrq.gov/qual/psoact.htm.

Alliance for Health Reform. (December 2006). Linking Providers via Health Information Networks. Washington, DC: Alliance for Health Reform.

American Association of Colleges of Nursing (AACN). (1998). *Essentials of baccalaureate education for professional nursing practice.* Washington, DC: AACN.

American Medical Informatics Association (AMIA) (July 25, 2007). AMIA 10x10™. Retrieved November 13, 2007, from http://www.amia.org/10x10/.

American Medical Informatics Association (AMIA) (May 3, 2007). Working Groups Consumer Health Informatics (CHI-WG). Retrieved May 31, 2007, from http://www.amia.org/mbrcenter/wg/chi/.

American Nurses Association (ANA). (2006). Essential nursing competencies and curricula guidelines for genetics and genomics. Retrieved November 6, 2007, from http://www.genome.gov/Pages/Careers/HealthProfessionalEducation/geneticsco mpetency.pdf.

American Nurses Association, Council on Computer Applications in Nursing. (1992). *Report on the designation of nursing informatics as a nursing speciality.* Congress of Nursing Practice unpublished report. Washington, DC: American Nurses Association.

American Nurses Association (ANA). (2007). *Scope and standards of nursing informatics practice.* Washington, DC: American Nurses Publishing.

American Nurses Association. (2001). *Scope and standards of nursing informatics practice.* Washington, DC: American Nurses Publishing.

American Nurses Credentialing Center (ANCC). (2007). Informatics Nurse Certification. Retrieved June 19, 2007, from http://www.nursecredentialing. org/cert/eligibility/informatics.html.

American Nurses Credentialing Center (ANCC). (2001). *Computer based testing for ANCC certification.* Retrieved December 11, 2002, from http://www.nursingworld.org/ancc/certify/cert/catalogs/CBT.PDF.

Anderson, S. (1992). *Computer literacy for health care professionals.* New York: Delmar.

Apoid, J., Daniels, T., & Sanneborn, M. (2006). Promoting collaboration and transparency in patient safety. *Journal on Quality and Patient Safety, 32*(12), 672–675.

Arnold, J. M. (1996). Nursing informatics educational needs. *Computers in Nursing, 14*(6), 333–339.

Association of College and Research Libraries (ACRL). (2002). *Information literacy competency standards for higher education.* Retrieved November 18, 2002, from http://www.ala.org/acrl/ilintro.html#ildef.

Ayer, A. J. (1966). *The problem of knowledge.* Baltimore, MD: Penguin.

Baldwin, G. (2006). The connected patient. *Healthcare Strategic Management, 24*(11), 11.

Ball, M. J. & Hannah, K. J. (1984). *Using computers in nursing.* Reston, VA: Reston Publishing.

Barton, A. J. (2005). Cultivating Informatics Competencies in a Community of Practice. *Nursing Administration Quarterly, 29*(4), 323–328.

Bauer, J. C. (2006). Patient safety: Getting it right by doing it backwards. *Journal of Healthcare Information Management, 20*(4), 5–7.

Bemmel, J. H. & Musen, M. A. (Eds.). (1997). *Handbook of Medical Informatics.* New York: Springer Verlag Publishing.

Blair, R. (2006). Putting Meat on the e-Prescribing Bone. *Health Management Technology, 27*(2), 52–55.

Booth, R. G. (2006). Educating the future ehealth professional nurse. *International Journal of Nursing Education Scholarship, 3*(1), 1–10.

Brennan, P. F. (2006). Nursing informatics and the NIH roadmap. In C. A. Weaver, C.W. Delaney, P. Weber, and R. L. Carr, (Eds). *Nursing and Informatics for the 21st Century: An International Look at Practice, Trends, and the Future.* Chicago: Healthcare Information and Management Systems Society, pp. 483–488.

Burgess, L. (2004). Marketing to meet today's consumer demands. *Nursing Homes: Long Term Care Management, 53*(12), 16–20.

Burroughs, T. E., Waterman, A. D., Gallagher, T. H., Waterman, B., Jeffe, D. B., Dunagan, W. C., et al. (2007). Patients' concerns about medical errors during hospitalization. *Journal of Quality and Patient Safety, 33*(1), 5–14.

Clauson, K. A., Marsh, W. A., Polen, H. H., Seamon, M. J., & Ortiz, B. I. (March 8, 2007). Clinical decision support tools: analysis of online drug information databases. *BMC Medical Informatics and Decision Making,7,* 7.

Consumer Influence on Technology Investments. (2006). *Healthcare Financial Management, 60*(9), 153–154,

Courey, T., Benson-Soros, J., Deemer, K., & Zeller, R. A. (2006). The missing link: Information literacy and evidence-based practice as a new challenge for nurse educators. *Nursing Education Perspectives,27*(6), 320–323.

Cousins, D. H. & Baker, M. (May 2004). The work of the National Patient Safety Agency to improve medication safety. *British Journal of General Practice,* 332–333.

Curtin, L. & Simpson, R. L. (2001). Standards of practice for nursing informatics. *Health Management Technology, 22*(4), 52.

Davenport, T. H., Thomas, R. J., & Cantrell, S. (2002). The mysterious art and science of knowledge worker performance. *MIT Sloan Management Review, 44*(1), 23. http://web.ebscohost.com/ehost/detail?vid=22&hid=22&sid=ed572e2c-ceb3–4e61–8144–2dbf9023e1ce%40sessionmgr2–bib4up#bib4up

Davidson, C. & Voss, P. (2002). *Knowledge management: An introduction to creating competitive advantage from intellectual capital.* Tandem Press, Auckland.

Desjardins, K. S., Cook, S. S., Jenkins, M., & Bakken, S. (2005). Effect of an informatics for evidence-based practice curriculum on nursing informatics competencies. *International Journal of Medical Informatics, 74*(11/12), 1012–1020,

DiCecco, K. L. (2005). Information literacy, part II: Knowledge and ability in the traditional resources. *Journal of Legal Nurse Consulting, 16*(4), 15–22.

Dreher, M. C. & Miller, J. F. (2006). Information technology: The foundation for educating nurses as clinical leaders. In C. A. Weaver, C. W. Delaney, P. Weber, and R. L. Carr, (Eds). *Nursing and Informatics for the 21st Century: An International Look at Practice, Trends, and the Future.* Chicago: Healthcare Information and Management Systems Society, pp. 29–34.

Donley, R. (2005). Challenges for nursing in the 21st century. *Nursing Economics, 23*(6), 312–318.

Doucette, J. N. (2006). View from the cockpit: What the airline industry can teach us about patient safety. *Nursing 2006, 36*(11), 50–53.

Educational Testing Service (ETS) (2007). iSkills™ assessment. Retrieved June 1, 2007, from http://www.ets.org/portal/site/ets/menuitem.1488512ecfd5b8849a77b13bc3921509/?vgnextoid=fde9af5e44df4010VgnVCM10000022f95190RCRD&vgnextchannel=cd7314ee98459010VgnVCM10000022f95190RCRD#WhatProficiency.

Engelhardt, H. T., Jr. (1980). Knowing and valuing: Looking for common roots. In H. T. Engelhardt and D. Callahan (Eds.), *Knowing and valuing: The search for common roots* (Vol. 4, pp. 1–17). New York: Hastings Center.

Eysenbach, G. (June 24, 2000). Consumer health informatics. *British Medical Journal.* Available online at: http://www.findarticles.com/cf_0/m0999/7251_320/63563322/p1/article.jhtml?term=%22consumer+ health+informatics%22. Accessed January 7, 2003.

Food and Drug Administration (FDA). (2004). FDA Issues Bar Code Regulation. Retrieved June 19, 2007, from http://www.fda.gov/oc/initiatives/barcode-sadr/fs-barcode.html.

Fischman, J. (July 31, 2006). The good and the wired. *U.S. News & World Report, 141*(4), 66.

Garde, S., Harrison, D., & Hovenga, E. (2005). Skill needs for nurses in their role as health informatics professionals: A survey in the context of global health informatics education. *International Journal of Medical Informatics, 74*(11/12), 899–907.

Gingrich, N. (June 21, 2006). Accelerating the adoption of health information technology, FDCH Congressional Testimony.

Gluck, J. & Baltes, P. B. (2006). Using the concept of wisdom to enhance the expression of wisdom knowledge: Not the philosopher's dream but differential effects of developmental preparedness. *Psychology and Aging, 21*(4), 679–690.

Gooch, J. J. (October 1, 2006). Providers and payers work to ease into e-prescribing. *Managed Healthcare Executive,* Retrieved November 13, 2007, from http://www.managedhealthcareexecutive.com/mhe/Technology/Providers-and-payers-work-to-ease-into-e-prescribi/ArticleStandard/Article/detail/376826.

Graves, J. R. & Corcoran, S. (1989). The study of nursing informatics. *Image: Journal of Nursing Scholarship, 21,* 227–231.

Guenther, J. T. & Caruth, M. P. (2006). Mapping the literature of nursing informatics. *Journal of the Medical Library Association, 94*(2) Supplement, E92–E98.

Gugerty, B. (2006). The state of informatics training and education for nurses. *Journal of Healthcare Information Management, 20*(1), 23–24.

Haase-Herrick, K. S. & Herrin, D. M. (2007). The American Organization of Nurse Executives' Guiding Principles and American Association of Colleges of Nursing's Clinical Nurse Leader: A lesson in synergy. *JONA, 37*(2), 55–60.

Halamka, J. (2006). Early experiences with positive patient identification. *Journal of Healthcare Information Management, 20*(1), 25–27.

Hart, K. A. (2007). The Aging Workforce: Implications for Health Care Organizations. *Nursing Economics, 25*(2), 101–102.

Hasman, A. (1998). Education and training in health informatics: the IT-EDUCTRA project.*International Journal of Medical Informatics, 50*(1–3), 179–185.

Hannah, K. (1985). Current trends in nursing informatics: Implications for curriculum planning. In K. Hannah, E. Guillemin, and D. Conklin (Eds.), *Nursing uses of computer and information science.* Proceedings of the IFIP-IMIA International Symposium on Nursing Uses of Computers and Information Science. Amsterdam: Elsevier Science.

Harsanyi, B. E., Lehmkuhl, D., Hott, R., Myers, S., & McGeehan, L. (1994). Nursing informatics: The key to managing and evaluating quality. In S. J. Grobe and E. S. P. Puyter-Wenting (Eds.), *Nursing informatics: An international overview for nursing in a technological era.* Proceedings of the Fifth IMIA International Conference on Nursing Use of Computers and Information Science, San Antonio, TX, pp. 655–659.

Hatcher, B. J. (ed), Bleich, M. R., Connolly, C., Davis, K., Hewlett. P. O., & Hill, K. S. (2006). *Wisdom at Work.* The Robert Wood Johnson Foundation.

Healthcare Information and Management Systems Society (HIMSS). (2002). *Using innovative technology to enhance patient care delivery.* A report delivered by the Improving Operational Efficiency through Elimination of Waste and Redundancy Work group at the American Academy of Nursing Technology and Workforce Conference in Washington, DC. Retrieved January 1, 2003, from http://www.himss.org/content/files/AANNsgSummitHIMSSFINAL_18770.pdf.

Hebert, M. (1999). *National Nursing Informatics Project discussion paper.* Retrieved June 24, 2003, from http://www.cna-nurses.ca/pages/resources/nni/nni_discussion_paper.doc.

Heller, B. F., Oros, M. T., & Durney-Crowley, J. (June 24, 2003). The future of nursing education: Ten trends to watch. *NLN Journal.* Retrieved June 24, 2003, from http://www.nln.org/nlnjournal/infotrends.htm.

HIMSS Nursing Task Force. (2007). The TIGER update: Facilitating collaboration among participating organizations to achieve the TIGER vision. Retrieved June 27, 2007, from http://www.himss.org/handouts/TIGER_PhaseII_Collaboratives.pdf.

HITS: Health Information Technology Scholars Program. (2007). Retrieved November 13, 2007, from http://www.hits-colab.org/index.htm.

Hobbs, S. D. (2002). Measuring nurses' computer competency: An analysis of published instruments. *Computers, Informatics, Nursing, 20*(2), 63–73.

Hohenhaus, S., Powell, S., & Hohenhaus, J. T. (2006). Enhancing patient safety during hand-offs. *AJN, 106*(8), 72A–72D.

Hulford, P., Gough, K., & Krieger, M. Making business intelligence 'End-user friendly' with Cognos 8 Go! Search and the Google Search Appliance. A Ziff Davis Webcast sponsored by Cognos. Accessed February 17, 2007, from http://www.Eseminarslive.com.

The Institute for Healthcare Improvement (IHI). (2007). Protecting 5 Million Lives From Harm. Retrieved June 11, 2007, from http://www.ihi.org/IHI/Programs/Campaign/Campaign.htm?TabId=1.

Institute of Medicine (IOM). (2007). The Learning Healthcare System: Workshop Summary. Washington, DC: National Academy Press.

Institute of Medicine (IOM). (1999). *To err is human: Building a safer health system.* Washington, DC: National Academy Press.

Institute of Medicine (IOM). (2001). *Crossing the quality chasm: A new health system for the 21st century.* Washington, DC: National Academy Press.

Institute of Medicine (IOM). (2006). Rewarding provider performance: Aligning incentives in Medicare. Washington, DC: National Academy Press.

International Medical Informatics Association. (2003). The Special Interest Group on Nursing Informatics. Retrieved April 7, 2004, from http://www.IMIA. org/NI/.

International Medical Informatics Association Working Group I: Health and Medical Informatics Education. (2000). *Recommendations of the IMIA on Education in Health and Medical Informatics.* Retrieved November 13, 2007, from http://www.imia.org/pubdocs/rec_english.pdf.

Johnson, K. & Maultsby, C. C. (2007). A plan for achieving significant improvement in patient safety. *Journal of Nursing Care Quality, 22*(2), 164–171.

The Joint Commission for Accreditation of Healthcare Organizations (JCAHO). (2007). About The Joint Commission. Retrieved June 13, 2007, from http://www.jointcommission.org/AboutUs/.

Joint Commission International Center for Patient Safety. (2007). World Alliance for Patient Safety. Retrieved June 11, 2007, from http://www.jcipatientsafety.org/14685.

Kisilowska, M. (2006). Knowledge management prerequisites for building an information society in healthcare. *International Journal of Medical Informatics, 75* (Issue 3/4), 322–329.

Krizner, K. (February 1, 2006). Health plans offer IT grants to encourage more provider adoption. *Managed Healthcare Exeutive.* Retrieved November 13, 2007, from Health plans offer IT grants to encourage more provider adoption.

Kuznar, W. (2001). E-prescribing aims to improve care, overcome prior authorization shortcomings. *Managed Healthcare Executive, 11*(3), 32.

Kyle, M. K. & Ridley, D. B. (2007). Would greater transparency and uniformity of health care prices benefit poor patients? *Health Affairs, 26* (5): 1384–1391.

Lang, R. D. (2006). Patient safety and IT: A need for incentives. *Journal of Healthcare Information Management, 20*(4), 2–4.

Manno, M., Hogan, P., Heberlein, V., Nyakiti, J., & Mee, C. L. (2006). Patient-safety survey report. Nursing, *36*(5), 54–63.

Mantas J. (1998). Developing curriculum in nursing informatics in Europe. *International Journal of Medical Informatics, 50*(1–3), 123–132.

McBride, A. B. (2006). Informatics and the future of nursing practice. In C. A. Weaver, C. W. Delaney, P. Weber, and R. L. Carr, (Eds). *Nursing and Informatics for the 21st Century: An International Look at Practice, Trends, and the Future.* Chicago: Healthcare Information and Management Systems Society, pp. 5–12.

McCoy, M. J. (2006). Advanced clinician order management—A superset of CPOE. *Journal of Healthcare Information Management, 19*(4), 11–13.

McDowell, D. E. & Ma, X. (2007). Computer literacy in baccalaureate nursing students during the last 8 years. *Computers, Informatics, Nursing, 25*(1), 30–36.

McNeil, B. J., Elfrink, V. L., Pierce, S. T., Beyea, S. C., Bickford, C. J., & Averill, C. (2005). *International Journal of Medical Informatics, 74*(Issue 11/12), 1021–1030.

Monegain, B. (November 2, 2007). Countries unite on patient safety. *Healthcare IT News.* Retrieved November 6, 2007, from http://www.healthcareitnews.com/story.cms?id=8073&fromRSS=true

Murray, A. J. (2000). Knowledge management and cousciousness. *Advances in Mind=Body Medicine, 16*(3), 233(5p).

Nath, C. (2007). Literacy and diabetes self-management. *AJN, 107*(6 supplement), 43–49.

National Advisory Council on Nurse Education and Practice (NACNEP). (1997). *A national agenda for nursing education and practice.* Rockville, MD: US Department of Health and Human Services, Health Resources and Services Administration.

Nugent, C., Wallace, J., Kernohan, G., McCreight, B., Mulvenna, M., & Martin, S. (2007). Using context awareness within the 'Smart home' environment to support social care for adults with dementia. *Technology & Disability, 19*(2/3), 143–152.

Newbold, S. K. (2002). FAQs about nursing informatics. *Nursing 2002, 32*(3), 20.

Nursing Informatics: Special Interest Group of the International Medical Informatics Association (IMIA-NI). (1998). Proceedings of the General Assembly Meeting, Seoul, Korea.

Ornes, L. L. & Gassert, C. (2007). Computer competencies in a BSN program. *The Journal of Nursing Education. 46*(2):75–78.

Panniers, T. L. & Gassert, C. A. (1996). Standards of practice and preparation for certification. In M. E. Mills, C. A. Romano, and B. R. Heller (Eds.), *Information management in nursing and health care.* Springhouse, PA: Springhouse Corporation, pp. 280–297.

Parker-Oliver, D. & Demiris, G. (2006). Social work informatics: A new specialty. *Social Work, 51*(2), 127–134.

Pesut, D.J. (2006). 21st century nursing knowledge work: Reasoning into the future. In C. A. Weaver, C. W. Delaney, P. Weber, and R. L. Carr, (Eds). Nursing and Informatics for the 21st Century: An International Look at Practice, Trends, and the Future. Chicago: Healthcare Information and Management Systems Society, pp. 13–21.

Pravikoff, D. S., Tanner, A.B., & Pierce, S.T. (2005). Readiness of U.S. Nurses for evidence-based practice. *AJN, 105*(9), 40–51.

Rabinowitz, A. B. K., Clarke, J. R., Marella, W., Johnston, J., Baker, L., & Doering, M. (2006). Translating patient safety legislation into health care practice. *Journal on Quality and Patient Safety, 32*(12), 676–681.

Roark, D. G. & Miguel, K. (2006). Bar coding's replacement? *Nursing Management, 37*(2) 28–31.

Rogers, G., Alper, E., Brunelle, D., Federico, F., Fenn, C. A., Leape, L. L., et al. (2006). *Joint Commission Journal on Quality and Patient Safety, 32*(1), 37–50.

Saba, V. & McCormick, K. (1996). *Essentials of computers for nurses.* New York: McGraw-Hill.

Saba, V. K. (2001). Nursing informatics: Yesterday, today and tomorrow. *International Nursing Review, 48*(3), 177.

Sandars, J. & Heller, R. (2006) Improving the implementation of evidence-based practice: A knowledge management perspective. *Journal of Evaluation in Clinical Practice, 12*(3), 341–346.

Saranto, K., Weber, P., Hayrinen, K., Kouri, P., Porrasmaa, J., Komulainen, J., et al. (2006). Citizen empowerment: Ehealth consumerism in Europe. In C. A. Weaver, C. W. Delaney, P. Weber, and R. L. Carr, (Eds). *Nursing and Informatics for the 21st Century: An International Look at Practice, Trends, and the Future.* Chicago: Healthcare Information and Management Systems Society, pp. 489–500.

Scholes, M. & Barber, B. (1980). Towards nursing informatics. In D. A. Lindberg and S. Kaihari (Eds.), *Medinfo, 80* (pp. 70–73). London: North-Holland.

Schwirian, P. (1986). The NI pyramid—A model for research in nursing informatics. *Computers in Nursing, 4*(3), 134–136.

Sensmeier, J. (2007). The future of IT? Aggressive educational reform. *Nursing Management, 38*(9—Supplement: IT Solutions), 2, 4, 6, 8.

Sensmeier, J. (October 2006). Survey says: Care, communication enhanced by IT. *IT Solutions,* 2, 4, 6, 30.

Shendell-Falik, N., Feinson, M., & Mohr, B. J. (2007). Enhancing Patient Safety. *JONA, 37*(2), 95–104.

Sidlow, R. & Katz-Sidlow, R. J. (2006). Using a computerized sign-out system to improve physician-nurse communication. *Journal On Quality and Patient Safety, 32* (1), 32–33.

Simpson, R. L. (2005a). Error reporting as a preventive force. *Nursing Management, 36*(6), 21–24, 56.

Simpson, R. L. (2005b). Practice to evidence to practice: Closing the loop with IT. *Nursing Management, 35*(9), 12, 17.

Simpson, R. (2006). Automation: The vanguard of EBN. *Nursing Management,* (June), 13–14.

Simpson, R. (2007). Information technology: Building nursing intellectual capital for the information age. *Nursing Administration Quarterly, 31*(1), 84–88.

Singh, S. P., Hummel, J., & Walton, G. S. (2005). Consumer driven healthcare: Strategic, operational, and information technology implications for today's healthcare CIO. *Journal of Healthcare Information Management, 19*(4), 49–54.

Skiba, D., Carty, B., & Nelson, R. (2006). The Growth in Nursing Informatics Educational Programs to Meet Demands. In C. A. Weaver, C. W. Delaney, P. Weber, and R. L. Carr, (Eds). *Nursing and Informatics for the 21st Century: An International Look at Practice, Trends, and the Future.* Chicago: Healthcare Information and Management Systems Society, pp. 35–44.

Skiba, D. J. (2005) Preparing for evidence-based practice: Revisiting information literacy. *Nursing Education Perspectives, 26*(5), 310–311.

Snyder-Halpern, R., Corcoran-Perry, S., & Narayan, S. (2001). Developing clinical practice environments supporting the knowledge work of nurses. *Computers in Nursing, 19*(1), 17–23.

Spurr, R. (2007). Portal to a Golden Age. *Health Management Technology, 28*(4), 44–43.

Staggers, N., Gassert, C. A., & Curran, C. (2001). Informatics competencies for nurses at four levels of practice. *The Journal of Nursing Education, 40*(7), 303–316.

Staggers, N. & Thompson, C. B. (2002). The evolution of definitions for nursing informatics: A critical analysis and revised definition. *Journal of the American Medical Informatics Association, 9*(3), 255–261.

Steyn, G. M. (2004). Harnessing the power of knowledge in higher education. *Education, 124*(4), 615–630.

Strachan, H., Delaney, C. W., & Sensmeier, J. (2006). Looking to the future: Informatics and nursing's opportunities. In C. A. Weaver, C. W. Delaney, P. Weber, and R. L. Carr, (Eds). *Nursing and Informatics for the 21st Century:*

An International Look at Practice, Trends, and the Future. Chicago: Healthcare Information and Management Systems Society, pp. 507–516.

Styles, M. (1989). *On specialization in nursing: Toward a new empowerment.* Kansas City, MO: American Nurses Foundation.

Tallberg, M., Saba, V. K., & Carr, R. L. (2006). The international emergence of nursing informatics. In C. A. Weaver, C. W. Delaney, P. Weber, and R. L. Carr (Eds). *Nursing and Informatics for the 21st Century: An International Look at Practice, Trends, and the Future.* Chicago: Healthcare Information and Management Systems Society, pp. 45–51.

Thompson, C. A. (2005 August 1). JCAHO views medication reconciliation as adverse-event prevention. *American Journal of Health-System Pharmacology, 62,* 1528, 1530, 1532.

Technology Informatics Guiding Education Reform (TIGER) (2007). The TIGER Initiative. Retrieved May 31, 2007, from www.tigersummit.com.

Troester, S. (2006). Drive nursing activities to the bedside with a closed-loop system. *Nursing Management, 37*(12), 18–20.

Trossman, S. (2006a). Staying power? Retaining mature RNs in the workforce. *American Journal of Nursing, 106*(7), 77–78.

Trossman, S. (November-December 2006b). Show us the data! NDNQI helps nurses link their care to quality. *The American Nurse,* 1, 6.

Trossman, S. (2005). Bold new world: Technology should ease nurses' jobs, not create a greater workload. *American Journal of Nursing, 105*(5), 75–77.

Turley, J. P. (1996). Toward a model of nursing informatics. *Image: Journal of Nursing Scholarship, 28*(1), 309–313.

Waegemann, C. P. (2001). Leading edge: An electronic record for the real world. *Healthcare Informatics, 18*(5), 55–56, 58, 60.

Warman, A. R. (1993). *Computer security within organizations.* London: Macmillan.

Watson, M. (2007). Knowledge management in health and social care. *Journal of Integrated Care, 15*(1), 27–33.

Weiner, E. & Trangenstein, P. (2006). Preparing our public health nursing leaders with informatics skills to combat bioterrorism in the United States. *Studies in Health Technology & Informatics, 122,* p. 215–219.

Wertenberger, S. (2006). Veterans Health Administration Office of Nursing Services exploration of positive patient care synergies fueled by consumer demand: Care coordination, advanced clinic access, and patient self management. *Nursing Administration Quarterly, 30*(2), 137–146.

Wickham, V., Miedema, F., Gamerdinger, K., & DeGooyer, J. (2006). Bar-coded patient ID: Review an organizational approach to vendor selection. *Nursing Management, 37*(12), 22–26.

Windsor J. (2006). Nursing and knowledge work: Issues regarding workload measurement and the informatics nurse specialist. *Journal of Healthcare Information Management, 20*(4):54–59.

Winter, N. (2006). The magnetic draw of information technology. *American Nurse Today, 1*(1), 40, 42.

Wojcik, J. (2007). Electronic Rx program helps cut health care costs at General Motors. *Business Insurance, 41*(5), 6.

World Health Organization (WHO) (2007). Patient Safety. Retrieved June 11, 2007, from http://www.who.int/patientsafety/solutions/patientsafety/en/index.html.

Yee, C. C. (2002). Identifying information technology competencies needed in Singapore nursing education. *Computers, Informatics, Nursing, 20*(5), 209–214.

Zolot, J. S. (1999). Computer-based patient records. *AJN, 99*(12), 64, 66, 68–69.

Zurlinden, J. (2003). FDA bands importing certain high risk prescription drugs using the Internet. *Nursing Spectrum, 4*(2), 12.

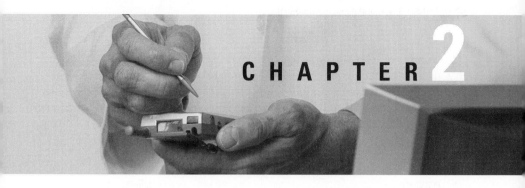

CHAPTER 2

Hardware, Software, and the Roles of Support Personnel

After completing this chapter, you should be able to:

1 Explain what computers are and how they work.

2 Describe the major hardware components of computers.

3 Understand what networks are, and list the major types of network configurations.

4 Explain some considerations for choosing and using a computer system.

5 List the advantages and disadvantages of mainframe, client server, and thin client technology.

6 Compare and contrast mobile and wireless devices, including personal digital assistants (PDAs), cell phones, MP3 players, iPods, iPhones, and the BlackBerry® in terms of basic technology and implications for use.

7 Understand the major types of software commonly used with computer systems.

8 Discuss the roles and responsibilities of various computer support personnel.

A **computer** is an electronic device that collects, stores, processes, and retrieves data. Information output is provided under the direction of stored sequences of instructions known as computer programs. The physical parts of a computer are frequently referred to as **hardware,** and the instructions, or programs, are collectively known as **software.** A computer system consists of the following components:

- Hardware
- Software
- Data that will be transformed into information
- Procedures or rules for the use of the system
- Users

Rapid advances in technology reshape computer capabilities and user expectations. Many changes have occurred since the introduction of the first computers in the 1940s. In general, computers have become smaller but more powerful and increasingly affordable. This is particularly evident with current notebook, tablet, PDA, and hybrid devices.

HARDWARE

Computer hardware is the physical part of the computer and its associated equipment. Computer hardware consists of many different parts, but the main elements are input devices, the central processing unit, primary and secondary storage devices, and output devices. These devices may be contained within one shell or may be separate but connected via cables or infrared technology. Figure 2–1 describes the relationship among these components.

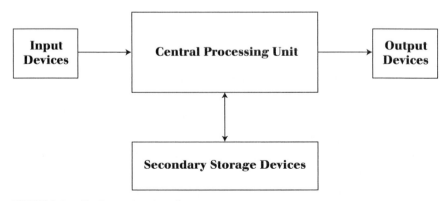

FIGURE 2–1 • Basic components of a computer

Input Devices

Input devices allow the user to feed data into the computer. Common input devices include the keyboard, mouse and trackball, touch sensitive screen, stylus, microphone, bar code reader, Fax modem card, joystick, image scanner, fingerprint scanner, digital camera, and Webcam.

Central Processing Unit

The **central processing unit (CPU)** is the "brain" of the computer. It has the electronic circuitry that actually executes computer instructions. The CPU can be divided into the following three components:

- The **arithmetic logic unit (ALU)** executes instructions for the manipulation of numeric symbols.
- **Memory** is the storage area in which programs reside during execution. Memory is subdivided into two categories: read-only memory and random access memory. **Read-only memory (ROM)** is permanent; it remains when the power is off. It typically cannot be changed by the user unless additional memory is installed. ROM contains start-up instructions that are executed each time the computer is turned on. **Random access memory (RAM)** is a temporary storage area that is active only while the computer is turned on. It provides storage for the program that is running, as well as for the data that are being processed.
- The **control unit** manages instructions to other parts of the computer, including input and output devices. It reads stored programs one instruction at a time and directs other computer parts to perform required tasks.

The CPU is located inside the system cabinet, which is the box that many people think of as "the computer." The CPU and memory are found on the main circuit board of the personal or desktop computer, which is known as the motherboard. The cabinet contains other components as well. Figure 2–3 will show some items that may be inside a computer cabinet.

Secondary Storage

Secondary storage provides space to retain data in an area separate from the computer's memory after the computer is turned off. Common mechanisms for secondary storage include **hard disk drives, USB flash drives, digital versatile** or **video discs (DVDs),** and **high density optical disc format,** which is the successor to DVD. Hard disk drives store digitally encoded data and rotating platters with magnetic surfaces. USB flash drives are portable, fairly inexpensive devices slightly smaller than a cigarette lighter that plug in to a USB port and can easily be transported from one computer to another. DVDs resemble the CDs that are used to record and play music but offer a larger amount of storage. Some older machines may still have **compact discs (CDs), floppy drives** and **diskettes,** and **Zip drive disks,** but these are not found on current computers. The CDs used for computers resemble those used for music. Floppy diskettes and zip diskettes come in a square plastic cases. **Magnetic tape drives** are still used for some large computers.

Output Devices

Output devices allow the user to view and possibly hear processed data. Terminals or video monitor screens, projectors, printers, speakers, and Fax modem boards are examples of output devices.

COMPUTER CATEGORIES

Computers vary in size, purpose, capacity, and the number of users that can be accommodated simultaneously. The main categories of computers are:

- Supercomputers
- Mainframe computers
- Minicomputers
- Personal computers (also known as PCs or desktop computers)
- Laptop or notebook computers
- Tablet computers
- PDAs and other handheld combination devices such as the iPhone, iPod, and BlackBerry®
- Embedded

The PDA has become a very popular device that is revolutionizing information access in healthcare. Table 2–1 provides a brief description of the various types of computers and some advantages and disadvantages associated with each.

Supercomputers are the largest, most expensive type of computer. They are complex systems that can perform billions of instructions every second. Prohibitive cost limits use primarily to government and academic settings.

Mainframes, which are large computers capable of processing several million instructions per second, are used for quickly processing large amounts of data. Mainframe computers support organizational functions and therefore were the traditional equipment in hospital environments until recently. Software for mainframes supports many customized functions, and this level of specialization results in its high cost.

A **minicomputer** is a scaled-down version of a mainframe computer. Minicomputers are slightly less costly than mainframes but are still capable of supporting multiple users as well as the computing needs of small businesses. Because they have become more powerful, minicomputers may be used in hospitals.

Personal computers (PCs) are also known as desktop computers and were previously referred to as **microcomputers.** This computer category provides inexpensive processing power for an individual user. A PC may stand alone or be connected to other computer systems through a network, dial-up or wireless connection, or cable service. Improved reliability, availability, manageability, and processing capabilities allow PCs to assume responsibilities once associated

TABLE 2–1	Types of Computers		
Type	**Description**	**Advantages**	**Disadvantages**
Supercomputer	Designed and used for complex scientific calculations	Performs complex calculations very quickly	Expensive Limited functionality
Mainframe	Used to support organizational information systems Multiple processors Varies in size	High-speed transactions Supports many terminals and users simultaneously Large storage capacity	Expensive Software expensive and inflexible
Minicomputer	Smaller version of a mainframe Designed for multiple users Supports corporate computing for smaller organizations	Less expensive than a mainframe Supports many terminals and users simultaneously	Relatively expensive
Personal computer (PC) or desktop computer	A single-or dual-processor machine intended for one user	Inexpensive processing Can connect to other systems through a network, dial-up, cable, or wireless connection	High support costs Somewhat slower response with fewer capabilities than larger systems
Laptop or notebook computer	Streamlined, portable version of a PC or desktop system	Provides portable computer capability	Limited battery life More expensive than a comparably equipped PC Generally has a smaller keyboard than a PC
Tablet computers	Smaller than a notebook computer Weighs 2–3 pounds	Small size makes it easy to carry Generally accepts handwriting or keyboard input May receive and transmit data from and to other systems	Limited battery life Slightly more expensive than a desktop system Cannot receive transmissions in some areas known as "deadzones"

(continued)

TABLE 2–1 *(continued)*

Type	Description	Advantages	Disadvantages
Handheld/personal digital assistant (PDA)	Small special-use device	Small, lightweight Inexpensive Quick learning curve Easily taken to the point of care Increases access to information Can improve productivity May accept handwriting, voice, or keyed input May download data from information systems and transmit data to other service May incorporate the functionality of more than one device (i.e., PDA, e-mail terminal, cell phone)	Small screen size Offers less functionality than desktop and notebook computers Limited battery life Limited speed and processing ability May not hold up to rough use Synchrony with other computers may require special equipment E-mail connectivity/telephone service requires wireless systems Small size makes it easy to steal Information security concerns related to theft May not be able to receive transmissions in some areas known as "deadzones"
Hybrid	Small, multipurpose device	Often combines telephone, text and/or e-mail messages, other Internet services, address book, and calendar functions	Small screen and keys can be difficult to use
Embedded	Small, special purpose	Easily transportable Integral part of many appliances, automobiles, other devices such as intravenous infusion pumps	Limited functionality

with mainframe computers. Some variations of the microcomputer are the notebook or laptop, tablet PC, and handheld computers. These devices all offer portable computer capability away from the office or desktop. The **notebook** or **laptop** computer is a streamlined version of the personal computer, using batteries or regular electric current. These devices are more expensive than comparable desktop computers. The **tablet PC** can be carried in one hand like a clipboard and is smaller and lighter than a notebook computer but rivals notebook capability. It accepts handwritten input via a stylus but also incorporates a keyboard and supports Windows-based applications. The stylus can be used like a mouse. Devices may also be configured to accept dictation. Handheld computers are special-use devices that offer portability and many of the features found in laptop and tablet PCs. Advances in technology add to the functionality of these devices. Some can accept handwriting and voice input, as well as send and receive data.

PDAs are a well-known type of handheld computer. These small devices were once used to keep appointment calendars, addresses, and telephone numbers. Advances in processing capability, memory, and design make PDAs attractive for a wide variety of functions, including many common software applications and data collection. PDAs can store extensive reference materials and have the ability to access patient information and transmit and receive information such as electronic prescriptions.

Hybrid or combination devices comprise another category of handheld devices. Hybrids may combine PDA capability with cell phones, MP3 players, or other functions. The BlackBerry®, iPhone, and iPod are hybrid devices. A MP3 player is a small handheld digital music player. It received its name from the audio file extension that it supports. MP3, also known as MPEG audio layer 3, compresses audio signals without sacrificing sound quality resulting in small, easily transferred files. MP3 players often support other file types as well. The iPod is a portable music player that supports MP3 and other file types. Its large capacity allows it to download, store, and play songs, movies, games, and photo slideshows from a computer or wireless connection. The iPod supports games, can also function as a portable hard drive, and offers contact and calendar functions that can synchronize with personal computers.

The iPhone is a multimedia, Internet-enabled mobile phone with touch screen and virtual keyboard and buttons. Functions include a camera-phone, text-messaging, visual voice-mail, and a portable medial player It also supports the following Internet services: e-mail; Web browsing; and local Wi-Fi connectivity. The BlackBerry® is a handheld device that supports wireless services that include a mobile telephone, push-mail, text messaging, Internet faxing and Web browsing. It also supports address books and calendars.

Work is underway at several universities on a quantum computer, which will break away from the binary mold used for current digital computers. Quantum computers will harness the power of quantum states and encode information as qubits. A **qubit** is a measurement similar to the bit but allows for a superposition of both 1 and 0.

PERIPHERAL HARDWARE ITEMS

Peripheral hardware or, more simply, a **peripheral,** is any piece of hardware connected to a computer. Examples of peripheral devices include:

- Monitors
- Keyboards
- Terminals
- Mouse and other pointing devices such as trackballs and touchpads
- Secondary storage devices such as external CD and DVD drives and memory sticks
- Backup systems
- External modems
- Printers
- Scanners
- Digital and Web cameras (Webcams)
- Multifunction devices that combine functions such as printers that also scan, copy, and Fax

The **monitor** is the screen that displays text and graphic images generated by the computer. PC monitors use LCD or CRT technology. **LCD (liquid crystal display)** technology uses two sheets of polarizing material with a liquid crystal solution between them. An electric current sent through the liquid causes the crystals to align so that light cannot pass through them. Each crystal acts like a shutter, either allowing light to pass through or blocking the light. LCD displays may be monochrome or color. Monitors that accept handwriting via a stylus use an electromagnetic field under or over an LCD to capture the movement on the screen. The monitor may be housed separately from the CPU or contained within the same box. Touch screens offer another variation in monitor technology. Touch screens are sensitive to contact; this allows users to enter data and make selections by touching the screen. Laptops and flat monitors use LCD technology. LED-backlit LCD panels are available but are a more expensive variant of the technology. LCD monitors requires less desktop real estate, weigh less than CRT devices, are more energy efficient, and provide a brighter picture with crisper text, less glare, and no flicker—thereby reducing eye strain. CRT (cathode ray tube) monitors use old television technology to generate colors by combining amounts of red, green, and blue. **Refresh rate** and **resolution** are terms that refer to monitor characteristics. The refresh rate is the speed with which the screen is repainted from top to bottom. Early monitors had a slow refresh rate that caused the screen to flicker. Higher refresh rates eliminate flicker. **Resolution** is the number of pixels, or dots, that appear horizontally and vertically on the screen, making up the image. Resolution is expressed as the number of horizontal pixels by vertical pixels. Higher resolution numbers provide a better screen image. CRT monitors are bulky but can display a greater number of colors and may be preferred by graphic artists for that reason.

Keyboards are input devices with keys that resemble those of a typewriter. Keyboards allow the user to type information and instructions into a computer.

A **terminal** consists of a monitor screen and a keyboard. It is used to input data and receive output from a mainframe computer. Untike a personal computer, the terminal itself does not process information, thus giving rise to the expression "dumb terminal." Very few terminals remain in operation due to the fact that it is expensive to find and replace parts for outdated technology.

The **mouse** is a device that fits in the user's hand and can be moved around on the desktop to direct a pointer on the screen. It is often used to select and move items by pressing and releasing a button. A mouse pad optimizes function by providing a surface area with the proper amount of friction while minimizing the amount of dirt that enters the mouse.

Some other examples of pointing devices include joysticks, touchpads, and trackballs. A **joystick** allows the user to control the movement of objects on the screen and is primarily used with games. A **touchpad** is a pressure- and motion-sensitive surface. When a user moves a finger across the touchpad, the on-screen pointer moves in the same direction. A **trackball** contains a ball that the user rolls to move the on-screen pointer. Touchpads and trackballs work well when available space is limited, as with laptop computers.

Secondary storage devices are generally provided via the hard disk drive, flash drive, DVD, or Blu-ray drives. Older computers and large mainframe computers may make use of technology that is not found on new personal computers. The hard disk drive allows the user to retrieve and read data as well as save, or write, new data. Data are stored in the hard drive magnetically on a stack of rotating disks known as *platters*. The amount of information that can be stored on disk is known as its *capacity*. Capacity is measured in bytes. Hard disk drives generally offer a larger capacity than do secondary storage devices. Home and office PCs offer hard disk drives with a capacity that is measured in gigabytes. One gigabyte is equivalent to 1,073,741,824 characters.

Unlike the CD drives that they replaced, DVD drives can read or play CDs as well as DVDs but access data more quickly. Most DVD drives now read and write data storing up to seven times more data than a CD. A DVD (digital versatile or video disc) is similar to a CD (compact disc) used to record music and is commonly used to store multimedia or full-length movies. A few older computers may still have floppy disk drives. A **floppy disk** is a thin plastic platter within a plastic cover. The amount of storage provided was small compared to a DVD. DVD drives are generally located within the system cabinet but may also be external and connected using cables. Other options for secondary storage particularly on larger computers include optical disk drives, magnetic disk or tape drives, and RAID. **Optical disk drives** rely on laser technology to write data to a recording surface media and read it later. The advantage of this technology is its large storage capacity. A **tape drive** copies files from the computer to magnetic tape for storage or transfer to another machine. In a virtual tape system data is saved as if it were stored on tape but is actually stored on a hard drive or another storage medium. Virtual tape systems offer better backup and retrieval times at a lower operating cost. A **file** is a collection of related data stored and handled as a single entity by the computer. The tape drive uses tiny electromagnets to write data to a magnetic media by altering the surface. A **redundant array of inexpensive or independent disks (RAID)** is precisely what the name indicates: duplicate disks with mirror copies of data. Using RAID may be less costly than using one large disk drive. In the event that an individual disk fails, the remaining RAID would permit the computer to continue working uninterrupted.

Backup systems are devices that create copies of system and data files. These systems use secondary storage device technology or take advantage of on-line backup options. The copies are generally kept at a location separate from the computer. A backup system is an important measure for protection against computer failure or data loss.

A **modem** is a communication device that allows computers to transmit information over telephone or cable lines. Faster modems transfer information more quickly. This, in turn, saves time and telephone charges. Modem speed is measured by the number of bits that can be transferred in 1 second of time, or **bits per second (bps)**. A **bit** is the smallest unit of data that can be handled by the computer. In actuality, transfer occurs in thousands of bits per second, or **kilobits (kbps)**. Many PCs include modem and Fax capabilities via a Fax modem board. A **Fax modem** board allows computers to transmit images of letters and drawings over telephone lines. **Wireless modems** allow users to send and receive information via access points provided with a subscription to wireless service. The **DSL modem** allows users who have this service available to them both by virtue of location and subscription to access high-speed service via telephone lines.

A **printer** produces a paper copy of computer-generated documents. Several types of printers are available. Laser printers offer the highest quality print by transferring toner, a powdered ink, onto paper like a photocopier does. Ink-jet printers heat ink and spray it onto paper to provide a high-quality output. Dot matrix printers create letters and graphics through the use of a series of metal pins that strike a ribbon against paper. Color is an option with all three printer types. Prices vary according to quality and capability with prices starting under $100 and ranging upward. Overall operating costs are based on purchase, supplies, and power consumption. Ink-jet printers were once considered cost effective but ink costs over time make laser printers a viable option. Printers that also scan, copy, and Fax are available. Users should base their selection on need. Laser printers are the office standard because they are quiet and provide a high-quality print. Ink-jet printers are suitable for some settings but are slow, and ink may smear when exposed to moisture. Dot matrix printers are noisy, provide a poor-quality print, and are rarely found now.

The **scanner** is an input device that converts printed pages or graphic images into a file. The file can then be stored and revised using the computer. For example, a printed report can be scanned, stored in the computer, and sent electronically to another output device. **Digital cameras** offer a means to capture and input still images without film. Digital images may be downloaded to a computer, manipulated, and printed. A **Webcam** is a small camera used by a computer to send images over the Internet. **Multiple function devices** combine functions such as printers that also scan, copy, and Fax.

NETWORKS

A **network** is a combination of hardware and software that allows communication and electronic transfer of information between computers. Hardware may be connected permanently by wire or cable, or temporarily through modems, telephone lines, or infrared signals. This arrangement allows sharing of resources, data, and software. For example, it may not be practical to have a printer for every PC in the house or office. Instead, several PCs are connected to one printer through a network. Common use of hardware requires consideration of overall needs, convenience of location, priority by user and job, and amount of use. Figure 2–2 depicts a network.

Networks range in size from **local area networks (LANs),** with a handful of computers, printers, and other devices, to systems that link many small and large computers over a large geographic area. For example, some LANs provide support for **client/server** technology. In client/server technology, files are stored on a central computer known as the **server.** Any type of computer may act as a server, including mainframes, minicomputers, and PCs. One current trend is to combine servers by partitioning the hard drive to act as more than one server. This is known as a virtual server. **Client** computers can access information stored on the server. One major advantage of a LAN is that only one copy of a software program is needed for all users since it can be stored on the server. The client computers then access the server to use the software. This contrasts with the need to supply a separate copy of a software program for each PC user. The primary disadvantage to client/server technology is vulnerability. If the server fails, the network fails. Multiple servers circumvent this problem. Larger, more expansive systems are known as **wide area networks (WANs).**

Thin client technology, also known as **server-based computing,** represents another networking model that relies on highly efficient servers. All system processing occurs on the server, rather than on the client or local PC, as seen in

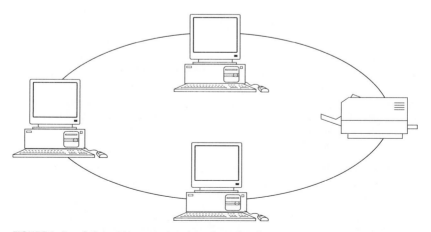

FIGURE 2–2 • Schematic representation of a network

traditional client/server technology. The thin client is primarily a display, keyboard, and mouse or other pointing device. It sends keystrokes and mouse movements to the server over the network and the server sends back changes in the display. Any PC can serve as a thin client. The minimal hardware requirements for this model give rise to the name "thin client" as opposed to "fat client," as seen in traditional client/server technology. This model helps to reduce hardware costs; older equipment can be used longer and new thin clients cost less than traditional PCs because no local drives or storage devices are required. The absence of local drives and storage also reduces maintenance and administrative costs and facilitates software upgrades. Software resides on the server requiring one upgrade at the server rather than a physical visit to each PC or client. Security is enhanced because users cannot run foreign disks locally that may contain a virus.

The largest and best known network in the world is the **Internet,** also known as the **Net.** The Internet actually consists of thousands of interconnected networks. The Internet was once limited to individuals affiliated with educational institutions and government agencies, but access is now available to the public. Variations of Internet technology are available via intranets and extranets. Both intranets and extranets use software and programming languages designed for the Internet. **Intranets** are private company networks that are protected from outside access. **Extranets,** on the other hand, apply Internet technology to create a network outside of the company system for use by customers or suppliers.

HOW COMPUTERS WORK

Computers receive, process, and store data. They use binary code to represent **alphanumeric** characters, which are numbers and alphabetic characters. **Binary code** is a series of 1s and 0s. All 1s are stored on the disk as magnetized areas and 0s are stored as areas that have not been magnetized. Each 1 or 0 is called a **bit.** Eight bits make up one **byte.** The unique code for each character is eight bits long. In the code for numeric characters, each position corresponds to a specific power of 2. Box 2–1 provides a binary representation of the number 13.

BOX 2–1 **Binary Representation of an Arabic Number**

The Arabic number 13 is represented using the binary system as 00001101. Each bit (0 or 1) represents a particular power of 2, depending on its position. If the position is taken by a 0, then it has no value. If a position is taken by a 1, it has the value of the associated power of 2. The Arabic number represented is the total of the powers of 2 represented by the 0s and 1s.

Binary representation of 13:	0	0	0	0	1	1	0	1
Powers of 2 by bit location:	2^7	2^6	2^5	2^4	2^3	2^2	2^1	2^0
Arabic value of position:	128	64	32	16	8	4	2	1
Actual value of bit:	0	+ 0	+ 0	+ 0	+ 8	+ 4	+ 0	+ 1	= 13

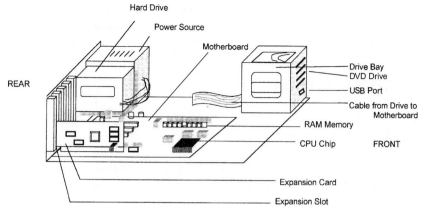

FIGURE 2–3 • Internal view of a PC

Computer programs, or software, use binary code to provide the instructions that direct the work computers do. PCs, notebooks, and PDAs differ slightly from supercomputers, mainframe computers, and minicomputers in the structure of their CPU. The CPU in larger computers is generally composed of one or more circuit boards, while smaller computers rely on a **microprocessor chip,** which contains the electronic circuits of the CPU etched on a silicon chip, mounted on a board, otherwise known as the **motherboard.** All electrical components, including the main memory, connect to this board. Figure 2–3 depicts the internal components of a PC. The motherboard also provides slots for network interface cards and peripheral device interface cards. The **network interface card** physically connects a computer to a network, controlling the flow of information between the two. Likewise, **peripheral device interface cards** connect equipment such as printers to the computer and control the exchange of information. The slot arrangement on motherboard allows users to change or add computer system components easily. Portable or laptop computers can be connected to networks or peripheral devices through the use of a **PCMCIA (Personal Computer Memory Card International Association) card.** These cards can be inserted into a slot, in the case of the laptop computer, to add increased functionality such as additional memory or network connections. PCMIA is an international association founded to establish standards for integrated circuit cards and promote interchangeability among mobile computers (PCMIA 2007). The organization also promotes interchangeability in other devices that include cameras, cable television, and automobiles.

Processor speed on personal computers is measured in **gigahertz.** A gigahertz (GHz) represents 1 billion cycles per second. The processor speed determines how rapidly instructions are handled. In general, each new PC model offers a faster CPU speed.

Whenever the power to a PC is turned on, the computer performs a start-up process. The program code for this test is stored in permanent memory and is known as **BIOS (basic input/output system).** The BIOS confirms that information about component parts is present and that this information coincides with existing hardware.

SELECTION CRITERIA

Equipment selection should be based on needs and expectations. When selecting a computer system and related hardware, it is important to consider the following:

- *The types of applications required.* For example, some people use primarily word processing programs, while others need applications to perform numeric calculations.
- *The program execution time and computer capacity needed to process jobs.* Complex jobs require higher processor speed and more memory for timely execution.
- *The number of workers who need computer access at any one time.* Single-user access demands can be met by a PC. Multiple demands for access may be better served by a network.
- *Storage capacity.* Storage needs are determined by the amount of information that must be kept and the length of time that it must be retained.
- *Backup options.* When information stored and processed on computers is critical to conduct daily business, another copy should be available to restore normal services after a crash.
- *Budget considerations.* The cost of hardware and software for various options should be considered in relation to the benefits and limitations associated with each.
- *Maintenance considerations.* There are several issues related to maintenance. These include durability, battery life and time required for recharging batteries, and the ability to easily disinfect or clean equipment to minimize the chances of spreading infection (Neely & Sittig 2002). Infection control may be accomplished via placement of computer equipment in areas away from splatter, the use of hand washing and antimicrobial hand cleaners, keyboard skins, and designated cleaning procedures with periodic cultures of equipment.

These factors will help to determine which type of computer or network is the best option, as well as the required hardware features. Advance planning ensures that current and future computer needs are well served.

User Needs and Ergonomic Considerations

Human factors should be considered in every work environment. Human factors, otherwise known as **ergonomics,** involves the study and design of a work environment that maximizes productivity by reducing operator fatigue and discomfort. Ergonomics considers physical stresses placed on joints, muscles, nerves, and tendons as well as environmental factors that can affect hearing and vision. Poor set-up of computer equipment leads to somatic complaints including headaches, eye strain, irritation, stress, fatigue, and neck and back pain. Even though the number of reported occupational injury claims has declined, failure to consider ergonomics is costly in terms of lost productivity (Bernhart 2006; Body Knowledge 2007; Brewer et al. 2006; Imrhan 2006; Visual ergonomics 2006). Ergonomics should receive the same attention given to other workplace education particularly since workplace injuries do not always start in the workplace. Additional research is also needed on the efficacy of interventions performed given that few quality studies have been done in this area. Ergonomics are especially important for users of laptop computers because these devices are designed for portability rather than good ergonomics. On a laptop computer, the keyboard and screen are too close together, causing eyestrain, and poor hand position and perching the computer on one's lap leads to poor posture (Gorman 2006; Holzer 2006; Tessler 2006). Whenever possible plug-in keyboards and laptop stands should be used to foster good ergonomics. Two health problems associated with poor ergonomics include computer vision syndrome and repetitive motion disorders.

Computer vision syndrome (CVS) is a term the American Optometric Association (AOA) uses to describe eye and vision problems that result from work done in close proximity such as occurs when using a computer for long periods of time (Anshel 2006). Eye and vision problems comprise the most frequently reported health problems and do impact productivity but receive less attention than do the musculoskeletal disorders primarily because vision problems are largely symptomatic and fleeting. Special consideration must also be given to the needs of the aging employee in designing work spaces. CVS symptoms include eyestrain, headaches, blurred distance or near vision, dry or red eyes, neck and/or backache, double vision, and light sensitivity. Poor lighting conditions, poor posture, and existing refractive errors contribute to the development of CVS in up to 90% of all computer workers.

Repetitive motion disorders or **repetitive stress injuries (RSIs)** result from using the same muscle groups over and over again without rest (National Institute of Neurological Disorders and Stroke 2007). One well-known example of a repetitive motion injury is **carpal tunnel syndrome.** Carpal tunnel syndrome occurs when the median nerve is compressed as it passes through the wrist along the pathway to the hand. This compression results in sensory and motor changes to the thumb, index finger, third finger, and radial aspect of the ring finger. Other repetitive motion injuries may involve the neck and shoulders. Good ergonomics helps to avoid occupational injuries and keeps employees productive. Box 2–2 provides a checklist to ensure good ergonomic design when designing and working at computer workstations. Another aspect of ergonomics addresses worker concerns about alleged health risks associated with computer use. The list of alleged health risks includes, but is not limited to, the following: cataracts, conception problems, miscarriage, and/or birth defects. Research has not established any clear links between computer use and these

BOX 2–2 Measures to Ensure Good Ergonomics When Using a Computer Workstation

Determine how a workstation will be used. Choose optimal settings for the chair, desk, keyboard, and monitor for the person who will use the area or that can easily be adjusted for each user. Adjustments are appropriate when wrists are flat and elbow angle is 90 degrees or more to prevent nerve compression.

Determine the length of time the user will be at the workstation. Individual adjustments are less critical if use is occasional or for very brief periods.

Configure work areas for specific types of equipment. Most workstation desks are designed for PCs rather than notebooks. Use a docking station or plug-in keyboard and stand if needed to ensure proper monitor and keyboard height.

Select sturdy surfaces or furniture with sufficient workspace. Desks should have room to write and use a mouse.

Provide chairs with good lumbar support. Relaxed sitting requires chairs that allow a reclined posture of 100 to 110 degrees.

Educate all workers on the need for good body mechanics when working with computers. Good posture is essential to reduce physical strain whether the individual works from a standing or sitting position.

Position monitors just below eye level approximately one arm's length away. The monitor should be about 30 inches from eye to screen and 20–40 degrees below the line of sight. This will help to prevent neck strain, especially for bifocal wearers.

Adjust screen resolution, font size, and brightness as needed. Sharp screen images help to reduce eye strain.

Periodically look away from the monitor to distant objects. This helps to avoid eye-focusing problems.

Minimize screen glare. Purchase nonglare monitors or place monitors at right angles to windows. Provide blinds or draperies, or adjust area lighting as needed.

Take frequent breaks. Intersperse computer work with other activities to avoid repetitive stress injuries.

Avoid noisy locations. Noise is distracting and stressful.

Place the workstation in a well-ventilated area. Fresh air and a comfortable temperature enhance working conditions.

Use ergonomic devices with caution. Select items that have been researched. Do not continue use if it remains uncomfortable after a trial period. Just because an item carries the label "ergonomic" does not mean that it is beneficial.

Use optical prescriptions designed for computer work. Everyday visual correction does not always work well for extended periods of computer work.

Provide lighting that can be adjusted to the needs of the individual. Older individuals need more light than younger persons to clearly view a task. Too little light contributes to eye fatigue and decreased productivity.

TABLE 2–2	Examples of Ergonomic Devices
Device	**Purpose**
Glare filter	Reduces eyestrain related to glare or light reflected from a monitor and may help make images appear sharper and text easier to read
Negative tilt keyboard	Tilts away from the user with the keyboard below elbow height to allow the user to rest arms, shoulders, neck, and back during pauses in typing
Document holder	Keeps documents at the same height and distance from the user as the monitor, limiting head and neck movement and tension
Ergonomic mouse	Various designs that aim to reduce wrist and hand pain
	No consistent research findings to support its use
Lumbar support	Maintains the natural curves of the back, minimizing back pain
Wrist rests	May actually increase carpal tunnel pressure unless a broad, flat, firm surface provides a place to rest the palm, not the wrist
Support braces/gloves	May relieve carpal tunnel symptoms when worn at night
	There are no consistent research findings to support use while typing
Ergonomic keyboards	Split keyboard designed to improve posture
	Research fails to support the benefit of this device
Foot rest	Encourages proper posture and supports the lower back to keep the pelvis properly tilted

risks. Table 2–2 lists several examples of commercially available ergonomic devices. Some controversy exists regarding the degree to which these devices benefit the user and prevent injury. Young (2006) suggests that organizations provide an area where employees can test ergonomic devices before bulk purchases are made. This would also be helpful for employees who need assistance to adapt to new types of devices (Armbrüster et al. 2007).

Physical Constraints

Space is a chronic problem in healthcare settings. For this reason, workstation planning is less a function of good ergonomics and more a function of finding a place to put the equipment. Ergonomics rarely receives high priority in planning. Provisions should be made for adequate numbers of computers in the clinical setting, located in quiet areas such as conference rooms.

Another major constraint to the installation of computers and networks in any institution centers on wiring and cabling. Adding power lines and cables for network connections to a current work space may prove to be more expensive than building a new work area. This is one reason for the growing popularity of wireless systems.

MOBILE AND WIRELESS COMPUTING

The terms **mobile** and **wireless** are often used interchangeably but are not the same. A device can be mobile without being wireless. **Mobile computing** uses devices that can be carried or wheeled from place to place. These devices may or may not have the capability to transmit and receive information while mobile. When mobile devices do not have a wireless connection the user must reestablish a connection periodically to receive updated information or to send collected information to a large computer on the network. This connection may be achieved by plugging into a network port, docking port, or, in the case of some handheld devices, the use of a special cable to communicate with a computer that is connected to the network. Mobile devices may include desktop, specialized workstations or notebook computers on carts, as well as some PDAs. **Wireless devices** are equipped with a special card enabling the broadcast and reception of signals that reach the network via access points. That network may be wireless or ultimately a traditional network connected by cable. Wireless devices are not tethered by a physical connection such as a cable or telephone line. Wireless devices can continually receive and transmit up-to-date information. Increasingly the term *mobile* is used to refer to wireless devices. Mobile and wireless computing offer the following advantages:

- *Both technologies bring computing to the bedside.* Point-of-care access allows healthcare providers and clients to view relevant information at the location where it is needed and eliminates the need to return to a workstation at the nurses' station, which might be in use.
- *Cost.* Mobile and wireless technology reduce the number of computers needed because the healthcare worker takes the device with him or her to where it will be used rather than needing to use the device at a fixed location. Mobile and wireless systems also reduce the costs associated with connecting a traditional network with cables. Installing cable is labor intensive, disrupts care, and can be difficult to accomplish, particularly in older buildings.
- *Improved data collection.* Computers at the point of care facilitate data collection. Care providers collect and input data once rather than taking handwritten notes for later entry into a computer.
- *More efficient work processes.* Wireless technology and redesign of work processes enable healthcare professionals to work more efficiently. A graphic example is seen with online prescription of drugs where the physician or nurse practitioner quickly accesses allergy and drug interaction information and instantly sends prescriptions to the hospital or patient's pharmacy without problems with interpretation of handwriting.

- *Error reduction.* Wireless technology is hailed as a means to prevent errors because it can deliver up-to-date information, provide decision support, access reference materials, and even provide electronic prescription application access at the point of care.

Until recently, wireless technology was plagued by a lack of interoperability. This obstacle was removed by the adoption of a standard for wireless data transmission, making it possible for all wireless devices manufactured after the adoption of the standard to communicate. Recent advances in processing capability make the PDA particularly attractive because it is small, lightweight, and easy to use.

The advantages associated with mobile and wireless technology also raise concerns that include:

- *Theft and loss.* These devices are more subject to theft and easy to lose because they are mobile and small enough to carry away. This requires the implementation of safeguards to protect information contained on stolen devices.
- *Threats to data security.* The security of data may be compromised when devices are stolen. The technology used to protect data on wireless networks has been less secure than technology used to encrypt information on traditional, hardwired networks. Vendors have been working on this issue.
- *Battery life.* Battery life varies according to use patterns and processing demands. Around-the-clock use requires close attention to the use of charge units and/or spare batteries.
- *Data loss.* Mobile devices are used to collect and send information to another computer system. Damage to devices, theft, loss, or downtime related to dead batteries may lead to loss of data before it can be shared.
- *Memory limitations.* While advances continue to add to the capability of handheld devices, memory limitations remain an issue, particularly when users expect additional features and capabilities.
- *Limited ability to display and see information.* Small screen size limits the amount of information that can be viewed at one time.
- *Deadzones.* Wireless devices may not be able to transmit and receive information in certain locations.
- *Lack of a means to readily exchange data between hospital information systems and handheld devices.* Physicians typically want clinical information systems available to them on their PDAs. The ability to provide clinical data to handheld devices can be arduous and expensive to develop.

Another concern related to the use of PDAs is that organizations need to develop a comprehensive strategy for their use and support if they do not already have one in place. Many physicians and other healthcare providers are purchasing their own PDAs but cannot fully realize benefits associated with their use without organizational plans for PDA use and support. Purchase recommendations from Information Services (IS) staff can help to avert disappointment. Useful information related to PDA use and available applications and databases can be found through the publications and Web sites of professional organizations as well as *PDA Cortex,* an online journal for mobile computing for healthcare professionals.

SOFTWARE

Software is a set of instructions that tells the computer what to do. **Programs** and **applications** are forms of software. All software is written in **programming languages.** Each programming language provides a detailed set of rules for how to write instructions for the computer. Numerous programming languages exist. A few examples are listed here. COBOL (Common Business Oriented Language) remains popular for business applications. MUMPS (Massachusetts General Hospital Utility Multi-Programming System) has been used for healthcare applications. Ada is a high-level, general-purpose programming language originally developed for the defense department. Ada supports real-time applications. C is a flexible language that is particularly popular for PCs because it is compact. C++ is a descendent of C. Unlike its predecessor it supports object-oriented programming, which allows reuse of some instructions. C++ is favored for graphical applications in the Windows and Macintosh environments. BASIC (Beginners All-Purpose Symbolic Instruction Code) is widely found in home computing. Java is a popular language for the development of programs for use on the Internet. Visual Basic is a programming language used for the development of graphical user interfaces. Structured Query Language (SQL) is an example of a programming language that allows the user to query or search a database for specific information.

Several categories of software exist; each has a different purpose. Some major software categories include operating systems, application software, and utility programs.

Operating Systems

The most essential type of software is the **operating system.** The operating system is a collection of programs that manage all of the computer's activities, including the control of hardware, execution of software, and management of information. *Control of hardware* refers to the ability of different parts of the computer to work together. Operating systems allow users to manage information through the retrieval, copying, movement, storage, and deletion of files.

The operating system also provides a user interface. The **user interface** is the means by which the individual interacts with the computer. For many years PC users had to enter specific text commands. Microsoft Windows provided a **graphical user interface (GUI).** A GUI provides menus, windows, and other standard screen features intended to make using a computer as intuitive as possible. GUIs decrease the amount of time required to learn new programs and eliminate the need to memorize commands. Work is underway on natural interfaces. The most natural user interface is the voice. Natural user interfaces are expected to free the user from conventional constraints such as mechanical keyboards, pointing devices, and GUIs, thereby making computers easier to use. Significant progress has occurred in recent years. Wireless technology, a highly mobile lifestyle, and advances in interactive voice recognition contribute to the increased use of voice recognition in call centers and for dictation. Voice recognition will not replace keyed data for some time yet. There are still limits to the number of words that are recognized and it is necessary to create a model of the user's voice before use. There also is an issue with accuracy, which is less than 100 percent.

Operating systems exist for all categories of computers. Windows and Linux are operating systems for PCs. Windows has been through several versions. Current versions include XP and VISTA. **Macintosh computers,** or **Macs,** have their own operating systems. Macs are commercial computers that offer a graphical interface and are available for home and office use. Macs are produced by Apple Computer Incorporated. Fewer software programs are available for Macs, but adaptations are available that permit Macs to run PC software. UNIX is an operating environment developed in the 1970s that is frequently found on large, commercial mainframe computers.

Application Software

Application software is a set of programs designed to accomplish a particular task such as word processing, financial management, or drawing. Application software builds on the foundation provided by the operating system. Box 2–3 lists some common types of software applications.

BOX 2–3 Common Types of Software Applications

- **Word processing.** Allows the creation of documents, utilizing features such as spelling and grammar correction, thesaurus, and graphics or pictures.
- **Presentation graphics.** Supports the preparation of slides and handout materials.
- **Spreadsheet.** Performs calculations, analyzes data, and presents information in tabular format and graphical displays.
- **Database.** Helps to manage large collections of information, such as payroll information, phone directories, and product listing. Performs calculations and produces reports from the stored information. Allows the user to find specific information.
- **Desktop publishing.** Offers expanded features that may not be commonly found in word processing programs. Useful for the creation of newsletters and other publications.
- **Web design.** Allows the user to create or revise Web pages and content that can then be posted to a Web site.
- **Specialized software**

Project management. Supports the management of projects with identification of tasks and time frames for completion, including PERT (program evaluation review technique) charts.

Personal information managers. Enhance personal productivity with time management tools, including an appointment calendar, telephone directories, and reminder lists.

Personnel scheduling. Automates the process of scheduling staff.

Report software. Allows database use for queries and to discern trends without the need to write code in computer programming languages.

Another factor that facilitates computer use is the development of software tutorials and online help. Most software packages now offer tutorials for review before application use, making software much more accessible to first-time users. Help screens are available while the program is running.

Utility Programs

Utility programs help to manage the computer and its data. Early operating systems offered few utility options such as optimization of the hard disk, system backup, or virus checks. To fill this need, a separate category of software evolved. Many utility programs are now included as part of the operating system. However, users may still choose to install and use utility programs that are independent of their operating systems.

ROLES OF SUPPORT PERSONNEL

Even though PCs bring computers closer to users, many people remain blissfully ignorant of computer technology beyond what they absolutely need to know. As a result, support is extremely important to maintaining user productivity. For example, PC support costs for large organizations typically range in the thousands of dollars for each computer. Support costs include time spent planning system upgrades, installation of upgrades for operating systems and various applications, troubleshooting, and user education. With help from support personnel, users can benefit from computers without knowing or understanding how they work.

In addition to personnel who support the computer user, many other positions are needed by hospitals and healthcare organizations that use computers and information systems. A **healthcare information system (HIS)** consists of a computer, including associated hardware and software that is dedicated to the collection, storage, processing, retrieval, and communication of information relevant to patient care within a healthcare organization. Staff are needed to create and maintain networks, customize and maintain software, and provide administration and leadership related to the HIS.

Supervisor/Manager

The size and complexity of information services departments requires a coordinated effort on the part of many different professionals, each with a different focus and set of talents. For this reason each team generally has a leader to help maintain this focus; this leader then reports to the chief information officer or vice-president of information services.

Superuser

The **superuser** has additional computer experience over the average employee and serves as a local resource person. In the hospital setting, the superuser is generally someone who knows the clinical area well and is able to answer most questions from users about the hospital computer system. The superuser often assists with information system training and support and may participate in the selection or design process.

Call Desk and Help Desk Personnel

The **call** or **help desk** is the first line of user support within an organization. These individuals require good communication skills as well as technical knowledge. A formal process exists for users to contact the call or help desk, usually by telephone or pager. All problems are logged to ensure that proper follow-up and resolution have occurred. If the problem cannot be resolved via telephone, then someone is sent to assist the user. Remote support tools have revolutionized help desk support in recent years largely eliminating the need for on-site, one-to-one support (Kane 2007). These tools allow help desk staff to see the same screens as the user and take over the user's computer if necessary. Remote capabilities also allow outsourcing of help desk functions often extending hours to 24-7. Help desk staff are more effective if they have an appreciation for the work of the organization.

Microcomputer or PC Specialist

The **PC specialist** provides information and training on commonly used productivity software and helps to acquaint users with new equipment including notebooks, PDAs, and aspects of mobile computing. These specialists often have technical training or an associate or a baccalaureate degree in computer science or a related area. PC specialists provide valuable services, but their salaries tend to be lower than those of other support personnel.

Clinical Information Analyst (CIA)

According to Versage (2006) the role of the **clinical information analyst** emerged out of the need to synthesize data and interpret its relationship to clinical interventions. It was made possible by electronic documentation using aggregate information stripped of patient identifiers. The work of the CIA supports process improvement and safety projects and quality initiatives that previously relied upon time and labor-intensive manual paper chart audits. The CIA can look at an infinite number of areas including patient satisfaction, wait times for treatment, medication use, and adverse events. This role supports evidence-based practice and is well suited to nurses, although other disciplines can use the same processes to monitor their respective areas.

Clinical Liaison

Clinical liaisons are clinicians who represent the interests and needs of the users and work with the information system team to address these issues during system design and implementation. They may or may not have formal computer or information system training or an informatics background. Liaisons sometimes continue their clinical role while fulfilling this responsibility.

Programmer

Programmers actually write the code, or instructions, that tell the computer what to do. They often lack a clinical background. For this reason, analysts are responsible for communicating user needs to programmers. In some institutions, one individual may serve as both analyst and programmer.

Network Administrator

Network administrators are responsible for the planning, management, and expansion of networks. Network administrators must decide whether to contract with outside agencies for network services and support or to educate in-house personnel for these functions. Unfortunately, many organizations lack a mechanism to coordinate equipment selection among different departments but expect the network manager to get the resulting hodgepodge of equipment linked together. This is particularly true as more users purchase their own devices and expect them to work seamlessly with an existing network. Organizations should involve network administrators in equipment decisions when the ultimate goal involves the creation or expansion of a network. It is possible to become a certified network engineer via special course work and an examination. Network administrators can access all data no matter who owns it. The salaries of network administrators typically exceed those of the personnel discussed thus far.

Trainer

Trainers are responsible for educating clinical users in one or more applications and may also be required to define and monitor user competencies. Trainers may or may not have a clinical background but have knowledge of the specific computer application that they are teaching. This role may be filled as a permanent position or may be done by other information systems or clinical staff, as needed. Some organizations have a separate trainer for common office applications and PC use and another for information systems training.

Security Officer

Security officers are responsible for ensuring that measures exist to protect information privacy. This usually includes a process for assigning and monitoring system access identification codes and passwords as well as paper-based information. In some cases the security officer may be responsible for protecting the physical equipment and data stored there. Federal legislation and interest in data security make this an important role, although there are few full-time security officers at the present. Strategic planning, risk management, and the development of corporate wide policies and procedures are increasingly a part of the security office role. Security officers also need to educate administrators, physicians, and staff about security issues. The use of the Internet in healthcare means that the security officer must protect corporate information systems from outside threats in addition to protecting information found solely on desktop systems.

Chief Information Officer

The **chief information officer (CIO)** should have a broad view of the needs of the institution and the design, implementation, and evaluation of information systems. Responsibilities include strategic planning, policy development, budgeting, information security, recruitment and retention of information services staff, and overall management of the enterprise's information systems. In some agencies the information services department is responsible for all computers and computer training. In recent years there has been a shift from chief technology officer to CIO as more CIOs play a greater role in developing their organization's strategies. The CIO is at the top of the compensation heap for computer-related positions. Preparation is usually at a master's or doctoral degree level.

Webmaster

The **Webmaster** is generally responsible for the design, maintenance, and security of materials placed on the Internet, intranet, and/or extranet. Growing concerns over information security, expanded use of Internet technology, and federal mandates require increased collaboration with other roles. The emphasis upon a well-designed Web page that is easy to navigate makes this an important position in any organization. Some facilities opt to outsource this function.

Chief Privacy Officer

Federal legislation mandates that each patient care organization name a **chief privacy officer (CPO)** to protect the personal health information of patients. This includes paper and electronic information. The time required to fulfill these responsibilities will vary according to the size of the organization, allowing for the combination of the roles of chief privacy and chief security officers in some cases or the integration of these duties into other existing positions such as an information services manager. The American Health Information Management Association (AHIMA) posted a sample job description on their Web site. AHIMA proposes that the health information management professional is uniquely qualified to serve as privacy officer through his or her professional preparation, experience, commitment to patient advocacy, and professional code of ethics. Grove and Dempster (2007) concur with this view in their privacy and security toolkit. Abundant information is available to assist the individual assuming these responsibilities through government and professional sites such as AHIMA and the Healthcare Information Management Systems Society (HIMSS).

Chief E-health Officer

The **chief e-health officer (CeO)** role was created in some organizations as part of a strategy for expanding their use of the Internet beyond informational Web sites to encompass a range of new services electronically. There were questions as to whether the creation of this role was a fad. There has been no mention of this role in recent literature, leading one to assume that the responsibilities have been delegated to other personnel.

Compliance Officer

The role of **compliance officer** is emerging in many organizations as one person is designated to ensure that state and federal regulations and accrediting requirements are met both via paper and automated records and systems. It may or may not be assumed by a member of the information services department but the professional preparation and experience of information services professionals provides an advantage. Many information services personnel believe that compliance is more of an educational issue than a systems issue.

Continuity Planning

Continuity planning is an essential component of strategic planning that needs to extend beyond the walls of any one institution. To ensure that plans are up-to-date and that business operations can be maintained despite extreme situations, one person should be designated to coordinate and update plans for all situations including natural and man-made disasters, and acts of terrorism.

Interface Engineer

Any healthcare organization is typically composed of many different information systems. The majority of these systems were not specifically designed to work with other systems. The interface engineer ensures that information is exchanged between disparate systems and isolates and corrects problems behind the scenes invisible to the users of the individual systems.

Clinical Systems Analyst

Healthcare information system analysts are responsible for a wide range of activities related to the successful automation of information management. They may be clinicians who became involved in system selection and training. Many learned their role on the job and furthered their education by taking computer or information science classes. Analysts interview staff, determine user needs, write specifications for software performance, participate in some computer programming and debugging, implement new automated functions, and document program specifications and changes.

FUTURE DIRECTIONS

Technology is a pervasive part of everyday life. It is an integral part of home appliances and is found throughout the healthcare delivery system. It is frequently invisible to the user but does require a bevy of behind-the-scenes people to ensure both its ongoing and optimal use. Technology will continue to develop and evolve in ways that are difficult to imagine today. Devices will become smaller and easier to use. This process will extend the capabilities of providers and create new disciplines. One area that is expected to have a large impact in the near future is nanotechnology. **Nanotechnology** is the science and technology of engineering devices at the molecular level (Gulson & Wong 2006; Health and Medicine 2006; Knowles 2006; McCauley 2005). Nanotechnology is already used in cosmetics and sunscreens and other industries. Work is underway to create electrical circuits that would allow the development of smaller computers, the design of new monitoring technologies, and the development of smart drug delivery systems. At this time the effects of nanotechnology on human health are not known and will need to be monitored over time.

CASE STUDY EXERCISES

2.1 You are appointed to the hospital's information technology committee as the representative for your nursing unit. The charges of the committee include the following:
- Identify PC software that is needed to accomplish unit work, such as word processing, spreadsheets, and databases.
- Determine criteria for the selection and placement of hardware on the units.

Discuss these issues and how they affect patient care and workflow.

2.2 Your committee is charged with setting up a computer system that will automate transcription of physician orders and reporting of results. Identify the support personnel that you need at this point and write job descriptions for each identified position.

2.3 The infection control nurse has traced the spread of a nosocomial infection to a computer keyboard on a hospital unit. It is located in a work area adjacent to four patient rooms. This computer is routinely used by staff for documentation, to check laboratory and radiology results, and to access reference materials. The infection control nurse has asked the unit director and staff to identify strategies to eliminate this problem. Identify measures that can help to eliminate this problem.

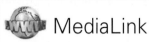

MediaLink

Additional resources for this content can be found on the Companion Website at www.prenhall.com/hebda. Click on "Chapter 2" to select the activities for this chapter.

- Glossary
- Multiple Choice
- Discussion Points
- Case Studies
- MediaLink Application
- MediaLink

SUMMARY

- Computers are machines that process data under the direction of a program, or stored sequence of instructions.
- The major hardware components of computers are input devices, the CPU, secondary storage, and output devices.
- The major categories of computers are: supercomputers, mainframes, minicomputers, PCs or desktop systems, laptop or notebook computers, tablet computers and handheld devices such as PDAs, the BlackBerry®, iPod, and iPhone.
- Peripheral hardware items, such as the keyboard, mouse, monitor, modem, and printer, help the user put data into the computer, read output, and communicate with other users.
- Networks are linked systems of computers. LANs, WANs, and the Internet are all types of computer networks.
- Networks may use various technologies including cabling, radio signals, client/server, and thin client.
- In choosing a computer system, one must consider current and future information processing needs, budget, and human factors.
- Good ergonomics reduces physical discomforts and injury associated with computer use.
- Mobile and handheld computer technology provide the promise of efficiency, improvements in the safety of care delivery, cost savings, and work redesign.
- Software is the set of instructions that make a computer run and control its resources. Operating systems, applications, utility programs, and programming languages are all types of software.
- Support personnel are essential to help people use PCs and information systems effectively and to maintain and upgrade hardware and software.

REFERENCES

Anshel, J. (2006). Visual Ergonomics in the Workplace: Improving eyecare and vision can enhance productivity. *Professional Safety, 51*(8), 20–25. Retrieved December 27, 2007, from Business Source Elite database.

Armbrüster, C., Sutter, C., & Ziefle, M. (2007). Notebook input devices put to the age test: The usability of trackpoint and touchpad for middle-aged adults.

Ergonomics, 50(3), 426–445. Retrieved December 27, 2007, from CINAHL with Full Text database.

Bernhart, H. (2006). Ergonomics offers preventive approach to musculoskeletal problems. *Employee Benefit News, 20*(13), 55–58. Retrieved December 27, 2007, from Business Source Elite database.

Body Knowledge: Improved Ergonomics = Improved Productivity. (2007, February). *Material Handling Management*, Retrieved December 27, 2007, from Business Source Elite database.

Brewer, S., Van Eerd, D., Amick, B., Irvin, E., Daum, K., Gerr, F., et al. (2006). Workplace interventions to prevent musculoskeletal and visual symptoms and disorders among computer users: A systematic review. *Journal of Occupational Rehabilitation, 16*(3), 325–358. Retrieved December 27, 2007, from CINAHL with Full Text database.

Gorman, R. (2006, January). Pain relief for laptop-lovers: Notebook computers are easy to adore—but hard on your body. Here are 5 easy fixes. *Health, 20*(1), 97–98. Retrieved December 27, 2007, from CINAHL with Full Text database.

Grove, T. & Demster, B. (January 2007). HIMSS Toolkit: Managing information privacy & security in healthcare administrative requirements for privacy. Healthcare Information and Management Systems Society. Retrieved December 31, 2007, from http://www.himss.org/content/files/CPRIToolkit/version6/v6%20pdf/D73_Admin_Requirements.pdf.

Gulson, B. & Wong, H. (2006). Stable Isotopic Tracing—A Way Forward for Nanotechnology. *Environmental Health Perspectives, 114*(10), 1486–1488.

Hall, M. (2006, May 8). A Focus on 'Proper' Ergonomics. . . . *Computerworld, 40*(19), 10. Retrieved December 27, 2007, from Business Source Elite database.

Health alert: Never overlook ergonomics. (2006, April). *Quill*, Retrieved December 27, 2007, from Business Source Elite database.

Health and Medicine. (2006). *Futurist, 40*(6), Special section, p. 4–5.

Holzer, L. (2006, April). Good piano technique: The key to healthy computer keyboarding. *Positive Health*, Retrieved December 27, 2007, from CINAHL with Full Text database.

Imrhan, S. (2006). Health alert: Never overlook ergonomics. *Quill, 94*(3), 40.

Kane, C. (2007), Trends in IT Outsourcing. *Associations Now, 3*(10), Special section, p. 8–9.

Knowles III, E.E. (2006). Nanotechnology. *Professional Safety, 51*(3), 20–27.

McCauley, L. A. (2005). Nanotechnology: Are occupational health nurses ready? *AAOHN Journal, 53*(12), 517–521.

National Institute of Neurological Disorders and Stroke. (February 14, 2007). NINDS Repetitive Motion Disorders Information Page. Retrieved December 29, 2007, from http://www.ninds.nih.gov/disorders/repetitive_motion/repetitive_motion.htm

Neely, A. N. & Sittig, D. F. (July 23, 2002). Basic microbiologic and infection control information to reduce the potential transmission of pathogens to patients via computer hardware. *Journal of the American Medical Informatics Association, 9*, 500–508.

Personal Computer Memory Card International Association (PCMCIA). (December 29, 2007). About PCMCIA. Retrieved December 29, 2007, from http://www.pcmcia.org/about.htm.

Tessler, F. (2006, January). Laptop Ergonomics. *Macworld, 23*(1), 85–86. Retrieved December 27, 2007, from Business Source Elite database.

Versage, B. (2006). The clinical information analyst. *Pennsylvania Nurse, 61*(2),15.

Young, W. (2006). You're Invited to an Ergo Room. *Journal of Accountancy, 202*(6), 39. Retrieved December 27, 2007, from Business Source Elite database.

Visual Ergonomics. (2006, May). *T+D*, Retrieved December 27, 2007, from Business Source Elite database.

CHAPTER 3

Ensuring the Quality of Information

After completing this chapter, you should be able to:

1 Define *data integrity* and its relevance for healthcare.

2 Discuss the relevance of data management for data integrity.

3 Identify strategies to ensure the accuracy of data.

4 Differentiate between online and offline data storage.

5 Explain how storage conditions can affect data integrity.

6 Debate the relative merits of outsourcing data storage.

7 Discuss factors that should be addressed when planning for data retrieval.

8 Identify characteristics associated with quality information.

9 Discuss the significance of data cleansing for data warehousing and data mining.

10 Define *data mining* and recognize its uses within healthcare.

11 Examine the relationship between data mining, knowledge discovery in databases, and evidence-based practice.

12 Explore the role of the nurse with *knowledge discovery in databases*.

Data provides the building blocks in the formation of knowledge. For this reason it is essential to understand the concepts of data integrity, principles of good data management, the characteristics of quality data, the significance of data mining, and knowledge discovery in databases. The amount of data collected and stored has grown exponentially in all sectors in recent years. According to Berger and Berger (2004 p. 123), "The shift toward evidence-based practice and outcomes research presents significant opportunities and challenges to extract meaningful information from massive amounts of clinical data to transform it into the best available knowledge to guide nursing practice." This process, however, requires the collection of the right information in its entirety, no compromises to the quality of collected data and special analysis using statistics, artificial intelligence, and machine learning technologies to provide useful information about patterns and relationships that might not otherwise be obvious.

DATA INTEGRITY

Data integrity refers to the ability to collect, store, and retrieve correct, complete, and current data so it will be available to authorized users when needed. Data integrity is one of the most important issues related to computing and information handling in healthcare because treatment decisions are based on information derived from data. If the data are faulty or incomplete, the quality of derived information may be poor, resulting in decisions that may be inappropriate and possibly harmful to clients. For example, if the nurse interviewing a client collects data related to allergies but fails to document all reported allergies, the client may be given drugs that cause an allergic reaction. In this case, the data were collected but not stored properly.

Ensuring Correct Data Collection and Entry

Computer systems facilitate data collection but may increase the potential for entry of incorrect data through input errors. These errors may include hitting the wrong key on a computer keyboard, selecting the wrong item from a screen using touch or a mouse, or failing to enter all data collected. Several measures can be taken to decrease the likelihood of input errors, including educating personnel, conducting system checks, and verifying data.

Educating Personnel Staff who are proficient in the use of the input device and computer system are less likely to make data collection and entry errors (Wright & Bartram 2000). All personnel should attend classes that emphasize appropriate system access, input device use, potential harmful effects associated with incorrect data, data verification techniques, and error correction. On the completion of classes, all employees should demonstrate competence in system use. Even after staff display competence, continuing education should occur on a routine basis and as indicated by problems such as increases in data errors.

System Checks to Ensure Accurate Data Entry and Data Completeness Data entry systems should be easy to use and provide periodic checks to ascertain that data are correct and complete. A **system check** is a mechanism provided by the computer system to assist users by prompting them to complete a task, verify information, or prevent entry of inappropriate information. Computer systems facilitate data collection and verification in several ways. Examples of computer system safeguards and generated prompts include the following:

- *Data cleansing technology.* Information technology (IT) can help an organization to derive improved information and generate knowledge from data stored on different information systems (Gudea 2005). Originally software was developed to eliminate variations in name and address information for direct mail campaigns used by businesses as a means to eliminate multiple mailings for the same party. Used at the point of data entry, it serves to prevent data input errors. This is best illustrated when the system asks the user to confirm whether there is a match already in the database for a patient, thereby eliminating duplicate entries with several variants in name or address.
- *Requesting information about a client's allergies when no entry has been made regarding allergies.* In the absence of an entry regarding allergies, the system may not accept medication and radiology orders.
- *Informing the user that an order already exists when the user attempts to enter a duplicate order.* The system requests verification before processing the duplicate order. This can prevent unintentional repetition of expensive diagnostic tests. For example, a physician previously ordered a complete blood count (CBC) to be drawn on the current day. Another physician has ordered a hemoglobin and hematocrit (H & H), also to be drawn on the current day. When the order for the H & H is entered into the computer, the system will alert the user that this is a duplicate order, because the H & H is part of the CBC.
- *Producing printouts alerting the nurse that a prescribed medication has not been documented as given.* This improves the quality of client care and documentation.

Data Verification Techniques Another means to ensure data accuracy is to have clients verify data that are collected during the admission and assessment processes (Brennan 1996). The active participation of the client in the data verification process remains a relatively new concept in relation to healthcare computer systems. This verification may be accomplished through one of the following methods:

- Verbal confirmation
- Asking clients to review data on selected screens
- Asking clients to review printouts of entered data

Each of these methods has potential problems. For example, with verbal confirmation clients may answer "yes" without actually hearing or understanding what was said to them. Screen review is difficult for the visually impaired or may be done too quickly for the client to scan all information. Finally, reading print-outs is impractical for the visually impaired or illiterate. It also creates the additional problem of papers that must be disposed of with consideration for their confidential nature. All methods may be problematic for the individual who does not speak English.

Although the initial data collection and entry process provides an excellent opportunity to verify data accuracy and completeness, it should not be the only time that this is done. Healthcare consumers should be able to review their records at any time and furnish additional information that they believe is important to their care or to dispute portions of their record with which they do not agree. Recent federal legislation ensures these rights (Hicks 2001).

How to Minimize Fraudulent Information Another concern in the concept of data integrity is the entry of fraudulent information. Fraudulent information can lead to financial loss to the provider and third-party payer as well as sully the credit rating of an innocent victim whose identity and insurance information were used. It may also result in treatment errors. At present, admitting clerks and physician office staff ask for the client's insurance card at the time of treatment. This request should also include proof of identification, preferably photograph identification, as a means to decrease claims filed under another person's identity. Clients should be informed of the purpose of this request and sign a statement indicating that they are aware that insurance fraud is a criminal act and that use of another person's insurance data may result in bodily harm secondary to treatment decisions based on someone else's health record.

DATA MANAGEMENT

The changing healthcare delivery system provides the driving force for improved data management. **Data management** is the process of controlling the collection, storage, retrieval, and use of data to optimize accuracy and utility while safeguarding integrity. Computers are an essential tool in this process. Good data management is essential for organizational decision making and is sometimes referred to as business intelligence (BI) (Kolar 2001). One important part of decision making is the distribution of information via reports. Good data management involves knowing who needs report information, what reports are generated and what they are called, and when reports are available (Liebmann 2000).

Several levels of personnel are involved in data management. Personnel at the point of data entry include employees and, in some cases, clients. System analysts help the users to specify the data that are to be collected and how this will be accomplished. Programmers create the computer instructions or program that will collect the required data. They also build the **database,** a file structure that supports the storage of data in an organized fashion and allows data retrieval as meaningful information. Some facilities may also employ a

database administrator (DBA), who is responsible for overseeing all activities related to maintaining the database and optimizing its use.

A **relational database** is designed using data that are represented as tables. This type of database is easily updated and can provide specific information to answer a query. Additional types of databases may be used as well. A **data warehouse** provides an even more powerful method of managing and analyzing data. A data warehouse is a repository for storing data from several different databases so that it can be combined and manipulated to provide answers to complex analytic questions (Benander & Benander 2000).

Costs and benefits are additional considerations in the management of data. Storage and management of paper and film records are labor intensive and expensive. Retrieval of paper and film records must be done manually, and information may not be available when and where it is needed. Physical records are also subject to loss. One current solution is **document imaging,** which involves scanning paper records onto computer disks or other media to facilitate electronic storage and handling. Converting paper records to other storage media may facilitate management, but a better solution is to move away from paper, with data entered directly to automated records. Although automated solutions may also be costly, they provide increased efficiency and improved access.

Automation of healthcare records creates new issues related to data storage and retrieval. Recent estimates project that PC, network, and mainframe storage requirements will grow 50% per year. Along with an increase in volume and types of materials for storage, data storage and retrieval require special conditions to ensure data integrity.

Data Storage

There are two basic types of data storage: online and offline. **Online storage** provides access to current data. Online storage is rapid, using high-speed hard disk drives or storage space allocated on the network. **Offline storage** is used for data that are needed less frequently, or for long-term data storage, as may occur with old client records. Offline storage can be done on any secondary storage device. Access to data stored offline is slower than with online storage. Immediacy of need for particular data is a key factor in determining whether it is stored online or offline. Table 3–1 describes various types of storage media, along with their advantages and disadvantages.

To protect computerized information, organizations need a storage strategy that addresses the following issues (Digital Preservation Coalition 2002):

- *Environmental conditions and physical hazards.* These include temperature, humidity, shock, dust control, and protection from damage by fire, water, or electromagnetic fields. Some media are more sensitive to environmental factors than others. Strict environmental controls protect the storage media and the data it contains. In general, temperatures in the 10°C range in conjunction with ideal environmental conditions help to maximize the shelf life for media.

TABLE 3–1	Storage Media		
Type	**Description**	**Advantages**	**Disadvantages**
Optical media	A laser is used to alter the recording surface, which is then read as data	High data capacities Two major types: WORM (write once read many) and rewritable WORM: Does not use previously written sectors Difficult to alter Provides good data protection Identification is stamped into disks at production Sets aside corrupt data sectors May be accessed repeatedly over 30-year shelf life	Readable only in specific drives Disc swaps may be time-consuming Use of high-capacity discs decrease number of swaps and increases retrieval performance Limited expectations for future use as the price and performance for other media continue to improve Media subject to damage through poor handling or storage
Removable/portable hard drives	Easily removable from computer "docking bays"	Quick	Requires plug-and-play
Compact disc read only memory (CD-ROM)	CD-R uses a light-sensitive dye layer as the data layer CD-ROM uses a series of pits and plateau in a metallic layer	Requires little storage space May have a shelf life of up to 75 years assuming ideal storage conditions and limited use	Not feasible for large-scale data storage CD-R technology less stable than CD-ROM
DVD	Inexpensive Can store up to 18 GB	Large storage capacity Requires little storage space Affords backward compatibility with CD-ROM discs Suitable for storage of data, images, and sound May have a shelf life of up to 75 years contingent on storage conditions and use	Standardization in devices not reached

(*continued*)

TABLE 3–1 (*continued*)

Type	Description	Advantages	Disadvantages
Redundant array of disks (RAID)	Uses two or more hard drives connected together to mirror data on duplicate drives	Very safe storage method Provides better performance at a better price than optical technology	Requires purchase of twice the needed storage
Magneto-optical	Uses a special alloy layer modified by a magnetic field later read by laser	Durable and transportable Rewritable Thirty-year shelf life	Slow search time
Magnetic tape or cartridges	The magnetic field on the media surface is altered using tiny electromagnets to "write" the data	Traditional mainframe storage media Inexpensive Available in several formats Can store large amounts of information Easy to duplicate and move to another location Reusable 1 to 75-year shelf life contingent on storage conditions and use	Slow May be difficult to use Backup requires verification Tape drives require maintenance Can be damaged by exposure to dust, electromagnetic fields, moisture Store under climate-controlled conditions, 20° to 22° C Minimize unnecessary handling to reduce wear

- *Control of equipment and media.* This refers to who may access computer equipment and data and is supported through a combination of physical and logical restrictions. Physical restrictions maintain a secure locked environment for the computer hardware and operations areas. Logical restrictions limit data access to only those staff who require this information. For example, admission clerks might be restricted from accessing clinical information such as test results but might be able to access demographic and insurance information.
- *Contingency planning.* A secondary or backup copy of the data is created as a safeguard in the event of loss or damage to the primary data. This backup copy should be stored at another location separate from the computer, reducing the danger that a disaster will affect both the computer and the storage area.
- *Storage period for each record type.* The minimum length of time that client records must be stored is dictated by state laws. An organization may

choose to retain records indefinitely, but cost and physical storage constraints must be considered.

- *Plans to transfer data to new media before degradation occurs.* For example, data stored on magnetic tape may degrade after 1 to 50 years, depending on storage conditions. If the organization intends to retain records indefinitely, the data must be transferred to other media.
- *Recognition that most electronic media will be threatened by the obsolescence of the hardware and software needed to access them.* Rapid advances in technology lead to the discontinuation of formats and media as more efficient storage modalities are introduced.
- *Maintenance of access devices.* Problems with access devices are one of the most common causes of damage to magnetic storage media. Consideration should be given to writing and reading archive copies from different devices as a means to protect against data loss from malfunctioning devices.

Outsourcing Data Management and Storage

Internal data storage is costly in terms of human resources and space that can be allocated for other purposes. Storage costs include the purchase price for devices and the costs of media, maintenance, and environmental control. These costs may consume a significant portion of the information services budget. Storage can be handled internally or outsourced. **Outsourcing** is the process by which an organization contracts with outside agencies for services. Outsourcing provides a means to cut costs that would otherwise be required for the physical space, special conditions, and support personnel needed to maintain storage media and data.

Outsourcing companies specialize in all aspects of data management for multiple customers, providing services at a lower cost than if the customers performed the tasks themselves. It is important to review the contract to ensure that the outsourcing company can meet all of the institution's requirements for data storage and retrieval.

Data Retrieval

Data retrieval is a process that allows the user to access previously collected and stored data. Data retrieval most commonly occurs as a function of a software application in conjunction with secondary storage media. Recent developments in technology have cut storage costs and improved access and capacity. In addition to new options in storage media, a variety of automated devices are available that provide access to stored data. Automated magnetic tape has been used to archive healthcare data for many years.

The significance of data retrieval may be seen in the development of an automated client record that covers the client's life span. Although these advances are critical to the development of a birth-to-death health record, many providers are still in the first phases of developing systems for each client visit and have limited archival access. Furthermore, present hospital data storage systems save data but often lack the ability to manipulate data to demonstrate patterns. For example, it should be possible to easily extract demographic data on the population served, individual and aggregate responses to specific treatment modalities, or abnormal laboratory values for a given client.

The following factors should be considered when planning for data retrieval:

- *Performance.* Performance refers to the ability of the system to respond to user requests for data retrieval. Some of the specific factors that define performance include acceptable retrieval response time and the ability to accommodate numerous simultaneous requests for data.
- *Capacity.* Capacity is the number and size of records that can be stored and retrieved.
- *Data security.* Data must be protected against unauthorized access and retrieval.
- *Cost.* The costs include hardware, software, and support personnel. Data storage and retrieval costs overlap in many cases.

Retrieval needs are frequently underestimated. For example, some systems sharply limit the amount of archival data available to users and may impede treatment. Determination of system performance requirements helps data management personnel and administrators choose storage and retrieval strategies for user needs. Generally, record demand is highest soon after data are collected, with the number of access requests and need for rapid retrieval diminishing with the passage of time.

Data Exchange

In the past, data retrieval was primarily performed for use within a single institution. Changes in the healthcare delivery system now mandate exchange of client information between institutions. For example, a client may have surgery at a major medical center but have follow-up appointments at a satellite location. The client's record must be accessible to clinicians at both sites. Several other factors contribute to the need to send client records in a timely fashion from one provider to another and to submit reimbursement claims in a timely fashion. These factors include, but are not limited to, a highly mobile population and consumer demands for efficiency. **Electronic data interchange (EDI)** streamlines the flow of clinical and financial data from one location to another. EDI is the communication of data in binary code from one computer to another. As the number of automated client record systems increases, so does the need to establish standard record structure and identifiers for individual data items to facilitate data exchange.

Although EDI facilitates record exchange, there are problems associated with it. A major problem is that different computer systems use different formats for data. The data format from the sending system may not be understood by the receiving system. One solution to this problem is the development of a standard data format for EDI. At the present, no agreement exists among healthcare groups in the United States regarding a common EDI standard. Several groups are currently working toward a common standard. One proposed solution is **Health Level 7 (HL7)**. HL7 is both the name of the group and a standard for the exchange of clinical data. HL7 has an extensive set of rules that apply to all data sent.

Data Cleansing

The first step in data cleansing is determining the extent of the problem. This can help users to decide where to focus their efforts for quality improvement for the input of new data as well as data that have already been collected. Manual review and correction of poor-quality data are extremely labor intensive. **Data cleansing** or **scrubbing** is a procedure that uses software to improve the quality of data to ensure that it is accurate enough for use in data mining and warehousing. It uses technology to reconcile data inconsistencies that arise from different systems as well as duplicate entries in one system. These inconsistencies may include typographical errors, misspellings, and various abbreviations as well as address changes. According to Boyle and Cunningham (2002), data errors may be found in nearly one third of clinical records. The fact that abbreviations can have totally different meanings in different systems becomes a major problem with data warehousing. Another problem is the use of automatic defaults, which fill in blanks with information that is not accurate. One example is seen when the name of the ordering physician is "defaulted in" for the primary physician when it is not the same. Data cleansing is essential to data warehousing. Data inconsistencies that did not pose problems for daily operations do create a problem for data warehousing because it requires a higher quality data.

The use of Internet technology for data entry by employees as well as clients serves to minimize some problems but accentuate others. This is because employees can be trained in data entry and can be called back for additional training if problems are noted. Clients have not had the benefit of system training to know what constitutes acceptable entries, and they may not have the incentive to correct errors in some cases. The use of data cleansing technology was once limited by its high costs and difficulties in implementation but improvements in the quality of data can improve safety and save money through elimination of duplication (Gilhooly 2005).

Data Disposal

Appropriate disposal of electronic and print data that is no longer required is an important aspect of data management (Hoffman 2006). Print media can be discarded in special receptacles designated for confidential materials. Data destruction may be achieved through physical destruction and software destruction. Physical destruction may be accomplished by deforming storage media or using a magnet to destroy contents. Special equipment is available to destroy hard drives. Commercial software may be used to overwrite data by filling the hard drive with zeros. Destruction may be done internally or outsourced. Factors in the selection of vendor services should include:

- Procedures used to determine that destruction has occurred as planned.
- Vendor security to protect data and/or equipment.
- Errors and omissions insurance in the event that some data is accidentally disclosed.

It is important to ensure that disposal occurs as planned to avoid violating legislation intended to safeguard patient privacy.

CHARACTERISTICS OF QUALITY INFORMATION

If the recommended procedures for data collection, validation, storage, management, and retrieval are followed, then the end result is quality information. The significance of quality information is its potential impact on client care. High-quality information is needed by clinicians to make appropriate clinical decisions. In addition, quality information supports the ability of researchers to contribute to nursing science and the ability of healthcare administrators to perform outcomes analysis as a means to capture cost savings (Dakins 2001). The following characteristics describe quality information (Burke 1992; Kahn 1995; Tozor 1994; Zorkoczy & Heap 1995):

- *Timely.* Information is available when it is needed. The ability to access the client's insurance information at the time of an outpatient visit allows timely verification of coverage for specified procedures.
- *Precise.* Each detail is complete and clear. An example of a lack of precision is the client's report of previous "abdominal surgery." Precise data would be the identification of the specific surgical procedure, such as appendectomy.
- *Accurate.* Information is without error. An example of inaccurate data is documentation of the wrong leg in a below-the-knee amputation.
- *Numerically quantifiable.* The ability to measure data improves quality. An example is seen with the ability to measure and stage a decubitus ulcer, which aids the subsequent assessment of its status by other professionals.
- *Verifiable by independent means.* Two different people can make the same observation and report the same result. If two people listen to a client's apical heart rate simultaneously, they should both report the same rate.
- *Rapidly and easily available.* For example, the nurse can quickly retrieve a client's allergies from a past medical record stored by the computer system when a critically ill patient arrives in the emergency department.
- *Free from bias, or modification with the intent to influence recipients.* Data should be based on objective rather than subjective evaluation. Documenting that a client is depressed represents subjective interpretation. A better approach is to document observations about the client's activity level and interactions with others. These are quality data.
- *Comprehensive.* Required information is present. When a nurse asks a client for a list of current medications, it should include medication name, dosage, and frequency taken.
- *Appropriate to the user's needs.* Different users have different data needs. The appropriate data must be available for each user. For example, the nurse must be able to access data related to a client's previous diabetic teaching.
- *Clear.* Information is free from ambiguity, reducing the likelihood of treatment errors. An example is seen in the client's report of an allergy to eggs.

On questioning, the nurse determines that the client only dislikes eggs and does not wish to be served them but has never had a truly allergic response.

- *Reliable regardless of who collects it.* There may be certain data that multiple professionals collect. Client allergies may be documented by the nurse, physician, and pharmacist. All documentation of allergies should agree.
- *Current.* All files should contain the most current information available to the healthcare team. For information to be kept current, a regular system for updating must be put in place. Having current information available on the computer will help avoid errors that could be harmful to clients. For example, data retrieved at an outpatient setting should include all recent inpatient data that is pertinent, not just the most recent outpatient data.
- *In a convenient form for interpretation, classification, storage, retrieval, and updates.* The user must be able to access and use the data without difficulty.

Quality is also an issue when large amounts of data on different computer types and using different formats must be extracted for storage or analysis (Faden 2000). Format variations can accentuate inaccuracies and erode data quality, particularly as the number of databases and the age of the stored data increase. For example, a client may have been registered and treated at one hospital a number of times, using a slightly different version of the client's name for each registration. One registration may have been created using a client's legal name, another using a nickname, and another omitting a middle initial. There also may have been a change in address during this period. It can be difficult in this instance to verify that all records belong to the same person; until recently, each record had to be examined individually for error. Software tools can now perform this task. The data source that is most likely to be correct is used for this purpose. Box 3–1 lists a summary of threats to quality, availability, and confidentiality of information.

BOX 3–1 Threats to Information Quality, Availability, and Confidentiality

Threats to Information Quality

- **Alteration of files.** The accidental or intentional addition or change of data erodes the quality of the information. Accidental changes are known as data corruption. Intentional changes are viewed as forgery.
- **System alteration.** When systems are changed, the way that data are processed may be affected. For example, the addition of a new function may result in the loss of data due to planning or programming deficiencies.
- **Introduction of viruses, Trojans, or worms.** Viruses, Trojans, and worms are unwanted programs, created with malicious intent, that can damage, steal, or destroy data. These programs may be inadvertently introduced to a computer via infected disks or downloaded from another system or the Internet.

Threats to Information Availability

- **Destruction of hardware, software, and/or data.** This may occur through natural or manmade disasters or through lack of attention to environmental conditions and security.

(continued)

BOX 3–1 (*continued*)

- **Interruptions in power or radiofrequency disruption.** Interruptions in the processing of data may result in data loss.
- **Denial of service.** Malicious programs can overwhelm Web sites with the result that access to Internet-based healthcare information is impaired.
- **Sabotage.** Sabotage is the intentional destruction of hardware, software, or data. Potential sabotage should be considered in the design of security measures.

Threats to Confidentiality

- **Failure to adhere to information policies.** Misuse of computer access and inappropriate disclosure of information threaten confidentiality.
- **Eavesdropping.** Eavesdropping may involve unauthorized access to information, either looking at the system directly or reading confidential printouts. Security measures must limit computer access to authorized persons and provide appropriate guidelines for the handling and disposal of confidential printouts.
- **Unauthorized reception of wireless network technology transmissions.** The reception of radiofrequency transmission used in some wireless networks may provide another opportunity to eavesdrop. The use of technology safeguards, including coding data and changing frequencies, may minimize this threat.

DATA MINING

Data mining is a technique that uses software to look for hidden patterns and relationships in large groups of data (Berger & Berger 2004). It relies upon statistical analysis, artificial intelligence, and machine learning to analyze huge amounts of data to find patterns and relationships that may have been missed otherwise. Data mining has been used in business to identify customer interests and marketing trends and has subsequently been embraced in the healthcare industry. Data mining is used in healthcare for health resource planning, research, and surveillance, and to identify successful standardized treatments for specific diseases and pay-for-performance, track performance, chart quality improvement, and determine clinical system usage (de Lusignan, Hague, van Vlymen, & Kumarapeli 2006; Hersh 2007; Teasdale, Bates, Kmetik, Suzewits, & Bainbridge 2007). Data mining is used to provide a competitive edge by analyzing trends of referring physicians, decreasing costs, and increasing revenues (Andrews 2006). It allows users to sort and compare data in many different ways to discover relationships. One large advantage of data mining is that it can help to capture significant cost savings. Its power as a tool makes data mining a key component in business planning. While data mining is now easier to use, the lack of standardized clinical language and work processes serve as roadblocks because both contribute to a lack of clean data needed for effective mining. TrendStar is an example of a data mining application used in healthcare. It is a product of the McKesson HBOC corporation, a major vendor of health information systems. Data mining is a step in the knowledge discovery in databases process.

KNOWLEDGE DISCOVERY IN DATABASES (KDD)

Knowledge discovery is defined as "the non-trivial extraction of implicit, unknown, and potentially useful information from data" (Frawley, Piatetsky-Shapiro, & Matheus 1991). Data mining provides extracted trends and patterns that are transformed into useful data (Wright 1998). Clinical databases hold huge amounts of information about patients and their medical conditions. The potential to discern patterns and relationships within those databases that would contribute to new knowledge was recognized some time ago but efforts were hampered by the paucity of methods to discover useful information until recently (Prather, Lobach, Goodwin, Hales, Hage, & Hammond 1997; Mullins et al. 2005). New tools offer the capability to expand research. Clinical repositories are now available for research and utilization purposes. According to Berger and Berger, nurses, particularly nurse researchers, are ideally situated to discover information in patterns and trends extracted by data mining, which can then be used to apply new knowledge to guide practice, encourage collaboration, and stimulate interdisciplinary research. Knowledge discovery in databases is an expanding field.

FUTURE DIRECTIONS

The adoption of standard data exchange models and standards will facilitate research as researchers stand to benefit from interoperability with access to yet more databases, assuming that barriers to the acquisition of data mining tools are removed (Anderson 2007). Most commonly these barriers are related to costs and lack of institutional support. Improved access to basic data mining tools will further aid research. Data mining and knowledge discovery in databases will become routine, allowing better resource utilization, contributing to evidence-based practice, and providing the tools providers need to compete in tight markets. Volrathongchai (2005) demonstrated via a study that KDD could be used to generate nursing knowledge by creating models that identified clients at risk for falling using Minimum Data Set (MDS) data. Additional work will follow, contributing to the body of evidence supporting care.

CASE STUDY EXERCISES

3.1 Agnes Gibbons was admitted through the hospital's emergency department with congestive heart failure. During her admission she was asked to verbally acknowledge whether her demographic data were correct. Ms. Gibbons did so. Extensive diagnostic tests were done, including radiology studies. It was later discovered that all of Ms. Gibbons' information had been entered into another client's file. How would you correct this situation? What departments, or other agencies, would need to be informed of this situation?

3.2 A non-English-speaking Vietnamese man was admitted through the emergency department with suspected tuberculosis (TB). The system carried information under his name. Mr. Nguyen nodded his head when the admitting clerk pointed to the demographic screen. Mr. Nguyen was tested and treated for TB. When the public health nurse went to Mr. Nguyen's address for follow-up, the man there was not the Mr. Nguyen who had been treated for TB. How would you address this problem? Explain your rationale.

3.3   You volunteered to serve on a committee to identify information from prior admissions that would be helpful to staff caring for current inpatients. What information, if any, would you select for ready access, and how long would you recommend that it remain active in the system? Remember that your system has limited capacity so that items must be carefully selected and prioritized. Identify the priority assigned to each item and provide your rationale for this priority.

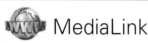 MediaLink

Additional resources for this content can be found on the Companion Website at www.prenhall.com/hebda. Click on "Chapter 3" to select the activities for this chapter.

- Glossary
- Multiple Choice
- Discussion Points
- Case Studies
- MediaLink Application
- MediaLink

SUMMARY

- Data can be managed using a database application.
- A data warehouse is a collection of several databases that can be manipulated to provide complex data analysis.
- Information quality is ensured when measures to protect it are an integral part of its collection, use, storage, retrieval, and exchange.
- Data integrity strategies should provide safeguards against data manipulation or deletion, and entry of fraudulent facts.
- Data storage measures should provide safe, accessible storage to authorized persons through a plan that considers provider, client, and third-party payer needs; physical threats to information and media; performance requirements; pros and cons of on-site versus off-site storage; technological advancements; and future needs.
- Performance, capacity, data security, and cost should be considered when planning for data retrieval.
- Electronic data interchange standards provide timely access to providers at distant sites and computer systems.
- Quality information is essential to the delivery of appropriate client care.
- Data mining uses software to look for hidden patterns and relationships in large groups of data such as performance information and successful treatments for specific diseases. It allows users to sort and compare data in many different ways to discover relationships.

- Data cleansing uses software to improve the quality of data to ensure that it is suitable for all purposes including data mining and warehousing.
- Knowledge discovery in databases uses data mining to derive knowledge from trends and patterns discovered in data mining.
- Nurses are well-situated to make good use of knowledge discovered in databases.

REFERENCES

Anderson, N. R. (2007). Issues in biomedical research data management and analysis: Needs and barriers. *Journal of the American Medical Informatics Association, 14*(4), 478–488.

Andrews, J. (September 2006). Digging down deep for useful information. *Healthcare IT News*, p. 40.

Benander, A. & Benander, B. (2000). Data warehouse administration and management. *Information System Management, 17*(1), 71.

Berger, A. M. & Berger, C. R. (2004). Data mining as a tool for research and knowledge development in nursing. *CIN: Computers, Informatics, Nursing, 22*(3), 123–131.

Bizzell, K. (2002). A giant step forward. *Health Management Technology, 23*(10), 56.

Boyle, D. I. R. & Cunningham, S. G. (2002). Resolving fundamental quality issues in linked datasets for clinical care. *Health Informatics Journal, 8*(1), 73.

Brennan, P. (1996). *Nursing informatics: Technology in the service of patient care.* Continuing education activity of West Virginia University Hospital, Morgantown, WV.

Burke, J. G. (1992). *System analysis, design, and implementation.* Boston: Boyd & Fraser.

Dakins, D. R. (2001). Center takes data tracking to heart. *Health Data Management, 9*(1), 32, 34, 36.

de Lusignan, S., Hague, N., van Vlymen, J., & Kumarapeli, P. (2006). Routinely-collected general practice data are complex, but with systematic processing can be used for quality improvement and research. *Informatics in Primary Care, 14*(1), 59–66.

Digital Preservation Coalition. (2002). *Media and formats.* Available online at http://www.dpconline.org/graphics/medfor/media.html. Accessed February 9, 2003.

Documented savings. (October 2001). *Health Management Technology, 22*(10), 56.

Faden, M. (April 10, 2000). Data cleansing helps e-businesses run more efficiently. *Informationweek.com* (781), 136, 138, 140, 144.

Frawley, W. J., Piatetsky-Shapiro, G., & Matheus, C. Knowledge Discovery In Databases: An Overview. In *Knowledge Discovery In Databases*, eds. G. Piatetsky-Shapiro and W. J. Frawley. AAAI Press/MIT Press, Cambridge, MA., 1991, pp. 1–30.

Gilhooly, K. (2005). Dirty data blights the bottom line. *Computerworld, 39*(45), 23–24.

Gillespie, G. (2000). There's gold in them thar' databases. *Health Data Management, 8*(11), 40.

Gudea, S. (2005). Data, information, knowledge: A healthcare enterprise case study. *Perspectives in Health Information Management, 2.*

Hersh, W. (2007, June). Adding value to the electronic health record through secondary use of data for quality assurance, research, and surveillance. *American Journal of Managed Care, 13*(6 Part 1), 277–278. Retrieved November 14, 2007, from CINAHL with Full Text database.

Hicks, G. T. (April 16, 2001). With privacy rule in effect, hospitals face two years of compliance actions. *AHA News, 37*(15), 1.

Hoffman, B. (2006). Data disposal. *Healthcare Informatics, 23*(11), 54–55.

Kahn, M. G. (1995). The computer-based patient record and Robert Fulghum's 16 principles. *M.D. Computing, 12*(4), 253–258.

Kolar, H. R. (2001). Caring for healthcare, *22*(4), 46–47.

Liebmann, L. (April 10, 2000). ERP's second act: Online access. *Informationweek.com* (781), 146.

Mullins, I. M., Siadaty, M. S., Lyman, J., Scully, K., Garrett, C. T., Miller, W. G., et al. (2006). Data mining and clinical data repositories: Insights from a 667,000 patient data set. *Computers in Biology and Medicine, 36*(12),1351–1377.

Prather, J. C., Lobach, D. F., Goodwin, L. K., Hales, J. W., Hage, M. L., & Hammond, W. E. (1997). Medical Data Mining: Knowledge Discovery In *A Clinical Data Warehouse. Proceedings: A Conference of The American Medical Informatics Association (AMIA). A Fall Symposium*, pp. 101–105.

Teasdale, S., Bates, D., Kmetik, K., Suzewits, J., & Bainbridge, M. (2007). Secondary uses of clinical data in primary care. *Informatics in Primary Care,15*(3), 157–166.

Tozor, G. V. (1994). *Information quality management.* Cambridge, United Kingdom: Blackwell.

Volrathongchai, K. (2005). Predicting falls among the elderly residing in long-term care facilities using knowledge discovery in databases. University of Wisconsin–Madison, Doctoral dissertation.

Wright, P. & Bartram, C. (2000). Text entry on handheld computers by older users. *Ergonomics, 43*(6), 702.

Wright, P. (1998). Knowledge Discovery In Databases: Tools and Techniques. Retrieved Nobember 18, 2007, from   http://www.acm.org/crossroads/xrds5-2/kdd.html.

Zorkoczy, P. & Heap, N. (1995). *Information technology: An introduction,* (4th ed.). London: Pittman.

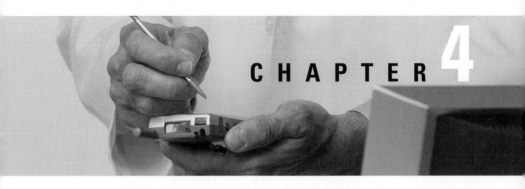

CHAPTER 4

Electronic Communication and the Internet

After completing this chapter, you should be able to:

1 Define *electronic communication* and compare and contrast e-mail, instant messaging, and text messaging.

2 Differentiate between the Internet and the World Wide Web.

3 Identify the process required to access both the Internet and the World Wide Web.

4 Discuss services available on the Internet and the World Wide Web.

5 Relate the advantages and disadvantages that the Internet and the World Wide Web have over traditional means of communicating information.

6 Identify examples of Internet and World Wide Web resources that may be useful to nurses and other healthcare professionals and consumers.

7 Compare and contrast a Web *page*, a Web *portal*, a *blog*, and a *wiki*.

8 Discuss the terms *search index*, *search engine*, and *search unifier*.

9 Evaluate the quality of a health information Web site.

10 Recognize the role that consumer informatics plays in the healthcare delivery system.

11 Compare and contrast the purpose and use of intranets and extranets to the purpose and use of the Internet.

12 Discuss the advantages and disadvantages of the Internet as a platform for healthcare applications.

13 Understand the concepts of *e-health*, *e-business*, and *e-commerce* and their role in the healthcare arena.

Computers and the Internet have revolutionized the way that we communicate. **Electronic communication** is the ability to exchange information through the use of computer equipment and software. This may be accomplished through fixed network connections, a **modem,** or mobile devices such as cell phones, PDAs, and wireless networks. A modem is a communication device that transmits data over telephone, cable lines, or satellite from one computer to another. This process allows individual users to communicate and share hardware, software, and information, and is otherwise known as **connectivity. Online** is a term that indicates a connection to various computer resources, such as the Internet and World Wide Web, that provide forums to encourage electronic communication and have revolutionized the way that information is shared. Computers can expedite the location and retrieval of information. This ability is particularly useful when material is difficult to obtain or quickly outdated.

THE INTERNET

The **Internet,** also called **the Net,** is a worldwide network that connects millions of computers. This technology first began as a United States government project to encourage researchers at different academic sites to share their findings. It now links government, universities, commercial institutions, and individual users. Content and information exchanged on the Internet are relatively free from the control of any government or single organization, although several nations would prefer more local jurisdiction, and China actually limits what its citizens can access (Governmental delegations 2005). Leaders at the United Nations (UN) and the European Union proposed that Internet control go to the UN Working Group on Internet Governance (WGIG), noting that the present system unfairly favors the United States. WGIG identified the following areas of concern: rights of nations to control Internet assets; the desire for developing nations to have a voice in the work of international bodies; control over the Internet domains; spam; and Internet crime (The need for global policies 2005; UN to control 2005). Still others propose that Internet administration occur under a multilateral treaty (Cukier 2005). No major changes have resulted from this dialog as yet. The United States has provided oversight and coordination of the Internet in four critical areas: domain names, Internet protocol numbers, root servers, and technical standards. The U.S. government established the non-profit Internet Corporation for Assigned Names and Numbers (ICANN) in 1998. The ICANN allocates top-level domain names and settles domain name disputes and is contracted by the U.S. government to do so through 2011 (Cukier 2005; McCarthy 2006). ICANN also assigns Internet protocol numbers that are needed by every machine on the network for recognition by other machines.

Governments are looking at jurisdictional problems created by the Internet and ways to harmonize laws related to hacking, fraud, and child pornography. The Council of Europe drafted the Cybercrime Treaty in an attempt to provide common definitions. The U.S. Senate ratified this treaty in 2006, joining 40 other nations in fighting crimes committed via the Internet (Senate ratifies treaty 2006). Acceptance has not been unanimous (Newly nasty 2007). The 14 nations of the South African Development Community (SADC) have also been working to harmonize their cybercrime laws to make it easier to prosecute criminals across boundaries (Malakata 2005).

The Internet Society has the greatest overall influence on the Internet. This nonprofit, professional organization provides direction when issues arise that can impact the Internet. The Internet Society also serves as a home for groups responsible for the promulgation of Internet infrastructure standards. These groups include the Internet Engineering Task Force (IETF) and the Internet Architecture Board (IAB). The IAB is chartered both as a committee of the Internet Engineering Task Force (IETF) and as an advisory body of the Internet Society (ISOC). Its responsibilities include architectural oversight of IETF activities and Internet Standards Process oversight and appeal.

The Internet Society serves as a global clearinghouse for information about the Internet and facilitates and coordinates Internet-related initiatives. The Society sponsors several events including the annual International Networking (INET) conference as well as training workshops, tutorials, research, publications, public policy, and trade activities for the benefit of people throughout the world (Internet Society 2007).

The Internet expands the range of available healthcare information through e-mail, discussion lists, blogs, wikis, file transfer protocol (FTP), Telnet, and World Wide Web resources. Many materials are no longer published on paper but are available only electronically. Some examples include research reports, journals, practice guidelines, educational materials, and conference proceedings.

The Internet is the largest, best-known wide area network in the world. Its exact size is difficult to estimate because of its rapid growth, but its users number in the millions. One major factor in the growth of the Internet is the development of companies known as **Internet service providers (ISPs),** which furnish Internet access for a fee. Some well-known examples of ISPs include America Online (AOL), Microsoft Network (MSN), and EarthLink. Many other ISPs exist as well. ISPs opened the Internet to small business and home users. Internet access through an ISP requires computer access, a modem, and communication software. Several variations for connectivity exist, including telephone dial-up, wireless, or high-speed access through digital subscriber line (DSL), cable, fiber optic, or satellite. Dial-up is slow but may be the only option available to some customers. DSL uses existing copper telephone wires but differs from the traditional dial-up connections in that it requires a special modem and is always "on." DSL is limited to customers who fall within a certain distance of the telephone switching station. Cable service has relied on coaxial cable to transmit television signals. Cable service also requires a special modem. Fiber optic cable service can be used for high speed Internet service as well as an alternative cable television service. While fiberoptic may be used in combination with cable it can also be provided all the way into the client's home or business for speeds several times faster than standard cable or DSL (Fiber: Friend or foe 2007; Hesseldahl 2007). Satellite service has been plagued with a reputation of difficult and expensive installations, poor service, and suspect performance. For these reasons it is less common except in areas where neither DSL nor cable is available. Other options for connectivity that are in various stages of development include the use of the existing electrical power grids and encoded light transmissions (Dunn 2006; Kavehrad 2007).

ISPs provide software and directions on how to access the Internet and a special account that provides Internet and World Wide Web access. Customers generally pay their ISP a monthly fee; in some cases there is an additional charge for access time. Some hotels, coffee shops, parks, hospitals, and even communities provide free Internet connections for their customers. Most ISPs provide a local telephone number for customer use.

The Internet offers many types of services and resources, including the following:

- *Electronic mail or e-mail.* **E-mail** is the use of computers to transmit messages to one or more persons. Delivery can be almost instantaneous. Text messages may be accompanied by attachment files. E-mail can be sent anywhere in the world as long as the individual has an Internet address. Internet addresses are based upon a domain name, which is based on the type of institution or ISP provider. For example Jane Doe, a nurse at St. Francis Medical Center, might have jdoe@stfrancismc.edu as her work e-mail address. Jane Doe can check her e-mail while at work or may be able to log on to her e-mail account from outside locations on her days off to check for announcements of upcoming meetings and new procedures and other pertinent messages.
- *Instant messaging (IM).* This feature allows interactive, real-time discussions that may take place on computers, cell phones, or other mobile devices. Messages are typed. IM has given rise to its own language or set of abbreviations as a means to allow communication in an expeditious manner. IM has gained some acceptance in the workplace but does not replace formal communication. The Internet supports voice but both users must be online at the same time. Instant messaging was known as *Internet relay chat (IRC)* in the past. One current widespread application of instant messaging is its use to notify large numbers of persons simultaneously that a state of emergency is in effect and precautions that should be taken.
- *File transfer.* This capability allows users to move files from one location to another directly over a network. The benefit of file transfer is that users can capture, view, edit, or use work developed by others rather than starting anew. It is particularly useful for large files that exceed the size allowed by e-mail systems such as a procedure manual or student handbook.
- *Database searches.* This feature allows users to conduct comprehensive literature searches online in a shorter period of time than could be accomplished manually. Access is obtained through universities, public libraries, or on a subscription basis using Internet connections. Previously searches were done via hardcopy manuals or periodic database increments on disc. In addition to literature databases there are databases that contain information about particular patient populations such as cancer patients, those that had cardiothoracic surgery, and many more groups.

- *Remote log-on.* This feature allows use of computer facilities at other locations to access directories, files, and databases. Most systems such as the Virginia Henderson International Nursing Library require an account, identification, and a password for user access.
- *Discussion and news groups.* The Internet provides a place where specialty interest groups can address concerns, discuss solutions, and exchange information in a timely fashion. One example of an international resource for student nurses is SNURSE-L. Groups provide specific instructions on how to participate and can be found through professional publications, conferences, word-of-mouth or a Web search.

INTERNET SERVICES

E-mail

E-mail is one of the most frequently used Internet applications. It is commonly found in private organizations, colleges, universities, corporations, hospitals, and private homes. It is a powerful connectivity tool and often is the feature that first attracts users to the Internet. E-mail encourages networking among peers, yields helpful tips and shared resources, and saves time and money that would otherwise be spent on printing and postage and individual problem solving. E-mail is a convenient way to contact employees, colleagues, students, and recruiters. It allows users to participate in educational offerings and send announcements and resumes. Box 4–1 lists some advantages and disadvantages associated with e-mail and instant messaging. The next few paragraphs explain the composition and management of e-mail.

An **e-mail application** is a computer program that assists the user to send, receive, and manage e-mail messages. Most have basic text editing and spell checking capability. Popular commercial e-mail applications include Microsoft's Outlook Express, Lotus Notes, and Eudora. Individuals who work in an environment supported by large mainframe computers may use other e-mail programs. Despite its popularity, some healthcare workers still do not have e-mail accounts. E-mail applications may reside locally on the user's computer or may be Web-based. Many organizations and ISPs allow users to access their accounts via a Web-page, affording them the opportunity to check their messages from almost any location. There are also Web sites that supply free e-mail accounts.

As e-mail popularity grows, so do concerns related to its use. These concerns include threats to data integrity and security, confidentiality, verification that messages emanate from the identified source, spam, and HIPAA (Health Insurance Portability and Accountability Act) compliance. Data integrity may be threatened by **computer viruses** and other malware. Viruses are malicious programs that can disrupt or destroy data and sometimes overwhelm networks with traffic. Viruses are not transmitted via e-mail messages themselves but may be found as file attachments sent with messages or launched when infected files are opened. The best way to minimize the threat of viruses is to scan all attached files

BOX 4–1 E-mail and Instant Messaging (IM): Advantages and Disadvantages

E-mail Advantages

Eliminates phone tag. Provides the ability to contact someone whose phone is busy. or to leave a written message.

Convenient. Can be sent or retrieved from multiple locations, including work, home, or while traveling. Can be used on a 24-hour basis.

Easy to prepare and send. Requires less effort to prepare and send than the traditional means of written communication.

Saves time and money. Eliminates postage and paper expenses

Delivery can eliminate the time lag associated with traditional mail.

Messages are time- and date-stamped. Provides documentation of the actual time of the mail transaction. Can also provide a log of when the message was received, read, and answered. Is searchable.

Instant Messaging (IM) Advantages

Bypasses phone use. Allows instant communication without wasted time for trivial communication.

Convenient. Can be sent or retrieved from multiple locations, including work, home, or while traveling.

Easy to prepare and send. Requires less effort to prepare and send than the e-mail and traditional means of written communication.

Saves time and money. Eliminates unnecessary social chit chat. Provides immediate responses.

Presence technology. Shows whether the desired recipient is online.

IM can be time and date stamped. May also provide a log of conversation.

E-mail Disadvantages

Interpretation of messages without the benefit of voice inflection or facial expression.

High volume of messages sent and received. E-mail's popularity and ease of use make it easy to generate large numbers of messages, including copies, forwarded messages, and "junk mail."

Malware contamination can occur via attached files. Attached files that contain a virus or worm or other malware may contaminate the recipient's computer.

Security concerns related to maintaining confidentiality. Message may be intercepted and read by unintended parties. Employers may read all messages. Employees may read messages not intended for their eyes. Deleted messages may be retrieved during system backups.

Instant Messaging (IM) Disadvantages

Interpretation of messages without the benefit of voice inflection or facial expression.

Message sent and received in an abbreviated language.

Malware contamination can occur via attached files. Attached files that contain a virus or worm or other malware may contaminate the recipient's computer.

Security concerns related to maintaining confidentiality. Message may be intercepted and read by unintended parties. Employers may read all messages on company systems. Employees may read messages not intended for their eyes. Deleted messages may be retrieved during system backups.

with the latest version of an antivirus software before opening. One can also delete e-mail and attachments from unknown sources at the risk of deleting wanted materials. When content needs to be kept secure and confidential, **encryption** is recommended. Encryption uses mathematical formulas to code messages. Message recipients decode content with special software known as an encryption key. Encryption may be done at the desktop or at the server level. Encryption is a feature with many commercial e-mail packages. Encryption serves to protect the individual computer and its network.

Methods to validate e-mail author identity include **public key infrastructure (PKI)** and digital credentialing. PKI provides a unique code for each user that is imbedded into a storage device. User information is stored in a database by the organization that created the code. Identity is confirmed when the storage device and a password or other form of identification match information stored in the database. A simpler alternative to PKI is the digital signature or credential. The digital signature is a unique identifier issued to the individual that can be verified against the sender's public key. Intel and the American Medical Association worked collaboratively to develop digital credentialing for physicians. Physician digital credentials are routed through a firewall to the Intel Internet Authentication Service (ITAS) to validate user identity and create an audit trail. This same process is available for other healthcare workers. Although the digital credential does not require biometric measures to verify identity, there is increased interest in the use of biometric measures as a means to ensure that only authorized users access private health information.

Another issue that has been raised about the security of health information transmitted via e-mail is the security of the mail server, or the computer on which e-mail messages reside, both coming into an organization and leaving. Use of the health provider's e-mail for nonwork purposes can open up the server to viruses and hackers. Secure e-mail applications ensure that all information remains available to enterprise servers when it is needed. The use of a secure e-mail service provider is likened to using a private postal carrier, which helps to maintain data integrity as well as provide audit trails and proof of receipt. This arrangement usually requires that servers on both ends are registered, so it is best suited for organizations that communicate regularly. Yet another safeguard of confidentiality is the ability to screen outgoing messages for appropriate content and to block them if they are going to unknown or suspect addresses.

Other issues surrounding e-mail focus on its increasing volume; the time required to sift through e-mail messages; unwanted or "junk" e-mail, also known as **spam;** accurate interpretation of messages; and HIPAA compliance. The number of legitimate e-mail messages has grown exponentially, but so have the number of unwanted messages. A significant portion of all e-mail traffic is now spam. Spam is a problem because thousands of messages may be sent at one time. Spam spreads advertisements and may be used to collect personal and credit card information. Spam is constantly evolving to use new approaches to avoid filters. Spammers forge return e-mail addresses and domain names, making it difficult to track and prosecute them when they engage in fraudulent claims and illegal activity. Efforts to block spam include lawsuits, state and federal legislation, industry initiatives, establishing separate e-mail accounts for different purposes, e-mail rules for incoming mail and filtering software, and challenge response tools. Additional proposals for dealing with spam have called for the establishment of a "do not e-mail" list, limiting the number of messages that can be sent out per day via free e-mail accounts, and a requirement that advertisement be labeled. Spam is costly in terms of user time to delete unwanted messages, costs for filtering and challenge software, and higher costs for ISP service.

Challenge response software works by asking the e-mail sender to answer a question or complete a task that requires human intervention. No mail is accepted unless its validity has been confirmed by a human being. Challenge response software is sometimes referred to as **CAPTCHAS,** which stands for Completely **A**utomatic **P**ublic **T**uring Test To Tell **C**omputers and **H**umans Apart. Challenge response tools are effective in filtering out spam, but they create additional network traffic. Box 4–2 provides some informal rules to guide e-mail and IM use.

BOX 4–2   Informal Rules for E-mail and Instant Messaging (IM) Use

- Change passwords for e-mail access immediately upon assignment and frequently thereafter.
- Limit e-mail copies to the people who need the information. This keeps the number of messages manageable. When sending a copy to the boss, list his or her name first if the e-mail package permits this action; some applications automatically alphabetize all recipients.
- Choose an accurate description for the e-mail subject line. This practice helps recipients to determine which messages should be read first.
- Avoid the use of Blind Copy (BC). It is considered unethical in many circles.
- Do not use e-mail or IM as a means to criticize or insult anyone.
- Use e-mail priority status and read receipts sparingly. Misuse may be found insulting.
- Check the e-mail list of recipients before pressing "send" to be certain that it is appropriate.
- Give e-mail and IM the same consideration given to business correspondence. Messages may be seen by parties other than intended recipients. Write nothing that would not otherwise be said or posted publicly. Consider how your message might be interpreted before sending it.
- Make messages clear, short, and to the point. Include original messages, or a portion, with your reply to provide context.
- Avoid the use of all capital letters. This is difficult to read, and may be perceived as shouting, according to e-mail etiquette.
- Limit abbreviations to those that are easily understood.
- Read mail, file messages in categories, and delete messages no longer needed on a regular basis. This frees storage space and helps to optimize system function, as well as making it easier to find and retrieve messages later.
- Try to reply to e-mail within 24 hours.
- Consider using mechanisms to prevent unwanted mail.
- Limit the use of emoticons in professional communication.
- Do not reply to messages that do not require a reply unless adding relevant information.

Like other Internet services, e-mail is based on a client/server system. In client/server technology, files are stored on a central computer known as a **server.** In this case, the server receives mail from other Internet sites and stores it until it is read, answered, or deleted. The client computer requests mail access from the server and generates new mail that will be handled by the server.

Components of an E-mail Message Every e-mail message has several standard components. These components include a header, body, attachments, and possibly a signature. The **header** lists who sent the message, when, to whom, and a subject line. Message copies may also be copied to others through either a "cc," which stands for carbon copy, or "bc," which stands for blind carbon or blind carbon copy. Persons designated to receive blind carbon copies will not have their names displayed on the e-mail copies sent to either the primary recipient or individuals receiving carbon copies. The subject line allows a brief phrase to describe the subject of the e-mail. While it is possible to send a message without completing the subject line many recipients will not bother to read such a message. The **body** of the e-mail contains the main contents of the message as typed by the sender. Most e-mail systems allow the sender to create a standard ending for all messages, which is known as the signature and typically includes the sender's name, address, and other contact or identifying information. E-mail software allows the sender to send messages with files. The attached files are known as **attachments** and are considered an easy way to share files.

Designated recipients of e-mail are listed in the to:, cc:, and bc: fields by their e-mail addresses. The user may see either the address or the person's name because it is stored along with that address in the e-mail system. E-mail addresses are created using a standard format that includes a user's name followed by the @ symbol and the location or computer where that person's e-mail account can be found. In the example thebda@chatham.edu the user is found at Chatham University. Additional information may be included to identify a subdivision within an organization. General information is listed first followed by more specific information separated by periods or back slashes. The last portion of an e-mail address indicates the type of organization and is known as the domain. Box 4–3 lists some common e-mail organizational domains.

E-mail can be composed online or in advance. In this case, "online" refers to the period that one computer is actively connected to another. Composing messages ahead of time can decrease costs for connection time and improve the organization of expressed thoughts. E-mail prepared in advance may be saved in e-mail draft form or done in another application and later pasted into an e-mail message. Mail received may be read while online or downloaded to the recipient's computer for later review.

Suggested Use and Netiquette E-mail is now a widely accepted form of communication. It is fast and convenient. It should not be used in lieu of

BOX 4-3   E-Mail Organizational Domains

The last portion of an e-mail address indicates the type of organization that provides the e-mail service used by the addressee. For example, thebda@chatham.edu indicates that a user named thebda is located at an educational organization. Country codes are two characters. Following is a partial list of some common organizational domains.

.com   commercial organization
.edu   educational organization
.gov   government
.mil   military
.net   networking organization
.org   nonprofit organization
.ca   Canada
.th   Thailand
.uk   United Kingdom

face-to-face meetings to convey unpleasant news such as work lay-offs or a bad diagnosis. It has evolved its own set of conventions and abbreviations. The appropriate and courteous use of e-mail is known as **netiquette.** The following list contains general standards for online communication.

- *Do not make assumptions.* Avoid one-word responses. Do not assume that the recipient remembers the original question or statement. Avoid abbreviations that are not commonly known.
- *Do not be judgmental.* Be professional and careful in what is written. E-mail is easily forwarded to others and can be printed. Instant messages may be shown to other people as well. Word statements carefully to prevent misinterpretation. Flaming is the use of angry and insulting language directed at a particular person or group.
- *Proofread messages.* Poor grammar and spelling reflect badly on the sender.
- *Reply in a timely fashions.* This is simple courtesy.
- *Use attachments wisely.* Check with recipients before sending a file to determine if they have the software to access it. For example, large files may take a long time to download and the recipient may prefer to receive this information in a compressed format. Special software is required by the sender to compress a file. The recipient must use the same software to restore the file for use. The process to attach a file is the same whether it is compressed or not.
- *Make postings brief and to the point.* Recipients may not read lengthy e-mail messages or postings.
- *Use online communication appropriately.* Do not send chain letters. Mass mailing of unsolicited "junk" mail is annoying for recipients and uses network resources. Do not copy or forward mail unless there is a "need-to-know."

- *Avoid the use of all capital letters.* This is known as shouting and is considered rude.
- *Respect others.* Read the frequently asked questions (FAQ) before participating in listserv or other group discussions to avoid unnecessary repetition.

Managing E-mail Because e-mail is popular it is easy to become inundated with incoming mail. For this reason it is wise to develop some strategies for handling e-mail. The subject line should describe the contents in the message to help the reader evaluate its urgency and decide whether to read it or delete it unread. E-mail should be read frequently to prevent large numbers of messages accumulating. Once read, messages should be deleted or organized into electronic folders for future reference. Most ISPs and e-mail applications include features to limit the number of spam messages, block messages from unwanted senders, and automatically delete some messages. It is important to consider whether recipients really want to receive copies or forwarded mail. Some organizations automatically delete e-mail after a specified time.

E-mail software programs allow users to develop lists of recipients for mailing and to set their preferences for how incoming mail is displayed. These preferences can include chronological or reverse chronological order, by sender or date. Read messages may appear differently than unread messages. It is also possible to search e-mail to find particular content, subjects, or senders.

The large number of e-mail messages can decrease productivity rather than enhance it if users are not careful to set limits. It has extended the work day for many persons who feel compelled to check messages before leaving for work, after coming home and on weekends and holidays. Some work places now forbid the use of e-mail one day a week and encourage telephone calls and face-to-face meetings as a means to foster productivity. Another management strategy is to turn off new e-mail alerts and change the number of times the system checks for new messages to once or twice per day. Recipients may not receive all of their messages if their message box is full.

Instant Messaging (IM)

IM requires a connection to the Internet, an account with one of the IM services, and IM client software. IM services offer the capability for one-on-one or multiparty text chat and file transfer. IM operates on a real time basis sending a text message immediately to the intended recipient. Users can limit access to a select few individuals or a larger community. Voice and videoconference may also be supported. IM relies upon presence technology to determine whether the recipient is available and informs users of their status. No time is wasted trying to communicate with persons who are not there. Public IM systems do not capture transcripts of messages. IM has come into the workplace primarily through free public networks such as AOLs Instant Messenger, MSN's Live Messsenger, and Yahoo Messenger (Bisconti 2007). It is easier to use than e-mail because it is not necessary to type an address and is widely perceived as more time efficient than either telephone or face-to-face conversations because it eliminates social chit chat and provides almost immediate responses. Disadvantages associated with the public versions include privacy concerns, the possibility that messages may be intercepted, lack of central administration, and **SPIM.** SPIM refers to unsolicited messages often containing a link to a Web site that the spimmer is attempting to market. Secure versions are available for corporate use at a cost. Commercial IM requires central administration. Both free and commercial versions may distract employees, waste time, and may spread malware via file transfer (IM threats proliferate 2006). On the other hand, IM readily lends itself to use for virtual office hours, class discussion, guest lectures, and mentoring. IM can take place between two or multiple participants. Earlier IM software was not interoperable, meaning that users could not communicate without anyone having different software. That situation has changed.

Text messaging is similar in many ways to instant messaging but exhibits some differences. Text messaging is the popular term for Short Message Service (SMS), which originated as a means to send short messages to and from mobile phones and handheld devices. Original messages were limited to 160 characters giving rise to its heavy reliance upon abbreviations. Text messaging is private, less intrusive than a phone call, and supports automatic messages without typing each one individually. Recipients may respond in real time or at their leisure. Text messages are less expensive than regular phone calls and less prone to spam than e-mail. Messages are stored and may be reread. Text messages can support all languages and support binary data, ring tones, pictures, and even animation. Recipients may not receive all of their messages if their message box is full.

Database Searches

This feature allows users to conduct comprehensive literature searches over a shorter period of time than could be accomplished via a manual approach. Most universities and public libraries offer online databases for review. In this instance, "online" refers to databases that are available through Internet connections.

File Transfer

File transfer is the ability to move files from one location to another across the Internet. Users may download archived files that they find interesting or give their files to others. Transferred files can include graphics, text, or shareware applications. One means to achieve the actual movement of data is through the **file transfer protocol (FTP).** FTP is a set of instructions that controls both the physical transfer of data across the network and its appearance on the receiving end. The benefit of file transfer is that users can preview work developed by others rather than starting anew. FTP may be available with World Wide Web software. Internet etiquette traditionally calls for the transfer of large files after peak business hours to prevent slow response times.

Listservs

A **Listserv** is actually an e-mail subscription list. A mailing list program copies and distributes all e-mail messages to subscribers. All mail goes through a central computer that acts as the server for the list. Some groups have a moderator who first screens messages for relevance. Listservs are sometimes referred to as *discussion groups, mailing lists,* or *electronic conferences.* Listservs provide information on thousands of topics. Subscription may be open to anyone with an e-mail address or restricted. A complete list of listservs may be obtained by visiting the Tile.net site (www.tile.net).

To subscribe to a listserv, individuals must send the e-mail message "sub" or "subscribe," followed by their first and last names. Exact commands may vary slightly. Most listservs provide help and instructions on request. Subscribers may participate in discussions or just monitor them. Listserv participants should read their mail frequently and skim messages for subjects of interest to keep up with discussions. Subscribers may terminate their participation at any time by sending an "unsubscribe" message.

Newsgroups

Usenet news groups are another available Internet feature. Usenet groups are similar to listservs in content and diversity. More than 100,000 discussion groups exist, each dedicated to a different topic. These groups provide a forum where any user can post messages for discussion and reply. Users do not subscribe to these groups, nor do they receive individual messages. Instead, they may participate at any time free of charge. ISPs do not carry every news group. ISP administrators decide which news groups will be available to their customers and how long messages will be stored. Only messages that are currently stored on the user's ISP computer may be read. Some ISPs restrict access to usernet groups or restrict the length of time that messages are saved. It may be necessary to subscribe to a usernet service to view older postings. Special browser programs called **news reader software** are needed by the individual users to read messages posted on the news group. Many different news readers are available. News readers come bundled with Web browsers. A list of Usenet groups may also be found at the Tile.net site. Some examples of nursing Usenet groups are the following:

- *sci.med.nursing.* This is a general forum for the discussion of all types of nursing issues. A review of discussion topics reveals current concerns in the profession by country and practice area. Individual nurses may request assistance with particular problems and receive help from people across the globe.
- *bit.listserv.snurse-l.* This is a group for international nursing students.

No single person is in charge of universal Usenet procedures, but informal rules and etiquette for participants have developed. The first rule is that all new users should read the **frequently asked questions (FAQ)** document before sending any messages of their own. The FAQ file serves to introduce the group, update new users on recent discussions, and eliminate repetition of questions. Additional Usenet guidelines call for:

- *Short postings.* This helps to maintain interest while preventing any individual or subgroup from monopolizing the group.
- *No sensationalism.* The intent of Usenet groups is the sharing of information, not gossip.
- *No outright sales.* Usenet originated in academia and relies on a cooperative environment. Advertising, by custom, is kept at a minimum.
- *Respect for the group focus.* Posting messages that are not relevant wastes time and resources.

News groups may be discovered through any of the following methods: searching the Web by topic, word of mouth from individuals with like interests, conferences, professional publications, or searching through lists of all available news groups. If no news group exists for a given topic, instructions on how to start one can be found on the Internet. Some groups that started as usenet groups may now be accessed through a Web address.

Bulletin Board Services

Bulletin board systems (BBSs) started out as a computerized dial-in meeting and announcement system for users to make statements, share files, and conduct limited discussions. The original BBS did not require Internet access, just a computer and modem. Some BBS were free while others required a subscription fee. The term *BBS* is sometimes used to refer to any online forum or message board. These sites may have moderators who determine what messages will be posted.

Remote Access

This feature allows individuals to use their computer to access directories, files, and databases housed on a distant computer via a secure connection or virtual private network. This type of access requires an account, identification, and a password. Typically users go to the home Web page of their company or school, then follow the links.

THE WORLD WIDE WEB

The **World Wide Web** is an information service that accesses data by content instead of file names. The Web supports a multimedia approach that includes text, images, sound, and links to other documents. The easy-to-use graphical user interface (GUI) makes it simple to learn and use. Users may search by specific words or move from one link to another. Links are displayed by highlighted keywords, text, or images. Selection of information in highlighted areas is accomplished through a click of the mouse button. The Web was first developed at the European Center for Particle Physics in Geneva for scientists to

BOX 4–4 The World Wide Web: Advantages and Disadvantages

Advantages

- Browser software is available for all types of computers.
- Browser software is easy to use.
- Text, pictures, video, and sound are supported.
- The amount of information available on the Web is constantly expanding.
- Internet overload is decreased because it links to other documents instead of including them as attachments.
- The need to hold a line open while a document is read is eliminated because the document is transferred to the host computer and the connection is terminated.
- Document transfer is facilitated.
- Voice communications can be supported.
- Information is available in real time.

Disadvantages

- The quality of available information varies widely.
- Documents may not supply sufficient depth in content.
- Not all Web pages display a date of authorship or credentials of the source.
- Web sites may change without providing a "forwarding address."
- The Web is vulnerable to hacker attacks.
- The large amount of available information may be overwhelming.
- Excessive company time may be spent exploring sites that are not work-related.
- Obsolete information may be out there.

publish documents while linked via the Internet. The Web provides a forum for the exchange of ideas, free marketing, and public relations. It now serves as a platform for a growing number of businesses. Box 4–4 lists advantages and disadvantages associated with using the World Wide Web.

Web pages frequently change as content is revised and new technologies are incorporated. This results in a different appearance for the page the next time the user accesses it. The use of new technology and software in Web page design may leave some users unable to access certain features or content. Periodic browser updates and the use of additional applications that can be downloaded from the Web or purchased in stores help to address this situation. It may also be necessary to evaluate, upgrade, and replace hardware and software to access and use desired Web features and applications.

One particularly popular Web feature is the **home page,** the first page seen at a particular Web location. The home page presents general information about a topic, a person, or an organization. Pages are written in hypertext markup language (HTML) or extensible markup language (XML). Markup languages include text as well as special instructions known as *tags* for the display of text and other media. HTML also includes highlighted references to other documents that the user may choose if additional information about that topic is desired. World Wide Web software interprets HTML tags for display. Tags specify formatting information such as the type of heading, font size, and alignment of type. Tags also indicate the location of other media such as graphics or even music. HTML can include links to other documents and may incorporate text, graphics or video, and sound files. Despite the fact that HTML is considered a standard, some variations exist to allow information to be displayed on personal digital assistants and other devices. XML was developed by the World Wide Web Consortium. The Consortium is a group of companies dedicated to the development of open standards to ensure the development of the Web.

Links are words, phrases, or images distinguished from the remainder of the document through the use of highlighting or a different screen color. Links allow users to skip from point to point within or among documents, escaping conventional linear format. Clicking on links with the mouse establishes a TCP/IP (transmission control protocol/Internet protocol) connection between the client and server, which sends a request in the form of a hypertext transfer protocol (HTTP) command. The TCP/IP connection is closed after the information is sent, while the user is seamlessly transported to another area of the document or another Web site.

HTTP supports hypermedia information systems, including the Web. The initial portion of Web site addresses, "http," refers to this protocol. Links are associated with a **uniform resource locator (URL),** a string of characters similar to a postal address. The URL identifies the document's Web location and the type of server on which it resides, such as HTTP or other Web server, FTP, or news server. Addresses that include an "s" (https) indicate secured sites, such as those that request entry and submission of credit card numbers.

Box 4–5 lists some steps required to create, post, and maintain a home page. Web sites may consist of a single page or hundreds of pages of information. They vary in complexity from simple text to sites with elaborate graphics, sound, and videos. The person responsible for putting a Web site together and maintaining it is known as the Web editor. One type of Web site is the blog. **Blog** is an abbreviation for Web and log (Anderberg 2007; Schloman 2006). The blog provides a forum for individuals to maintain an online journal on the Internet. Entries are time stamped. Simple blogs are regularly updated Web pages with the most recent entries appearing at the top of the page. Content varies widely from personal diaries, requests for contributions, and special interest blogs organized by topics. Blogs may not display credentials. Many blogs function as monologs but may also serve as discussion forums, news digests, classroom tools, and promotional devices. Blogs can support text, images, MP3 files, and RSS (Really Simple Syndication). MP3 files are compressed without sacrificing quality for users. MP3 is primarily used to facilitate the exchange of music over the Internet. RSS is a markup language for the delivery of Web content to users. Its use is well suited for rapidly changing online newsletters. Blogging software and providers are available to help create and maintain blogs. Many blogs have been abandoned in recent years as their creators tire of the work associated with their ongoing maintenance.

BOX 4–5   Steps in Creating, Posting, and Maintaining a Home Page

Content and Design Considerations

- **Determine purpose, intended audience, and content.** A well-designed Web page starts with good planning.
- **Select a Web developer or an authoring tool.** A Web developer can help ensure the success of a site. A variety of tools can be used to create Web pages, including word processors, browsers, and dedicated Web-authoring tools. The complexity of design, user comfort, and experience are factors in tool selection. Basic knowledge of html markup commands is helpful but not essential.
- **Determine page layout.** Do not crowd pages with information and images. Limit introductory page information so that essential data are visible without scrolling. Review existing Web pages for pleasing appearance and useful features.
- **Readability.** Use high-contrast backgrounds for easy reading, such as black print on white. Dark backgrounds can cause fatigue. Use 12-point fonts or larger.
- **Choose links.** Links can make the site more interesting and useful. Organize links to help users find what they are looking for. Use specific link references rather than the phrase, "click here."
- **Include contact information.** Contact information, such as name, organization, credentials, an e-mail link, and a postal address, provides the appearance of credibility and a means to establish contact.
- **Update/revision information.** A date helps the user to determine whether posted information and links are current. Updates and revisions also maintain interest, giving users a reason to come back. Consider the addition of icons to identify new or recently revised materials.
- **Download time.** Lengthy download times can frustrate users, causing them to move to other sites.
- **Check the page for errors.** Spelling, grammar, and content errors reflect poorly on the author or site. Review all materials prior to posting.
- **Do not include a counter.** Visitors do not need to know how many people visited a site.
- **Consider including activities for users.** Users want more than just information.
- **Consider copyright issues.** Request permission prior to using work developed by others. Register original work with the U.S Copyright Office and place a copyright notice with year next to protected material. Develop a written agreement that identifies copyright ownership when working with a Web developer.

Posting and Maintenance Considerations

- **Test the page before posting.** Ensure that it looks and performs as conceived. Use different browsers to view results. Pages that do not load properly or that have a sloppy appearance make a poor impression.
- **Gather information on Internet service providers and Web servers.** Compare service, cost, and support when selecting an ISP and home for Web pages.
- **Establish Internet access.** Internet access is essential for periodic review of Web materials and to receive mail generated by the site.
- **Find a Web server.** Many ISPs and Web sites offer space for home pages. Determine which service provider can best meet the requirements for the page being posted.
- **Obtain a Web or domain site.** An address provides a location to post pages. A domain name refers to one or more IP addresses. Domain names are used in URLs. Suffixes

(continued)

BOX 4–5 (*continued*)

provide information about the type of affiliation. Memorable names help users to find and return to pages. Initial cost to obtain a domain name may be minimal unless it presents a commercial interest.

- **Review and revision procedures.** To remain timely, pages should include review or revision dates.
- **Security issues.** Use mechanisms to protect against unauthorized changes in posted materials.

Another type of Web page is a **wiki** (Fichter 2005). Wikis are sites created with a Web application that allow anyone to collaboratively write and edit documents without any special technical knowledge. Unlike blogs there is no attribution for individual contributions. Wikipedia, the free online encyclopedia, is an example of this type of site. The open editing capability raises concerns about misuse, abuse, and reliability of information. Wikis work best in an environment with a high level of trust when control can be delegated to the users. Wiki software recognizes URLs and creates hyperlinks easily. Sites provide information for new visitors, helping them to learn how to use the site. Wikis are particularly valuable as an online workspace, allowing individuals to contribute knowledge and pertinent comments. Wikis can also be used in organizations to foster collaboration where access is restricted to internal use. Wikis are well-suited for the storage of committee work and minutes and as a log book of complaints and actions. Unlike IM there is no indication of who is currently online.

A **Bliki,** sometimes known as a WikiLog, Wog, WikiWeblog, Wikiblog, or Bloki, combines the concepts of Web-based collaboration and publishing from blogs and wikis. It incorporates posts or articles in reverse chronological order but allows editing in wiki style with a version history for each page. Permission to edit is at the discretion of the administrator(s). The bliki aims to make the blogging experience more interactive while promoting quality and accuracy of posts. Blikis may be adopted by organizations to organize internal information centrally and in a format that is always accessible.

Nurses and other healthcare professionals may use the World Wide Web to learn more about any of the following topics:

- *Undergraduate, graduate, and doctoral nursing programs.* School Web pages provide information about their philosophy, curriculum, and application process, and often allow candidates to complete an application online.
- *Professional associations.* Groups such as the American Nurses Association maintain Web sites that provide information about the purpose of the group and advantages of membership. This increases visibility for the group and serves as a recruitment strategy to attract new members.

- *Nursing informatics.* Announcements of upcoming meetings and calls for papers about nursing informatics can be found on the Web.
- *Online nursing journals.* Many traditional journals offer electronic versions of their publications in addition to the printed version. Some restrict general access to the electronic format to paid subscribers or allow for the purchase of specific articles for a fee.
- *Continuing education offerings.* Program announcements and even entire courses may be found on the Web.
- *Disease-specific information and recommended treatment modalities.* This content may be directed to the healthcare consumer and/or the healthcare professional.
- *Pharmacological information.* The most current information about drugs can be found for healthcare professionals and consumers.
- *Consumer education.* The American Heart Association and the National Cancer Institute are among the growing list of groups that maintain Web sites.

A list of nursing Web sites and related sites of interest can be found on the Companion Website at www.prenhall.com/hebda.

Browsers

A **browser** is a retrieval program that allows access to hypertext and hypermedia documents on the Web by using HTTP. The computer, acting as server, interprets the client's HTTP request and sends back the requested document for display. Browsers can also use Telnet FTP protocols. Browsers may be obtained free from an ISP, as a download over the Internet, or purchased. The National Center for Supercomputing Applications (NCSA) developed Mosaic, the first Web browser. Web use increased after the introduction of Mosaic. Examples of popular browsers include Microsoft's Internet Explorer, AOL's Netscape, Apple's Safari, and the alternative browsers Opera and Firefox from Mozilla. Internet Explorer has dominated the market but alternative browsers are expected to increase in popularity. Browsers may distribute advertisements or be available without ads for a fee. Browsers use the URL to request a document from the server.

Browsers are available for many types of systems and frequently offer features that extend their utility. However, there are still some things that browsers do not do. **Helper programs** and **plug-in** programs evolved to fill this void. Helper and plug-in programs are computer applications that have been designed to perform tasks such as view graphics, construct Web pages, play sounds, or even remotely control another PC over the Internet. The main difference between helper and plug-in programs is that the first does not require the browser to be running to function, while the second does require the browser to be running. Both are typically available on the Web at no cost and are often written in **Java.** Java is a programming language that enables the display of moving text, animation, and musical excerpts on Web pages. Java is popular for the following reasons:

- Applications will run on any Java-enabled browser.
- Actual code can reside on the server until it is downloaded to the client computer as it is needed.
- Java reduces the need to purchase, install, and maintain on-site software.

An alternative to Java for the development of Internet-enabled tools and technologies is Microsoft's ActiveX.

Search Tools

The overwhelming amount of data available on the Web requires the use of tools to locate specific information. Several types of search tools are available to help users find information on the Web. Most users are familiar with Google, Yahoo!, and MSN but there are other many other tools and techniques that are less well known (Hawkins 2005; Notess 2007; Pike 2007). Knowledge workers, persons who primarily earn a living by developing or using knowledge, spend an estimated 9.5 hours per week searching for information. This makes awareness of different tools and techniques important. The distinction among the types of tools is blurred. Some sites, such as Yahoo, index links by broad subject categories. **Search indexes** are appropriate when general information is requested. **Search engines** use automated programs that search the Web, compiling a list of links to sites relevant to keywords supplied by the user. The search may also include Usenet discussions. Search engines are indicated when it is necessary to find a specific topic. Google and AltaVista are examples of search engines. Each search tool maintains its own list of information on the Web and uses its own method to organize materials. Because of this variation in organization, searches conducted with different engines yield different results. Although subtle differences exist among each, all permit the user to enter a search word or phrase. Web sites that contain the search item are then displayed. The number of hits or Web sites that carry this word or phrase varies according to the search engine used and the time the search is done, since new sites are constantly being indexed. Search engines also weight the pages. Weighting is designed to display the most useful links first. There are several ways to weight pages, but the best-known method is based on the popularity of each site as is represented by the number of other sites that link to it. Enclosing key phrases in quotation marks is recommended as a way to obtain better results with some, but not all, search tools; otherwise, all documents containing portions of the key phrase will be identified. Help pages are available to aid the user in conducting searches. It may also be necessary to use more than one tool for the best results. The newer browsers, search tools, and several Web sites make it easier to switch from one tool to another. Internet Explorer, Mozilla, and Opera all have a search box in the upper right corner that allows the user to access additional search engines (Notess 2007). The relevance of results is determined by whether the search engine is sponsored by advertisements. Many results contain links that advertisers have paid the search engine to display. Paid links are not always labeled as advertisements. Consumer groups have asked the Federal Trade Commission to look at this issue. It is also possible to search a particular Web site or type of site, find a definition, or hunt for a particular type of file. To search a site the user must enter the URL and the search term. A definition may be located by typing "define:" followed by the word. Google Scholar helps users to locate scholarly works on the Internet. While it may be suitable as a starting point users still need to resort to major database services for a thorough review of referred scholarly works (Kent 2005).

Despite the success of search engines, important information is frequently missed. This occurs for several reasons. Search engines have interfaces in the major languages but may miss results that are not in any of those languages. Another reason that information is missed is that it may be password-protected or stored in formats that are not indexed. Yet another reason that information is missed is that the incorporation of multiple concepts makes indexing difficult. There are also problems with filters designed to block pornography that may block access to health information sites. Search tools are still evolving.

Search engine unifiers, also known as metasearch tools, can shorten search time by using several engines at one time. Some of these tools allow searchers to create their own personalized list of resources or to switch back and forth between searches of the Web, blog, and news. Some examples of search unifiers include Dogpile (www.dogpile.com), Search (www.search.com), and WebSeeker. Some are available at no cost while others require purchase. Users should try several search tools to determine what provides the best results for their needs.

OmniMedicalSearch (www.omnimedicalsearch.com/) was created to bring the best sources of medical information together in one easy-to-use platform for consumers and healthcare professionals. It selects sources deemed as reliable. Medical World Search (www.mwsearch.com) is a search tool for selected medical sites that requires a subscription fee. It uses indexing and a thesaurus of uniform healthcare terms, which users can view before conducting a search.

Portals, Intranets, and Extranets

The terms *portal, intranet* and *extranet* received considerable attention when they were introduced. All three concepts remain viable but the terms intranet and extranet are used less frequently. Instead it is more common to speak of portals.

Portals **Portal** is a term that refers to some Web sites. Portal sites require registration and collect information from the user that can be used to personalize features for individual users. Services such as e-mail, news search capability, and online shopping may also be available. Portals organize data with different formats from multiple sources into a single, easy-to-use menu. Portals started as entry points to the Web that added additional features to attract and maintain user interests. AOL and Yahoo represent general portal sites. There are also special interest or niche portals. Some examples of nursing portals include The Nursing

Portal (www.nursing-portal.com) and http://nurses.info/. Physician's Briefing—Today's News, WebMD, HealthAtoZ.com, Healthfinder.gov, and HealthCentral provide services for physicians, consumers, nurses, and office managers. CVS and other commercial pharmacies also have portal sites that provide information for consumers and allow prescriptions to be filled online. A portal for a health organization typically contains links to individual member organizations, physicians, educational material, and possibly scheduling capability for consumers; many contain separate links for employees to access continuing education, policies, internal phone numbers, and other relevant information. Employees can access this information independently at times convenient for them to complete required education. Other uses for portal technology include providing secure Web access to patient care systems or information contained within these systems. This includes making results available to physicians, as well as digital images and monitor strips, and the opportunity for electronic review and sign-off of medical records. Basic portals furnish information in a static fashion. More sophisticated sites are interactive, allowing users to complete and submit forms online, complete health assessments, schedule appointments, and perform other activities. There are variations on the portal theme. Active portals focus on a specific topic and use a customized search agent that automatically updates searches. Enterprise portals provide access to information quickly and easily, extending user access across departments and organizations.

Intranets As mentioned earlier, the terms *intranet* and *extranet* garnished attention when they were introduced, and although the concepts remain viable, the terms themselves are used less frequently. Instead it is more common to speak of portals. **Intranets** are private computer networks that use Internet protocols and technologies, including Web browsers, servers, and languages, to facilitate collaborative data sharing. They were first developed in response to concerns over slowdowns, security breaches, and fears of Internet collapse. Intranets sit behind firewalls or other barriers and may not normally be available to people outside of the organization. In some cases authorized users may be able to access content from remote sites.

Intranets allow integration of disparate information systems. Intranets can save money by providing an easy-to-use, familiar interface that is intuitive and therefore requires little training. Most organizations use the corporate intranet first for publication of internal documents. This cuts down on paper and distribution costs, and makes materials available more quickly and widely. It also provides a mechanism to ensure that all parties view the most recent document, which does not always occur when hard copies are distributed. This type of intranet application may be used to distribute policy and procedure manuals or other reference materials. It also acclimates employees to using the intranet as the single source of information. Additional features may include the ability for employees to view and enroll in benefits, request vacation days, and apply for internal jobs. Intranets are also an effective tool for marketing and advertising. Intranets in healthcare enterprises may also be used for mail and messaging, conferencing, and access to clinical data once the infrastructure is in place to bring together clinical systems and authenticate authorized users. In some cases, clients may be able to view their own health information, schedule appointments, and register for the hospital online. The concerns associated with intranet use mirror those discussed earlier; these include data security, the need to develop and implement strong organizational policies on appropriate intranet use, and the development of the infrastructure to support an intranet. Remote access may present additional issues for users because intranet content is generally designed to take advantage of fast network connections.

Extranets Extranets represent another variation of the Internet. **Extranets are networks** that sit outside the protected internal network of an organization and use Internet software and communication protocols for electronic commerce and use by outside suppliers or customers. Extranets are more private than a Web site that is open to the public but are more open than an intranet, which can be accessed only by employees. Many extranets offer information that is a byproduct of the organization's main business either gratis or for a fee. Customers benefit because information is available 24 hours a day. For example, a vendor may develop an extranet that customers can use to obtain prices and place orders for merchandise. Security measures can be used to restrict access and secure information, making extranets more private than the Internet. Extranets may be subject to viruses, worms, and hacker attacks. One example of an extranet in use is the U.S. Navy Medical Information Management Center's initiative to share medical and benefit information, newsletters, and e-mails with more than 100,000 users worldwide (Simpkins 2003). Hospitals and physician offices also use extranets to share data (Silkey 2004).

Healthcare Information and Services

Internet and Web resources provide another means to increase access both to information for professionals and healthcare consumers and to select healthcare services. Much of this information is free. Federal agencies, healthcare institutions, physicians, nurses, psychologists, dentists, online journals, drug companies, equipment manufacturers, and discussion groups all offer information and advice. Information may be located by symptom, disease, drug interaction, nutrition, common injuries, or support group. Users can post inquiries, read documents of commonly asked questions and answers, or search by keyword or subject. Some services, such as consults and disease management, involve costs. The Institute of Medicine called for healthcare organizations to provide care whenever needed, including the use of the Internet where appropriate (IOM 2001; Tang, Black, & Young 2006). Third-party payers, commonly referred to as insurance providers, have been asked to consider payment for some Web-based services; a small number of private payors are moving in this direction (Whitten & Buis 2007).

The Internet encourages timely sharing of information among professionals, healthcare organizations and alliances, vendors, federal agencies, schools, and students. It decreases geographic isolation and allows professionals in remote areas to keep informed of the latest discoveries, treatment modalities, regulations, trends, drugs, and adverse reactions or interactions. Nurses benefit from communication with experts, listservs and discussion groups, online literature searches, and access to Web sites. These resources offer tutorials, multimedia instruction, online journals, and continuing education. Electronic communication disseminates information quickly, allowing clinicians to learn about revisions in practice guidelines and new study findings. The Internet provides teleconferencing capability for distance learning and continuing education. Electronic communication facilitates networking among nurses, saves labor through the sharing of useful tips and policies, and facilitates collaborative research and writing.

Consumer Informatics

Consumer health informatics is the branch of medical informatics that studies the use of electronic information and communication to improve medical outcomes and the healthcare decision-making process from the patient/consumer perspective (AMIA May 3, 2007). As more consumers become active participants in their care the Internet provides a vital tool to research their healthcare problems, find information about providers, schedule and even receive services, and seek out support. Due to the rapid development and dissemination of new knowledge, consumers often hear about discoveries and treatments before the professional does. Consumers may even consult the same source as their healthcare providers. Online resources can aid in diagnosis, present new treatment options, and help consumers locate support groups. The Web also presents another medium for health teaching. Some examples of Web sites that furnish client education materials include the American Heart Association and American Cancer Society. Figure 4–1 shows a page from the American Heart Association Web site explaining heart attack, stroke, and cardiac arrest warning signs. Some organizations and individual practitioners also provide information on the Web as a public service, although disclaimers are included stating that this advice does not replace a visit to a practitioner. The American Academy of Family Physicians is one organization that provides health information online. Other sites, such as MyPhysician.com and Askyourfamilydoc.com, offer individual consultations for a fee.

In their study Good, Stokes, and Jerrams-Smith (2007) noted that some informational Web sites are plagued with issues of poor accessibility and usability, which are particularly important for novice and elderly users. These issues must be factored into the instructional design of consumer-oriented Web sites. Cited problems included small font size, low contrast between background and font colors, too much text on one page, inappropriate reading levels, unclear navigational links, pop-up ads that obscure screen content, and limited user control over how the site can be used.

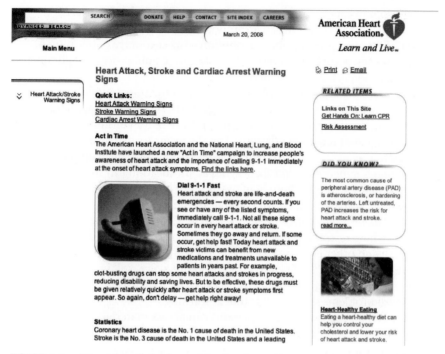

FIGURE 4–1 • "Heart Attack, Stroke, and Cardiac Arrest Warning Signs." Reprinted from American Heart Association Web Site http://www.americanheart.org.presenter. jhtml?identifier=3053 by permission of Heart and Stroke Encyclopedia.

Online Publications and Journals

Soaring costs for paper, layout, printing, distribution, and the time that it takes to get materials to press make traditional publication an expensive process. Online publication does not eliminate the costs associated with the collection, writing, and editorial processes, but it does offer several advantages over traditional approaches that include the following:

- *A shorter time frame between writing and publication.* This is particularly important when material is quickly outdated, as occurs in healthcare. Individuals can place information on the Internet as soon as it is written rather than wait until a formal article or manuscript is accepted for publication. Peer-reviewed publications expedite the publication process when reviews are done electronically. Timely articles can be published almost immediately rather than sit in a queue once accepted. This shortens the traditional period of 4 months or longer from the time that an article is submitted until it appears in print.
- *Lower printing and distribution costs.* Electronic publication eliminates the need for paper, postage, and handling costs. Instead, documents are transferred from computer to computer in binary code. This transfer process is known as **electronic document interchange (EDI).** EDI also

lowers publication costs because information is typed only once. An example of EDI is seen when an author submits an article for publication via FTP. Lower printing and distribution costs encourage publication of diverse viewpoints and small studies. Electronic publication also eliminates the need to curtail article length.

- *Instant revisions.* For example, recommended treatment modalities often change with the latest research findings. Texts, professional standards of practice, nursing procedure manuals, and advice for consumers must reflect current recommendations. The electronic format also eliminates the need to replace and discard large volumes of out-of-date print materials.
- *Facilitates joint authorship.* Colleagues at any location can share ideas and revise manuscripts without actually meeting in one physical location or spending scarce resources for travel or telephone charges.
- *Rapid identification of knowledge deficits.* FAQ on the Internet may indicate areas where research is needed. Surveys can be conducted quickly via e-mail and other electronic means.
- *Supports multimedia.* The inclusion of sound, voice, still images, and video permits the inclusion of links and allows comprehensive simulation of clinical problems that can aid student learning.
- *Improved access to materials.* Persons can access materials at any time and from any location as long as they have online access. There is no need to wait until a library is open. As a consequence, users can view literature previously unavailable to them. Many publishers allow access by subscription only, whereas others permit purchase on an article-by-article basis.
- *Facilitates electronic document searches for keywords or phrases.* Users can locate relevant information more quickly.
- *Lower subscription and storage costs for libraries.* Electronic publications can save libraries monies otherwise spent on higher costs for hard copies and physical management and storage.

Several nursing and allied health journals and health-focused publications for consumers are currently available online. Some are published in both print and electronic format, whereas others are available only electronically. The existence of online journals may be researched through many of the same methods discussed earlier to find discussion groups and Web sites.

Despite the many advantages of electronic publication, there are some disadvantages. Electronic documents lack the same type of portability provided by print media. Reading lengthy documents online can cause eye strain and take longer because of the time that it takes for documents to download. Plagiarism is easier to commit and more difficult to find as the volume of online materials soars. There are also unresolved issues about archiving electronic publications. Excessive use of links may confuse the reader. Consideration must also be given to the fact that there are still large numbers of persons who have no online access.

Blogs represent another source of online health information. It is possible to locate health-related blogs of interest through the use of search tools or following links from other sources. Some examples include the Ehealth blog, code blog: tales of a nurse, and The Health Care Blog.

Marketing Services

Web sites are a cost-effective public relations tool in healthcare. This is particularly true for sites that attract return visitors through the incorporation of interactive features. The Internet and Web can provide a competitive edge in the healthcare delivery system in the following ways:

- *Job postings.* Both employers and persons who are job hunting can use the Web to advertise positions and find new opportunities. Several sites offer help in locating job opportunities. Nursing World is one site that offers job search capability. Several employment services make it possible to complete resumes online, and some employers incorporate employment applications into their Web sites for electronic completion.
- *Virtual tours of educational institutions.* Some schools use their Web sites to introduce their facility and key people as well as allow the potential student to view available resources and complete an application online.
- *Support groups.* Emotional support and information is available for professionals and healthcare consumers. For example, International Nurses Anonymous (intnursesanon.org) is a support and advocacy group for nurses involved in a 12-step recovery program. The newsgroup alt.support.arthritis is a support group for the lay population. The presence of these resources on the Internet makes them readily available to a large number of people 24 hours a day.
- *Advertisement of services and consumer education.* Many healthcare providers furnish information about their services, assist with finding a physician or dentist, and provide general healthcare information via Web sites.
- *Dissemination and revision of product information.* Pharmaceutical companies and hospital equipment suppliers may also maintain Web sites that provide additional information about their products.
- *Online risk assessments.* Some healthcare providers post tools that users may complete to determine their risk for developing a particular health problem. Basic advice for follow-up care may be provided along with names of area providers.
- *Completion of forms.* The time spent in the healthcare delivery system can be shortened when online prescreening forms are completed at the same time that appointments are requested.
- *Benchmarking information.* Many providers and educational facilities include information that notes how their services compare with like entities in recent surveys. The Centers for Medicare and Medicaid Services (CMS)

Hospital Compare database provides information to consumers on the quality of care at most of the nation's hospitals (Rousch 2005).

E-health

There is a lack of consensus over a precise definition for **e-health** but it has been commonly used to refer to health information, services, and products provided via the Internet (Oh, Rizo, Enkin, & Jadad 2005). The definition has been expanded to encompass the technology used for education, research and administration, marketing and customer service (Harrison & Lee 2006). The Internet is already used for business transactions, electronic prescriptions, online hospital registration, consumer education and support via Web sites, and information about clinical trials and communication among professionals. It offers the potential to increase access to health care information, empower consumers, educate practitioners, and transmit information quickly, efficiently, and safely. E-health is also known as e-healthcare. The eHealth Initiative (Foundation for eHealth Initiative 2007) is an effort to drive improvement in the quality, safety, and efficiency of healthcare through information and information technology. This initiative represents multiple stakeholders including healthcare organizations, providers, consumers and various vendors. **E-business** and **e-commerce** refer to services, sales, and business conducted over the Internet. This can include procurement, electronic claims processing, eligibility authorization, and electronic purchase of prescription drugs and health insurance. Benefits associated with e-business and e-commerce include real-time responses to inquiries, clinical alerts, authorization and eligibility information, tracking, and the ability to quickly submit claims. These may also be found with e-health. E-health is changing the relationships between healthcare professionals and consumers as well as the way that the healthcare industry is conducted as consumers become empowered to select and impact their own care (Saranto et al. 2006). Browsers and the Web provide a user-friendly environment that allows users to focus on their needs rather than the technology. The Web provides the framework to expedite the delivery of services and revolutionize the way that care is delivered. Web portals help to create virtual communities both for professionals and consumers. Educated consumers come for treatment armed with knowledge that empowers them and may lead them to question treatment modalities. Full realization of the benefits of e-health requires good strategic planning, financial commitment, redesign of processes, consideration of regulatory demands, physician acceptance, and adequate data protection.

E-health affords the opportunity for providers and insurers to offer new services as well as use their strengths and bargaining powers to lower costs and increase the efficiency of services delivered. **E-care** is another term used to refer to the automation of all parts of the care delivery process across administrative, clinical, and departmental boundaries. Examples of e-health include wellness tips found on Web sites, e-mail reminders of appointments, follow-up e-mail from healthcare practitioners to consumer questions, electronic prescriptions, centralized storage of health records on the Web, regional telemedicine networks on the Web, consults, and long-term management of chronically ill patients. Another major application is electronic submission of claims and payment. Electronic claims submission reduces time and costs for claims submission and results in fewer rejections.

Another service that ultimately benefits the consumer is the electronic prescription. Electronic prescriptions eliminate the problem of lost or unreadable prescriptions while providing access to Web-based personal health information, drug interaction warnings, formularies, and verifications that reduce the incidence of medication errors. Handheld prescribing devices facilitate the electronic prescription process. The use of the Web to store healthcare information makes it available from different locations and to practitioners with different computer systems.

A number of current sites allow consumers to store personal health information and modify it for access when it is needed. One Web-based application that holds great promise for improved patient outcomes and lower long-term costs is disease management. Chronic illness now accounts for the majority of healthcare costs. Web-based management provides a way to monitor large numbers of clients efficiently on a daily basis. Client participation is stimulated through the development of health goals and recording improvements. A device may be used to measure overall health. In this case, readings are obtained and sent for review by a healthcare practitioner. For example asthmatics and persons with congestive heart failure have equipment that input data into monitoring systems, which then warn practitioners of abnormal findings that require intervention. The simplicity of the Web allows the addition of features easily and relatively inexpensively. E-health is expected to increase particularly as technology improves and becomes more prevalent. Nursing support is critical to its utilization and realization of benefits (Harrison & Lee 2006).

CONCERNS RELATED TO THE USE OF THE INTERNET AND WORLD WIDE WEB

The single largest concern related to the Internet is the quality of online information followed by security of client data, collection of personal information, worries over slowdown, collapse, and the ability to transact business smoothly. Lesser concerns include viral contamination and a lack of adherence to Internet standards among some products.

Quality of Online Information

The Internet offers unprecedented access to healthcare information. While reports of the numbers of persons who access the Internet for information vary, Harrison and Lee (2006) noted that almost 90% of people with Internet access have used it to search for health information at some point. Unfortunately, the accuracy, readability, depth, diversity, and presentation of this content vary greatly from site to site. Some online information can even be harmful. The lack of a controlling body over the Internet makes it impossible to regulate the quality of information before posting. For this reason, healthcare professionals and consumers must be wary.

Evaluating Online Information As the number of consumers who independently access health information online increases, it is essential that all healthcare professionals critically evaluate the quality of online materials and assist consumers to judge what they find. Many consumers do not examine the quality of information that they locate while others rely upon their provider to help them find credible sources (Doctors now writing "Info" Prescriptions 2005; Fox 2006). Online resources should be evaluated according to the following criteria:

- *Credentials of the source.* Large professional associations, such as hospitals, universities, government, and official health organizations, tend to have the most reliable sites. In some cases the source is not readily apparent. For example, it is important to consider whether the information provided mirrors the focus of professional education and expertise.
- *Ability to validate information.* Validation of information can be difficult unless the source can be traced back to a reputable university or other agency. Many messages and Web sites identify a person or persons to contact for further information. When facts and studies are cited, the original source should be stated so users can review it and draw their own conclusions. It should also be possible to corroborate information from independent sources.
- *Accuracy.* Because no single person controls information that is placed on the Internet, the mere existence of information does not indicate that it is accurate. Postings should identify contact persons or cite references that may be checked to allow evaluation of posted information.
- *Comprehensiveness of information.* If the site professes to provide information about medications, it should discuss indications, contraindications, protocols, and dosages. If the user must go elsewhere to find relevant information, the site is not comprehensive. Sites with broad generalizations or poorly referenced research should be considered suspicious. The user should continue to use caution because the information could be biased.
- *Date of issue or revision.* One problem with the Internet and World Wide Web is that not all pages contain dates indicating when material was written, revised, or reviewed, making it difficult to determine whether information is current. Publication, review, and revision dates help the user to determine if material is current or outdated.
- *Bias or sponsorship.* Commercial uses of the Internet are growing daily. The consumer must consider whether information is biased in favor of a particular product or commercial service. One means to consider bias is to look for a funding and advertising policy.
- *Ease of navigation.* Content should be well organized with the appropriate use of hyperlinks. All links should be to current Web pages and load easily.

- *Intended purpose and audience.* Sites should indicate the intended audience and use terminology and a reading level appropriate to that population.
- *Disclaimers.* Sites that express individual opinions should contain a statement to that effect to help users distinguish between fact and opinion.
- *Site accreditation.* Several groups have been working to ensure the quality of information found on health-related Web sites. As a consequence of these efforts, some sites display a "seal" that indicates that their sites meet a set of predetermined standards for the quality of information posted. Compliance is purely voluntary.
- *Privacy policies.* Sites that collect personal information need to identify how that information may be used so that visitors can determine whether they choose to disclose information.

Organizations A number of groups are concerned with the quality of posted materials, including most professional organizations, the Health Internet Ethics (Hi-Ethics) Alliance, the Health on the Net Foundation (HON), HealthWeb, Healthfinder, the Healthcare Coalition, the American Accreditation HealthCare Commission (URAC), the European Council, and the World Health Organization. None of these groups impose mandatory controls over quality. Hi-Ethics published a set of 14 principles in 2000 that forms the basis for URAC accreditation. Sites that have URAC accreditation display a seal. The seal indicates that the site meets more than 50 standards that include disclosure, site policies and structure, content currency and accuracy, linking, privacy, security, and accountability. The accreditation process is one way to quickly identify posted content that meets quality standards. Accreditation also fosters trust (D'Andrea 2002). URAC accreditation also considers HIPAA security accreditation standards (Kohn 2003).The European Union has also developed criteria for evaluation of Web content that largely mirror those already defined by URAC (Commission of the European Communities, 2002). HON has partnered with Google to provide data on each accredited site (Google Co-op 2006). When users type in a broad disease condition Google allows them to refine their search by treatment, symptoms, and other appropriate areas. Results from accredited sites show that they are labeled by HON. Sites may receive approval from other partners as well.

Overload

The Internet consists of many interconnected networks. Actual collapse is improbable, although vendor and facility outages and problems will likely continue as the number of users increases. Many first-time providers are undercapitalized or have poorly trained staff, so periodic overload or slow service can be expected. These problems raise interesting questions about maintaining data availability and integrity for the healthcare institution that uses the Internet to transport health data.

The majority of overload and collapse problems result from technical problems such as traffic jams, transmission difficulties, attacks by malware, and poor Web site design. These problems may occur on the user's network or an outside network. The popularity of the Internet makes it difficult to accommodate the needs of all of the users. Two initiatives that emerged to address these concerns were Internet2 and the Next Generation Internet. Internet2 (Internet2 2007; Matlis 2006) is a collaborative effort of universities, government, industry, and various research and educational groups. The purpose of the Internet2 effort is to build and operate a research network capable of enhancing delivery of education and other services, including healthcare. This includes the development and support of advanced applications and standards. The National Science Foundation Next Generation Internet project was launched by the Clinton Administration (Rapoza 2002). This program conducted research but did not actually build a secure, newer Internet.

Security

Most organizations focus security efforts on their internal networks, for the obvious reason that any disruption in computer operation affects service. As a consequence of this action, Web sites traditionally received less attention. Web sites are also vulnerable to attack and subsequent disruption can affect business operations. Hacker changes to Web pages may prove embarrassing, endanger consumers who follow altered advice, and/or result in libel charges. This recognition brings with it a heightened awareness of the need to safeguard Web sites as well as internal networks. At the same time, Webmasters are being encouraged to put their organizations on the Web so the world can access them, but they must also protect the organization from intruders.

The following measures can protect Web sites and their information:

- *Construct a separate firewall for the Web server.* Firewalls provide the same level of protection for Web servers as they do for private networks with Internet access. Some, if not all, hacker attacks can be prevented with a firewall for each Web server.
- *Limit access to Web page content or configuration.* The risk of internal attacks or accidental damage is directly related to the number of persons with authority to change Web information or setup.
- *Isolate Web servers.* Web servers should not have direct connections to other agency systems, nor should they be located at a site subject to attack. This action minimizes the chance of Web site damage.
- *Heed security advisories.* Updates on hacker attacks and warnings on new breach techniques are posted by several sites on the Web, including the WWW Security FAQ and commercial sites such as Symantec.com. Webmasters should anticipate attack and take proactive measures.
- *Keep antivirus systems up-to-date and install intrusion detection systems to hail attacks.* Webmasters or network administrators need to maintain up-to-date virus detection to avoid having their site(s) being brought down by the latest virus or worm. Alarms and tracking mechanisms alert administrators or Webmasters to attacks early so that action can be taken to minimize Web site damage.

Contamination by Viruses, Worms, and Other Malware

Viruses can be spread when files are imported for use without subjecting them to a viral scan. The danger of contamination cannot be eliminated, but it can be reduced through the following measures:

- *Strict policies on Internet use.* These policies should include scanning all files before use, including FTP files, and deletion of files with unfamiliar file extensions. Viruses may be included in materials available for public consumption. Consider deleting all attachments with unfamiliar file extensions.
- *Use the latest version of antiviral software.* New viruses are created daily. Older releases of antiviral software cannot recognize new viruses; therefore, it is important to frequently update the virus files for antiviral software. This can usually be done using downloads from a Web site and may or may not require a fee.
- *Download and install software security patches.* Security patches for operating systems and applications are available from the vendor once problems have been identified.
- *Install or enable a computer firewall.* Some operating systems come with a firewall. A firewall provides a barrier against outsiders infiltrating a computer or network.
- *Use security features that come with software.* Word and Excel documents may contain macros that open automatically. This can be controlled by setting the security level to "high."

Firewalls

The open design of the Internet invites security abuse, particularly for private networks with Internet access. Most organizations with an Internet connection are under continuous attack by human attackers and automated software applications. Any of these attacks have the potential to pose a serious security breach or a launching pad for large-scale attacks on other computers. For this reason, private networks need a gateway to intercept and examine Internet messages before they are permitted to enter the private network. A **gateway** is a combination of hardware and software used to connect local area networks with larger networks. A **firewall** is a type of gateway designed to protect private network resources from outside hackers, network damage, and theft or misuse of information. It consists of hardware and software that can use one of several mechanisms to protect data. A firewall should be transparent to users. A firewall does not preclude the need for a security plan or periodic security testing; outside intruders may still be able to penetrate firewall protection.

Not all threats to a network arise from outside sources; firewalls alone do not protect against internal attacks or prevent viral contamination. Strong security policies for employees can minimize these threats as long as users are aware of the policies, their responsibilities, and the implications for policy violations. Another key factor in network protection is knowledge. Network administrators must educate themselves about attacks on Internet sites and protective measures recommended by the federally funded Computer Emergency Response Team (CERT) Coordination Center and Usenet groups. Subsequent work by a coalition of federal and private organizations produced a set of security configurations entitled "Consensus Baseline Security Settings." This effort was geared toward the protection of government Windows-based workstations from external and internal attacks, but it is expected to help other systems administrators to protect their systems and provide guidance for the future development of network protocols and systems.

Institutional Policies

All organizations with an Internet connection need policies that address the following areas:

- *E-mail privacy.* The organization has the legal right to read employee e-mail unless stated otherwise. Employees should be aware of their organization's e-mail policy. Some organizations may permit a limited amount of personal e-mail.
- *Encryption.* Potentially sensitive data should be coded or encrypted to prevent unauthorized people from reading it. Any client data are sensitive and should be encrypted for transmittal over the Internet.
- *Transmission of employee data or photographs.* Employers should obtain consent before the transmittal of employee pictures or personal data over the Internet.
- *Intellectual ownership.* Guidelines should establish how issues of intellectual ownership are determined for network postings and other communications. In other words, it is important to resolve who owns the information: the employee who developed it or the employer.
- *Free speech.* The organization's stance on ideas or images that it considers offensive or inappropriate should be plainly delineated. This helps to protect the organization from liability for inappropriate statements made by employees. Pornographic or sexually explicit or otherwise offensive materials are not acceptable.
- *Acceptable Internet uses in the workplace.* Permissible Internet uses must be identified and communicated to employees. Violations of accepted use may constitute grounds for dismissal. One example of unacceptable use is the downloading of pirated music or software. One means to enforce this policy is the inclusion of a section on acceptable Internet use in the employee's annual performance evaluation.
- *Citation of sources and verification of information downloaded from the Internet/Web.* Authors of materials on the Internet and Web deserve the same recognition as authors of any other media. Failure to cite sources is plagiarism. Guidelines for the citation of online resources can be found at the American Psychological Association and the Modern Language Association Web sites as well as at most college and university sites.

- *Monitoring policies.* Employees need to be aware that e-mail and Internet use may be monitored and that inappropriate use can be cause for dismissal.
- *Acknowledgment of receipt of Internet policies.* Employees should sign a statement that they have read and understand the organization's Internet policies at the time of hire and on yearly review.

FUTURE DIRECTIONS

Electronic communication is here to stay. Its impact upon healthcare will continue to increase and evolve. As more consumers become connected and Internet savvy more e-health applications will be seen. Nurses have an obligation to prepare for these changes and to assist healthcare consumers along in this journey.

CASE STUDY EXERCISES

4.1 As the representative for your medical center's Better Care Initiative, a project with the purpose of identifying ways that services can be delivered in a more efficient manner, you have suggested that the Internet be made available to clinicians at the point of care. Develop a report listing both the potential uses as well as potential problems of using the Internet.

4.2 One of your clients has a rare genetic defect. The client is requesting additional information about this defect from you, but no reference books on the unit describe this condition. Discuss strategies for how you might obtain quality information using the Internet and electronic communication.

4.3 The e-health committee at your facility is looking at ways to provide greater client involvement in accessing their own health information. What ramifications must be considered for this to occur in terms of security, interpretation of results, and training?

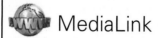 MediaLink

Additional resources for this content can be found on the Companion Website at www.prenhall.com/hebda. Click on "Chapter 4" to select the activities for this chapter.

- Glossary
- Multiple Choice
- Discussion Points
- Case Studies
- MediaLink Application
- MediaLink

SUMMARY

- Electronic communication is the ability to exchange information through the use of computer equipment and software, using network connections or a modem.
- The Internet is a network of networks, connecting computers worldwide. It offers a wealth of information about many topics, and can be extremely useful for the exchange of healthcare information.
- The World Wide Web (Web or WWW), a popular Internet feature, allows users to find information more easily by conducting word searches using browser software or locating a specific Web site or address. It is characterized by a GUI that makes it easy to use.
- A popular Web feature is the home page, the first page seen at a particular Web location. The home page provides general information about a topic, a person, or an organization.
- Links are words, phrases, or pictures that are distinguished from other parts of a WWW home page, usually by color, and enable users to move directly to another Web location.
- Nurses, other clinicians, and consumers may use the Web to obtain information regarding clinical topics, diseases, treatments, and healthcare agencies.
- Electronic mail, or e-mail, is the use of computer technology to transmit messages from one person to another. Delivery can be almost instantaneous. The Internet allows e-mail to be sent anywhere in the world, as long as the recipient has an Internet address.
- File transfer is the ability to move files from one location to another across a network.
- Other forms of electronic communication include instant messaging (IM), blogs, wikis, listservs (electronic mailing lists), and usenet groups (message discussion groups). These forums provide information and support.
- E-commerce, or e-business, uses Internet technology to provide healthcare organizations with mechanisms to safely and quickly exchange information with other business entities.
- E-health refers to online availability of health information, products, and services.
- E-care is a broad term used to refer to the automation of all parts of the care delivery process, including purchasing and patient management.
- Evaluation of online information entails consideration of the source of the information, validation, accuracy and depth, dates for publication or review and revision, possible bias or sponsorship, organization and linkage, intended audience, presence of disclaimers and privacy policies, and accreditation or sponsorship by reputable organizations.
- Security is a major concern surrounding the use of the Internet and electronic communication. Firewalls and encryption are two prevalent strategies for safeguarding information.

- Internet technology is used internally in an organization in systems known as intranets, or external to the organization in systems known as extranets. Increasingly, these applications are referred to as Web portals.
- Consumer health informatics is the use of electronic information and communication to improve medical outcomes and the healthcare decision-making process from the patient/consumer perspective.

REFERENCES

American Medical Informatics Association (AMIA) (May 3, 2007). Working Groups Consumer Health Informatics (CHI-WG). Retrieved May 31, 2007, from http://www.amia.org/mbrcenter/wg/chi/.

Anderberg, K. (February 2007). Patience is OK. *Communication News,* p. 4.

Bisconti, K. (January 1, 2007). IM: Ready for the enterprise? *Communications News,* 44(1), 44–45.

Commission of the European Communities. (2002). EEurope 2002: Quality criteria for health related Websites. *Journal of Medical Internet Research,* 4(3), e15.

Cukier, K. N. (November/December 2005). Who will control the Internet? *Foreign Affairs.* Retrieved June 27, 2007, from http://www.foreignaffairs.org/20051101facomment84602/kenneth-neil-cukier/who-will-control-the-internet.html.

D'Andrea, G. (2002). Health Web site accreditation: Opportunities and challenges. *Journal of Healthcare Information Management,* 16(3), 9–11.

Doctors Now Writing "Info" Prescriptions. (February 1, 2005). *USA Today Magazine,* 133(2717), 4.

Dunn, D. (2006 May 22). Power Line Broadband Expands. *InformationWeek,* Issue 1090, 19.

Foundation for eHealth Initiative. (2007). About: eHealth Initiative Strategy. Retrieved July 11, 2007, from http://www.ehealthinitiative.org/about/priorities.mspx.

Fichter, D. (2005). Intranets, wikis, blikis, and collaborative working. *Online,* 29(5), 47–50.

Fiber: Friend or foe To DSL? (3/29/2007). *Electronic Design,* 55(7), 55.

Foundation for eHealth Initiative. (2007). About: eHealth Initiative Strategy. Retrieved July 11, 2007, from http://www.ehealthinitiative.org/about/priorities.mspx.

Fox, S. (October 29, 2006). Online Health Search 2006. Washington, DC: Pew Internet & American Life Project. Retrieved July 13, 2007, from http://www.pewinternet.org/pdfs/PIP_Online_Health_2006.pdf.

Good, A., Stokes, S., & Jerrams-Smith, J. (2007). Elderly, novice users and health information websites. *Journal of Healthcare Information Management,* 21(3), 72–79.

Google Co-op. (November 10, 2006). Retrieved July 12, 2007, from http://www.hon.ch/Project/GoogleCoop/.

Governmental delegations to watch in Tunis. (November 2005). *InformationToday,* 49.

Griffiths, K. M. & Christensen, H. (2005). Website quality indicators for consumers. *Journal of Medical Internet Research,* 7(5).e55.

Harrison, J. P. & Lee, A. (2006). The role of e-health in the changing health care environment. *Nursing Economics,* 24(6), 283–289.

Hawkins, D. T. (2005). The latest on search engines. *Information Today,* 22(6), 37–38.

Hesseldahl, A. (2007, May 30). More Bandwidth Than You Can Use? *Business Week Online,* 26.

IM threats proliferate. (2006). *Communication News,* 43(1), 10.

Institute of Medicine. (2001). *Crossing the Quality Chasm: A New Health System for the 21st Century.* Washington, D.C: National Academy Press.

Internet Society. (2007, June 7). *About the Internet Society.* Retrieved June 27, 2007, from http://www.isoc.org/isoc/.

Internet2. (2007). Internet2 Network. Retrieved July 12, 2007, from http://www.internet2.edu/network/.

Kavehrad, M. (2007). Broadband Room Service By Light, *Scientific American, 297*(1), 82–87.

Kent, M. L. (2005, Winter). Conducting better research: Google Scholar and the future of search technology. *Public Relations Quarterly,* 35–40.

Kohn, C. (2003, June 2). URAC board approves HIPAA security accreditation standards. *Managed Care Weekly,* 25.

Malakata, M. (2005, May 16). South African nations to standardize cyberlaws. *Computerworld,* 14.

Matlis, J. (2006, August 28). Quick Study: Internet 2. *Computerworld, 40*(35), 30.

McCarthy, K. (2006, August 16). ICANN awarded net administration until 2011. *The Register.* Retrieved June 27, 2007, from http://www.theregister.co.uk/2006/08/16/icann_awarded_iana/.

The need for global policies. (2005, November). *InformationToday, 383*(8530), 63–64.

Newly nasty. (2007, May 26). *Economist, 383*(8530), 63–64.

Notess, G. R. (2007, June). Switching your search engines. *Online.* 44–46.

Oh, H., Rizo, C., Enkin, M., & Jadad, A. (2005). What is eHealth?: A systematic review of published definitions. *World Hospitals and Health Services, 41*(1):32–40.

Pike, S. (2007). Use a colon. *PC Magazine, 26*(13), 107.

Rapoza, J. (2002, July 15). It's time for next Internet. *EWeek, 19*(28), 58.

Saranto, K., Weber, P., Häyrinen, K., Kouri, P., Porrasmaa, J., Komulainen, J., et al. (2006). Citizen empowerment: eHealth consumerism in Europe. In C. A. Weaver, C. Delaney, P. Weber, & R.L. Carr, eds. *Nursing and Informatics for the 21st Century. An International Look at Practice, Trends and the Future.* Chicago: HIMSS, p. 489–500.

Schloman, B. F. (2006, October 20). Is it time to visit the blogosphere? *OJIN: Online Journal of Issues in Nursing.* Retrieved July 13, 2007, from http://www.nursingworld.org/ojin/infocol/info_21.htm.

Senate ratifies treaty on cybercrimes. (2006, August 4). *CongessDaily,* p.8.

Silkey, R. C. (2004). Extranet helps practices keep their business connected. *Ophthalmology Times, 29*(19), 31–32.

Simpkins, A. (February 2003). Navy secures healthcare network. *Communications News, 40*(2), 20.

Stebbins, L. (2007). Email Is Evolving—Are You? *Searcher, 15*(2), 8–12.

Tang, P. C., Black, W., & Young, C. Y. (2006). Proposed Criteria for Reimbursing eVisits: Content Analysis of Secure Patient Messages in a Personal Health Record System. In AMIA Annual Symposium Proceedings, 764–768.

The need for global policies. (November 1, 2005). Information Today. Retrieved January 2, 2008, from http://www.allbusiness.com/technology/telecommunications/948099-1.html.

U.N. to control use of Internet. (February 22, 2005). WorldNetDaily. Retrieved January 2, 2008, from http://www.worldnetdaily.com/news/article.asp?ARTICLE_ID=42982.

Whitten P. & Buis, L. (2007). Private payer reimbursement for telemedicine services in the United States. *Telemedicine and e-Health, 13*(1),15–23.

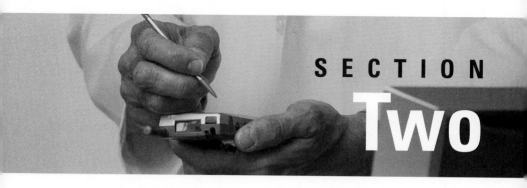

SECTION Two

Healthcare Information Systems

CHAPTER 5

Healthcare Information Systems

After completing this chapter, you should be able to:

1 Identify the various types of information systems used within healthcare institutions.

2 Define the terms *healthcare information system, hospital information system, clinical information system, nursing information system, physician practice management system, long-term care information system, home care information system*, and *administrative information system*.

3 Explain the functions of a nursing information system.

4 Differentiate between the nursing process and critical pathways/protocol approaches to the design of a nursing system.

5 Review the key features and impacts on nursing and other healthcare professionals associated with order entry, laboratory, radiology, and pharmacy information systems.

6 Describe the functions of client registration and scheduling, and coding systems.

7 Explain the purpose of decision support and expert systems.

8 Identify ways that mobile devices such as personal digital assistants, tablet computers, and iPods can improve the utility of healthcare information systems.

An **information system** can be defined as the use of computer hardware and software to process data into information to solve a problem. The terms **healthcare information system** and **hospital information system** (**HIS**) both refer to a group of systems used within a hospital or enterprise that support and enhance healthcare. The HIS comprises two major types of information systems: clinical information systems and administrative information systems. **Clinical information systems** (**CISs**) are large, computerized database management systems that support several types of activities that may include provider order entry, result retrieval, documentation, and decision support across distributed locations (Clinical Information Systems 2002; Sittig et al. 2002). Clinicians use these systems to access client data that are used to plan, implement, and evaluate care. CISs may also be referred to as *client care information systems.* Some examples of CISs include nursing, laboratory, pharmacy, radiology, medical information systems, emergency department systems, physician practice management systems, and long term and home care information systems. **Administrative information systems** support client care by managing financial and demographic information and providing reporting capabilities. This category includes client management, financial, payroll, and human resources, and quality assurance systems. Coding systems use clinical information to generate charges for care. Figure 5–1 shows the relationships between various components of a hospital information system.

Clinical and administrative information systems may be designed to meet the needs of one or more departments or functions within the organization. In recent years the trend has been to adopt vendor-based solutions with little, if any, customization, allowing implementation to occur more quickly (Conn 2007a). Either clinical or administrative systems can be implemented as standalone systems, or they may work with other systems to provide information sharing and seamless functionality for the users. Any one healthcare enterprise may use one or several of the clinical and administrative systems but may not use all of them. Increasingly, organizations are looking at the need to improve productivity, improve safety, increase the quality of care, and reduce costs across the enterprise. Information technology is seen as the means to achieve these ends through the application of evidenced-based care, improved work flow, and better management of resources. Realizing the full potential of patient safety initiatives requires healthcare facilities to first establish a culture of safety in which problem areas are identified, then measure the culture periodically, share findings, and solicit feedback for change (Smetzer & Navarra 2007).

CLINICAL INFORMATION SYSTEMS

Although many CISs are designed for use within one hospital department, clinicians and researchers from several areas use the data collected by each system. For example, the nurse documents client allergies in the initial assessment. The physician, the pharmacist, the dietician, and the radiologist can then use these data during the client's hospital stay. The goal of CISs is to allow clinicians to quickly and safely access information, order appropriate medications and treatments, and implement cost-effective, evidence-based care while

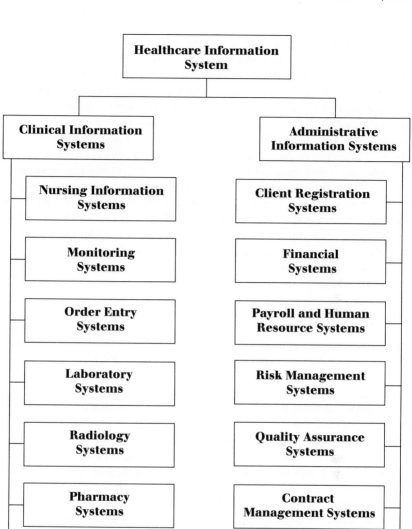

FIGURE 5–1 • Relationship of the healthcare information system components

avoiding duplicate services. Several tools help clinicians to achieve these goals. These include electronic health records, clinical decision support systems, bedside medication administration using positive patient identification, computerized provider order entry (CPOE), patient surveillance, and the clinical data warehouse (CDW) (Harrison & Palacio 2006; Hastings 2006; Mangalampalli, Chakravarthy, Raja, Jain, & Parinam 2006; Solovy 2005). While large teaching hospitals are generally better able to afford the investment in information technology to make use of these tools, forces calling for cost containment and returns on investments have all healthcare providers looking at information technology solutions (Kelley 2007). Mobile and wireless technology are used with CISs to allow information entry and retrieval at the point of care or wherever it is needed by the healthcare professional. Most often this is at the bedside, but it may be in another hospital department. This is best illustrated by the healthcare professional who can view client lab results while walking. This type of access enhances worker productivity because healthcare professionals do not need to walk back to a central location to view test results, and it improves client service because treatments can be ordered and initiated in a more timely fashion. Internet technology is also changing the way that users interact with CISs. This capability allows a physician to view client test results from the comfort of his or her home or office or even while on the golf course or at the mall. Despite the fact that the technology exists to permit this type of access, not all facilities can provide it at this time. The following descriptions of CISs address those that are most frequently seen in the hospital setting.

Nursing Information Systems

A **nursing information system** supports the use and documentation of nursing processes and activities, and provides tools for managing the delivery of nursing care (Hendrickson 1993). An effective nursing information system must accomplish two goals. The first goal is that the system should support the way that nurses function, allowing them the flexibility to use the system to view data and collect necessary information, provide quality client care, and document the client's condition and the care that was given. Necessary information includes past health medical history, allergies, test results, and progress notes, among other things. The second goal of an effective nursing information system is that it should support and enhance nursing practice through improved access to information and tools. These tools include online literature searches such as the Cumulative Index of Nursing and Allied Health Literature (CINAHL) and MEDLINE, and automated drug information and hospital policy/procedure guidelines. Consideration of these two goals in the selection and implementation of a nursing system will ensure that it benefits nursing. The challenge for nursing is to identify and implement technology and information systems solutions that provide more breadth, depth, flexibility, and standardization (Hughes 1997). Bao and Lin (2005) noted improved quality and efficiency in their observation of a nursing information system.

In general, there are two approaches to nursing care and documentation using automated information systems: the *traditional nursing process* approach and the *critical pathway,* or *protocols,* approach. The traditional nursing process approach allows documentation of nursing care using well-established formats such as admission assessments, problem lists, and care plans. A more organized version of this approach incorporates **standardized nursing languages (SNLs)** accepted by the American Nurses Association (Prophet, Dorr, Gibbs, & Porcella 1997). The SNLs include nursing diagnoses defined by the North American

Nursing Diagnosis Association (NANDA), Nursing Interventions Classification (NIC), Nursing Outcomes Classification (NOC), and several other languages. SNLs provide a common language across the discipline of nursing that allows all nurses to describe nursing problems, treatments, and outcomes in a manner that is understood by all nurses. SNLs facilitate data collection and research that can be replicated and shared across all of nursing (Powelson, McGahan, & Wilkinson 2000). The University of Iowa Hospitals and Clinics have been working for 20 years on the development of a clinical database to support patient care planning and documentation via their INFORMM NIS (Information Network for Online Retrieval & Medical Management Nursing Information System) (Prophet 2000). The recent adoption of the first international standard for nursing, *The Integration of a Reference Terminology Model for Nursing*, at the International Organization of Standardization Technical Committee for Health Informatics represents an important step in representing nursing diagnosis and other key concepts in a manner suitable for computer processing (Health Informatics Standards 2003). Despite this progress in representing nursing language in automated systems, the use of interdisciplinary pathways remains popular. These protocols suggest specific treatments related to the client's diagnosis and outline the anticipated outcomes. The advantages of using a nursing information system are listed in Box 5–1.

Nursing Process Approach The nursing process approach to automated documentation is based on the paper forms traditionally used by nurses. The nursing diagnosis often serves as the organizational framework. Many current information systems follow this format.

- *Documentation of nursing admission assessment and discharge instructions.*
  A menu-driven approach to the admission assessment ensures capture of

---

BOX 5–1 Advantages of an Information System

- Better access to information
- Enhanced quality of documentation through promps
- Improved quality of client care
- Increased productivity
- Improved communications
- Reduced errors of omissions
- Reduced hospital costs
- Increased employee satisfaction
- Compliance with agency regulations
- Common clinical database
- Improved client perception of care
- Enhanced ability to track records
- Enhanced ability to recruit/retain staff
- Improved hospital image

essential information. A **menu** lists related commands that can be selected from a computer screen to accomplish a task. For example, the menu may include selections such as past medical history, advanced directives, organ donation status, psychosocial history, medications, and review of body systems. This approach can also be used to ensure that all necessary information is covered in the client's discharge instructions, including follow-up appointments and diagnostic studies; diet and activity restrictions; wound care; and medication information such as drug names, instructions for administration, and common side effects that the client should report. The system should generate printed copies of these instructions for clients to review on discharge and for their use at home, as well as for use by the Home Health staff.

- *Generation of a nursing worklist that indicates routine scheduled activities related to the care of each client.* These activities can be grouped according to scheduled time or skill level.
- *Documentation of discrete data or activities such as vital signs, weight, and intake and output measurements.* The automation of this type of data promotes accuracy and allows the data to be readily available to all care providers at any time.
- *Documentation of routine aspects of client care, such as bathing, positioning, blood glucose measurements, notation of dietary intake, and/or wound care in a flowsheet format.*
- *Standardized care plans that the nurse can individualize for clients as needed.* This feature saves time yet allows flexibility to address the client's needs while promoting quality care.
- *Documentation of nursing care in a progress note format.* The nurse may accomplish this through narrative charting, charting by exception, or flowsheet charting. Regardless of the method, automated documentation can improve the overall quality of charting by prompting the nurse with predefined selections. Box 5–2 describes three of these traditional formats and some typical automation approaches.
- *Documentation of medication administration.* This multi-step feature may be performed through the nursing information system, but increasingly it is instead performed through a separate medication administration application. When this feature is used there are worklists that specify the administration times and medications for each patient; the nurse can use the worklist for preparation and administration of medications with subsequent documentation through the system.

Recent initiatives to improve patient safety and decrease medication errors call for the use of barcode medication administration systems. While these are not considered to be a part of a nursing documentation system, barcode systems are designed to prevent common medication administration errors at the bedside, document medication administration, and capture charges. These systems require the nurse to scan the barcodes found on his or her identification, the patient's identification bracelet, and on all prescription medications

---

BOX 5–2   Automation of Traditional Nursing Documentation Methods

Many forms of nursing documentation have been automated by various nursing information systems. Some of these formats are listed below.

- **Narrative charting.** Traditionally, nurses complete charts using narrative text. In a nursing information system, this may be accomplished using free text entry or menu selections.
- **Charting by exception.** Client-specific documentation addresses only the client's exceptions to normal conditions or ranges. Automated documentation should provide all normal standards and allow the nurse to easily document any exception observed. This may involve menu selections or free text entry.
- **Flowsheet charting.** Routine aspects of care are documented in tabular form. This format is most effective when presented in a personal computer–based graphical user interface. A pointing device such as a mouse is used to make menu selections or text entries. One form of flowsheet charting is the automation of medication administration records.
- **Standardized nursing languages.** This approach uses NANDA nursing diagnoses as well as the Nursing Interventions Classification and Nursing Outcomes Classification languages. It removes the ambiguity of meaning found in other documentation systems.

---

during the medication administration process. These systems are designed to help the busy nurse to ensure that the right medication is given in the correct dosage and form at the correct time for the right patient. Barcoding systems often include warnings for high-risk drugs, medications with sound-alike names, dosage discrepancies, and maximum dosages.

Critical Pathway or Protocols The critical pathway or protocol approach to nursing documentation is another approach used in automated nursing information systems, particularly with the onset of managed care. This approach is often used in a multidisciplinary manner, with many types of care providers accessing the system for information and to document care. Nurses, nursing or patient care assistants, dietitians, social workers, respiratory therapists, physical and occupational therapists, case managers, and physicians all use these systems for documentation. Critical pathway systems include the following features:

- *The nurse, or other care provider, can select one or more appropriate critical pathways for the client.* If more than one path is selected, the system should merge the paths to create one "master" path or protocol.
- *Interaction with physician orders.* Standard physician order sets can be included with each critical pathway and may be automatically processed by the system.
- *Tracking of protocol variances.* The system should identify variances to the anticipated outcomes as they are charted and provide aggregate variance data for analysis by the providers. This information can be used to fine tune and improve the critical pathways, thereby contributing to improved client outcomes.

Despite the many reasons to establish a nursing information system and the fact that nurses constitute the majority of workers in healthcare, most systems are designed for use by all clinicians.

Standardized Nursing Languages

Standardized healthcare languages and reference terminology are important in the development of the electronic health record, which forms the foundations of information content in the electronic health record and provides data for research, public health reporting, and reimbursement (AMIA & AHIMA Terminology and Classification Policy Task Force 2006; AMIA NIWG letter 2006). Murphy (2005) notes that measuring nursing's contribution is essential particularly since there is inadequate evidence to link nursing care to outcomes at present, leading nurses to draw upon experience rather than prove best practice. Measuring contributions can instead create referential knowledge and transform into executable knowledge with the help of alerts and links to references built into information systems. Standardized nursing languages (SNLs) provide visibility to the work done by nursing (Saba & Taylor 2007). SNLs recognized by the American Nurses Association have been integrated into the larger structure for standardized languages, the Systematized Nomenclature of Medicine (SNOMED). SNLs are meant to provide a common language for all nurses in all locations. While the majority of SNL terms have counterparts in SNOMED there are occasional problems in mapping terms and translation to and from other languages that require attention to avoid confusion and prevent errors in aggregate data (Burkhart, Konicek, Moorhead, & Androvich 2005; Lu et al. 2006; Park, Konicek, & Delaney 2007). Box 5–3 lists SNLs accepted by the American Nurses Association.

BOX 5–3   American Nurses Association Recognized Standardized Terminologies

North American Nursing Diagnosis Association International
Nursing Interventions Classification
Omaha System
Clinical Care Classification
Nursing Outcomes Classification (NOC)
Nursing Management Minimum Data Set (NMMDS)
Patient Care Data Set (PCDS)
PeriOperative Nursing Data Set (PNDS)
Systematized Nomenclature of Medicine—CT
International Classification for Nursing Practice
Logical Observation Identifiers Names & Codes

Monitoring Systems

Monitoring systems are devices that automatically monitor biometric measurements in critical care and specialty areas, such as cardiology and obstetrics. These devices may send information to the nursing documentation system. For example, a monitoring system would directly enter measurements such as blood pressures, eliminating the need for the nurse to enter these data manually. Another example may be seen with blood glucose monitors that send client readings to the laboratory system for display with other laboratory tests. Box 5–4 describes some additional features of monitoring systems.

Order Entry Systems

With **order entry systems,** orders for medications and treatments are entered into the computer and directly transmitted to the appropriate areas such as the pharmacy, laboratory, radiology, social service, or another area. The preferred method is direct entry of orders by the physician, nurse practitioner, physical therapist, or other provider because this eliminates issues related to illegible handwriting and transcription errors, checks orders for accuracy and completeness, speeds the implementation of ordered diagnostic tests and treatment modalities, can enhance staff productivity, save money, promote safety, and improve outcomes when used in conjunction with evidence-based practices (Kuiper, McCreadie, Mitchell, & Stevenson 2007; Simon, Rundall, & Shortell 2007). This process is known as **computerized physician, provider,** or **prescriber order entry (CPOE)** (Hastings 2006). CPOE represents a major initiative on the part of the Institute of Medicine and Leapfrog Group to improve the quality of care and reduce medication errors (Conn 2007b). While most CPOE is found in inpatient settings, its benefits apply to outpatient and ambulatory settings as well, where it also plays a critical role in the prevention of prescription errors (Varkey et al. 2007). The safety of CPOE systems is enhanced through the incorporation of built-in reminders and alerts that help the

---

BOX 5–4 **Some Common Features of Monitoring**

- **Alarms alerting the nurse of significant abnormal findings.** Sophisticated systems provide different alarms indicating various abnormalities. For example, the nurse may be able to hear a specific alarm sound that indicates which cardiac arrhythmia the client is experiencing.
- **Portable monitoring systems.** These allow easy transportation of the client throughout the facility without loss of data or functionality.
- **Records of past abnormal findings.** The system maintains a record of all past abnormal findings during this monitoring episode. The system allows the user to find trends in data using graphical displays and to focus on specific details.
- **Download capabilities.** The system may be able to transfer patient data to a separate system in another facility to provide a continuous patient record.

prescriber to select the most appropriate diagnostic test or medication for a particular patient as well as the appropriate dose and form. Challenges to the implementation of CPOE include buy-in by busy clinicians, significant changes to work processes, difficult system sign-on, limited system access or response time, funding constraints, inadequate access to clinical data to support the expert decision-making features of CPOE, and the perception by many physicians that CPOE affords them few advantages (Kelly 2007). Successful CPOE implementation requires significant expertise in healthcare processes, information technology, and change management as well as careful planning and building that includes input from nurses, pharmacists, and other stakeholders (McBroom et al. 2006; Knowles, Cornish, & Etchells 2006; Kravet, Knight, & Wright 2007; Lehmann & Kim 2006; Subramanian et al. 2007). At present, full implementation of CPOE exists in a limited number of institutions, although most have plans for its use (Hillman & Given 2005). In some settings, transcription of physician orders into the clinical information system is still done by a nurse or by ancillary personnel. When entries are made by ancillary personnel, nurses are responsible for ensuring that entries are correct.

Entry of an order into a clinical information or order entry system *alerts all departments* to carry out orders. For example, when a physician orders a barium enema, the order entry system can automatically notify the dietary department to hold the client's breakfast, the pharmacy to send the appropriate medications, and the radiology department to schedule the test. These systems prompt the clinician to provide the information necessary for carrying out the order.

Another feature of an order entry system is *duplicate checking.* When an order is entered, the system checks to see if a similar order has been placed within a specified time frame. If this is the case, the system can alert the user with a message, or automatically combine the two orders, permitting only one execution of the order.

The order entry system can reflect the *current status* of each order. For example, the status may be listed as pending, complete, or canceled. This allows the user to see a comprehensive list of the client's orders at any point in time. It can also afford a mechanism for the entry of charges for a procedure once it has been completed.

One mechanism that is used in some order entry systems uses rules-based or knowledge-based programming. Rules provide guidelines to assist physicians to select the preferred and most cost-effective medication along with the best route and dose for a particular patient problem. Rules can also provide prompts for when patients should be seen next and diagnostic tests that should be performed. These automated reminders help to improve the quality of care by reducing reliance upon memory, providing evidence-based practice guidelines, and informing the prescriber when a more cost-effective oral medication is available in lieu of an intravenous form (Rogoski 2005; Saleem et al. 2007).

Despite the many advantages associated with CPOE it may also introduce new problems and errors related to new work processes (Ash et al. 2007; Bradley, Steltenkamp, & Hite 2006; Knowles, Cornish, & Etchells 2006; Weant, Cook, & Armistead 2007). These unintended consequences may include an increase in medication errors even if the level of harm related to errors does not increase.

Pharmacists can help identify potential problem areas and needed modifications prior to implementation. Some examples include reminders or alerts to:

- Prescribe laxatives for patients prescribed opiods
- Order drug levels for therapeutic levels
- Avoid lapses in medications
- Avoid prescribing drugs that are contraindicated for certain medical conditions such as impaired renal function

Pre-implementation planning should address unintended consequences. It is important not to underestimate the time required for training or the impact of CPOE on nursing practice as nurses are called upon both to assist physicians struggling to learn the system and to execute more verbal orders by physicians unwilling to use the system (Hastings 2006). Verbal orders are subject to errors, defeating the safety checks built into CPOE. Nursing leaders must provide sufficient resources to manage the additional workload as staff and physicians make the transition to CPOE and ensure that no verbal orders will be accepted except during emergency situations.

Laboratory Systems

Laboratory information systems (LISs) can provide many benefits, including a shorter turnaround time for results, prevention of duplicate testing, decreased likelihood of human error, and identification of abnormal results according to age, sex, and hospital standards. Systems have the capability to alert providers when new or stat tests results are back or values are critical (Goedert 2007). Additional features can include the automatic entry of repeating tests at the time of the original order. An example might include the order "troponins x3," which would automatically schedule the first troponin level, with the second 8 hours later and the third level 8 hours after the second and which would subsequently bundle serial tests into one claim for reimbursement. Systems may also allow providers to enter orders without leaving the patient's electronic record. In addition, microbiology culture and sensitivity testing can provide treatment suggestions for the physician.

Automatic generation of specimen labels should occur when an order is placed either directly into an LIS or passed to an order entry system. Labels may include client demographic identifiers, the name of laboratory studies to be performed, and any special instruction for handling, such as "place on ice." Labels may be configured to print immediately at the client location for stat or nurse-collected specimens or in the laboratory in batch mode for laboratory-collected specimens. *Batch mode* allows the labels to be printed in groups for standard collection times, either on demand or at predefined times.

When specimens are processed by the laboratory instrumentation, the results are automatically transmitted to the LIS. The results can be viewed directly from the LIS or transmitted to another information system, such as the nursing or medical information system. Laboratory values are available immediately on completion of the testing process. If desired, printed paper copies of the results may be produced immediately at predefined locations, such as the nursing unit or physician's office, or can be printed in cumulative format for permanent chart copies. Another feature of many laboratory systems is automatic client billing for tests completed. This information may be communicated to the client billing system.

Another feature seen in many laboratory systems is the ability to integrate results collected at the bedside using portable devices. This is seen with the performance of blood glucose monitor tests in the clinical area. Results are then sent to the laboratory system immediately or sent when the blood glucose monitor is docked. This affords clinicians an integrated view of patient results and the ability to compare glucose readings taken at the bedside with glucose readings from blood specimens sent to the laboratory. While this feature is widely used and appreciated more commonly, the demand is to have LIS results available at the bedside or via mobile devices such as personal digital assistants (PDAs) in which results are passed either through the laboratory or clinical information system to the PDA for review.

Another feature of some laboratory systems is the ability to use rules-based testing. A **rule** is a predefined function that generates a clinical alert or reminder. **Arden syntax** is the standard language used in the healthcare industry for writing rules. A rules-based LIS could automatically order a second test based on the results of an initial test. For example, if a client has an abnormal complete blood cell count value, the system will perform a differential, which is a more specific second test. Rules-based testing could also eliminate unnecessary testing after several consecutive normal results have been obtained, as when physicians order daily laboratory work. These measures save costs and the staff time of assessing the need for and performing the tests. The incorporation of rules-based technology may require the user to enter all of the information needed for specific tests. An example is weight for a creatinine clearance test to determine whether the client's renal function falls within the normal range. Another example of rules-based technology is seen when labels are printed with collection instructions such as tube color, amount needed, and directions such as "place on ice." Rules can also be used to limit tests to those covered by Medicare or other third-party payers or to determine how and where test results will be sent (Rogoski 2003).

Laboratory systems also have the potential to provide more meaningful information such as genetic predisposition toward certain diseases based on information that already exists in the hospital or laboratory database, information that can be useful in the diagnosis and procurement of payment from third-party payers (Rogoski 2003).

One traditionally weak area in the collection and processing of laboratory results is patient identification. Handwritten labels may be illegible for reasons of poor handwriting or spills. The use of barcoding in conjunction with an LIS to track specimens helps to eliminate this type of problem. Barcodes are either printed directly onto collection labels or affixed at the time of processing to help improve specimen tracking. This process results in improved patient safety and productivity (Marietti 2003).

Although many institutions are moving toward a paperless record, it has been common practice for staff and students to print out copies of laboratory findings for their personal reference and to communicate to other staff. The ability to send results directly to secure PDAs helps to ensure the privacy of health information because it eliminates the need for large numbers of print-outs and the need to Fax sensitive information. This feature helps healthcare providers to comply with government requirements to safeguard client health information (Schuerenberg 2002).

Radiology Systems

A **radiology information system (RIS)** provides scheduling of diagnostic tests, communication of clinical information, generation of client instructions and preparation procedures, transcription of results and impressions, and file room management such as tracking of film location. Orders may be entered directly into the radiology system or transmitted from an order entry system. Radiology clerical staff use order information to schedule patients for testing. Once the test is complete, the radiologist interprets the findings and dictates a report. This report can be transcribed using the radiology system or a separate transcription system. The radiology system generates billing information that can be sent to the billing system. The reports are then stored within the radi-ology system. They may also be Faxed to the physician's office or viewed through the clinical or nursing information systems.

One example of how a radiology system might be used is seen with magnetic resonance imaging (MRI) orders. As the first step in placing an MRI order, the system generates a questionnaire that asks questions pertinent to the MRI pro-cedure. For example, it asks whether the client is cooperative or claustrophobic, and if there are any metal foreign bodies related to previous surgeries or injuries. The nurse reviews these questions with the client, then enters the answers to each question and the order requested into the system. A radiologist reviews the order request and the questionnaire answers, and determines if the client is appropriate for testing. This procedure allows scheduling of appropriate clients only, and eliminates the time-consuming and costly scheduling and attempted testing of inappropriate clients.

More recent developments in radiology information systems include digital, filmless images as a replacement for traditional radiology films. These **picture archiving and communication systems (PACS)** allow images to be electronically transmitted and viewed using sophisticated, high-resolution monitors. The en-hanced quality of these images over traditional films may result in fewer repeat procedures and improved diagnostic capability. The use of digital filmless imaging is also an integral component in the evolution of the electronic client record. Use of this technology may allow hospitals to do away with radiology images captured on film. This reduces or eliminates the large expense of radiology films, as well as handling and storage of the x-rays. In addition, PACS can provide the physician with a radiology image viewed on a computer screen within seconds after the completion of the procedure. Another benefit of a PACS is that more than one physician can view an image simultaneously in multiple locations (Gillespie 2001).

Other benefits of this technology are seen when these images are transmitted to high-acuity areas, such as emergency departments and intensive care units, where quick turnaround and immediate availability of images are critical to providing optimum client care. The use of this technology can facilitate client care in remote rural healthcare facilities where a radiologist may not be on-site. Images can be transmitted to a major medical center for evaluation by radiologists and other physicians. Benefits are realized in terms of cost, because it is not necessary to staff a radiologist, and improved client care when a radiologist is on staff but not available.

Implementation of a PACS system should include consideration of the following issues (Tabatabaie 2001):

- *Systems standards base.* The system should be operable without proprietary software that makes it difficult to use or upgrade.
- *Access to previous studies.* On-demand access to all prior client studies is preferable.
- *Required infrastructure.* Can the system be used with existing computers and the electronic medical record system?
- *System performance.* Are records available quickly and of sufficient quality for diagnostic purposes?

Pharmacy Applications and Systems

The inpatient pharmacy process is complex and the source of many medication errors given the large number of drugs on the market, sound-alike names, high patient acuity levels, and large number of medication orders processed (Kuiper et al. 2007). The National Coordinating Council for Medication Error Reporting and Prevention, a group comprised of more than 20 national organizations, including the Food and Drug Administration (FDA), defines a medication error as "any preventable event that may cause or lead to inappropriate medication use or patient harm while the medication is in the control of the healthcare professional, patient, or consumer." Several other groups are also working on strategies to reduce errors. In 2001 the Patient Safety Task Force was formed to improve data collection on patient safety. The lead agencies in the Patient Safety Task Force are the following:

- FDA
- Centers for Disease Control and Prevention
- Centers for Medicare and Medicaid Services
- Agency for Healthcare Research and Quality

Data is then reviewed. The FDA reviews reports that come from drug manufacturers through the agency's safety information and adverse event reporting program, MedWatch. The FDA now rejects all applications for similar drug names by using a computer program that searches for similar sounding names. The Institute for Safe Medication Practices accepts reports from consumers and health professionals using collected information to publish a consumer newsletter on medication errors. Hospitals report medication errors via the MedMARX error-reporting program.

Combining pharmacy information systems with barcode technology, as described in Box 5–5, can drastically reduce medication errors. Information

BOX 5–5 Using Information Systems to Reduce Medication Errors

Order entry, pharmacy, and BCMA systems, along with automated medication supply management systems, can be used to assist healthcare providers in reducing the occurrence of medication errors. These systems interact to provide checks and alerts throughout the medication ordering and administration process, as directed in the following examples:

1. A physician enters a medication order into the order entry system.
2. The information is automatically transmitted to the pharmacy system.
3. The pharmacy system integrates laboratory values and uses rules to ask the physician if he or she chooses to change or add medications based on laboratory values or dose for patient size or age.
4. The pharmacy system checks the patient's history and alerts the physician to any drug interactions or allergies. The physician can change the order at this time, if indicated.
5. The pharmacy system issues a warning when sound-alike medications are ordered, forcing the physician and care giver to consider which drug the patient is actually to receive.
6. The order creates a requisition in the pharmacy that contains a barcode indicating the correct medication, as well as a barcode identifying the patient.
7. A robot in the pharmacy fills the medication order by matching the medication barcode on the requisition to the barcode on the medication. The medication is transported to the nursing unit.
8. The nurse scans a barcode on the patient's identification band and the barcode on the medication, administers the medication only if there is a match, and documents medications given in the barcode medication administration system. A warning will appear if insufficient time has passed since the drug was last administered.
9. The system prompts the nurse to enter pain scale, blood pressures, and pulses where appropriate.
10. The system automatically adds the nurse's electronic signature.
11. The barcode medication administration system can generate the following reports:
    • A medication due list, showing medications that need to be administered within specific time parameters, including one-time, on-call, continuous, PRN orders, and regularly scheduled medications
    • PRN effectiveness list that prompts the nurse to record the effectiveness of PRN medications
    • Medication administration history, which records nurse initials and times for medications given in a traditional medication administration record format
    • Missing dose report—prints in pharmacy to alert staff when a dose needs to be reissued; done at the time the nurse was administering meds with essentially no disruption in work flow
    • Medications not given report—lists all missed doses according to the documentation on the medication administration record
    • Variance log—captures meds given more than 60 minutes early or late

systems can provide checkpoints at each phase of the medication ordering and administration process using evidence-based medication selection and dosing guidelines (Kuiper et al. 2007). Other checkpoints may include alphabetizing drugs by chemical name; decreasing the amount of floor stock so that staff are less likely to accidentally choose the wrong drug, dose, or form for administration; improved unit dose availability from the pharmaceutical companies; final preparation of drug admixtures such as antibiotics in the pharmacy, thereby eliminating drug errors and compatibility problems with the admixture solution; availability of online drug references; delivery of only one dose at a time; and delivery of single-dose packages only (Summerfield & Lawrence 2002).

Integration of the various clinical information systems with subsequent exchange of information decreases medication errors and improves therapeutic drug monitoring in patients with compromised renal function and those receiving drugs with narrow therapeutic ranges through the use of CDS alerts (Mahone, Berard-Collins, Eleman, Amaral, & Cotter 2007). Pharmacy systems offer many benefits that promote cost containment, improve the quality of care, and decrease medication errors. These systems can be used by a variety of healthcare professionals who perform activities related to the ordering, dispensing, and administration of medications. A hospital pharmacy may use an information system to access client data such as demographics, health history and diagnosis, medication history, client allergies, laboratory results, renal function, and potential drug interactions. Traditionally, pharmacists reviewed each client's medication profile, laboratory values, medical history, and progress notes manually to monitor medication disbursement and effectiveness (Amsden 2003). This is a time-intensive, laborious process. Automated systems pull in laboratory results and client information from the HISs more quickly and accurately identifying allergy and interaction problems than a manual process. This integration of information allows pharmacists to recommend changes in parenteral nutrition formula based on laboratory abnormalities, verify that medication dosages are appropriate based on serum drug levels, avoid drugs that may impair renal function, and monitor laboratory values for possible drug toxicity. Pharmacy systems can also provide automatic alerts that can save lives. Automation of previously manual processes can result in significant cost savings. Kuiper et al. (2007) notes that successful technologies reduce the potential for error by automating tasks that require high levels of accuracy and repetition.

Another benefit offered by pharmacy systems is the tracking of medication use, costs, and billing information. Automation of these functions generally improves accuracy and is more cost-effective than manual methods. In addition, this information can be manipulated and analyzed more easily for executive decision making when it is available as a computer file.

Physicians and other direct care providers may also use pharmacy systems. These systems provide on-line access to client and drug information that is critical in the drug prescription process. Pharmacy systems can provide easy access to clients' health and medication history, as well as their allergies and demographic information. Access to formulary information and on-line drug reference information helps physicians determine the most effective drug and the appropriate doses for clients. In addition, these systems can provide comparisons of costs and drug effectiveness, particularly important in the managed care arena. Pharmacy information systems provide data for BCMA systems.

Creating a culture of safety is a critical first step to making changes needed to reduce medication errors. There are many opportunities to use technology to prevent medication errors but the implementation of some of these applications has been delayed (Schneider 2007). The Institutes of Medicine recommend the use of pharmacy systems, BCMA, smart infusion pumps, and decision support software to improve safety (McCartney 2006; IOM 1999, 2001).

Pharmacy Dispensing Systems Pharmacy systems can automatically dispense each client's medications in unit dose format, creating labels for each dose with the client's name and other demographic identifiers. The actual dispensing of the medications may be accomplished either with or without the intervention of the pharmacist. Some systems automatically dispense ordered medications in unit dose packages, which the pharmacy staff place in the client's medication drawer. This process can be streamlined by using robotic systems, which both collect the appropriate medications and place them in the drawers. Robotic dispensing systems are seen as a mechanism to prevent medication errors as well as reduce inventory and labor costs (Kohn, Walton-Brooks, & Henderson 2003). These systems serve to support rather than supplant the pharmacist (Barcia 1999).

Unit-based Dispensing Cabinets Another aspect of pharmacy systems is the use of automatic dispensing systems for use by the nurse. These systems provide a medication dispensing unit in the clinical area, generally for use by nurses who administer medications. The system is usually secured by requiring a user ID and password or biometric measure for access to the system and the actual medications. Features include menu-driven prompts for identifying the client, medication, dose, and number of unit doses removed. The user can also be prompted to count the current number of doses on hand when removing narcotics or other controlled substances. Automatic dispensing systems provide accurate records of medicines given in terms of what was taken from the unit and the date, time, and user who performed this activity. These records can be accessed centrally in the pharmacy to determine when supplies in the clinical area dispensing units must be replenished. In addition, this information can be used to efficiently and accurately bill clients for medications used (Barcia 1999). Nurses must recognize that there are limitations to these safety devices and still carefully check medications before removing them from the cabinet, avoid returning unused doses, take only one dose for a single patient when it is needed, and avoid unsafe practices such as overriding the system (McCartney 2006).

Barcode and RFID Medication Administration Applications Bar Code
Medication Administration (BCMA) is a quality initiative identified by the
Leapfrog Group and the Veterans Administration's National Center for Patient
Safety (Educating Patients 2007; Barcode Implementation 2007). BCMA is a
system that uses the barcode found on the unit-dose medication package and on
a patient's identification patient to ensure that nurses administer the right drug
to the right patient in the right dose at the right time and by the right route
(Cummings et al. 2005; Medication safety issue brief 2005). It prevents errors at
the point of care, where they can do the most harm. It also helps hospitals comply
with the Joint Commission standards and patient safety goals. Specifically, it
helps hospitals meet requirements to verify orders and patients before
medication administration. The reductions in medication errors provides a
return on investment (Medication safety issue brief 2005). BCMA systems may
exist as stand-alone systems or as a part of a complete hospital information
system. Typically the nurse uses a portable scanner to scan a barcode on his or her
identification badge to log on to the software application. Next the patient's
identification bracelet is scanned. The system displays a list of the patient's
medication orders and times for administration. Medications due for
administration are scanned as the nurse checks them. Documentation is
automated with the process. Successful BCMA implementation eliminates
loopholes that allow nurses to bypass key features such as scanning the patient's
identification bracelet (Cummings et al. 2005). The extent of the benefits accrued
from BCMA will be influenced by several factors, including adherence to
standardized dispensing practices and human factors such as ergonomics
associated with the medication cards (Mills et al. 2006). When discussing the
prevention of medication errors Manno (2006 p. 60) notes that technology that is
used to enhance health, and delivery systems "should be designed to make it easy
to do the right thing and hard to do the wrong thing." Pairing BCMA with CPOE
further decreases errors (Comeaux, Smith, & Stern 2006). Adding CDS to the
combination drastically lowers mortality and the harm rate associated with
adverse drug reactions and errors (Reifsteck et al. 2006). Additional features, such
as prompts when pain assessments are past due, improve documentation. Other
BCMA benefits include more consistent patient identification, fewer missed
medication doses, and fewer adverse effects since system alerts warn the nurse of
allergies and possible drug interactions (Mills et al. 2006). Radio Frequency
Identification (RFID) technology offers the same benefits. It is slightly more
expensive but is not subject to read errors with smudges or obscured visibility.
The disadvantages associated with BCMA include poorly functioning scanners,
identification bracelets that do not read consistently, and the need to transport
equipment (McCartney 2006). Smart IV pumps that contain special drug error
reduction software may integrate with BCMA.

E-Prescribing *E-prescribing* is a process that allows the physician to enter a
prescription into an information system. This information is electronically
communicated to the client's pharmacy. This may be done using a variety of
devices, including personal digital assistants (PDAs), wireless computers, or other

handheld devices that allow prescriptions to be easily sent from the physician's exam room or the patient's bedside. Electronic prescriptions provide the following benefits:

- Elimination of telephone authorization for refills
- Review of clients' drug histories before ordering drugs
- Reminders to order home medications for the hospitalized client
- Alerts about drug interactions
- Checking of formulary compliance and reimbursement
- Provision of a longitudinal prescription record

Electronic prescriptions require direct links between physician offices, hospitals, pharmacies, and third-party payers. Some state laws must also be changed to accommodate electronic prescription writing.

Some healthcare systems offer a unified view of information drawn from several systems into a clinical dashboard. Figure 5–2 exemplifies such a view.

Physician Practice Management Systems A recent survey (Mattocks et al. 2007) revealed that practice management systems comprised the most commonly used type of technology in physician offices. Features typically include the ability

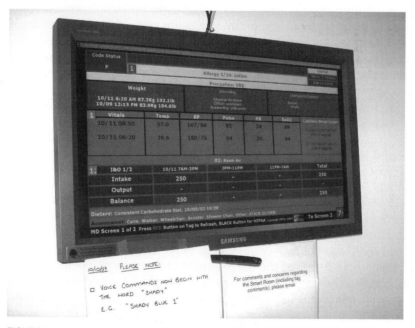

FIGURE 5–2 • Reprinted by permission of University of Pittsburgh Medical Center

to capture some demographic information, schedule appointments, maintain lists of insurance payers, perform billing tasks, track outcomes and generate reports. There may, or may not, be a connection to electronic patient records. For practices that do not connect to hospital electronic records practitioners may still opt to maintain patient records electronically entering data themselves or having patients input information (Bachman 2007). Patient records in paper format are expensive to maintain, unwieldy to handle and relevant information may be difficult to locate contributing to the overall fragmentation of individual health records. For this reason many hospitals now provide hardware and software for physician offices to access and use their information systems with the hope that records will be more accurate, quality of care improved and fewer errors will occur. Automation of physician office records help to maintain client confidentiality and HIPAA compliance because health information is contained within the information system rather than loose papers which can easily be viewed by unauthorized clinical and nonclinical office staff.

Long-term Health Information Systems The adoption of information technology (IT) has been slow in long-term care for many reasons, including fragmentation among facilities, limited operating budgets, high implementation costs, and multiple providers in one facility. The integration of clinical information systems in this area is imperative for the improvement of quality of care, better management of the complex needs of the population, and a decrease in adverse drug effects (Alexander et al. 2007; Brandeis et al. 2007; Gillespie 2007; Shugarman, Nishita, & Wilber 2006; Subramanian et al. 2007). The adoption of information systems is also critical to the business survival of long-term health facilities given the constantly changing managed care environment and Medicare Prospective Payment System (Nahm, Mills, & Feege 2006). Integration must extend beyond the walls of a single long-term care facility to best serve the needs of the patients. Boston Medical Center and University Geriatric Services partnered with several area nursing homes to provide the hardware and software that subsequently improved communication between providers, hospital, and nursing home staff. This is particularly important given the fact that many nursing home patients have multiple transfers from one facility and set of providers to another. Long-term care information systems include documentation and financial information. Ideally, features include order entry, results retrieval, and medication administration. One particular example of improved communication is the use of the electronic record to document patient preferences about advanced directives. Lindner et al. (2007) note that modification of admission orders at a Veterans Affairs nursing home improved completion of resuscitation status by physicians.

IT also promises to ease the heavy burden of paper-based documentation in this setting. While doubts have been voiced about the acceptance of computerized documentation in long term care, Yu, Qiu, and Crookes (2006) found that the majority of workers surveyed in nursing homes are willing to adopt electronic documentation. The cost of widespread adoption of IT in long-term healthcare must be carefully considered. The reality is that costs must be borne by facilities and physicians. Financial incentives may be required to encourage and expedite the use of technology in this arena (Subramanian et al. 2007)

Home Care Information Systems Braunstein (1994) noted that home care nurses were ideally situated to be early adopters of electronic systems because of their mobility, front-line role in the healthcare system, their lack of a support structure at the point of care, and the excessive demands for documentation. McBride (2006) notes that systems can be tailored to streamline the work of nurses, improve quality of care delivery, and improve payment for services because billing personnel can find needed information more quickly, allowing them to send out bills earlier. The adoption of technology for home care will increasingly make use of monitoring technology, which integrated into information systems as a way to care for an aging population at home (Cheek, Nikpour, & Nowlin 2005). At best home care systems can communicate with hospital information systems for access to test results, medication lists and allergy information, and possibly order entry.

Other Clinical Systems

A number of other clinical systems address the needs of specific departments within the healthcare setting. Box 5–6 lists some of these systems. The rapidly changing healthcare environment has resulted in several requirements on the part of the clinical information system vendor. The vendor's initial support services and ability to provide ongoing support are critical success factors as the healthcare paradigm continues to shift.

Westbrook (2005) summarized research that found that the successful implementation of clinical information systems is determined by the complex

---

BOX 5–6   Other Common Clinical Systems

- **Medical records/abstracting systems** facilitate the abstracting, or coding, of diagnoses and chart management processes. Client records may also be stored on optical disk.
- **Operating room systems** may be used to schedule procedures, manage equipment setup for individual physicians, facilitate inventory control, and provide client billing.
- **Emergency department systems** provide ready access to independent systems such as poison control. They also provide tracking capability, alerts, and the capability to print specific discharge and follow-up instructions based on the client's diagnosis.
- **Home care systems** allow the healthcare provider to access information on clients and outpatient resources, and to document care provided.
- **Long-term care systems** help to ensure continuity and quality of care in a population with complex needs by automating documentation and providing the capability to exchange information with key systems such as order entry, pharmacy and medication administration, and diagnostic systems

interaction between the technical features of the system and human, social, and organizational factors that determine whether the system will be used and whether it will prove to be safe and effective.

Administrative Systems

Various administrative systems may be used in healthcare organizations to support the process of providing client care. Box 5–7 provides a brief review of many of these systems.

Registration Systems

The client registration system is critical to the effective operation of many other systems within the healthcare setting. This system is used to collect and store client identification and demographic data that are verified and updated at the time of each visit. For this reason, these may also be known as *admission/discharge/transfer(ADT) systems*. CISs use these data for the management of client care and billing purposes. The information is shared with those clinical systems that communicate directly with the registration system.

An important aspect of a registration system used in a multi-entity health system network is the development of a unique client identifier. This number or identification code is used to identify the client in all information systems across the organization and across all entities. This enables accurate client identification, supporting the development of a longitudinal client record that contains all clinical information available for the client.

BOX 5–7   Administrative Information Systems Used in the Healthcare Setting

- Financial systems provide the facility with accounting functions. Accurate tracking of financial data is critical for enabling the organization to receive reimbursement for services.
- Payroll and human resource systems track employee time and attendance, credentials, performance evaluations, and payroll compensation information.
- Contract management systems manage contracts with third-party payers.
- Risk management systems track and plan prevention of unusual occurrences or incidents.
- Quality assurance systems monitor outcomes and produce reports that are used to guide quality improvement initiatives.
- Physician management systems support patient registration, scheduling, coding, and billing in the physician's office and may support results retrieval. These systems also provide better protection of patient privacy than paper records.
- Executive information systems provide administrators with easy access to summarized information related to the financial and clinical operations of the organization.
- Materials management systems facilitate inventory control and charging of supplies.

Scheduling Systems

A scheduling system allows a healthcare organization to schedule clients and resources efficiently. Client demographic information must be available in the system either by direct entry or through electronic communication with a registration system. For the system to be used to schedule patient appointments, it must contain information regarding available resources. This resource information may include the following:

- Referral and authorization by patient's insurance
- Department
- Equipment
- Dates and times
- Room
- Staff
- Permits and preps
- Charging and billing information

The system uses predetermined rules for determining how resource and client information should be used to schedule a particular type of appointment. This provides the capability to schedule a patient in one location. In addition, scheduling across all facilities in an enterprise can be accomplished using one system. The benefits associated with using a scheduling system include increased staff productivity, increased client satisfaction, and cost savings to the organization (LeDonne 1997).

Contract Management Systems

Contract management (CM) software provides invaluable assistance to organizations to better manage their resources and improve efficiency. Healthcare institutions typically have multiple contracts with third-party payers as well as with vendors and various suppliers. CM software provides the visibility and control that allow organizations to negotiate better contracts, ensure that suppliers meet their contractual obligations, track compliance, save money, and accelerate the cycle times from sourcing through contract (Avery 2006). Anthes (2006) notes that, traditionally, organizations focus efforts to maximize profits on cutting costs and boosting sales. Pricing is based upon competitors' prices and production costs, plus a standard markup fee or value pricing, which segments buyers and sets prices based on each segment. Value pricing requires good use of data mining and modeling capabilities. Value pricing reflects different levels of charges set by sellers of services for patients in accordance with their insurance plan. CM software features support contract creation, report capability, e-procurement, alerts, and notifications on key business events and can even support automation of the entire contract process.

DECISION SUPPORT AND EXPERT SYSTEMS

Decision support and expert systems use data from both the clinical and the administrative information systems and can provide information related to clinical and administrative users. According to Turley (1993), little agreement exists on the definition of the terms *decision support systems* and *expert systems* except for the distinction of how much authority is placed in the computer system.

Decision support systems aid in and strengthen the selection of viable options using the information of an organization or a field to facilitate decision making and overall efficiency. Decision support software organizes information to fit new environments. It provides analysis and advice to support a choice. The final decision rests with the practitioner. Software can be off-the-shelf or homegrown. **Off-the-shelf software** is commercially available. The advantage to the consumer is that someone else has borne the cost for its development and testing. It is, however, geared to a general market and may not meet the needs of a particular party. **Homegrown** software has been developed by the consumer to meet specific needs usually because no suitable commercial package is available. The customer bears the cost of its development, testing, and communication with other software applications. Decision support software can provide a competitive edge and facilitate the move to managed care. **Clinical decision support** (CDS) provides clinicians with knowledge or specific information that is intelligently filtered, or presented at appropriate times, to enhance health and healthcare (Kawamioto & Lobch 2007; Mangalampalli et al. 2006; Osheroff et al. 2007). Tools may include clinical practice guidelines, alerts and reminders, order sets, patient data reports and dashboards, diagnostic support, workflow tools, and financial applications. CDS is effective in all phases of the clinical process. CPOE with CDS has been shown to decrease medication errors by as much as 80% (Cornish, Etchells, & Knowles 2006). An example of a decision support application is a program that assists nurses performing a skin assessment to review available alternatives, from which the best may be selected to maintain skin integrity. CDS is best used when available at the point of care. Access is facilitated through the use of wireless devices such as PDAs, tablet computers, and iPhones, which are easily transported and with the practitioner at the point of care. While CDS has been proven effective in improving outcomes at many sites it is not universally available or available at the same level at all locations (Simon, Rundall, & Shortell 2007). Strong external drivers are expected to change this situation. The American Medical Informatics Association has presented a roadmap for national action that calls for improved CDS capabilities and increased use throughout the U.S. health sector. Financial rewards for improved outcomes are expected to accelerate adoption of order entry with CDS.

Expert systems use artificial intelligence to model a decision that experts in the field would make. Unlike decision support systems that provide several options from which the user may choose, expert systems convey the concept that the computer has made the best decision based on criteria that experts would use.

FUTURE DIRECTIONS

Information technology applications will become more commonplace, easier to use, and offer additional features from this point forward. The drivers for this trend will include concerns for safety, worker retention, the need to expand evidence for evidence-based practice, and cost containment. McCartney (2006) notes that technology "can promote a safe environment for nursing practice by reducing negative exposure to risk and liability." Electronic databases offer the potential to facilitate retrospective analysis of errors.

CASE STUDY EXERCISES

5.1   You are a nurse participating in the customization and implementation of a barcode medication administration system. Analyze how the process will change from the current manual process. Include potential problem areas and solutions.

5.2   You are the physician liaison for the information system department. Recent federal initiatives call for the implementation of CPOE. You have the technology available, but you need to get administrative, nursing, and physician support. How would you go about this?

5.3   You are participating in the customization and implementation of the radiology system. Define the data that must be included in the order entry process. Define the information that the nursing staff would like to view or print from the radiology system.

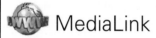 MediaLink

Additional resources for this content can be found on the Companion Website at www.prenhall.com/hebda. Click on "Chapter 5" to select the activities for this chapter.

- Glossary
- Multiple Choice
- Discussion Points
- Case Studies
- MediaLink Application
- MediaLink

SUMMARY

- A hospital or healthcare information system consists of clinical and administrative systems.
- Well-designed clinical information systems can improve the quality of client care.
- Clinical information systems can extend the capabilities of healthcare providers.
- A nursing information system using the nursing process approach should support the use and documentation of nursing processes and provide tools for managing the delivery of nursing care.

- The use of standardized nursing languages such as NANDA, NIC, and NOC supports automation of nursing documentation and expands the utility of collected information.
- The critical pathway/protocol approach to nursing information systems provides a multidisciplinary format for planning and documenting client care.
- Other clinical systems, including order entry, radiology, laboratory, pharmacy systems, and physician management systems, give the nurse and other heathcare providers the support and tools to more effectively care for clients.
- Administrative systems support the process of client care by managing nonclinical, client-related information, including demographics, codes for procedures, and insurance.
- Information systems enable decision makers to examine trends and make informed choices during these times of healthcare reform.
- Federal initiatives for patient safety call for the implementation of computerized physician order entry and barcode medication administration as methods to reduce error.
- Personal device assistants and wireless technology further enhance the capability of information systems to support the work of clinicians.

REFERENCES

Alexander, G. L., Rantz, M., Flesner, M., Diekemper, M., & Siem, C. (2007). Clinical information systems in nursing homes: An evaluation of initial implementation strategies. *Computers Informatics Nursing, 25*(4), 189–197.

American Medical Informatics Association and American Health Information Management Association Terminology and Classification Policy Task Force (2006). Healthcare Terminologies and Classifications: An Action Agenda for the United States. Retrieved November 28, 2007, from http://www.amia.org/inside/initiatives/docs/terminologiesandclassifications.pdf.

American Medical Informatics Association Nursing Informatics Work Group.(April 27, 2006). Letter to Dr. Patricia Grady, Council Chairperson, National Institute of Nursing Research with comments to the *Draft of Strategic Plan of NINR2006–2010*, Retrieved November 20, 2007, from http://www.amia.org/mbrcenter/wg/ni/education/cat1.asp.

Amsden, D. (2003). Push technology in the pharmacy. *Health Management Technology, 24*(1), 28, 30–31.

Anthes, G. (2006).The price point. *Computerworld, 40*(30), 33–35.

Ash, J. S., Sittig, D. F., Poon, E. G., Guappone, K. G., Campbell, E., & Dykstra, R. H. (2007). The extent and importance of unintended consequences related to computerized provider order entry. *Journal of the American Medical Informatics Association, 14*(4), 415–423.

Avery, S. (2005). How to use software to manage contracts. *Purchasing, Electronics & Technology, 134*(11), 39–41.

Bao, F., Yan, X., & Lin, P. (2005, April). Practice of nursing information system in management of nursing quality in wards. *Chinese Nursing Research, 19*(4A), 640–641. Retrieved November 19, 2007, from CINAHL with Full Text database.

Barcia, S. M. (1999). Man vs. machine. *Health Management Technology, 20*(9), 24.

Barcode Implementation Strategies. (2005). *H&HN: Hospitals & Health Networks, 79*(7), 65–66.

Bachman, J. (2007). Improving care with an automated patient history. *Family Practice Management, 14*(7),39–43.

Bradley, V. B., Steltenkamp, C.L., & Hite, K.B. (2006). Evaluation of reported medication errors before and after implementation of computerized practitioner order entry. *Journal of Healthcare Information Management, 20*(4), 46–53.

Brandeis, G. H., Hogan, M., Murphy, M., & Murray, S. (2007). Electronic health record implementation in community nursing homes. *Journal of the American Medical Directors Association, 8*(1), 31–34.

Braunstein, M. L. (1994). Electronic patient records for homecare nursing. *Computers in Nursing, 12*(5), 232–238.

Burkhart, L., Konicek, D., Moorhead, S., & Androwich, I. (2005). Mapping parish nurse documentation into the nursing interventions classification: A research method. *Computers, Informatics, Nursing, 23*(4), 220–229.

Cheek, P., Nikpour, L., & Nowlin, H. D. (2005). Aging well with smart technology. *Nursing Administration Quarterly, 29*(4),329–338.

Clinical Information Systems. (January 28, 2002). Where are we today, where do we need to be, and how do we get there? *Modern Healthcare, 32*(4), 73.

Comeaux, K., Smith, M. E., & Stem, L. G. (2006). Tech update. Improve PRN effectiveness documentation. *Nursing Management, 37*(9), 58.

Conn, J. (2007a). Starting out with a "bang." *Modern Healthcare, 37*(32), 32–33.

Conn, J. (2007b). More moving to entry level. CPOE adoption slowly gains ground, with larger number expecting installations. *Modern Healthcare, 37*(9), 41. Retrieved November 19, 2007, from CINAHL with Full Text database.

Cornish, P. E., Etchells, E. E., & Knowles, S. R. (2006). Pharmacists' role in assessing potential value of CPOE. *American Journal of Health-System Pharmacy, 63*(22), 2182–2184. Retrieved November 19, 2007, from CINAHL with Full Text database.

Cummings, J., Bush, P., Smith, D., & Matuszewski, K. (2005). Bar-coding medication administration overview and consensus recommendations. *American Journal of Health-System Pharmacy, 62*(24), 2626–2629. Retrieved November 19, 2007, from CINAHL with Full Text database.

Educating Patients. (2007). *H&HN: Hospitals & Health Networks, 81*(9), 82.

Gillespie, G. (April 2007). Erickson Health Takes Long View with Technology. *Health Data Management.* Retrieved November 29, 2007, from Erickson Health Takes Long View with Technology. Retrieved November 28, 2007, from http://www.mywire.com/pubs/HealthDataManagement/2007/04/01/3178636?extID=10037&oliID=229.

Gillespie, G. (November 2001). Filmless radiology brightens its image. *Health Data Management, 9*(11), 55–60.

Goedert, J. (2007). A new battery of tests for lab systems. *Health Data Management, 15*(9), 40–46.

Harrison, J. & Palacio, C. (2006, July). The role of clinical information systems in healthcare quality improvement. *HealthCare Manager, 25*(3), 206–212. Retrieved November 19, 2007, from CINAHL with Full Text database.

Hastings, C. (2006). Consider this. Reduce errors with computerized prescriber order entry. *Nursing Management, 37*(12), 68.

Health informatics standards illuminated under the northern lights. (2003). *HIMSS News, 14*(7), 5.

Hendrickson, M. (1993). The nurse engineer: A way to better nursing information systems. *Computers in Nursing, 11*(2), 67–71.

Hillman, J. M. & Given, R. S. (2005). Hospital implementation of computerized provider order entry systems: Results from the 2003 Leapfrog Group Quality and Safety Survey. *Journal of Healthcare Information Management, 19*(4), 55–65.

Hughes, S. (May 1997). Time for new thinking. *Healthcare Informatics,* 57–68.

Kelley, J. (2007, March 5). IT use in hospitals continues to grow, according to the AHA's annual survey. *AHA News, 43*(5), 3. Retrieved November 19, 2007, from Health Source: Nursing/Academic Edition database.

Kohn, C., Walton-Brooks, D., & Henderson, C. W. (February 17, 2003). Hospitals purchase robotic drug dispensing system. *Managed Care Weekly Digest,* 41.

Kravet, S., Knight, A., & Wright, S. (2007, February). Ten lessons from implementing a computerized provider order entry system. *Journal of Clinical Outcomes Management, 14*(2), 105–109. Retrieved November 19, 2007, from CINAHL with Full Text database.

Kuiper, S., McCreadie, S., Mitchell, J., & Stevenson, J. (5, January 2007). Medication errors in inpatient pharmacy operations and technologies for improvement. *American Journal of Health-System Pharmacy, 64*(9), 955–959. Retrieved November 19, 2007, from CINAHL.

LeDonne, J. (1997). Rehab facility saves $300,000 a year, reduces FTEs, with scheduling system. *Health Management Technology, 18*(7), 30.

Lee, T. (2007). Nurses' experiences using a nursing information system. *Computers, Informatics, Nursing, 25*(5), 294–300.

Lee, E., Lee, M., & Jung, O.B. (2006). Mapping of nursing records into the NIC and the ICNP in a Korean Oriental-Medicine Hospital. *Computers, Informatics, Nursing, 24*(6), 346–352.

Lehmann, C. & Kim, G. (2006, December). Computerized provider order entry and patient safety. *Pediatric Clinics of North America, 53*(6), 1169–1184. Retrieved November 19, 2007, from CINAHL with Full Text database.

Lindner, S. A., Davoren, J. B., Vollmer, A., Williams, B., & Landefeld, C. S. (2007). An electronic medical record intervention increased nursing home advance directive orders and documentation.*Journal of the American Geriatrics Society, 55*(7), 1001–1006.

Lu, D.F., Eichmann, D., Konicek, D., Park, H.T., Ucharattana, P., & Delaney, C. (2006). Standardized nursing language in the systematized nomenclature of medicine clinical terms: A cross-mapping validation method. *Computers, Informatics, Nursing, 24*(5), 288–296.

Mangalampalli, A., Chakravarthy, R., Raja, M., Jain, A., & Parinam, A. (2006). IT systems. Clinical systems: Using IT to improve care. *British Journal of HealthCare Management, 12*(9), 277–281. Retrieved November 19, 2007, from CINAHL with Full Text database.

Manno, M. (Mar2006). Preventing adverse drug events. *Nursing, 36*(3), 56–62. Retrieved November 19, 2007, from CINAHL with Full Text database.

Marietti, C. (2003). Vigilance in the lab. *Healthcare Informatics 20*(5), 58.

Mattocks, K., Lalime, K., Tate, J.P., Giannotti, T.E., Carr, K., Carrabba, A., et al. (2007). The state of physician office-based health information technology in Connecticut: current use, barriers and future plans. *Connecticut Medicine, 71*(1), 27–31.

McBride, M. (2006).The home healthcare pot of gold. *Health Management Technology, 27*(5), 22–3.

Mcbroom, K., Anderle, M., Mackowiak, L., Bride, W., Sawyer, T., Swartz, C., et al. (Apr2006). Computerized physician order entry: Nurse input is essential for success. *Critical Care Nurse, 26*(2), S3. Retrieved November 19, 2007, from CINAHL with Full Text database.

McCartney, P. (2006). Using technology to promote perinatal patient safety. *JOGNN: Journal of Obstetric, Gynecologic, & Neonatal Nursing, 35*(3), 424–431.

Medication safety issue brief: Barcode implementation strategies. (2005). *H&HN: Hospitals & Health Networks, 79*(7), 65–66.

Mills, P. D., Neily, J., Mims, E., Burkhardt, M. E., & Bagian, J. (2006). Improving the bar-coded medication administration system at the Department of Veterans Affairs. *American Journal of Health-System, 63*(15), 1442–1447.

Murphy, J. (2005). Using technology: Making evidence-based practice a reality. Retrieved November 28, 2007, from http://www.amia.org/mbrcenter/wg/ni/docs/ni2005/murphy.pdf.

Nahm, E. S., Mills, M.E., & Feege, B. (2006). Long-term care information systems: An overview of the selection process. *Journal of Gerontological Nursing, 32*(6), 32–38.

Osheroff, J. A., Teich, J. M., Middleton, B., Steen, E. B., Wright, A., & Detmer, D. E. (2007). A roadmap for national action on clinical decision support. *Journal of the American Medical Informatics Association, 14*(2), 141–145.

Park, H., Lu, D., Konicek, D., & Delaney. (2007). Nursing interventions classification in systematized nomenclature of medicine clinical terms: A cross-mapping validation. *Computers, Informatics, Nursing, 25*(4), 198–208.

Powelson, S. A., McGahan, S. A., & Wilkinson, J. M. (July–September 2000). Where to start? Introducing Standardized Nursing Languages in educational settings. *Nursing Diagnosis, 11*(3), 135.

Prophet, C. M. (2000). The evolution of a clinical database: From local to standardized clinical languages. *Proceedings of AMIA Symposium, 660*–664.

Prophet, C., Dorr, G. G., Gibbs, T. D., & Porcella, A. A. (1997). Implementation of standardized nursing languages (NIC, NOC) in on-line care planning and documentation. *Informatics: The Impact of Nursing Knowledge on HealthCare Informatics.* Amsterdam: IOS Press, 395–400.

Reifsteck, M., Swanson, T., & Dallas, M. (2006). Driving out errors through tight integration between software and automation. *Journal of Healthcare Information Management, 20*(4), 35–39.

Rogoski, R. (2003). LIS and the enterprise. *Health Management Technology, 24*(2), 20–23.

Rogoski, R. (2005). Putting patients first: Regardless of the application implemented, healthcare organizations are on a steadfast mission to improve patient safety with the use of IT systems. *Health Management Technology, 26*(2), 12. Retrieved November 19, 2007, from CINAHL with Full Text database.

Saba, V. & McCormick, K. (1996). *Essentials of computers for nurses.* New York: McGraw-Hill.

Saba, V. & Taylor, S. L. (2007). Moving past theory. *Computers, Informatics, Nursing, 25*(6), 324–331.

Saleem, J. J., Patterson, E. S., Militello, L., Anders, S., Falagiglia, M., Wissman, J. A., et al. (2007). Impact of clinical reminder redesign on learnability, efficiency, usability, and workload for ambulatory clinic nurses. *Journal of the American Medical Informatics Association, 14*(5), 632–640.

Schuerenberg, B. (2002). Lab systems are joining the team. *Health Data Management, 11*(9), 61–66.

Shugarman, L. R., Nishita, C. M., & Wilber, K. H. (2006). Building integrated information systems for chronic care: The California experience. *Home HealthCare Services Quarterly, 25*(3–4), 185–200.

Simon, J. S., Rundall, T. G., & Shortell, S. (2007). Adoption of order entry with decision support for chronic care by physician organizations. *Journal of the American Medical Informatics Association, 14*(4), 432–430.

Sittig, D. F., Hazlehurst, B. L., Palen, T., Hsu, J., Jimison, H., & Hornbrook, M. C. (2002). A Clinical Information System Research Landscape. *The Permanente Journal, 6*(2). Retrieved November 20, 2007, from http://xnet.kp.org/permanentejournal/spring02/landscape.html.

Schneider, P. J. (2007). Opportunities for pharmacy. *American Journal of Health-System Pharmacy, 64*(14), S10–S16.

Smetzer, J. & Navarra, M. B. (2007). Patient safety. Measuring change: A key component of building a culture of safety. *Nursing Economics, 25*(1), 49–51.

Solovy, A. (2005 July). The quality connection. *H&HN: Hospitals & Health Networks, 79*(7), 38–50. Retrieved November 19, 2007, from CINAHL with Full Text database.

Stablein, D. & Drazen, E. (2003). Getting the most out of CPOE. *HealthCare Informatics, 20*(2), 96–98.

Subramanian, S., Hoover, S., Gilman, B., Field, T., Mutter, R., & Gurwitz, J. (2007, September). Computerized Physician Order Entry with Clinical Decision Support in Long-Term Care Facilities: Costs and Benefits to Stakeholders. *Journal of the American Geriatrics Society, 55*(9), 1451–1457. Retrieved November 19, 2007, from Health Source: Nursing/Academic Edition database.

Summerfield, M. R. & Lawrence, T. (2002). Rethinking approaches to reducing medication errors: An examination of 10 core processes. *Formulary, 37*(9), 462.

Tabatabaie, H. (November 2001). Imaging and the enterprise. *Health Management Technology, 22*(11), 14–23.

Turley, J. P. (May 1993). The use of artificial intelligence in nursing information systems. Available online at: http://www.vicnet.net.au/vicnet/hisa/MAY93/MAY93-The.html.

Varkey, P., Aponte, P., Swanton, C., Fischer, D., Johnson, S., & Brennan, M. (2007, March). The effect of computerized physician-order entry on outpatient prescription errors. *Managed Care Interface, 20*(3), 53–57. Retrieved November 19, 2007, from CINAHL with Full Text database.

Weant, K., Cook, A., & Armitstead, J. (2007, March 1). Medication-error reporting and pharmacy resident experience during implementation of computerized prescriber order entry. *American Journal of Health-System Pharmacy, 64*(5), 526–530. Retrieved November 19, 2007, from Health Source: Nursing/Academic Edition database.

Westbrook J. (2005). Guest editorial: Exploring the interface between organisations and clinical information systems. *Health Information Management Journal* (4),102–103

Yu, P., Qiu, Y., & Crookes, P. (2006). Computer-based Nursing Documentation in Nursing Homes: A Feasibility Study. In Park, H., Murray, P. and Delaney, C. (Eds.). In *Consumer-Centered Computer-Supported Care for Healthy People—Proceedings of NI2006*, 570–574.

CHAPTER 6

Strategic Planning

After completing this chapter, you should be able to:

1 Define *strategic planning*.

2 Describe how strategic planning is related to an organization's vision, mission, goals, and objectives.

3 Identify the participants in the strategic planning process.

4 Understand the relationship between strategic planning for information systems and planning for the overall organization.

5 Explain the importance of assessing the internal and external environments during the planning process.

6 Discuss how potential solutions are derived from data analysis.

7 Review the benefits of using a weighted scoring tool when selecting a course of action.

8 Understand the importance of developing a timeline during the implementation phase of strategic planning.

9 List tools or processes that may be used to evaluate the outcome of and provide feedback to the planning process.

10 Discuss the relationship between strategic planning and information technology.

Strategic planning is the development of a comprehensive long-range plan for guiding the activities and operations of an organization (Brunke 2006; Crane 2007; Kaleba 2006). This process includes defining the corporate vision and mission, specifying achievable goals and objectives, developing strategies, and setting policy guidelines. The process entails a determination of what products and services to offer and to what markets, and is particularly important when organizations have more potential markets than available resources or there is a very competitive market. The organizational strategic plan should guide the planning for all areas within the organization. Hospitals and healthcare enterprises face increasing regulatory challenges, pay-for-performance, consumer demands, and technological changes, and they have mountains of data to analyze (Kaleba 2006). Typically organizations cut expenses in response to increased financial pressures, sometimes in the areas of personnel development or other areas that stifle creativity and development (Clarke 2006). All of these factors make good strategic planning ever more critical for long-term survival. For many businesses, including healthcare delivery, technology is transforming the strategic landscape and must be factored into the organization's strategic plan. Technology facilitates the collection of data that will help administrators determine whether objectives and goals are met (Willging 2007). Strategic planning is an outcome of strategic thinking. Strategic thinking is the broad process that an organization uses to determine what its future should look like. This is referred to as the vision of where the organization would like to find itself (Willging 2006). Strategic planning provides the focus for how that vision will be achieved. Successful strategic plans require the identification of a single vision and a single mission that fits within that vision, with all activities designed to meet the identified mission.

THE MISSION

The **mission** is the purpose or reason for the organization's existence and represents the fundamental and unique aspirations that differentiate the organization from others. The mission is often conveyed in the form of a mission statement that tells the organization's personnel and customers "who we are" and "what we do." The mission statement is an important tool when used to guide the planning process. An example of a mission statement is seen in Box 6–1.

The purpose of the St. Theresa Health System is clearly evident in its mission statement, which states that "the essence of our Mission and Philosophy is best depicted in our logo—St. Theresa and the words 'Healing Body, Mind and Spirit.'" This medical center's unique purpose is to provide healing for the mind and spirit, in addition to the expected purpose of physical healing. Its mission statement communicates this purpose effectively to both employees and customers.

The **scope** of an organization's mission defines the type of activities and services it will perform. The scope should be clearly identified in the mission statement so that employees and customers understand which aspects of organizational operation are most important. For example, a broad scope for a healthcare enterprise might be to "provide healthcare." The problem with such a broad scope is that the target client population is not identified, nor are the

> ### BOX 6–1 The Mission of St. Theresa Medical Center
>
> The Mission of St. Theresa Medical Center is the same as the Mission of St. Theresa Health System, which is:
>
> 1. To establish and maintain a hospital and other healthcare facilities for the care of persons with illnesses or disabilities that require that the patients receive hospital or long-term care, without distinction as to their religious beliefs, race, national origin, age, sex, disability, or economic status.
> 2. To carry on any educational activities related to rendering care to the sick and injured or the promotion of health which, in the opinion of the Board of Directors, may be justified by the facilities, personnel, funds or other requirements that are or can be made available, including, but not being specifically limited to, the conduction of schools for the education of registered nurses and practical nurses with power to grant diplomas to graduates and residency programs for physicians in training.
> 3. To promote and carry on scientific research related to the care of the sick and injured insofar as, in the opinion of the Board of Directors, such research can be carried on in or in connection with the hospital.
> 4. To participate, as far as circumstances may warrant, in any activity designed and carried on to promote the general health of the community.
>
> In working toward the fulfillment of these objectives, as members of the healthcare team, we strive to give generously of our efforts and work harmoniously together for the love of God and of our neighbor. As a result, we find that our own lives and the lives of those with whom we come in contact are being enriched and blessed.
>
> The essence of our Mission and Philosophy is best depicted in our logo—St. Theresa and the words "Healing Body, Mind and Spirit."

types of services that will be provided. A narrower scope provides the amount of detail necessary to appropriately guide administrators and managers in decision making. The scope of the St. Theresa Medical Center is also seen in the mission statement, which states, "the patients receive hospital or long-term care, without distinction as to their religious beliefs, race, national origin, age, sex, disability or economic status." The medical center's commitment to caring for the indigent population is clearly described in the mission statement. This scope is the basis for the development of certain goals and objectives that guide the decision makers in strategic planning.

GOALS AND OBJECTIVES

Identification of an organization's goals and objectives is a critical factor in fulfilling the mission. The goals and objectives explain how the mission will be realized. A **goal** is an open-ended statement that describes in general terms what is to be accomplished. Examples of goals include maintaining quality client care while promoting cost-effective operations, striving to increase market share by attracting a larger percentage of clients than their competitors, and broadening the scope of services offered. The ability to achieve defined goals is especially

TABLE 6–1 Areas of Potential Strategic Planning	
Goals and Objectives	**Strategy**
Improve organizational efficiency	Redesign work of processes so that tasks can be completed in fewer steps, more easily, and in a more cost-effective method.
Increase customer base	Target new populations within the already-defined geographic area as well as reaching out to rural and outlying communities with new programs.
Maximize the use of existing resources	Cross train workers so that they can perform several tasks.
Improve customer relationships	Create a Web site, or patient portal, that allows patients to find physicians, schedule appointments, e-mail providers, create and maintain a personal health record (PHR), access information on a variety of topics, and complete evaluations of services provided.

important in the rapidly changing healthcare environment as hospitals merge into large enterprises and services evolve to meet changing needs.

Objectives state how and when an organization will meet its goals. Some of the primary areas that goals and objectives may address are listed in Table 6–1. For example, objectives that support the goal of broadening the scope of services offered may include the following:

- *Development of clinics that support and promote wellness services.* Traditionally, clinics provide treatments for various medical problems. Expansion of these services to support wellness maintenance may attract a larger market share. Some additional services that may be offered are mammography, and blood pressure and cholesterol screening.
- *Expansion of home care services.* These services might be expanded to include routine postsurgical follow-up visits as well as occupational and physical therapy and special home monitoring programs to help keep the elderly in their own homes.

Prior to writing goals and objectives administrators need to communicate the vision and mission to employees in a manner that elicits understanding and buy-in (Willging 2006). Participant buy-in is critical to the success of the plan.

DEVELOPING STRATEGIES

An organization's **strategy** is a comprehensive plan that states how its mission, goals, and objectives will be achieved (Breene, Nunes, & Shill 2007; Kaleba 2006; Willging 2006). An examination of the mission and goals will help to define the steps that are necessary to attain them. A clear understanding of the end point is critical to the effective development of the plan. It is also important to review current strengths, weaknesses, opportunities, and threats. This includes the presence of competition. The strategic position for the organization can be determined by its reputation for quality of service and innovation, its access, the scope of services provided, and the demographics of the population served. An analysis of the current position of the organization in relation to these factors will help to determine available options. It is then possible for administration to select major initiatives to achieve their vision for the organization in light of available resources. Expediting the achievement of the mission and goals is the primary purpose of a strategic plan. It must be recognized, however, that strategy development is an ongoing task.

Strategic planning is led by members of the organization's upper management, including the board of directors and chief executive officer (CEO), who is ultimately responsible for the organization's strategic management (Breene, Nunes, & Shill 2007; Strategy officers 2007). Day-to-day responsibilities faced by CEOs often prohibit them from managing the incremental progress of the strategic plan, giving rise to the emergence of the role of chief strategy officer (CSO). The CSO must clarify the vision created by the CEO and leadership team for his or her own benefit and for all managers and employees. It is then up to the CSO to drive change and monitor the timelines and progress towards realization of the strategic plan. CSOs may also face the potential challenge of conflict with the chief financial officer. Typically there is no clear career path or title for the CSOs although they share a wide skill set and prior experience in planning. Many organizations choose to bring in a dedicated project leader instead, particularly when there is no margin for error and success is critical and time constraints exist (Clark 2006; Kodjababian & Petty 2007). Dedicated project leaders generally have extensive experience working in multiple settings and are characterized by their ability to:

- Motivate a diverse group of staff to follow them
- Build consensus on important decisions
- Identify issues that must be dealt with by their immediate team to keep the project on track
- Anticipate and resolve interpersonal conflicts that can derail the best-managed projects
- Communicate progress to key executives
- Identify and manage project and business risks

Physicians should also have representation at this level.

The next level of management, those who report to the CEO such as vice presidents, are also major participants in strategic planning. This should include the chief information officer (CIO). The CIO must ensure that executives understand the role that information technology plays in the organization as well as how information technology can be used to advance the goals of the organization. There must be a strong link between the organization's strategic plan and the information technology plan (Glaser 2006). It is the CIO's responsibility to see that upper management sees information technology as a tool to achieve organizational goals rather than just another cost center. This involvement will help to provide direction for all information technology initiatives, establish priorities, eliminate the duplication of information systems, and ensure the wise use of information technology resources. Other lower-level managers within the organization, such as department heads, are responsible for supporting the planning process by providing information related to the current operations as well as insight into future needs of the organization. This information enables the planning team to balance the present reality against the future vision and goals. Changing economics, resources, and markets make planning more difficult, but a well-crafted strategic plan makes provisions for these changes as well as for the expenditure of time, money, and resources to carry out the plan. Consumer demands represent a major driver in the current market, forcing providers to analyze the actual costs for every service rendered, prepare for the scrutiny of comparison shopping, develop competitive prices, make prices and payment options available to consumers, and restructure billing statements for increased clarity (Bauer & Hagland 2006). These changes require extensive input from administrators, clinicians, and information services.

STRATEGIC PLANNING FOR INFORMATION SYSTEMS

Although the broader scope of strategic planning concerns all areas of the healthcare institution, one important component is the plan for information systems. Without a plan that points information systems in the right direction and helps the organization to use information systems to execute its business strategies, the organization will not be able to effectively meet its overall goals (Glaser 2006).

The strategic planning process is often initiated by other changes that are taking place within the organization. For example, suppose a healthcare enterprise plans to purchase a client monitoring system to be used throughout its facilities. Other organizational changes—such as plans for construction and unit relocation, infrastructure upgrades including computer wiring and cabling, and updating the client care information systems in general—may have initiated the plans for obtaining the monitoring system. Once administrators realize the need for strategic planning for the monitoring system, they must identify the goals of the plan. These goals should be developed in accordance with the mission and goals of the organization. External factors that impact planning include changing standards and technology.

Some of the goals of information systems strategic planning are discussed next. Each goal is followed by a brief explanation of how it applies to the previously described example of selecting a new client monitoring system.

- *To support business and clinical decisions.* Data management supports better decision making by providing timely and accurate information. In the example of planning for a new monitoring system, a driving force behind these plans is the need to provide physicians and nurses with accurate and complete data regarding the client's condition.

- *To make effective use of emerging technologies.* New technologies can create administrative efficiencies and attract physicians and clients. A perfect example of this can be seen with the use of PDAs and other wireless devices to collect, view, and transmit patient information from the point of care. The Internet and e-health represent other developments that change the access to and delivery of healthcare because patient results can be made available online from any location and patient questions addressed. These developments must be included in the strategic planning process. An increasing number of customers also expect Internet access at the bedside.
- *To enhance the organization's image.* The effective use of information technologies enhances how the organization is perceived by physicians, clients, the community, and other external groups. This is especially critical in these times of competitive healthcare. For example, achieving state-of-the-art technology for cardiac monitoring will provide efficient and effective client care, which will enhance the organization's image.
- *To promote satisfaction of market and regulatory requirements.* Effective information systems strategic planning must include those issues related to meeting market and regulatory requirements, such as e-health, payer requirements, the Joint Commission guidelines, client confidentiality, and data security. For example, when selecting a monitoring system, it is also important to determine that the system complies with safety regulations such as protection against damage from defibrillation.
- *To be cost-effective.* Cost-effectiveness is achieved when redundancies are eliminated. In the monitoring system example, this advantage is evident. If all of the critical care and monitored bed areas in the enterprise use the same monitoring system, training is cost-effective, because nurses need to be trained on only one system to work in any monitored area of the hospital. Other cost benefits are seen in the need to maintain only one type of backup monitor for replacement of nonoperational equipment, as well as increased efficiency for the biomedical technicians who must maintain the monitoring equipment.
- *To provide a safer environment for patients.* There is strong initiative for patient safety at this time. A number of organizations, including government agencies, regulatory bodies, consumer groups, and professional organizations, are looking into ways to improve patient safety.

STEPS OF THE STRATEGIC PLANNING PROCESS

The first step of the strategic planning process is the realization that there is a need for change (Glaser 2006). Each department in the organization should have its own long-range plan that fits within the larger organizational plan, and most departments within the organization are dependent on the management of information systems. As a result, each department comes to the information services department with its own requirements related to strategic planning. The IT strategic plan must support and enable the organization's goals. It is the responsibility of the CIO and information systems department to prioritize and merge these ideas together, helping to develop a master strategic plan for the organization. This task is complicated by the rapidly changing nature of information technology, consumer demands, and clinician expectations for information availability at the bedside—whether that occurs via PDAs, blackberries, iPODs, tablet computers, or other devices. The fast pace of evolving technology requires periodic review and revisions of both the organization's strategic plan and the information systems department's strategic plan.

The CIO is ultimately responsible for IS strategic planning. The need to create administrative efficiencies through e-commerce, mergers and acquisitions, and requests for outcomes reporting forces CIOs to look at ways that information technology can be used to achieve strategic and operational changes (Glaser 2006). The CIO generally selects a project manager or chairperson for each major project within the overall strategic plan. Project management is a set of practices that if executed well will raise the likelihood that a project will succeed. Project management practices entail:

- Defining the scope and results of the project
- Identifying the tasks within the project, when they must occur and any interdependencies
- Defining who will be responsible for each task
- Establishes timelines for task and project completion
- Establishing how project decisions will be made
- Ensuring that stakeholders receive appropriate communication about the status of the project

The project manager may help to develop an advisory board or a strategic planning team. The strategic planning team is generally composed of top-level managers who devise the plan and present it to the CIO, who in turn presents it to the board of directors. One particularly important aspect of this process is the ability to prioritize all projects for the next 2 to 5 years. This requires estimating benefits, resources, costs, and timelines for each and then reevaluating the priority of each as new developments come into play. Some developments that affect information technology in healthcare include legislation that involves patient privacy and billing as well as initiatives calling for the implementation of barcoding for medication administration, computerized physician order entry, a computerized patient record, concerns over bioterrorism, an emphasis upon customer relationship management, and consumer-driven demands (Bauer & Hagland 2006; Langer 2003; Briggs 2003; Magliore 2003; Young 2007). These developments impact information technology budgets. The IT plan should also include applications and systems that are under consideration, needed infrastructure changes, and any additional resources in the way of additional equipment, staff, or training.

Another level of strategic planning is performed by members of the project implementation team, which reports to the advisory board. This team is composed of representatives from the user departments, including managers and front-line employees who are most familiar with the activities of the department. The project implementation team should also include the analysts and programmers who will implement the system changes. The project team needs the active involvement of end users to succeed. This is particularly true when nursing staff and other clinicians are ambiguous about change (Gillespie 2002). Stakeholders need to know the potential contributions as well as the limitations of new technology (Glaser 2006). Frequent communication between the advisory board and the implementation team is imperative for the ongoing success of the strategic plan. This plan generally addresses a time frame covering between 3 and 5 years into the future.

Identification of Goals and Scope

Once the strategic planning teams have been identified, the actual planning process can begin. The first step is to identify the goals and scope of the project. The goals of the project must meet the needs of the users as well as support the mission and goals of the institution. The identified goals will then provide the direction for the remainder of the planning process.

In the example of selecting a cardiac monitoring system for a healthcare enterprise, the goals and scope of the project might be to implement a one-vendor solution. This should result in the selection of a single system that will meet the needs of all monitored areas in the organization. However, decisions should be made with input from key users. Good communication between information systems personnel and clinicians is critical to the success of any project. It is essential to elicit support from nurses and physicians in the selection of any system that they will use and to listen to their feedback (Gillespie 2002; Glaser 2006; Schuerenberg 2003). Nurses are resistant to change unless they see the potential benefits. Physicians will not use a system if it is not easy to access and use. More and more, that translates to the ability to access information at the bedside, office, or from home or other locations using a variety of devices including traditional computers, PDAs, and other devices. No system should hinder clinical staff.

Scanning the External and Internal Environments

The next step in the planning process is to **scan**, or gather information from, the external and internal environments. The **external environment** includes those interested parties and competitors who are outside of the healthcare institution, such as vendors, payers, competitors, clients, the community, and regulatory agencies. The **internal environment** includes employees of the institution, as well as physicians and members of the board of directors. The purpose of scanning the environment is twofold: to define the current situation and to identify areas of need.

Environment scanning is best accomplished by developing a detailed plan for collecting pertinent data. This step is often called the *needs assessment*. Information related to current trends in both healthcare and information technology should also be collected. Data may be collected from a variety of sources, including the following (McCormack 1996):

External Environment Scanning

- Published literature and reports
- Information from vendors
- Regulatory and accreditation requirements
- Information related to market trends

Internal Environment Scanning

- Interviews and questionnaires from managers and end users
- Observations of current technology and operations, as well as anticipated technological developments

When selecting a monitoring system, information may be obtained from vendors regarding the technologies that are currently available. All pertinent regulatory and accreditation requirements must also be investigated. A scan of the internal environment may include an inventory of equipment currently in use throughout the enterprise. Insufficient data comprises one of the pitfalls of strategic planning (Clark & Krentz 2006).

Data Analysis

After data have been collected during the internal and external environmental scans, the project implementation team must perform analysis, identifying trends in the current operations as well as future needs and expectations. Current trends in healthcare should be identified when considering future needs and may be related to topics such as consumer-driven healthcare, managed care and other financial healthcare coverage, and reimbursement considerations. Some trends to consider include the merging of hospitals into large enterprises and the growing focus on care outside of the acute hospital setting, which has resulted in an increased number of services related to wellness promotion and home care. Information technology trends such as e-health, the Internet, telemedicine, client/server technologies, and the computerized client record must also be addressed.

In selecting a universal cardiac monitoring system, the features of each vendor's system must be evaluated, including the desirable and undesirable features of each. For example, strengths may include an easy learning curve, vendor support, integration capability, transport monitor capabilities, and screen visibility. Weaknesses may include a large number of screens for each function, busy or hard-to-read screens, slow speed of initial data entry, and unsuitable cabling requirements.

Identification of Potential Solutions

The next step in the planning process involves the identification of potential solutions, which may be in the form of system upgrades or replacements. At this point, the strategic planning team should be aware of the information system needs of the end users.

When identifying potential solutions, healthcare organizations must address many issues, including the following:

- *Hospitals with differing information systems may be merged together into one enterprise.* In this situation, either each organization continues to use its previous system or one system is chosen for use throughout the enterprise as a means to build a cohesive information systems strategy. Several factors influence the decision to retain or adopt an information system, including costs associated with the purchase and use of software and hardware; site licenses; consulting fees; contract negotiation; maintenance and support agreements; expenses associated with training personnel to use a new system; and the availability of support staff.
- *Many hospitals use mainframe* **legacy systems,** older vendor-based systems that have often been highly individualized to meet customer specifications. As it is necessary to upgrade or replace these systems, CEOs and CIOs must weigh the advantages and disadvantages of alternatives that may better meet the needs of the organization. These might include retaining current systems, providing a new look and easier access to legacy software via a Web interface, new versions of vendor software, client/server or thin client technologies, outsourcing services, or using an application service provider (ASP). Box 6–2 lists several information technology considerations related to strategic planning. Box 6–3 identifies pros and cons associated with the outsourcing of services.

BOX 6–2   Information Technology Considerations for Strategic Planning

- Does the system use open architecture?
- Is the system based on personal computer, client/server, thin client, or Internet technology?
- Does it support the use of PDAs, iPODs, and other devices to retrieve data?
- Is it user friendly?
- Does the software comply with HL7 and other standards?
- Does it sufficiently safeguard individual patient data from unauthorized users?
- Does the system allow the user to query aggregate data and produce online reports?
- Does it support performance measurement?
- Does it support a customized view?
- Can it support expansion of features, increased numbers of users, and/or records?
- Does it allow other technologies such as smart cards, optical disks, interface engines, wireless technology, integrated services digital network (ISDN) communication, e-health or e-commerce, video conferencing, telemedicine, and fiberoptic networks?
- Does it support a paperless environment?
- How much will it cost for purchase, installation, training, and ongoing support?
- Have criteria been developed to measure successful implementation?

BOX 6–3   Pros and Cons Associated with the Outsourcing of Services

Pros

- Allows the organization to focus on its core competencies
- Can shorten the time frame to implement new applications or technology
- Better compliance with project implementation dates
- Easier to budget and manage because costs for development and implementation are shifted to the outsourcing agency
- May improve customer satisfaction because services can be delivered at the same or at a higher level as in-house services but at a lower cost
- Provides leading-edge technical skills when skilled labor resources are not available in-house
- Contract negotiations aid definition of project scope

Cons

- Limited control over data security and confidentiality
- Lack of control over application maintenance and downtime
- Insufficient advance notice of downtime
- Lack of control over when updates are implemented
- Customization may not be available
- Promises may exceed ability to deliver
- Costs can be much higher than anticipated
- Identification and resolution of system problems may be delayed
- Ability to change outsourcing services may be limited

Selecting a Course of Action

Once all of the potential solutions have been identified, they must be analyzed and compared. One way to accomplish this task is to measure the components of the plan in terms of their ability to meet identified current and future needs. This can be accomplished by listing these needs and weighting them according to their importance. For example, essential features may be given a weighting factor of 5, and desirable but not essential features may be given a weighting factor of 3. Weighting of each desirable system feature should be completed before the various systems are scored.

The next step is to score the features, or requirements, of each potential system. For example, each feature may be given a score from 0 to 5, with 0 indicating that the requirement is not met, and 5 indicating that the requirement is fully met. Finally, the score is multiplied by the weighting factor for each item to determine the weighted score. The overall score is the sum of weighted scores for all items.

Figure 6–1 illustrates using a weighted score as an evaluation tool to select a hospital-wide cardiac monitoring system. This figure lists only a minimal number of the features that would actually be evaluated in this situation.

Evaluation of the various potential solutions should also include a summary of pertinent findings that have been discovered during data analysis.

Selection of a Hospital-Wide Cardiac Monitoring System

Monitoring System: _____
Evaluator: _____

Ratings (How well does the system do this?):
   1 = Poor   2 = Fair   3 = Adequate   4 = Good   5 = Excellent

System Feature	Rating	×	Weighting Factor	=	Weighted Score	Comments
Operation						
1. Easy to learn and operate			5			
2. Easy to set up screen			3			
Alarms						
3. Easy to set alarms			3			
4. Alarm limits displayed continuously			5			
Bedside Monitors						
5. Does the bedside unit work exactly the same as the central station and transport monitors?			3			
6. Can you view, control, review, and record any parameter from any bed on the network?			5			
					_____	Overall system score (Total of weighted scores):

FIGURE 6–1 • Example of an evaluation tool for cardiac monitoring systems

Other factors that should be considered when making a final decision include the following:

- Purchase costs versus outsourcing costs
- Ongoing maintenance and support costs
- Time required for installation
- Number of employees required to install and maintain the system
- Vendor's history and stability
- Service considerations
- Existence of national user groups
- Time and staff resources required for training

The process of strategic planning and selecting a course of action may involve time, money, and personnel resources. Nonetheless, the resources expended during this process are well worth the value of the plan that is produced, because this plan will guide the decision making of the IS department and the healthcare enterprise.

Implementation

The next phase in the strategic planning process is implementation of the chosen solution. The first step in the implementation process is to identify the working committee for the implementation phase. Development of a timeline is one of the initial tasks the committee will perform. Once all of the individual components of the timeline have been identified, the tasks can be assigned and initiated. Other tasks during this phase include budgeting, procedure development, and execution of the plan.

When implementing a universal cardiac monitoring system, the working committee may include representatives from the IS, purchasing, and staff development departments, as well as physicians and nurse managers. This group would first develop a timeline, prioritizing the order in which units would begin using the system. They would also be active in developing a procedure and a plan for educating staff in the use of the new equipment. Box 6–4 lists some measures to ensure a successful experience when services are outsourced.

BOX 6–4   Measures to Ensure a Positive Outsourcing Experience

- Define information technology functions for possible outsourcing
- Research vendor availability and capabilities
- Establish outsourcing goals and objectives
- Select the vendor that meets the requirements
- Negotiate a contract that outlines the following:
  - Term of contract and provisions for termination and renewal
  - Management of the relationship
  - Vendor and client responsibilities
  - Liabilities
  - Warranties
  - Ownership issues regarding assets/intellectual property
  - Fee structure
  - The process for staff assignment
  - Performance measures
  - Resources key to success
  - Security safeguards
  - Back-up and disaster recovery measures
  - Service level agreements inclusive of availability, response times, service quality
- Develop and use oversight procedures
- Insure against losses related to poor work

Ongoing Evaluation and Feedback

Strategic planning is an ongoing process (Glaser 2006). Frequent evaluation of the current processes as well as the current and future needs must be performed. In this way, the organization is able to remain current with changing technology and healthcare trends. The process for identifying evaluation tools can be difficult. Measures must be adjusted to environmental changes and competitor actions as a means to help ensure success of strategic plans. One particular type of measure is benchmarking.

Benchmarking is the continual process of measuring services and practices against the toughest competitors in the healthcare industry. An example of benchmarking is to compare the number of IS staff required to support the clinical applications for the enterprise to that of other healthcare providers with similar demographic and volume statistics. When needs are no longer met, or the organization falls far below the benchmark, the process of identifying potential solutions and selecting the best option is begun again. Clinical examples of benchmarks might include the organization's cost for open heart surgery or length of stay. Benchmarking has become widespread throughout the healthcare industry.

FUTURE DIRECTIONS

Strategic planning for the next few years for health information technology will focus primarily upon implementation of the electronic health record, barcode medication administration, and the development of customer portals and customer-directed initiatives. Strategic planning for hospitals must address these needs.

CASE STUDY EXERCISES

6.1   You are a nurse manager in a hospital that has recently merged with two other hospitals, forming a large healthcare enterprise. Each of the three hospitals currently uses a different clinical information system. You are a member of the strategic planning committee, which is charged with the task of selecting which of the three systems will be used throughout the enterprise. Describe the process you would use to scan the internal and external environments, as well as the types of data you would collect.

6.2   Develop a tool to evaluate each of the three clinical information systems for the scenario described above.

6.3   Your facility belongs to one of three healthcare delivery systems in the city. Competition is fierce. You have been asked to serve on a committee to study and recommend the retention or deletion of certain clinical services. Develop a plan for how you would do that and for how information services might facilitate that task via the use of benchmarking.

6.4 Your facility recently acquired and closed a competing hospital. All paper medical records are stored at a distant site. Records are not readily accessible. Client documentation and results were online but no longer available after the hospital closure. Some physicians never received test results for clients at the time of shut down. This had a negative impact on client care and satisfaction. How might strategic planning prevent this type of situation from occurring again?

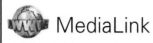 **MediaLink**

Additional resources for this content can be found on the Companion Website at www.prenhall.com/hebda. Click on "Chapter 6" to select the activities for this chapter.

- Glossary
- Multiple Choice
- Discussion Points
- Case Studies
- MediaLink Application
- MediaLink

SUMMARY

- Strategic planning is the development of a comprehensive long-range plan for guiding the activities and operations of an organization.
- Strategic planning is one of the most important factors in the selection, design, and implementation of information systems, because it can save valuable resources over time and ensure that the needs of the enterprise are met.
- The strategic plan should support the mission, goals, and objectives of the organization.
- The mission is the purpose for the organization's existence and represents its unique aspects.
- Strategic planning is guided by upper-level administrators, including the CIO and CSO, but requires participation from other levels of management as well.
- Strategic planning involves the following steps: definition of goals and scope, scanning of external and internal environments, data analysis, identification of potential solutions, selection of a course of action, implementation, evaluation, and feedback.
- Strategic planning is an ongoing process.

REFERENCES

Bauer, J. C. & Hagland, M. (July 2006). Consumer-directed health care: What to expect and what to do. *Health Financial Management, 60*(7), 76–78, 80, 82.

Breene, R. T. S., Nunes, P. F., & Shill, W. E. (2007), The Chief Strategy Officer. *Harvard Business Review, 85*(10), 84–93.

Briggs, B. (2003). Choose your battles wisely. *Health Data Management, 11*(4), 27–34.

Brunke, L. (2006). On reflection: Developing a strategic plan. *Nursingbc, 38*(2), 37.

Clark, F. C. (2006). IT Homecoming. *ADVANCE for Health Information Executives, 10(9)*, 47–48, 50–51.

Clarke, R. L. (2006). Managing the storm. *Healthcare Financial Management, 60*(7), 152.

Clark. C. S. & Krentz, S. E. (2006). Avoiding the pitfalls of strategic planning. (November). *Healthcare Financial Management,* Retrieved December 1, 2007, from CINAHL with Full Text database.

Crane, A. (2007). The New Era CFO. *Hospitals & Health Networks, 81*(6), 38–42. Retrieved November 30, 2007, from Business Source Elite database.

Cross, M. A. (1996). Building an I.S. strategy in the wake of a merger. *Health Data Management, 4*(10), 85–89.

Gillespie, G. (2002). IT a tough sell for nursing staff. *Health Data Management, 10*(4), 56–59.

Glaser, J. (Feb 2006). Wired for success. *Health Financial Management, 60*(2), 67–74.

Kaleba, R. Strategic planning getting from here to there. (2006). *Healthcare Financial Management, 60*(11), 74–78. Retrieved December 1, 2007, from CINAHL with Full Text database.

Kodjababian, J. & Petty, J. (2007). Dedicated project leadership helping organizations meet strategic goals. *Healthcare Financial Management, 61*(11), 130–134.

Langer, J. (2003). Prioritizing IT projects. *Healthcare Informatics, 20*(6), 110.

Magliore, M. (2003). Preparing business for biochemical attacks. *Contingency Planning and Management, 8*(4), 48–50.

McCormack, J. (1996). Strategic planning in changing times. *Health Data Management, 4*(12), 6–16.

Schuerenberg, B. (2003). Docs respond to group therapy. *Health Data Management, 11*(1), 34–38.

Strategy officers create new challenges for CFOs. (2007). *Financial Executive, 23*(9), 11.

Willging, P. (2007). Paul Willging says . . . You've got to construct your strategic plan. *Nursing Homes: Long Term Care Management, 56*(1),18. Retrieved December 1, 2007, from CINAHL with Full Text database.

Willging, P. (2006). You can't get there without a road map. *Nursing Homes: Long Term Care Management, 55*(11), 14, 16–17.

Young, T. (2007, October). Hospital CRM: Unexplored frontier of revenue growth? *Healthcare Financial Management, 61*(10), 86–90. Retrieved November 30, 2007, from Business Source Elite database.

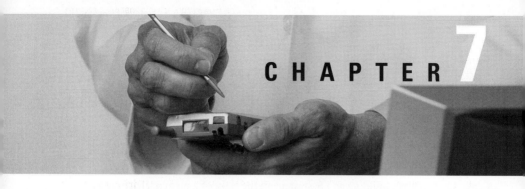

CHAPTER 7

Selecting a Healthcare Information System

After completing this chapter, you should be able to:

1 Define the term *life cycle* as it relates to information systems.

2 List the phases of the life cycle of an information system.

3 Recognize the purpose of the needs assessment.

4 Identify the typical membership composition of the system selection steering committee.

5 Explain the importance of using the mission statement in determining the organization's information needs.

6 Identify several methods for analyzing the current system.

7 Discuss the value of using a weighted scoring tool during the selection phase.

8 Review the system criteria that should be addressed during the selection process.

9 Describe the request for information and request for proposal (RFP) documents.

10 Evaluate request for proposal (RFP) responses from vendors.

11 Formulate a list of contract demands for a vendor once a system has been chosen.

The competitive advantages associated with health information systems are contingent upon the technology, the degree to which the technology meets the organizational needs, the strength of the information services staff, and the speed and method by which the system is implemented although the economic benefits may not be realized for at least 2 years after implementation (Costa & Marrone 2007; Glaser 2007; Havenstein 2007; Jusinksi 2007). Organizations that follow the implementation process of competitors may benefit from the mistakes of those who preceded them. This is particularly important given the high costs associated with implementation of new technology, which are driven higher if organizational needs are not met. For these reasons the selection and implementation processes are critical. Many options are available today, adding to the complexity of the task. No "right" solution exists for all facilities. The best starting point when considering the purchase or development of information technology is the strategic plan, given that it sets goals and determines technology needs. From this point the selection and implementation of an information system occur through a well-defined process known as the **life cycle.** This term describes the ongoing process of developing and maintaining an information system. This cycle can be divided into four main phases that cover the life span of information systems. These four phases are:

1. Needs assessment
2. System selection
3. Implementation
4. Maintenance

Figure 7–1 illustrates the relationship of these phases as circular, because needs assessment and evaluation are ongoing processes. As needs change, the organization may find it necessary to upgrade information systems periodically. The first two phases, needs assessment and system selection, are discussed in this chapter. Details regarding system implementation and maintenance are covered in Chapter 8. It is essential to develop a timeline that delineates the major events or milestones when working through the various phases of the information system's life cycle. For example, while it is desirable to complete the needs assessment and selection processes in less than 1 year, it is necessary to recognize that the process

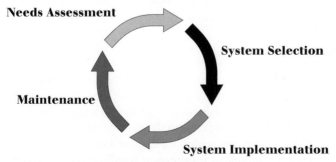

FIGURE 7–1 • The life cycle of an information system

Milestone	Person Responsible	Estimated Start Date	Completion Date
PHASE 1: **NEEDS ASSESSMENT**			
Develop steering committee			
Perform needs assessment:			
Identify system **requirements and** **weighting of criteria** Technical Administrative/general Registration Order entry/results reporting Medical records Accounting			
PHASE 2: **SYSTEM SELECTION**			
Develop the RFP Organization description System requirements Response evaluation procedures			
Evaluate RFP responses			
Conduct site visits			
Select the system for **purchase**			
Contract negotiations and **contract signed**			

FIGURE 7–2 • Sample template for developing a timeline or Gantt chart

may take 1 year to complete. Therefore, it is vital to organize responsibilities around a realistic timeframe. Figure 7–2 provides a template that may be used to develop a timeline or Gantt chart for the needs assessment and system selection phases of the information system's life cycle.

NEEDS ASSESSMENT

Needs assessment is the first phase in the information life cycle (Costa & Marrone 2007; Jusinski 2007; Teague 2007). This process is usually initiated by a person or group with a vision of the future. The needs assessment should analyze the overall needs of the organization with consideration to the strategic plan. After this is done it is appropriate to look at segments within the organization. A deficit in the current method of manual or automated information handling is often recognized by people from several different groups or disciplines, such as clinical and administrative personnel who use the information, as well as programmers and other technical staff who manage the information system. Once the deficit or need is realized, a more detailed understanding of the issues must be developed.

After the selection committee discusses the current deficits and needs, they brainstorm to generate a list of possible directions for action. These actions may include minor modifications to the current manual or automated system, major enhancements to the current system, or the purchase of a new automated information system.

The analysis of identified possible actions and the decision-making process must be a collaborative effort, and is often performed by a committee that includes clinical users, information systems specialists, and administration or executive board representatives.

The Steering Committee

The steering committee is an essential component of the assessment and selection processes. Its membership should include board members to ensure that information technology is aligned with the organization's overall strategy (Marshall & Heffes 2007). Too often a disconnect exists between the expressed importance that board members assign to IT and budget allocations and actual IT applications. A recent survey conducted by Deloitte Consulting suggests that a distinct and positive correlation exists between the attention paid to IT and corporate performance. Steering committee leadership may affect the success or failure of the project. The committee chairperson may be a manager or director of information services or have an administrative position elsewhere in the hospital, such as chief financial officer (CFO), chief nursing officer (CNO), or medical director. The committee membership must be multidisciplinary, including representation from all departments affected by the new system and incorporating the clinical, administrative, and information system divisions. This strategy is essential for identification of all pertinent issues and reduces the possibility of overlooking potential problems. In those healthcare organizations that include affiliations with other facilities, it is imperative that representation from these areas be included to address any additional needs. A general rule to follow is that any department or area that uses the information or is affected by it must have a voice in the selection process.

The structure of the steering committee must be defined early in the process. When designing the committee, it is important to consider the appropriate size of the group. The committee should be large enough to make a good decision but small enough to be effective and efficient. At this point, it is necessary to define who has the authority to make the final decisions. For example, decision-making power may be given to a particular department, shared among a group of administrators from various departments, or shared equally among all members of the steering committee.

One strategy that is effective in larger organizations is to develop a multilevel committee. The upper level or executive board of the committee is responsible for the final decisions regarding selection. This may be a small group of high-level executive chief officers, such as the CEO, CIO, privacy officer, vice presidents responsible for major departments, medical staff leadership and an informatics nurse specialist. This subcommittee is supported by a larger group of department managers and supervisors. Few guidelines exist for the selection of users to serve on the committee but it should include some frontline employees who will actually be using the system (Jusinski 2007; Saleem, Tran, & Moses 2006). These are the people who will be responsible for doing most of the groundwork and investigation during the assessment and selection processes. There should also be representation from information services, risk management, patient registration, and financial services to ensure that related issues are addressed. Selected committee members must be able to devote the necessary time and energy to the project. Their managers must be willing to provide them with time away from their normal responsibilities and support their involvement in the project. This requirement can be difficult to meet given that the shortage of experienced nurses reduces time available to participate in the selection process (CDW 2007). The CDW Healthcare second annual study of more than 1000 nurses found that the involvement of an informatics nurse and nurses in information technology decisions can accelerate IT integration. In general an effective strategy is to assign tasks to individual members or subgroups based on their expertise and knowledge. Their findings are then presented to the larger committee for discussion and approval. The lack of guidelines for users to serve on the committee may result in a less than optimal membership. Front-end users should demonstrate functional expertise, good communication, and ideally a computing background.

Consultants

Consultants may be hired for assistance in any phase of the selection process, including recommendations for the composition of the steering and selection committee, assessing the current information system, system planning, testing, security, policy and procedure development, and implementation (Hoch 2006; The future is now 2007). The effective use of consultants requires clear definition of the contractual relationship and expected outcomes as well as good communication throughout the association. The consultant should be provided with all available data regarding the current system and identified needs. The consultant's role is to analyze this information and make recommendations for action. Box 7–1 lists some of the primary qualities of an effective consultant or consulting service. On occasion, problems arise with the use of consultants, including limited experience, and adequate knowledge of the needs of hardware and software applications under consideration. Also, there may be a lack of incentive to work toward the most useful and cost-effective solution, and failure to keep promises made to clients. A good consultant always acts in the best interest of the client (Czerniawska 2006).

Developing a Common Vision

The needs assessment committee should start the process by examining the vision and mission statements of the organization as well as the strategic plan (Wickham et al. 2006). This will guide the committee in looking to the future

BOX 7–1   Qualities of an Effective Consultant

- Experience, including longevity and diversity
- Knowledge and understanding of the healthcare industry
- Consulting skill and a proven methodology
- Verbal and written communication skills
- Good project management skills
- Clearly defined work plan and deliverables
- Advice that will result in cost savings
- Flexibility and availability
- A fit with the corporate culture
- Leadership in a team environment
- Ability to manage expectations rather than results
- Dedication to the project at hand
- Credibility
- Always acting in the best interest of the client

and determining the organization's information needs while continuing to support the mission. From this, goals should be developed to guide the work of the committee. These goals must reflect the organization's purpose, scope of services, and customers. The primary goal of the committee is to identify how healthcare delivery can be enhanced to provide optimum client care; this can be accomplished by providing more meaningful and accurate client data. Some additional expectations of an information system might be to save time, increase productivity, contain costs, promote quality improvement, and foster staff recruitment and retention. In addition, the system must be able meet and support regulatory guidelines such as those related to Health Insurance Portability and Accountability Act (HIPAA) requirements. The committee should consider using brainstorming techniques when defining the expectations of an information system. An open-minded and creative approach will facilitate comprehensive exploration of all possibilities.

Understanding the Current System

A thorough understanding of how information is currently collected and processed is the starting point in performing a needs assessment. This is also known as assessing the internal environment. Methods for accomplishing this include questionnaires and observation of day-to-day activities (Saba & McCormick 1996). The goal is to determine what information is used, who uses it, and how it is used. Every data item used in the current paper or automated system should be analyzed. Some examples of data items include client name, sex, marital status, and diagnosis. Next, the committee must decide what information should be kept, what information is redundant, and what information is unnecessary. They should evaluate the strengths and weaknesses of the current manual or automated information system to determine the needs of the healthcare enterprise.

Determining System Requirements

To determine the appropriate course of action, the committee must first understand the organization's requirements for operation. One strategy for obtaining this information is to interview staff from each department or work area. The interviewer might ask what information is necessary to conduct business and what information is desired but not essential. These are often called the "musts" and the "wants." Some examples of essential information include client name, admitting physician, and insurance information. It is important to also consider those criteria that may not be necessary at the present time but might be important in the future, such as voice recognition technology. The information from numerous interviews is then compiled into a list of "musts" and "wants."

The next step is to prioritize or weight the list of "musts" and "wants" from high to low. To accomplish this task, selection committee members should develop a rating scale such as a 1 to 10 scale or rankings of low, medium, and high. Table 7–1 displays an example of some weighted "wants" and "musts" that could be identified when performing the needs assessment. The criteria should also be grouped into functional categories to present a comprehensive picture of the system requirements. Some of the common categories that may be considered are listed next.

Technical Criteria Technical criteria include those hardware and software components necessary for the desired level of system performance. Areas to consider are the following:

• *Type of architecture.* **Architecture** refers to the structure of the central processing unit and its interrelated elements. An **open system** uses protocols

TABLE 7–1 Sample of Criteria Defining "Musts" and "Wants" for Barcode Medication Administration System

Charting/Documentation Information Criteria	"Must" or "Want"	Weight*
Is capable of multidisciplinary charting	M	10
Provides positive patient identification	M	10
Provides list of right medications and routes for the time		10
Automatically records medications during scanning process.		
Generates reminders of outstanding medications and pain assessments as due	M	10
Automatically calculates charted IV products into intake and output	W	7
Automatically totals fluid balance by shift and 24-hour period	W	6
Able to easily switch between functions (such as charting and entering orders)	W	5

*1–10, where 10 = most important.

and technology that follow publicly accepted conventions and are used by multiple vendors, so that various system components can work together.

Examples of Criteria

1. System maintains an open architecture environment that can continue to evolve as new technology becomes available
2. Features ease of implementation and support of real-time integration to existing and future information systems

• *Amount of downtime.* **Downtime** refers to the period of time when an information system is not operational and available for use. Some systems have daily scheduled downtimes, during which maintenance and backup procedures are performed.

Examples of Criteria

1. Provides 24-hour system availability with no scheduled daily downtime
2. Does not have a history of prolonged or frequent unscheduled downtimes

• *Connectivity standards.* These standards help to maximize the connectivity between application and information files, supporting system integration.

Examples of Criteria

1. Provides for HL7–compliant interfaces
2. Includes the ability to interface from and to client care instruments such as monitors

• *Test environment separate from live environment.* A separate environment for the development and testing of updates and changes to the system must be available, so that the actual system (live system) can continue to operate without interference during these activities.

Examples of Criteria

1. Provides the ability to update the test environment without impacting the live system
2. Provides a training environment that is separate from the live and test environments

• *Response time.* **Response time** is the amount of time between a user action and the response from the information system. For example, after the user selects a laboratory test from a menu, the system requires a certain amount of processing time before that result can be viewed.

Examples of Criteria

1. Ensures acceptable response time for all online transactions (1 second or less)
2. Able to continuously track and monitor response time and provide reports containing this information

- *Support of electronic technologies.* The information system should support other technologies that will enhance client care and business operations.

  Examples of Criteria
  1. Supports various methods of data entry by the user, including touch-screen entry and voice recognition
  2. Allows the use of barcoding and scanning

Administrative/General Criteria Administrative criteria describe how the system may be administratively controlled for appropriate and effective use of the information.

- *Security levels to comply with regulatory and legal requirements.* The Joint Commission, for example, regulates the confidentiality, security, and integrity of hospital systems. The HIPAA imposes requirements for the protection of patient data and penalties for noncompliance.

  Examples of Criteria
  1. Allows various levels of security to be defined for different user groups; each group should have access to only the information required for its client care or job duties
  2. Provides an auditing utility to track and report what information has been accessed by which users

- *Online help screens.* Online help screens display instructions to assist the user with completing a specific function.

  Examples of Criteria
  1. Help screens must be available and easily accessed by the user
  2. Help screens must be concise and easy to understand

- *Purging and restoring data.* It is important to determine how long it is necessary to maintain online access to client data before sending it to other storage devices. Sometimes it becomes essential to restore these files for the purposes of audits, and the ease of performing these procedures must be considered. Advances such as the use of imaging technology to store diagnostic images and forms must be considered when purge criteria are defined.

  Examples of Criteria
  1. Includes a flexible client purge process, allowing both automatic and manual purge capabilities
  2. Process for restoring data that have been purged to storage to be convenient and readily accessible

- *Report capabilities.* The system should provide a report-writing software component that allows specific types of information to be extracted from the database and presented in a report.

Examples of Criteria

1. Predefined reports to be produced automatically on a set schedule
2. Users should be able to generate ad hoc reports on demand, with the capability to format them as desired
3. Reports should be available online, eliminating concerns related to printing costs, labor, distribution, storage, and disposal of confidential materials

Registration Criteria The registration criteria are essential for ensuring that the client is properly identified for all aspects of information management.

Examples of Criteria

1. Assigns each client a unique identifier across the organization
2. Supports multiple registration sites; clients may enter the health system at a number of points of service, including the physician's office, clinics, the emergency department, or the admissions office
3. Provides the ability to change or update registration information
4. Demonstrates the ability to track a client's location within the institution, as well as to track the use of system services
5. Prevents the user from omitting required data before completing a function

Order Entry/Results Reporting Criteria These criteria ensure that accurate entry of physician orders is accomplished in a timely and efficient manner, resulting in improved client care.

Examples of Criteria

1. Able to indicate details of orders such as frequency (for example, every six hours or daily) and priority (stat, routine, and so on)
2. Notifies the user when a duplicate order is entered, and requests verification before accepting the new order. For example, the client may have a previously ordered daily chest x-ray. If a new order for a chest x-ray is now entered, the system should alert the user and request verification that this additional test is necessary.
3. Through order entry and results reporting, produces an audit trail that identifies the person who entered the order, the date/time of order entry and execution, and the status of the order (such as pending or completed)
4. Supports documentation of medications and treatments, and relates this documentation to the appropriate order
5. Automatically generates client charges for specific orders or treatments as a result of entry or completion

Medical Records Criteria The medical records criteria should support the storage of all pertinent client data obtained from various information systems, allowing the user to access a longitudinal record of all client activities and events or visits. The system should allow inquiry about clients, using various identifiers, including social security number, name, medical record, or account number.

Examples of Criteria

1. Provides support for automatic coding, including verification of codes entered with narrative description (for example, *ICD-9-CM* and *CPT-4* codes)
2. Translates diagnosis and procedure terminology into numeric code
3. Produces deficiency lists on demand for individual records and individual physicians

Accounting Criteria These criteria facilitate reimbursement for services rendered and help to ensure the financial stability of the enterprise.

Examples of Criteria

1. Generates summaries or detailed bills on demand
2. Allows the user to enter the client's insurance verification data, insurance plan, and charges at any time during the stay and to change the client's financial class
3. Supports physician billing and captures data for linkage to physician billing services

SYSTEM SELECTION

If the decision is made to purchase a new information system, the life cycle proceeds to Phase 2: system selection. This phase is critical to the success of the project. High cost for purchase, installation, and maintenance for new or upgraded technology mean that the decision must be made carefully. The information gathered during the needs assessment phase is the basis for the system selection process and decision. Because it has been determined that a new system must be purchased, further information must now be gathered. Box 7–2 identifies some system selection considerations. The selection committee should also be aware of the amount of money available for the purchase, installation, and maintenance of a new system, as this influence will guide their questions and impact available choices (Costa & Marrone 2007).

Additional Sources of Information

Trade shows and conferences are beneficial sources of information. Attendance at these events provides the opportunity to examine systems from various vendors in an informal atmosphere, to compare and contrast system capabilities, and to view demonstrations.

Other potentially helpful sources of information include weekly publications, trade newspapers, and monthly journals that address information and

BOX 7–2   System Selection Criteria

- Overall costs
  Hardware, software, and network costs
  Implementation costs
  Support and maintenance costs
- Vendor characteristics
  Reputation
  Experienced staff and consultants
  Financial status
- Software features
  Ease of use
  Intuitive user interface, requiring minimal training
  Includes all functionality identified as "musts"
  Supports security requirements
  Supports interfaces with other applications
  Supports future growth options
- Environmental issues
  Energy consumption of equipment
  Recycling and e-waste options once equipment is outmoded

technology, and local user groups. Textbooks and reference books also provide discussions of system options. Published conference proceedings may provide insight into pertinent issues and solutions. Finally, communication via the Internet and World Wide Web can furnish additional information, including insights from other users of a given system. This avenue may provide the most current and candid responses to questions.

Request for Information

An information systems **vendor** is a company that designs, develops, sells, and supports systems. Consideration of vendor characteristics is crucial in choosing a system that will be responsive to current needs and unanticipated changes. Characteristics to examine include service, performance, and stability. A great deal of information can be gleaned from vendors who are eager to make a sale. The **request for information (RFI)** is often the initial contact with vendors. An RFI is a letter or brief document sent to vendors that explains the institution's plans for purchasing and installing an information system. The purpose of the RFI is to obtain essential information about the vendor and its systems to eliminate those vendors that cannot meet the organization's basic requirements. One method for obtaining names of appropriate vendors is to complete reader response cards following advertisements in professional journals.

The RFI should ask the vendor to provide a description of the system and its capabilities. Often the vendor responds to the request by sending written literature. More information can be obtained by asking additional specific questions of the vendor. Some topics to consider for questioning include:

1. The history and financial situation of the company, including the extent of its investment into research and development; this provides an indication of the company's commitment to enhancing and updating the product
2. The number of installed sites, including a list of several organizations that already use the product you are considering
3. System architecture, including the required hardware configuration
4. Use of state-of-the-art technology
5. Integration with other systems. Which other systems are currently integrated with the vendor's software in other hospital sites?
6. The methods of user support provided by the vendor during and after installation
7. Future healthcare provider development plans
8. Procedures for the distribution of software updates

Request for Proposal

At this point, the steering committee will probably be overwhelmed with information. The next step is to evaluate this information and prepare a formal document called the **request for proposal (RFP)**. An RFP is a document sent to vendors that describes the requirements of a potential information system. The RFP prioritizes or ranks these requirements in order of their importance to the organization. Preparation of this document can be daunting. Its purpose is to solicit proposals from many vendors that describe their capabilities to meet the "wants" and "needs." The vendors' responses may then be used to narrow the number of competitors under consideration.

Strategies for a Successful RFP Because of the importance of the RFP, it must be structured to ensure successful system selection (Hoch 2006). All aspects of the document must be detailed and precise to facilitate an accurate response from the vendor. If questions are vague or poorly written, they could easily be misinterpreted by the vendor. For example, an ambiguous question might lead a vendor to indicate that the system meets a requirement when in fact it does not. It is advantageous to limit the number of requirements to those that are most important and to produce a simple and straightforward document. If an RFP is too lengthy, it will cost both the organization and the vendor a great deal of time and money to prepare and evaluate. It is difficult to evaluate a long document that is not focused on the important issues. Finally, a well-written RFP provides a framework that allows the steering committee to more accurately evaluate the vendor's proposal.

The format of RFP questions and answers may influence the authenticity of vendor responses. For example, for each question about a system feature, the RFP might offer four response choices, such as:

1. *"Yes."* If the vendor indicates that this functionality is currently available, then the vendor must also provide a written explanation of how the system performs this function.
2. *"Available with customization."* The vendor must provide an estimated cost of customization and time frame for availability.
3. *"Available in the future."* The vendor must provide an estimated time frame for availability.
4. *"No."* No further information is required.

RFP Design Although the actual format of the RFP may vary from organization to organization, all RFPs must contain certain components that are essential for a complete and effective document. The RFP should include the following details:

- *Description of the organization.* The first objective of the RFP should be to familiarize the vendor with the organization. The RFP must describe the organization's overall environment, as well as the specific setting in which the system will function. The vendor needs to have enough information to facilitate proposal of appropriate systems and hardware configurations. The following information should be included:

  1. *Mission and goals.* The mission statement and any supporting documentation will provide the vendor with a view of the driving forces behind the selection process.
  2. *Structure of the organization.* The RFP should describe how the healthcare enterprise is structured, including all facilities and satellite areas that provide inpatient, outpatient, and home care services.
  3. *Type of healthcare facility.* The RFP should specify whether the facility is a profit or nonprofit organization and contain descriptors appropriate to the organization, such as community, university, government, or teaching facility.
  4. *Payer mix.* Additional information should quantify the proportion of clients for the various types of payers encountered. For example, the percentage of clients having private insurance, Medicare/Medicaid coverage, or health maintenance organization (HMO) membership should be indicated.
  5. *Volume statistics.* The RFP should provide volume statistics such as number of inpatient beds, average occupancy, annual outpatient visits, emergency department visits, volume of lab tests performed, number of operations annually, and number of various categories of staff, including physicians, nurses, and technicians and any plans for growth.

- *System requirements.* Following the description of the organization, the RFP should include a comprehensive list of the system requirements previously developed by the committee. One point to consider when defining system requirements is to avoid limiting the vendor to specific configurations, such as the type and number of devices, because the vendor may be able to suggest better solutions. The requirements should not necessitate the vendor to recreate a manual or current automated system. These limitations may prohibit the vendor from exploring improved methods of information use with the proposed technology (Metrick 2002).

- *Criteria for evaluation of responses.* Providing the vendor with an explanation of the RFP evaluation process may improve the quality of the vendor's response. If the vendors respond in the expected format, evaluating responses from multiple vendors can be more easily accomplished, and results more easily compared.
- *Deadline date.* Inform the vendor of the expected date of responses. Vendors who do not meet deadlines may be excluded.

Evaluation of RFP Responses Once responses from various vendors have been received, the process of evaluation begins. Some initial considerations are related to how the vendor approached the RFP. For example, some questions to ask are:

- Was the response submitted by the deadline date?
- Does it represent the work of a professional team and company?
- Were the vendor representatives responsive and knowledgeable?
- Does the proposal address the requirements outlined in the RFP, or does it appear to be a standard bid?

Further evaluation is centered around the specific responses of the vendors to the requirements listed in the RFP. The prioritization and ranking of the requirements that were previously developed by the steering committee now are used to weight each item in the RFP. This produces an overall score for each vendor response. This score allows the vendors to be ranked objectively, based on their ability to meet the requirements. Vendors that are unable to meet all of the "musts" should be automatically eliminated.

The remaining vendors must now be evaluated in terms of benefits and costs. Examining the scores for the "wants" and discussing the vendor's proposed costs are components of the final decision-making process. It may be helpful to narrow the list to three finalists and then examine these more closely.

Hoch (2006) suggests that the committee might want to consider writing a **Request for Quote (RFQ)** instead, stating that the RFP invites vendors to focus on marketing hype. The RFQ is a statement of need that focuses upon pricing, service levels, and contract terms. It should be written in precise, technical but vendor-neutral language. When customers are unclear about needs in a particular area they should request pricing for different solutions. The RFQ should ask for quotes based on present as well as projected levels of growth with consideration given to response times, stability, and monetary compensation for downtime and loss of business. Other issues for consideration include termination clauses and use of subcontractors.

Site Visits The use of site visits is very helpful in selecting a system. Site visits allow the system to be seen in action at a location that is comparable in size and services provided. Comparison of site visit evaluations for the top three vendors may provide additional information that will facilitate decision making.

A successful site visit often begins with the preparation of a list of questions. Asking the same questions at each site visit helps the committee draw meaningful comparisons. It is helpful to request a demonstration of the live system. This will allow observations regarding the response time. It is also beneficial to examine reports and printed documentation produced by the system, and to interview people who are actually using the system. Often, more candid information can be obtained if the vendors are not present during the interview process. Box 7–3 lists several questions that may be used during a site visit.

In addition, the vendor should provide a contact list of users from other organizations who are willing to be interviewed by phone. Representatives from hospital departments may ask their counterparts in other organizations about the performance of the information system. This will provide insight into how the systems actually operate, as well as the support that the vendor provides.

Contract Negotiations Once the decision has been made by the steering committee, the enterprise's legal and purchasing representatives carry out the actual contract negotiations. They may request the names of the three highest ranked vendors, as well as their RFP responses. In this way, the contract

---

BOX 7–3 Questions to Ask During a Site Visit

- How reliable is the system?
- How much downtime do you experience?
- What is the response time?
- How is the system backup accomplished, and how frequently is this done?
- Are there any problems with information exchange with other information systems?
- How do customizations or enhancements get made to the system (in-house or by vendor)?
- How much training was required for users to learn the system?
- What do you like most about the system?
- What things would you like to change about the system?
- What features would you like to see added to the system?
- How is information access restricted, and how is security maintained?
- What have your experiences been with vendor support?
- Is it easy to generate reports and can they be customized easily to meet user needs?

negotiations will be able to address issues not specifically included in the RFP responses, such as cost justification and expected implementation schedules. The end result will be the selection of one vendor and a system that will be implemented in the enterprise. After the contract is signed, the implementation phase begins.

FUTURE DIRECTIONS

The selection of healthcare information systems will occur many times in the future as manual processes are replaced by automated ones and as individual systems require upgrades, outlive their utility, or can no longer be supported for various reasons. As the process is repeated the body of knowledge required to support this practice will continue to grow, helping to ensure the choice of the best system for a given organization. At the same time this knowledge will allow the process to take place with greater efficiency over a shorter period of time. Melanson, Lindeman, and Jarolim (2007) note that at present it may take 14 months from the time that a committee is formed until a system selection is finalized. Individual users on the selection committee will also become more savvy, allowing them to be more discriminating in the selection process. Cortese and Smoldt (2007) share their vision of teams of professionals who use **information technology** and systems engineering to learn from each other and quickly disseminate and assimilate new evidence that can be used to benefit individual patients providing individualized, evidence-based care efficiently and at the lowest possible cost.

CASE STUDY EXERCISES

7.1 You are a member of the committee that will select a clinical documentation system for nurses. Prepare a timeline for the needs assessment and system selection phases. These processes should be accomplished over a 6-month period.

7.2 Develop a list of "musts" and "wants" and assign a weight to each item. Define what your weighting scale will be.

7.3 Create a list of questions related to this system selection process that you will ask at site visits.

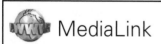 **MediaLink**

Additional resources for this content can be found on the Companion Website at www.prenhall.com/hebda. Click on "Chapter 7" to select the activities for this chapter.

- Glossary
- Multiple Choice
- Discussion Points
- Case Studies
- MediaLink Application
- MediaLink

SUMMARY

- The selection and implementation of an information system occur through a well-defined process called the life cycle of an information system.
- The four phases of the life cycle of an information system are needs assessment, system selection, implementation, and maintenance.
- The needs assessment process is often initiated when a deficit in the current method of manual or automated information handling is recognized.
- The system selection steering committee is an essential component of the assessment and selection processes, and leadership as well as membership of this group may impact the success or failure of the project.
- The needs assessment process should include an examination of the vision and mission statements of the organization, because these should guide the committee in looking to the future and determining the organization's information needs.
- A thorough understanding of how information is currently collected and processed is the starting point in performing a needs assessment.
- Determination of the system requirements should address criteria related to all aspects of system performance, including technical, administrative, registration, order entry, results reporting, medical records, and accounting criteria.
- The request for information is a letter or brief document sent to vendors that explains the institution's plans for purchasing and installing an information system. The purpose of the RFI is to obtain essential information about the vendor and its system capabilities to eliminate those vendors that cannot meet the organization's basic requirements.
- The request for proposal is a document sent to vendors that describes the requirements of a potential information system. The purpose of this document is to solicit from many vendors proposals that describe the capabilities of their information systems and support services.
- A weighted scoring strategy will facilitate the evaluation of complicated request for proposal responses from vendors and will improve the ability of the steering committee to make an informed decision.

REFERENCES

CDW Healthcare. (2007). Nurses Talk Tech 2007™: The catch-22 of nursing and information technology. Retrieved December 12, 2007, from http://webobjects.cdw.com/webobjects/docs/pdfs/healthcare/Nurses-Talk-Tech-2007.pdf.

Cortese, D. & Smoldt, R. (2007). A health system by design. *Modern Healthcare, 37*(38), 38.

Costa, M. & Marrone, B. (2007). What's the best approach to choosing IT? *Healthcare Financial Management, 61*(2), 108–112.

Czerniawska, F. (2006). Consultant: good consulting firm: bad. *Consulting to Management—C2M, 17*(2), 3–5.

Glaser, J. (2007). The competitive value of healthcare IT. *Healthcare Financial Management, 61*(7), 36–40.

Havenstein, H. (April 2, 2007). Hospitals Are Slow to Gain Benefits From IT Spending, *Computerworld*, 12.

Himiak, L. (2007). Building a Team for EMR Success, *ADVANCE for Health Information Professionals, 17*(6), 12.

Hoch, M. (2006). 3 1/2 RFP rules. *Communications News, 43*(9), 00103632.

Jusinski, L. (2007). EHR Selection Suggestions. *ADVANCE for Health Information Professionals, 17*(10), 19.

Maleshefski, T. (October 15, 2007). IT planner: 5 steps to green IT. *eWEEK*, 41–43, 46.

Melanson, S. E. F., Lindema, N. I., & Jarolim, P. (July 2007). Selecting Automation for the Clinical Chemistry Laboratory. *Archives of Pathology and Laboratory Medicine 131*(7), 1063–1069.

Marshall, J. & Heffes, E. M. (2007). Most Directors Fail to Link IT with Strategy, *Financial Executive, 23*(6), 9.

Metrick, G. (2002). Selecting a product or services using the request for proposal process. *Scientific Computing and Instrumentation, 19*(12), L-8–L-12.

Saba, V. K. & McCormick, K. A. (1996). *Essentials of computers for nurses.* Philadelphia: Lippincott.

Saleem, N., Jones, D. R., Tran, H. V., & Moses, B. (2006). Forming design teams to develop healthcare information systems. *Hospital Topics: Research and Perspectives on Healthcare, 84*(1), 22–29.

Teague, P.E. (March 1, 2007). 5 "musts" for justifying IT budgets. *Purchasing*, 41–42.

The future is now: Consultants spotlight. (November 2, 2007). *Pharmaceutical Executive, 27*, 11–34.

Wickham, V., Miedema, F., Gamerdinger, K., & DeGooyer, J. (2006, December). Bar-coded patient ID: Review an organizational approach to vendor selection. *Nursing Management, 37*(12), 22–26. Retrieved December 7, 2007, from Health Source: Nursing/Academic Edition database.

CHAPTER 8

System Implementation and Maintenance

After completing this chapter, you should be able to:

1 Describe how implementation committee members are selected.

2 Discuss the importance of establishing a project timeline or schedule.

3 Explain the differences between the test, training, and production environments.

4 List the decisions that must be addressed when performing an analysis of hardware requirements.

5 Review the issues that must be addressed when developing procedures and documentation for users.

6 Discuss the factors that contribute to effective training.

7 Discuss the "go-live" process and identify the components involved in planning for it.

8 Recognize several common implementation pitfalls.

9 Name several common forms of user feedback and support.

10 Explain the significance of providing ongoing system and technical maintenance.

11 Recognize that the life cycle of an information system is an ongoing cyclical process.

The previous chapter discussed the first two phases of the life cycle of an information system. This chapter explores system implementation and maintenance, which make up the third and fourth phases.

SYSTEM IMPLEMENTATION

Form an Implementation Committee

The implementation phase is planned prior to the purchase of the system. Once the organization has purchased the information system, the implementation phase continues. A project leader is identified and a team of hospital staff is selected to support the project as a working committee. The steering committee chairperson or another member of the steering committee may serve as the implementation project leader. Either the chief information officer, strategy officer, an informatics specialist, project manager, or a consultant experienced in this area may serve in this capacity. It is important, however, that the project leader be involved in the entire selection and implementation process and possess strong leadership and communication skills. This ensures that the project leader has a firm understanding of the vision, goals, and expectations for the system.

The committee membership should include technical staff from the information services department, informatics representatives, and clinical representatives who are familiar with current manual or automated procedures (Summers & Jerard 2006). Each group should include managers who have the authority to make the decisions and department staff who have knowledge and experience of day-to-day operations as well as an understanding of how those processes might be improved. Recruiting efforts should focus on people who display the characteristics that support effective group dynamics and represent all key stakeholders. In addition, the project leader should facilitate the development of effective group dynamics. Any effort that involves the implementation of a system for nurses or that will be used by nurses should include an informatics nurse specialist or informatics nurse, as these individuals are uniquely qualified to communicate the needs of clinical staff to information services personnel and have a working knowledge of regulatory and system requirements, strategic plans, and budgetary constraints. The informatics nurse specialist and informatics nurses are qualified to identify current problems or issues and help to choose or develop a solution. Organizations that have nursing informatics professionals are more likely to include a representative from the nursing team in decisions involving information technology selection and implementation (CDW 2007). The committee members and organizational issues are every bit as important as the technology itself when implementing a new system. Despite the qualifications of the committee members the group may not select the best system or create the best implementation plan (Summers & Jerard 2006). Box 8–1 lists some of the characteristics of a successful implementation committee.

BOX 8–1   Characteristics of a Successful Implementation Committee

Characteristics of Individual Members

- Communicates openly
- Uses time and talents efficiently
- Performs effectively and produces results
- Welcomes challenges
- Cooperates rather than competes

Group Characteristics

- Works toward a common goal
- Encourages members to teach and learn from one another
- Develops its members' skills
- Builds morale internally
- Resolves conflicts effectively
- Shows pride in its accomplishments
- Enhances diversity of its members

Plan the Installation

The initial work of the implementation committee is to develop a comprehensive project plan or timeline, scheduling all of the critical elements for implementation. This plan should address what tasks are necessary, the scope of each task, who is responsible for accomplishing each element, start and completion dates, necessary resources, and constraints (Figure 8–1). Questions asked at this stage focus on the background of the project, its goals and its sponsor, key stakeholders, benefits, and budget. Clear definition of this phase of the project requires time, energy, and lots of good communication. Failure to adequately address this phase jeopardizes successful implementation. Project planning software may be helpful in developing the project timeline or schedule and a hierarchical arrangement of all specific tasks. This type of plan is referred to as a **work breakdown structure (WBS).** After the project is defined, it is imperative to work on team building, control and execution, and review and exit planning. Inadequate attention to these phases can also jeopardize implementation success.

The committee members should first become familiar with the information system they will be implementing. This can be accomplished in several ways. The vendor can provide on-site training, hospital staff can receive training at the vendor's corporate centers, or third-party consultants may be hired. Vendor training should provide the opportunity to continue to update the skills of employees and to subsequently use them as a resource throughout the implementation process (Schuerenberg 2003). Once committee members have acquired an understanding of how the system functions, they will have the knowledge needed to analyze the base system as delivered from the vendor. Ideally the following issues are addressed during system selection but should be considered by the implementation

Milestone	Person Responsible	Estimated Start Date	Completion Date
PHASE 3: SYSTEM IMPLEMENTATION			
Develop implementation committee			
Analyze customization requirements			
Perform system modifications and customizations			
Analyze hardware requirements			
Develop procedures and user guides			
System and integrated testing			
Provide user training			
Go-live conversion preparation and backloading			
Go-live event			

FIGURE 8–1 • Sample template for a system implementation timeline

committee before the system is installed in the event that clarification or changes are necessary:

- *The technology.* It is important to consider whether the technology that is used is current and can be upgraded easily or is already obsolete. It is also necessary to have a good match between the system and the needs of the area.
- *Vendor standing.* Committee members need to consider vendor history of similar projects as well as financial solvency of the vendor for long-term service and dialog with other customers to determine the implementation issues and resolution (Vendor selection 2007).
- *Vendor compliance with regulatory requirements.* System customization for regulatory compliance can be expensive. It is essential to determine vendor responsibility for federal and state regulatory compliance.
- *Integration with other systems.* It is important to establish how easily the selected system exchanges information with other major systems such as medical records and financial systems (Vendor selection 2007).
- *Use for different types of patient accounts.* Does the system work equally well for inpatient, outpatient, and emergency care encounters?
- *Electronic medical record support.* Does the system support the electronic medical record?

- *Remote access.* Does the product permit secure access to patient data from all locations, particularly remote sites?
- *Clinician support.* Does the product support patient care?

The next step is to decide whether this system should be used as is or customized to meet the specific needs of the organization. This decision will act as the implementation strategy that will guide the committee through the implementation process.

Regardless of which implementation strategy is followed, the committee must next gather information about the data that must be collected and processed. Consideration must be given to the data that are pertinent to each function and available to the user for entry into the system. A **function** refers to a task that may be performed manually or may be automated; some examples include order entry, results reporting, and documentation. The output of the system should also be examined. For example, the format and content of printed requisitions, result reports, worklists, and managerial reports must be evaluated. A detailed analysis of the current work and paper flow will provide this information. Once decisions have been made regarding system design and modification, the appropriate department head should approve these specifications before the actual changes are made. Numerous changes delay implementation of the system and drive up costs.

At this point, the identified changes should be made to the system in the test environment. The **test environment** is one copy of the software where programming changes are initially made. After any changes are made, they must be tested to ensure that they display and process data accurately. Before this can be accomplished, the implementation team and all responsible managers agree on a test plan. This plan includes long-term goals and items to be tested. Testing is best accomplished by following a transaction through the system for all associated functions. In some cases vendors provide a significant cost reduction in product purchases if the buyer is willing to beta test the product. Beta testing occurs on-site under everyday working conditions. Software problems are identified, corrected, and then retested. This follows alpha testing, which is an intensive examination of new software features. An example of this testing procedure might be to enter a physician's order for an x-ray into the system for a particular client. The correct printing of the requisition should be verified. Next, the results of the x-ray are entered for this client. Both online results retrieval and printed report content should be verified. Finally, the system is checked to make certain that the appropriate charges have been generated and passed onto the financial system. It is important to realize that the test environment is not exactly the same as the live environment, because the live environment is much larger and more complex. As a result, the findings of the system test may not always indicate how well the system will perform in the live environment. To help ensure that testing is valid, it is essential to involve a number of people from information services, the implementation committee, or a quality assurance group. Select end-users must be involved to put the test environment through the same type of stresses and rigors as occur in daily work processes.

Analyze Hardware Requirements

A separate group of tasks related to the analysis of hardware requirements must also be addressed during the implementation phase. These tasks should be initiated early in the implementation phase and continue simultaneously while system design and modifications are being completed. Some of these items include the following:

- *Network infrastructure.* The determination of network requirements, cable installation, wiring and access points, and technical standards should be initiated early in the implementation phase. The processing power, memory capacity of network components, and anticipated future needs must be addressed by the technical members of the implementation committee or other information services staff. This is particularly important because the majority of current network outages and downtime now result from cabling issues and are costly in terms of lost productivity and customer dissatisfaction (Mouton & McNees 2003). Extensive changes to network configuration are expensive and should be avoided whenever possible. Wireless technology is not an alternative in some cases. Some functions that place a heavy demand on the network include digital imaging and archival, and telemedicine.
- *Type of workstation or mobile device.* The system may be accessed via a number of different devices. These may include a networked personal computer (PC), thin client, wireless or handheld device such as a personal digital assistant (PDA), or mobile laptop PC that uses radiofrequency technology. The committee must investigate the advantages of each option and make recommendations regarding the type of hardware for purchase and installation. Once a decision has been made regarding the type of workstation, the appropriate number of devices per area or department must be determined.
- *Workstation location strategy.* A related workstation decision is the strategy for locating and using the hardware. Several options are available. **Point-of-care** devices are located at the site of client care, which is often at the client's bedside in the emergency department, delivery room, operating room, and radiology. Another strategy involves a centralized approach, where workstations are located at the unit station. A third option is to use handheld or mobile devices that may be accessed wherever the staff finds it most convenient.
- *Hardware location requirements.* The area where the equipment is to be placed or used must be evaluated as to whether there are adequate electrical receptacles, cabling constraints, and/or reception and transmission capabilities. In addition, the work area may require modifications to accommodate the selected hardware. Another major consideration is the need to protect health information from casual view.
- *Printer decisions.* The various printer options should be examined, even though the need to print documents has decreased. The defacto standard is laser printer technology, but some label printers use dot matrix. Ink jet

printers appear occasionally in low traffic locations. Other decisions focus on features such as the number of paper trays and fonts. Printed output requires the same consideration for privacy of information.

Develop Procedures and Documentation

Comprehensive procedures for how the system will be used to support client care and associated administrative activities should be developed before the training process is begun. In this way, training can include procedures as well as hands-on use of the system. One approach is to examine the current nursing policy and procedure manuals and to incorporate new policies and procedures related to automation. System updates provide an opportunity to introduce new, more stringent policies that may not have been supported with the old system (Amatayakul 2007). Information should be included on backup procedures to be used in the event that the system is not running either for reasons of scheduled maintenance or unforeseen circumstances, so that staff is aware of what to do in the case of planned or unexpected system downtime. Scheduled downtime allows for the implementation of changes in the system. Unscheduled downtime may occur with server, application, network, or electrical problems. It may be beneficial to develop separate documentation that includes the downtime procedures and manual requisition forms and to have this located in an easily identifiable and accessible location.

System user guides should also be developed at this point. These documents explain how to use the system and the printouts that the system produces (Saba & McCormick 1996). User guides provided by the vendor may be adequate if a limited number of modifications were made to the base system. However, if significant modifications have been made, it is necessary to customize documentation to reflect the system as the users will see it. In this case, user guides cannot be completed until all modifications have been completed, tested, and approved for the live system.

Another important aspect of documentation is the development of a dictionary of terms and mapping terms from one system to another. This ensures that everyone has a clear definition of terms and uses them in the same way. Data dictionaries do not contain actual data but list and define all terms used and provide bookkeeping information for managing data. Data dictionaries help to ensure that data are of high quality.

Testing

The process of testing includes the development of a test plan, the creation of test scripts, system testing, and integrated testing. An effective test plan cannot be created until screens and pathways have been finalized and policies and procedures determined. Otherwise, the plan must be revised one or more times. The test plan prescribes what will be examined within the new system as well as all systems with which it shares data. Successful testing requires the involvement of staff that perform day-to-day work because they know the current process and expected outcomes. The test plan should include patient types and functions seen in the facility. A review is then done to identify whether functions are completed without error. Problem areas should be tested again before the person responsible for that area indicates approval and signoff. After system testing, integrated testing can start. Integrated testing looks at the exchange of data between the test system and other systems to ensure its accuracy and completeness.

Provide Training

Once all modifications have been completed in the test environment, a training environment should be established. A **training environment** is a separate copy of the software that mimics the actual system that will be used. Many organizations populate the training database with fictitious clients and make this database available for formal training classes during the implementation process and for ongoing education.

Training is most effective if the training session is a scheduled time independent from the learners' other work responsibilities and at a site separate from the work environment. This allows the learner to concentrate on comprehending the system without interruptions. Planning should address providing adequate resources to allow for the scheduling of training sessions as close as possible to the "go-live" date. In addition, learners should have a place to practice after the formal classroom instruction.

Go-Live Planning

The committee should determine the **go-live** date, which is when the system will be operational and used to collect and process actual client data. At this point, the **production environment** is in effect. The production environment is another term that refers to the time when the new system is in operation. Some of the necessary planning surrounding this event includes the following:

- *Implementation strategy.* It must be determined whether implementation will be staggered, modular, or occur all at once. An example of a staggered implementation strategy may be to go-live in a limited number of client units but in all ancillary departments. The remaining client units would be scheduled to go-live in groups staggered over a specified time frame. The term **roll out** is sometimes used to refer to a staggered, or rolling, implementation. It may also be used in a broader context to refer to both the marketing blitz leading up to implementation and the implementation itself.
- *Conversion to the new system.* Decisions must be made regarding what information will be **backloaded,** or preloaded into the system before the go-live date. This includes identification of who will perform this task and the methodology used to accomplish it. Plans for how orders will be backloaded must be developed. For example, a "daily x 4 days" order for a complete blood cell count should be analyzed to determine how many days will be remaining on the go-live date. This number should be entered when the backload is performed. Backloading may be needed to create

accurate worklists, charges, or medication administration sheets. Plans for verification of the accuracy of preloaded data should be considered.

- *Developing the support schedule.* It often is necessary to provide on-site support around the clock during the initial go-live or conversion phase. Support personnel may include vendor representatives, information system staff, and other members of the implementation committee.
- *Developing evaluation procedures.* Satisfaction questionnaires and a method for communicating and answering questions during the go-live conversion should be provided.
- *Developing a procedure to request post go-live changes.* Priority must be given to changes required to make the system work as it should. Additional changes should go before the implementation committee or hospital steering committee to determine necessity. This process helps to keep costs manageable.

SYSTEM INSTALLATION

Once the production system is turned on users are expected to switch from manual procedures or their prior information system. Generally it takes users longer to perform tasks during this transition period until they become acclimated to changes in workflow and the new system. This can cause stress, frustration, and treatment delays. Adequate support staff must be available 24-7 at the point of care to help users through this process for the first few weeks until they become adept at its use. Typically this is a time that unforeseen problems will surface; problems might include users who did not receive training, access issues, system errors, and failure of the system to perform as designed in all cases. Support staff at the point of care can resolve issues quickly on-site or refer them to appropriate information services staff for follow-up.

Common Implementation Pitfalls

There are several common pitfalls with system implementation. Perhaps the most common is an inadequate understanding of how much work is required to implement the system, resulting in underestimation of necessary time and resources. While figures differ slightly a typical system implementation generally requires 14–18 months (Lee 2007; Winsten 2005). If the initial timeline is not based on a realistic estimate of the required activities and their scope, the implementation process may fall behind schedule. Therefore, it is necessary to fully investigate the impact of the system and control the scope of the project in the early stages of planning.

Another serious problem that may occur during implementation is that of numerous revisions during design activities, creating a constantly moving target. This is sometimes known as "scope creep" or "feature creep." **Scope creep** is the unexpected and uncontrolled growth of user expectations as the project progresses. **Feature creep** is the uncontrolled addition of features or functions without regard to timelines or budget. As needed customizations and modifications are identified, it is imperative that the appropriate user department heads approve and sign off on them before programming changes are made. Frequent changes can become very frustrating for the technical staff and result in missed deadlines. Ultimately, this can be very expensive and emotionally draining for the implementation team.

The amount and type of customization that is done to the information systems can also result in problems. To guide the implementation team, the implementation strategy must address the degree of customization that will be done. One strategy is using the system as delivered by the vendor, with minimal changes. The advantage of this strategy, which is often called the "vanilla system," is an easier and quicker implementation. In addition, future software upgrades may also be implemented with greater ease and speed. The disadvantage of using this system is that user workflow may not match the system design.

The opposite implementation strategy is to fully customize the information system so that it reflects the current workflow. Although this may seem appealing, the disadvantages include a complicated, lengthy, and expensive implementation process. A further disadvantage is seen when system software upgrades are attempted. Many of the customizations may prohibit the upgrades from being installed without extensive programming effort. As a result, the present trend in the hospital information systems industry is to recommend use of the vanilla systems as delivered by the vendors.

Other common pitfalls include failure to consider annual maintenance contracts and related costs, providing insufficient dedicated resources to the implementation committee, and a hostile culture. The vendor's purchase price for a system is only a portion of overall costs. Vendors charge additional fees for annual technical support, customization, and license fees. These charges are levied on the size of the institution or the number of users, which may or may not be concurrent. Additional costs may include hardware, operating or report software needed to support the system, site preparation, uninterrupted power systems, installation, and ongoing operating costs such as maintenance, supplies, personnel, and upgrades. Clinical representatives of the implementation committee cannot be expected to manage a full-time clinical position while contributing significant time to the implementation project. Because the end result of effective implementation is improved client care, it may be cost-effective to temporarily reassign clinical staff to the project. Project success is impeded by a hostile culture, resistance to change, and refusal to see the benefits of technology.

There may also be problems with testing. These can include poorly developed test scripts, inadequate time to retest problem areas, and the inability to get other systems to exchange data with the test system. Inadequate testing can lead to unpleasant surprises at the time of roll-out or go-live.

All too often, training suffers from inadequate allocation of time and resources. The training environment should mirror the testing environment and later the production environment. Design may not be completed when training starts. This creates a negative impression of the system among end users, as well as confusion.

Finally, it is important to continually reinforce the concept that the implementation and the information system are owned by the users. If the users feel no ownership of the system, they may not accept the system or use it appropriately, nor will they provide feedback regarding potential system improvements. In the event that the implementation does not proceed as planned it is important to determine the problem (Alexander et al. 2007; Rodriquez 2005). Common problems include a lack of communication, insufficient support, and inadequate training for users and information technology staff. All stakeholders should receive frequent communication via newsletters, posters, banners, buttons, and informational meetings. Input from all stakeholders must be solicited and evaluated. It is important to work with the vendor to resolve issues rather than assign blame. Consider whether the scope of the project was clearly defined, responsibilities assigned, parties empowered to perform their jobs, and whether project milestones have been defined and tracked.

MAINTENANCE

After implementation of the system, ongoing maintenance must be provided.

User Feedback and Support

One important aspect of maintenance is communication. Soon after the go-live event, feedback from the implementation evaluation should be acted on in a timely manner. This is usually the first aspect of system maintenance to be addressed. The results should be compiled, analyzed, and communicated to the users and information services staff. Any suggested changes that are appropriate may then be implemented.

Continued communication is imperative for sharing information and informing users of changes. Communication can be accomplished in a variety of ways. For example, a newsletter or printed announcement can be sent to the users, on either a regular or an as-needed basis. System messages can be displayed on the screen or printed at the user location. Focus groups or in-house user groups can be formed for discussion and problem solving.

Another form of user support is the help desk. The **help desk** provides round-the-clock support that is usually available by telephone. Most organizations designate one telephone number as the access point for all users who need help or support related to information systems. The help desk is usually staffed by personnel from the information systems area who have had special training and are familiar with all of the systems in use. Often they are able to help the user during the initial telephone call. If this is not possible, the help desk may refer more complex problems or questions to other staff who have specialized knowledge. The help desk should follow up with the user and provide information as soon as it is available. The biggest problems during go-live occur with sign-on and passwords. Users may have missed training or may not remember how to sign on to the system.

Visibility of the support staff in the user areas is another important form of support. By making regular visits to all areas, the support staff is able to gather information related to how the system is performing and impacting the work of the users. In addition, users have the opportunity to ask questions and describe problems without having to call the help desk.

System Maintenance

Ongoing system maintenance must be provided in all three environments: test, training, and production. This enables programming and development to continue in the test region without adverse effect on the training or production systems. Therefore, training can continue without interruption and the training environment can be upgraded to reflect programming changes at the appropriate time. Actual client data and workflow will not be affected in the production system until the scheduled upgrade has been thoroughly tested in the test environment.

Requests submitted by users can provide input for upgrading or making necessary changes to the system. For example, a user might request changes to standard physician orders, such as a request to delete some lab tests to contain costs, or nursing documentation related to regulatory issues or the Joint Commission recommendations, such as adding advanced directives documentation. Advanced directives are used to convey whether the client wishes to be intubated, ventilated, or receive CPR or other lifesaving or life-sustaining measures in the event of a medical emergency. The requesters must provide a thorough explanation of the desired changes, as well as the reason for the request. One method of facilitating this communication is to develop a request form, to be completed by the requesting users and submitted to the information services department. On receiving this form, the information services staff should determine if the change is feasible and should consider whether any alternative solutions exist. Figure 8–2 provides an example of a request for services form.

Technical Maintenance

A large portion of ongoing maintenance is related to technical and equipment issues. This maintenance is the responsibility of the information services department. Some examples of technical maintenance include:

- Performing problem solving and debugging
- Maintaining a backup supply of hardware such as monitors, printers, cables, trackballs, and mice for replacement of faulty equipment in user areas
- Performing file backup procedures
- Monitoring the system for adequate file space
- Building and maintaining interfaces with other systems
- Configuring, testing, and installing system upgrades
- Maintaining and updating the disaster recovery plan

INFORMATION SERVICES REQUEST FOR SERVICES

Requested by: _____ Date: _____

Department: _____

Department Head (print) _____Telephone #: _____

Department Head (signature) _____

Priority: _____Routine _____Urgent Date Request Needed: _____

Requirement: _____

_____

_____

_____

_____

Reason for Request: _____Cost Reduction   _____ Service Improvement

_____ Client Care Improvement   _____ Organizational Requirement

_____ Regulatory Requirement   _____ Other (explain)_____

Please provide other supporting details related to the reason for the request:

FIGURE 8–2 • Request for information services form

FUTURE DIRECTIONS

As users and technical support staff work with the system, they may come to identify problems and deficiencies. Eventually, these faults may become significant enough that the need to upgrade or replace the system becomes evident, illustrating the cyclical nature of the information system's life cycle. Phase 1, the needs assessment phase, is initiated again, and the life cycle continues. In other words, the life cycle is an ongoing process that never ends. Some specific considerations that point to the need for a new system include poor performance, frequent down times, dated programming languages, no vendor support, a difficult user interface, outmoded technology, and inadequate growth capability (Winsten 2005). On the other hand if the system still meets business needs, is reliable, has little unscheduled downtime, is supported by vendors, can sustain growth, presents a high risk of operational disruption with replacement and if available replacements offer no substantial benefits, then it should be retained until these conditions change. One other major consideration for the implementation of a new system is the return on investment (ROI) that it can provide (Arthour 2007; Kaplin 2007; Kywi 2007; Russell & Slate 2007). These can include decreased costs for labor and nonlabor expenses such as maintenance, outsourcing of forms, alignment with business strategy, and increased revenue. Increasingly ROI is also measured in less tangible measures, such as increased patient safety and satisfaction, improved quality of service, system usage and compliance with regulations, and streamlined workflow with improved provider satisfaction, which helps to attract and retain caregivers. Patient and family acceptance are also key to the successful introduction of all health information technology (Wolf et al. 2007). Acceptance is tempered by perception. As staff adjust to new tools they must be reminded to maintain their focus on customer service and care to prevent their actions from being misconstrued as being inattentive. ROI can also be measured via increased gross revenue due to a shortened revenue cycle and better documentation and tracking (Rushnell & Slate 2007). It may take two or more years to realize ROI for IT investments.

The role of nursing A growing number of nurses are drawn to informatics, often as a result of their involvement working on an IT project or deployment (Rollins 2007; HIMSS Nursing Informatics Survey 2007). While not every clinical system is used by nurses directly, most clinical systems impact nurses and the systems that they use in some way. Systems development and implementation have been identified as the top responsibilities for nurse informaticists, followed by liaison, quality initiatives, strategic planning, education, and vendor communication, respectively. Nurse informaticists provide credibility for IT projects. The ability to fulfill these responsibilities is largely dependent upon a supportive environment created at the executive level. Implementation of information technology is a very political process, particularly in the cost-controlled healthcare delivery systems of today. The realization of a successful system for nursing requires a strong nurse leader who is politically savvy and technologically competent (Simpson 2007). The Chief Nursing Officer (CNO) must work with the Chief Information Officer (CIO) and other key players to develop strategies to transform care, prioritizing system design to maximize the value and benefits of a clinical information system, providing abundant bedside access, and re-allocating time saved in documentation and other efficiencies to improve patient care services (Ambrosini 2006; Nagle 2006; Summers & Jerard 2006). This requires executive leadership for change management, involvement of clinicians throughout every phase of the project, and commitment to extensive training of staff to ensure that everyone develops competencies in the use of the system

CASE STUDY EXERCISES

8.1 You are the project director responsible for creating an implementation timeline that addresses the training and go-live activities for a nursing documentation system that will be implemented on 20 units and involves 350 users. Determine whether the implementation will be staggered or occur simultaneously on all units, and provide your rationale.

8.2 Create the timeline for the training and go-live schedule for this implementation.

8.3   Your present manual medication administration record is being replaced by BCMA, an automated information system. Discuss the specifications you would recommend for reports that the system will generate to notify the nurse when medications are due. Determine how often the reports should print and what information they should contain.

8.4   You have been selected to develop test scripts for interface testing for a new patient care system. Develop a test script with multiple interfaces. Define the output that you should see for each system.

8.5   As the manager of the gastrointestinal laboratory in your facility, you are expanding the applications for your information system. At the present, it allows physicians to capture images and produce consults and referral letters in a timely fashion. You have been working with the vendor to expand its features to include capture of patient history. Consider the pros and cons of interchanging information collected by admitting nurses and physicians.

 MediaLink

Additional resources for this content can be found on the Companion Website at www.prenhall.com/hebda. Click on "Chapter 8" to select the activities for this chapter.

- Glossary
- Multiple Choice
- Discussion Points
- Case Studies
- MediaLink Application
- MediaLink

SUMMARY

- One important aspect of system implementation is the development of an effective implementation committee comprising the informatics specialists and the clinical and technical representatives.
- The first task for the committee is the development of a timeline for system implementation activities then stay with it.
- The implementation strategy must be determined by the committee. This strategy may call for using the system as it is delivered by the vendor or significantly customizing the system to match the current work needs.
- Identified modifications are made to the software in the test environment, so that actual client data and workflow are not affected.
- The following hardware considerations must be addressed during the implementation phase: server, type of workstation device, hardware location, printer options, and network requirements.
- User procedures and documentation are developed during the implementation phase, and provide support to personnel during training and actual use of the system.
- Training is a key element for a successful system implementation.

- Careful consideration must be given to planning the go-live conversion activities to minimize disruptions to client care.
- The implementation committee must be aware of the common pitfalls and problems that may negatively affect the implementation process.
- Maintenance, an ongoing part of the implementation process, includes user support and system maintenance.
- The information systems life cycle is a continuous cyclical process.

REFERENCES

Alexander, G. L., Rantz, M., Flesner, M., Diekemper, M., & Siem C. (2007). Clinical information systems in nursing homes. *Computers, Informatics, Nursing, 25*(4), 189–197.

Amatayakul, M. (2007). Updating Policies & Procedures. *ADVANCE for Health Information Executives, 11*(2), 12.

Ambrosini, R. (2006). Chief nursing officer's role in IT and the delivery of care. In C. A. Weaver, C. W. Delaney, P. Weber, & R. L. Carr, (Eds.). *Nursing and Informatics for the 21st century.* Chicago: Healthcare Information and Management Systems Society, 75–79.

Arthour, T. (2007). True value of IT. *ADVANCE for Health Information Executives, 11*(6), 35–38.

CDW Healthcare. (2007). Nurses Talk Tech 2007™: The catch-22 of nursing and information technology. Retrieved December 12, 2007, from http://webobjects.cdw.com/webobjects/docs/pdfs/healthcare/Nurses-Talk-Tech-2007.pdf.

Health Information Management Systems Society (HIMSS). (2007). HIMSS Nursing Informatics Survey. Retrieved December 17, 2007, from http://www.himss.org/content/files/surveyresults/2007NursingInformatics.pdf.

Kaplin, J. (2007). Predicting health. *Healthcare Informatics, 24*(7), 55–56.

Kywi, A. (2007). Connecting Care. *ADVANCE for Health Information Executives, 11*(6), 10–11.

Lee, T. (2007). Nurses'experiences using a nursing information system. *Computers, Informatics, Nursing, 25*(5), 294–300.

Mouton, A. & McNees, R. (July 2003). Does cabling need intelligent monitoring? *Communications News, 40*(7), 24.

Nagle, L. N. (2006). Nurses in chief information officer positions. In C. A. Weaver, C. W. Delaney, P. Weber, & R. L. Carr, (Eds.). *Nursing and Informatics for the 21st century.* Chicago: Healthcare Information and Management Systems Society, pp. 87–93.

Rodriquez, V. (2005). The second time around. *ADVANCE for Health Information Executives, 9*(2), 18.

Rollins, G. (2007, April). Nurses Find New Calling in Information Technology. *Hospitals & Health Networks, 81*(4), 16–18. Retrieved December 13, 2007, from Health Source: Nursing/Academic Edition database.

Rushnell, C. & Slate, J. (2007). Improved revenue cycle. *ADVANCE for Health Information Executives, 11*(6), 26–29.

Saba, V. K. & McCormick, K. A. (1996). *Essentials of computers for nurses.* New York: McGraw-Hill.

Schuerenberg, N. (2003). Going "live" in a hurry. *Health Data Management, 11*(2), 32–36.

Simpson, R. (2007, October). The politics of information technology. *Nursing Administration Quarterly, 31*(4), 354–358. Retrieved December 13, 2007, from CINAHL with Full Text database.

Summers, M. & Jerard, M. (2006). 12 simple rules for implementing clinical systems. *ADVANCE for Health Information Professionals, 10*(6), 47–49.

Winsten, D. (2005). Extending the life of an aging LIS. *ADVANCE for Health Information Executives, 9*(2), 50, 52, 54.

Wolf, D. M., Hartman, L. M., Larue, E. M., & Arndt, I. (2007). Patient first. *Computers, Informatics Nursing, 25*(2), 112–117.

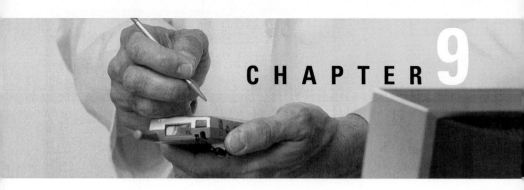

CHAPTER 9

Information Systems Training

After completing this chapter, you should be able to:

1 Describe how learning needs and objectives are determined for end users.

2 List content areas required for information system training.

3 Identify human factors related to information systems.

4 Understand training strategies and blended learning as an instructional approach.

5 Recognize factors that affect learning and knowledge retention.

6 Select training resources that match organizational requirements.

7 Compare two training evaluation methods.

8 Discuss issues associated with training, including scheduling, confidentiality, cost, technology, and training environments.

Information systems (IS) are prevalent in today's healthcare setting and provide software applications that assist clinical staff in the management of computerized client information. Healthcare settings have various needs for information systems (Hillestand et al. 2006). Smaller settings may need only basic support, such as a client database, appointment scheduling software, and the ability to process charges and perform billing functions. Larger institutions require complex financial and comprehensive clinical information systems that are able to support the **electronic health record.** The availability of desktop computers connected to an information system is an inevitable and integral part of the clinical environment. Workplace training activities designed for information systems play an important role in the adoption and integration of computer technology by healthcare workers. Nurses, allied healthcare professionals, and support staff learn to master computer skills in order to access client medical information and document the delivery of care (Duggan 2005). For most workers, information systems are a welcome change and the transition from paper to automation is a smooth one. Some are anxious about learning new skills and what they perceive as the forced use of computers to carry out their job duties. The emotional reaction to the infusion of workplace technology is not unfounded in some situations. As computer applications evolve and manual processes become automated, healthcare workers potentially face job loss or significant changes to work duties in order to meet client and institutional needs (Harvard Business School 2003). Organizations can minimize the perceived negative impact of information technology through a well-planned employee education program. Healthcare administrators need to recognize that education is a key to the successful use of any information system. While educational programs are costly and time consuming, the end result is a knowledgeable work force that can efficiently handle information technology and have a positive effect on the quality of healthcare (Thielst 2007).

THE TRAINING PLAN

An educational strategy aligns with the organization's strategic initiatives and defines the goals, objectives, and action plan for educating workers (Meister 1998). The educational strategy addresses work force training needs for information systems and provides the blueprint for how employees will learn new computer skills. **Training** focuses on acquiring practical knowledge and skilled behaviors and is an organized approach to providing large numbers of staff and healthcare workers with the knowledge needed to use an information system in a clinical setting. Trainers design structured lesson plans that include "learn by doing" activities and practice so that knowledge and skills that are taught can be discretely measured through class exercises and proficiency assessments.

Educators associated with healthcare settings tend to view the term *training* negatively because of its association with behavioral psychology and its focus on behavior change through skill acquisition. This is in contrast to the educational approach of cognitive psychology, which concentrates on learning, thinking, and problem solving as a way to change behavior (Fleming & Levie 1993). Organizations may adopt a more inclusive definition of training and use the terms *training* and *development* to help bridge philosophical differences between trainer and educator roles. Training and development focuses on workplace learning and improving performance using both behavioral and cognitive psychology concepts (Driscoll 2000).

Information system implementation projects require a tactical strategy to deliver training (Barritt et al. 2004). A **training plan** is designed and developed to help ensure instructional success and address the following areas:

- *Training philosophy.* Training is most effective when instruction occurs at a dedicated time, close to the **go-live** date, removed from the work area, and independent of other work responsibilities. The physical environment or classroom where training takes place should be free of work-related interruptions and distractions.
- *Identification of training needs.* There is a general acknowledgment of the importance of studying a training need before deciding upon a training solution. A needs assessment is performed in response to a training request in order to gather information to make a data-driven and responsive recommendation (Rosett & Sheldon 2001). A needs assessment is commonly done early in the implementation planning timeline and leads to the development of instruction. A needs assessment will help to determine who needs to be trained, the content area to be taught, the amount of instruction time needed to master the prescribed tasks, requested equipment, and when and where training will take place. Training needs are reviewed and revised at regular intervals during implementation and when new requests are submitted by the information systems team.
- *Training approach.* Once the initial needs assessment data are analyzed and the task analysis is performed, decisions need to be made about how to plan instructional interventions and deliver the training. Instructional decisions include content development and how the course will be taught. Organizations decide whether to create materials through internal resources, outsource or contract the development of content, or purchase class materials available through the software vendor. Materials purchased through the software vendor are developed for the base information system and may need to be tailored to match any customized build that the organization makes to the base system. Content development or tailoring starts once the detailed implementation plan is complete and clinical design of the system is under way and continues through implementation. Training delivery may include one or a combination of methods, for example, instructor-led, technology-based, or on-the-job training. Job aids and an **electronic performance support system (EPSS)** are integrated into the training methodology. A blended approach may prove to be effective and cost efficient because it has the capability to target different learning styles, enhance knowledge transfer, offer alternatives to classroom instruction, and deliver just in time training (Driscoll 1998).
- *Training resources.* The next step in the training plan is to identify the individuals or group who will coordinate or conduct information systems

training. The selection of training resources is usually completed 6 months prior to implementation. Administrators need to evaluate the availability and skill level of internal resources or decide to contract with outside or vendor-related training professionals. Internal training resources are preferred over external trainers because of their familiarity with the organization and its operational processes and ability to support a flexible training schedule.

- *Timetable and training schedule.* The training timetable is developed in coordination with the projected go-live date of the information system. The factors to consider include the number of users who will need training and the amount of time required to complete the training. The training schedule is designed to allow enough time for learning transfer, practice, and application of skills. The goal is to conduct training as close to implementation as possible. The timetable and schedule is a delicate balance; end user training conducted too early in the implementation process may require retraining before go-live. Individuals trained late in the implementation process may need additional support once the system is in use.

- *Budget and costs.* Training is consistently an under-budgeted item within an organization (Slater 1998). Gartner Research reports that each hour of effective training is worth 5 hours to the organization. Well-trained users reach required skill levels in less than a quarter of the time, require less assistance from peers and less calls to the help desk, and spend less time correcting errors (Aldrich 2000). Although training is time consuming and labor-intensive, it should be considered an investment in enhancing work force knowledge and as a measurement in the successful implementation of an information system. The considerations for estimating the direct cost of information system training include salary for training resources, trainee coverage or replacement during training, cost of materials, educational technology and equipment, travel expenses, and space allocation. Implementation training requires thoughtful planning and careful allocation of resources in order to stay within budget and to minimize indirect costs, such as trainee overtime and unanticipated retraining activities. Organizations interested in determining the overall value of training can use Return on Investment (ROI) metrics. ROI utilizes industry standard financial investment indicators that compare dollar costs to the value added benefits of an innovation. An ROI study done after the implementation of an information system may measure all direct training costs compared to reported reductions in medical errors, timeliness of charting, a decrease in staff turnover, and an increase in employee job satisfaction and productivity (Phillips & Phillips 2005).

- *Evaluation strategy.* The purpose of an information systems training evaluation strategy is to collect subjective participant feedback about the learning experience, identify pre- and post-training skill gaps, and measure knowledge and performance of the stated learning objectives. The ultimate success of training is measured by the ability of the participant to perform the targeted computer skills.

There are two popular program evaluation models, a traditional approach to training intervention evaluation and a process evaluation approach. The Kirkpatrick Level 4 Model is an example of a simple, intervention-based approach to evaluation. Many organizations have been interested in a process-based evaluation and have adopted the targeted evaluation process (TEP) as an evaluation methodology. TEP is a process approach that allows for a full range of evaluation tools, technology, and techniques (Combs & Falletta 2000).

Some organizations require proficiency testing and provide remediation so that all employees can achieve the necessary skill level. If instruction is delivered through the use of technology, it can often be set up to provide immediate feedback and supplemental practice for employees to learn the new skills. Technology based instruction can evaluate, measure progress, and track the acquisition of skills of each employee (Newbold 1996).

IDENTIFICATION OF TRAINING NEEDS

The training preparation process begins by identifying user needs, determining content, establishing learning objectives, and deciding upon the approach and evaluation strategy. The delivery process begins by creating the training timetable, allocating space, and defining hardware and software requirements. The training budget and all associated costs are monitored throughout the preparation and delivery process. Administrators review budget reports and may request adjustments to how training dollars are being spent at any point during implementation. Budgetary changes during the course of implementation may affect how training content is created and delivered; for example, an instructor-led approach may switch to a technology-based one, or external trainers may be replaced by internal training resources.

End User Training Needs

Healthcare workers who use an information system to view or document client information are called **end users.** End users are identified and grouped by job class responsibilities to guide what applications and level of access they will have in the information system. The training needs of each job class are determined according to what functions each will perform. Administrators decide what applications or modules will be automated first, and end user training is delivered respective to these decisions. The client database and registration modules for admissions, discharges, and transfers are usually implemented first, followed by clinical documentation and physician order entry.

Most end users have access to view client demographic data, allergies, diagnosis, emergency contacts, and recent medical history. Information systems are designed so that security levels can be set and access or functionality can be restricted for some job classes and not others. Access to sensitive client information and advanced system functionality may be given to physicians, nurses, and supervisors while restricted from administrative support personnel. Laws governing professional practice also help to determine the degree of access

BOX 9–1   Who Might Need Training?

Providers

- Physicians and Residents
- Nurse practitioners
- Midwives
- Physician assistants
- Dentists

Non-providers who provide care

- Registered nurses
- Licensed practical nurses
- Pharmacists
- Nutritionists and Dieticians
- Respiratory therapists
- Occupational therapists
- Speech therapists
- Physical therapists
- X-ray technicians
- Patient care and medical assistants

Students

- Students from all professional and technical healthcare programs
- Medical students

Support Personnel

- Admission clerks
- Dietary personnel
- Social service staff
- Home healthcare personnel
- Pastoral care staff
- Housekeeping personnel
- Central supply staff
- Case managers
- Unit clerks and secretaries
- Infection control and quality assurance personnel
- Persons who check insurance authorization; billers and individuals who enter charges

assigned to an end user. See Box 9–1 for a matrix of end users who may need information system training.

User class defines the level of access to an information system. A **user class** is defined and categorized as the personnel who perform similar functions. Representatives from clinical areas can help identify user classes based upon job descriptions. The user class refines the types of training classes needed for implementation. For example, provider training classes may include physicians, residents, nurse practitioners, and physician assistants as they use similar information. However, physicians would have additional security access to allow them to review and co-sign orders. Non-provider training classes may include registered nurses (RNs) and ancillary department staff. RNs are provided with a higher level of security in accordance with their scope of practice to include order entry, processing of physician orders, charting medication administration, and documenting client medical information. The licensed practical nurse (LPN) is another example; an LPN needs to view and document client information but may not perform order entry functions. Higher-level user classes, such as registered nurses, may perform functions assigned to lower-level classes to allow them to carry out functions assigned to support personnel when these personnel are unavailable.

Replacement staff and students who commonly rotate through institutions also need to use the information system. The degree of automation within the institution determines what groups require computer training. For example, if physician order entry is the only automated function, then neither replacement staff nor students may need training. In healthcare settings where system access is required for the retrieval of data or to document client information, training is necessary for replacement staff to perform their job. Students may opt to attend training as an educational experience in order to learn and acquire job related computer skills.

Training Class Content

Project scope is the information systems term used to describe the details of the system functionality that is slated for automation. Learning objectives and training class content are developed in accordance with the project scope document and when changes are made during implementation. Learning objectives reflect the information system functionality defined for the end users within a user class. For example, learning objectives for the documentation of vital signs by a nursing assistant would include the ability to: log in to the system, access the client record, accurately record and save the vital sign data, and retrieve the entered vital signs at the end of the training activity.

Training class content should address the following topics:

* *Computer-related policies.* The training class provides an excellent environment to discuss client confidentiality policies, ethical computing, and penalties for the inappropriate use and access to data within the information system. Most organizations require employees to sign confidentiality statements that advise against sharing user access codes and passwords. Employees may receive their user access code and password at the completion of training. In some organizations, the application for access to the information system is completed by the employee's supervisor. An **access code** or user ID is some form of unique identifier and provides authentication of the end user's identity within the information system. The entry point or log in to the information system may require both an access code and a password. Note that some information systems have a more sophisticated mechanism to identify an end user, such as biometric fingerprint authentication, iris or retinal scans, and voice

recognition technology (Woodward et al. 2002). Equipment will need to be available to support the training of these technologies.

- *Access privileges.* End users, such as students and other non-employees, may be required to sign additional documents regarding access to an information system. Organizations need to protect client information, and any misuse of privileges should result in loss of clinical privileges and possible legal action. Two examples of misuse might include viewing the medical record of a high profile client for no clinical reason or failure to properly handle and dispose of confidential paper reports.

- *Human factors.* The implementation of an information system presents a major disruption in the work setting, especially when an organization transitions from minimal automation to a complex computing environment (Harvard Business Review 2003). Organizations may use educational strategies to prepare the workforce for technology. Pre-implementation presentations, hands-on demonstrations, bulletin board messages, tent cards, newsletter articles, administrative role modeling, and unit level champions help to ease the associated anxiety and uncertainty of change. The classroom may provide a safe place for employees to learn about change, ask questions, and realize the benefit of automating their work processes.

- *Computer literacy.* Employees may lack fundamental computer skills and knowledge. A separate needs assessment may be required in the pre-implementation phase. This needs assessment may be completed through Human Resources so that basic job competencies can be identified and met before the introduction of an information system and its associated training. Organizations that need to provide basic computer literacy training may send employees to outside computer training classes, provide on-site sessions, or use computer based training software.

- *Workflow.* The transition from manual work to automation is considered a cultural change in the work setting (Harvard Business Review 2003). Employees are expected to learn new ways to carry out current job duties or accept new responsibilities in a technology enhanced work environment. Workflow diagrams that visually display new processes help end users to understand what is expected of them and eases their transition into the information age.

- *Scenario and step-by-step design of instruction.* Training content can be designed in formats that enhance end user knowledge retention and target different learning styles. Scenario-based content provides medical case studies in a realistic frame of reference in which trainees work through, for example, the client admission process (Guite et al. 2006). Another effective instructional technique is the use of step-by-step exercise and practice that can be used to demonstrate the electronic order entry process. For example, trainees can practice entering different types of orders and then view the expected results. The accurate completion of step-by-step exercises can serve as proof of skill acquisition.

- *Electronic help.* Reference documents, context level help screens, and online tutorials can be beneficial provided that they are accurate, easily accessible, user friendly, and that the end user knows of their existence. Reference documents are usually a minimum of 2 pages in length, provide topic specific help, and are saved in portable document format (PDF). Reference documents are most helpful if they can be accessed through a **hyperlink** within the information system, have a logical name, and are alphabetically organized on a list. **Context sensitive help** topics are available throughout the software and provide directions at the screen and field level to help end users to complete a particular task. **Online tutorials** provide computer animation or written instructions for how to use the software application or one of its features. Online tutorials are available for referral at any time. Training classes should introduce online help features, demonstrate their use, and provide directions for how to access them.

- *Error messages.* **Error messages** are generated by an information system to warn of missing information or data entry errors. Error messages alert end users that they need to correct or add information. Some examples include missing data in a required field or a medication order that needs one or more of the following fields completed or corrected: drug name, dosage, route, or administration schedule. Failure to satisfy the error message may prevent the end user from proceeding or completing an order, procedure, or documentation. Error messages are a safety feature designed to reduce or prevent client documentation or clinical charting related mistakes. Class content should address how error messages are generated, tips to prevent them, and how they can be corrected in the information system.

- *Error correction.* Data entry errors result from typographical or misspelled words within free text fields or by selecting an incorrect choice from selection boxes or drop-down menus. Corrections can be made at the time of entry and before saving or at a later date and time. For example, some clinical documentation systems provide an opportunity to review and correct information before processing the data. Data entry errors can be corrected after processing; however, the information system maintains an audit trail that records all changes made to the computer record. Quality assurance personnel may review the audit logs and track data entry errors for frequency, severity, and degree of risk to client safety. These audit trail error logs also provide information systems analysts with data. Trends in data entry errors can be studied so that changes to the information system can be made that would help to reduce these common data entry errors. Training content should include drill and practice exercises to familiarize end users with performing accurate data entry and completion of electronic forms.

- *Screen and system "freezes."* **Freezing** refers to a situation where the end user is logged in to the information system but is unable to enter or process data. Possible causes include a workstation malfunction, computer network overload, order queue processing issue, or a system crash. Depending on the root cause, a freeze may be a momentary slowdown or a more serious problem resulting in downtime. Training content should include basic troubleshooting guidelines and information about how to report a problem to the information systems help desk.

- *System idiosyncrasies.* Information system developers attempt to develop software applications that are intuitive and easy to use (Thielst 2007). System design, programming, and technical platform determine what an information system can and cannot do. One goal of software development is to provide automated solutions to manual processes. Automated solutions often handle information in a way that is very different from the manual process. This change in process may initially disrupt the **comfort zone** of the end user and seem counter-intuitive. Graphical user interfaces (GUI) help end users adjust to doing their work electronically. In some situations, major programming changes need to be done to accommodate complex workflows. Programming changes and customization are costly and require development time. Organizations may decide to delay or forego system enhancements. For this reason, healthcare workers need to understand the limitations of their information system.

- *Equipment maintenance and basic troubleshooting.* Some problems are easy to fix, such as a loose computer cable or unplugged electrical cord. Most printing issues stem from an empty paper tray or toner cartridge. Other problems are more complex and require some basic troubleshooting knowledge. Training content should include instructions for creating desktop shortcuts and icons and for adjusting computer settings, such as mouse speed and screen colors. Organizations may lock down workstations in order to limit end user changes to the desktop, for example, to prohibit changes to the display background or to the screen saver. The importance of logging out of both the workstation and the information system should be emphasized in the training session. End users who know how to troubleshoot and know who to contact for help will save time and maintain a high level of productivity (Regan & O'Connor 2000).

- *Downtime procedures.* Information systems personnel carefully plan **computer downtime** to perform system or code maintenance and upgrades. Planned downtime is scheduled at a time when few end users are routinely logged into the information system, usually during the early morning hours. Unplanned but scheduled downtime can happen at any time; for example, a software fix is necessary and needs to be installed immediately into the information system. Unplanned and unscheduled downtime can happen at any time when the network or computer hardware malfunctions. Downtime procedures are not implemented unless downtime is expected to last for several hours. The administrator on call usually decides when to start using downtime procedures. Paper medication administration records, clinical and lab reports, and manual requisitions are used during an information system downtime. Downtime procedures should be introduced during training and should be reviewed annually. It is also important to review downtime procedures if the system will be out of operation for an extended scheduled downtime.

- *Ability to retrieve and view clinical information.* An information system changes the way nurses and healthcare workers view clinical data. Data elements can be sorted, filtered, and displayed in different ways; for example, test results can be displayed by test, by date, or graphically on a flow sheet. Training activities should include hands-on activities to practice how to retrieve data. Table 9–1 displays sample screen options that permit review of a client's laboratory results using any one of a variety of data sorting and filtering options.

TABLE 9–1   Sample Screen Options for Retrieving Lab Result and Graphical Display

Screen Option	Training Activity	Information Retrieved
For the most recent tests	Filter on a date range or sort chronologically	Provides results of the most recent results
For today	Sort by date	Lists all laboratory results for the current date
For the previous 2 days	Filter on a date range	Shows laboratory results from the previous 2 days
From the time of admission	Column sort by order	Displays all laboratory results from admission to the present time, in either chronological or reverse chronological order
Previous admissions	Retrieval by admission date	Lists laboratory findings by dates of previous admissions
Department specific, e.g., chemistry, hematology, or microbiology	Filter or sort by department	Allows practitioners to quickly find a particular result, such as a wound culture
Glucose values for a date range	Graphical display	

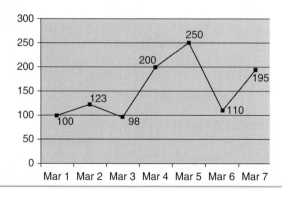

Class Schedules

The timing of end user training can be a challenge that requires careful planning and flexibility when scheduling class times. Factors to consider include trainee availability, class length, and location. Healthcare organizations are a 24×7 operation. Since employees may work rotating, flexible, or steady shifts, the class schedule must accommodate end user availability to attend classes. Class length depends on the amount of content that needs to be covered and can range from 1- to 8-hour sessions. It is often difficult for employees to leave their clinical area during a shift for training without disrupting patient care and ensuring adequate coverage. Conversely, scheduling classes before or after work shifts will contribute to fatigue, decreased concentration, and lack of attention to the training. Employees who are tired or distracted will not retain what they need to know regarding the use of the information system. Successful training strategies provide a plan that includes dedicated training days in which the participants are relieved of clinical duties and can focus on training activities.

Instructors need to be available to deliver training to accommodate employees working all shifts. Preparation time for each class must be factored into the training team schedule, as back-to-back classes may target different audiences. Planning and preparation in advance will make the training effort and classroom experience less stressful and more productive for both the trainers and trainees. As mentioned earlier in this chapter, the timetable for training should be developed to allow adequate days to reach all end users and should be scheduled as close to the go-live date as possible. Computer instruction is most effective when provided no more than one month before the actual anticipated use in the work setting (Craig 2002).

Hardware, Software, and Environment Requirements

The end user learning experience is most effective when the hardware, software, and computer training environment match what the end user will use in the clinical setting. Administrators who understand the importance of training will support these requirements. Ideally, each trainee will have a networked computer workstation that is connected to peripherals, such as printers, fax machines, scanners, hand-held devices, and any other specialized equipment. The **computer training environment** is defined as a software or application copy of the information system's production environment. The environment is stripped, which means that actual client or **live data** and employee data are removed after the copy process. This ensures that client and employee data are kept confidential. The copy of the production environment for the training environment is done close to the start of implementation training in order to capture as much of the customized application build as possible. Any additional changes made to the production environment must be replicated for training. The trainers are responsible for creating training data that will be uploaded into the training environment. Training data includes simulated client and employee databases, log in and access codes, orders and procedures, medications, alerts, admission history, and test results. Trainers design instruction and the training environment to meet the learning needs of the various user classes and disciplines employed within the organization. Since no training should occur on the actual system, the training and information system teams work together to coordinate and plan the creation, support, and maintenance of the training environment. The training team needs to be included in the information systems project team status meetings to keep up to date with application build and production environment changes, such as code and software updates that may impact the training environment.

Training Costs

The largest line item in a training initiative budget is salary for trainers, administrative support, and for replacement staff coverage, while end users attend training sessions. Training is considered expensive primarily because of the personnel hours required to support a training function (Filipczak 1996). For this reason, salary costs for the following staff must be considered:

- *Trainers.* Trainers are accountable for the development of training to support an information system implementation. Trainer time is spent assessing, developing, delivering, evaluating, and supporting training activities. External, contract, or vendor-supplied trainers may prove to be costly in the long run. Organizations may choose to hire trainers or recruit current employees for information system training.
- *Administrative support staff.* Staff is needed to support the trainers and training function through clerical support, typing, copying, collating materials, and registering and tracking attendees. Administrative support staff may also help with preparing class materials, such as using special-ized software to prepare job aids, create presentations, and convert files for electronic and Web applications.
- *Employee training.* End users can be either salaried or hourly employees. Compensation for time spent in training may be considered a "work" day for exempt employees and documented at the regular hourly rate for non-exempt staff. Employee overtime can be kept to a minimum if the training schedule is flexible and can accommodate the various shift and work schedules. Clinical and department supervisors should have access to the training schedule in advance in order to schedule employee training and plan for coverage or replacement staff. Training classes held on the weekend may accommodate exempt and weekday employees, who can use compensation time at a later date.
- *Replacement staff.* Implementation training is mandatory in most organ-izations. Unit and department supervisors must arrange coverage for employees attending training. Replacement staff may be needed during times when regular staff is not available to cover the clinical areas.

Some other line items in the training budget to consider include the purchase of training materials from the vendor and desktop software applications to support training and development, such as file conversion software, authoring packages, and Web development tools. Training materials, if purchased from the vendor, usually need to be edited due to information system customization. Some organizations may decide to develop training materials and not purchase them. In either scenario, trainer desktop workstations may need additional memory or disk space to support the training software applications.

Training Center

The training center or classroom space planning starts in the early phase of the implementation plan. As emphasized in this chapter, learning and knowledge transfer is most effective when instruction is conducted away from the work area and free of work-related interruptions and distractions. A dedicated training space allows for trainees to focus on what is being taught and encourages retention of information. Training conducted in the work areas should be limited to short in-services and just-in-time sessions to address critical issues. Classroom space located within the organization is recommended in terms of convenience, travel and parking, and closeness to technical support. In multisite facilities, temporary classrooms can be strategically set up for implementation training. When classroom space is not available within the organization, convenience of location, travel time, parking or shuttle service, and technical connectivity are considerations for the selection of an offsite facility. Box 9–2 lists some factors to consider when selecting a training site. The physical and learning environment of the classroom or facility should be a comfortable and calm learning space. The use of ambient lighting, a comfortable temperature and ventilation, and workstation ergonomics that allow chair, desk, and workstation adjustments minimize fatigue and prevent repetitive stress injuries.

Once the implementation training is complete, the classroom space may serve other purposes, for example, as the implementation system go-live command center, for one-on-one training and support, computer-based learning, and end user requests for space to practice and review the information system. The workstations can be set up to access either the training environment or the production system.

Training Approaches

The overall training approach should be consistent with the organization's philosophy and should consider the various disciplines that make up the workforce (Abla 1995; Fender & Jennerich 1997; Glydura, Michelman, & Wilson 1995). A blended approach to training may prove to be effective to target different learning styles and promote knowledge transfer (Horton 2001). A blended approach includes one or a combination of methods, for example, instructor-led, technology-based, or on-the-job training (Troha 2002). Job aids and an **electronic performance support system (EPSS)** are considered adjuncts to training and are integrated into the approach (Driscoll 1998). Classroom technology and teaching tools are welcome and necessary elements for supporting the training approach. The minimum equipment includes a separate instructor workstation connected to a printer, ceiling mounted data projector, wireless mouse, white boards, and laser pens. Classroom techniques that engage the

BOX 9–2 Selecting a Training Site: Factors to Consider

- **Classroom availability and cost.** Training is ideal if it can be delivered on-site. However, space within the organization may not be available. Off-site locations should be evaluated to ensure network access and classroom capacity requirements. Rental or leasing costs need to be considered in the decision-making process.
- **Network connectivity and power supply.** Network compatibility and an adequate power supply for workstations are considerations for creating a classroom in an existing space. Administration may need to do a cost comparison to determine if off-site alternatives are an appropriate choice.
- **Classroom capacity.** All trainees should have their own networked workstation and access to a printer and other peripherals as needed to learn the expected job skills.
- **Travel and parking.** An off-site training facility needs to be easy to find, accessible from major roadways, a short driving distance from the primary work site, and have adequate parking,
- **Communication access.** An on-site training location provides participants with the close proximity to their department or work unit. Telephones and other communication tools, such as access to e-mail, need to be available in the classroom so that participants can check voice messages, e-mail, or take calls for urgent clinical issues during the training session.
- **Training environment.** The classroom must have access to the computer training environment so that training can be conducted where there is no actual client or employee data.
- **Setup costs.** Setup costs include cabling and wiring at any location, office furniture, hardware, software, and peripheral equipment. Off-site facilities may also require construction to accommodate training requirements. Additional security measures may need to be added to protect equipment and data.
- **Maintenance costs.** Maintenance costs are driven by the decision to buy, remodel, build, or lease space and the need to maintain and service hardware, software, and office equipment.

participants, such as active participation, group activities, hands-on exercises, and other various instructional approaches, enhance attention and learning. The use of an **advanced organizer** is a way to guide the instruction, manage time, and allow for logical breaks in the classroom instruction (Fleming & Levie 1993). A sample scenario describing a blended approach is described as follows:

> The instructor welcomes the class, reviews housekeeping details, and introduces participants to each other through an icebreaker. A slideshow follows that explains the class content. A copy of the agenda is distributed in the advanced organizer format. The instructor demonstrates system access and log in through the trainer workstation and data projector. The participants practice logging with a training access code and password, following step-by-step instructions listed in their training manual. The instructor uses a slideshow and lecture to review confidentiality policies. There is a short break. The instructor proceeds with the training session using a combination of lecture, scenario-based demonstrations, and hands-on practice. A case study is presented and the participants work as a group to complete the assignment. After lunch, the participants log in

to the workstation and access a computer-based training (CBT) module located on the organization's intranet to learn about Order Entry. The CBT is completed at the learner's own pace. The learner completes an online evaluation of the CBT, which automatically provides feedback to the instructor and creates a computer generated report and proficiency assessment score of the participant's progress for Order Entry. After the afternoon break, the session continues with instructor-led lecture, drill and practice exercises, and step-by-step assignments that are reviewed one on one with the instructor. Another group exercise follows. At the end of the training session, the participants complete an online proficiency test, which is automatically scored. Participants return for remediation, as needed. The instructor records attendance and test scores, then prepares for the next class...

This use of blended delivery includes a combination of approaches to maximize retention, target learning styles, and allow the participant to actively participate in learning activities. See Box 9–3 for factors to consider when choosing training methods.

Many types of training delivery method options exist, including instructor-led classroom instruction, computer-based training, online multimedia or Web-based training, online tutorials, on-the-job training, peer training, videotaped sessions, job aids, and self-directed text-based exercises. Other options include threaded discussions, video conferencing, and simulation (Simonson et al. 2003). Instuctor-led instruction continues to be the most popular approach even though it is resource intensive (Zielstorff 1996). Box 9–3 provides specific factors to consider when selecting a training method, and Table 9–2 outlines advantages, disadvantages, and organizational tips for each instructional approach.

Blended learning has grown in popularity; however, adopting this approach for information systems training requires that it is appropriate for the content that needs to be taught (Rosett & Sheldon 2001) and that the organization's network infrastructure can support electronic training delivery. Web-based training may prove appropriate for information systems training. **Webcasts** are a popular push technology in which Web-based information is sent to

---

BOX 9–3 Selecting a Training Method: Factors to Consider

- **Time.** The time required to develop and present material using each instructional approach varies; for example, lectures can be written and revised quickly and content can be delivered to a large number of participants at one time.
- **Cost.** Initial content development time and subsequent revisions can be lengthy for computer based training. CBT may be cost prohibitive in terms of the number of personnel hours needed to develop, support, and revise this approach.
- **Learning styles.** Blended delivery includes a combination of approaches that target learning styles and allow learners to actively participate in training activities.
- **Learning retention.** Active participation through scenarios, case studies, practice exercises, and repetition provide opportunities for learning, applying job skills, and retaining knowledge.

TABLE 9–2 Advantages, Disadvantages, and Tips Associated with Various Training Approaches

Training Approach	Advantages	Disadvantages	Tips for Effective Organizational Use
Instructor-led class	Flexible Easy to update Can include demonstration Allows for individual help Can test proficiency	Often relies on lecture ↑ Class size ↓ effectiveness of demonstrations Consistency varies with trainer Difficult to maintain pace good for all	For each user group: • Keep a file with objectives and exercises • Use the same presentation order • Use generic examples unlikely to change over time Never rely on just one trainer—leaves no paper trail for others to follow
Computer-based training (CBT)	Self-paced Interactive ↑ Retention—uses technology to teach technology 24-hour availability Can be offered online or offline Can be done in increments Facilitates mastery learning Emulates "real" system without threat of harm	Time and labor intensive to develop and revise Requires great attention to accompanying materials Limited usefulness of vendor supplied materials that are not specific to customization Lacks the flexibility of access to an actual information system—only programmed options can be tried	Trainer serves as a facilitator Needs specific, well-prepared learning aids
Online multimedia	Interactive Stimulates multiple senses for ↑ retention May allow user to bookmark and return to the same spot Can test proficiency	Requires intense planning, resources for design, and revision Less flexible to revise	Use and revise carefully

Training Approach	Advantages	Disadvantages	Tips for Effective Organizational Use
Online tutorials	24-hour availability Allows immediate application of learning Can test proficiency May allow user to bookmark and return to the same spot	Design and revision more involved than instructor-led training	Must have access from all locations and availability must be known
E-mail	Provides individual feedback on entry errors Provides a mechanism for all users to ask questions	Too slow for actual training	Effective for announcements and updates
Video	24-hour availability Easily revised/ updated Extends resources	Not interactive Appropriateness limited to select content such as ethical issues—not actual training	Use on a limited basis
Web-based	Can be accessed from any networked PC Provides 24-hour availability Easily updated and revised May allow user to bookmark and return to the same spot Can test proficiency	Requires knowledgeable Webmaster Requires an existing intranet that can be accessed by all employees	Include online learner assessment
On-the-job training	Individualized Permits immediate application Can test proficiency	Trainer often does not know educational principles May lose productivity of two workers Seasoned employees may pass on poor habits Difficult to achieve with many interruptions	Trainer must know basic adult education principles May work well for unit clerks, working in pairs

(continued)

TABLE 9-2 (continued)

Training Approach	Advantages	Disadvantages	Tips for Effective Organizational Use
Peer training	Training specific to function Can test proficiency	Trainer often does not know educational principles Seasoned employees may pass on poor habits	Trainer must know basic adult education principles May work well for unit clerks, working in pairs or to learn PC applications
Super User	Acquainted with clinical area and the information system May come from any user class Serves as communication link between end users and information system personnel to help resolve issues	Spends time away from clinical responsibilities for additional information system training and meetings	May serve as resource persons particularly during off-shifts May assist with training other users
Job aids	↓ Need to memorize ↓ Training time ↓ Help requests Can be created quickly and inexpensively	Not effective if access is limited	Make accessible and user friendly
Self-directed text-based courses	Self-paced Can test proficiency Lacks interaction with training hospital/system	Requires high level of motivation	Need highly structured materials

participants. Webcasts can be live or recorded instruction. This format allows multiple learners to access a Web site to attend a scheduled class. The learners are able to view a slideshow or multimedia presentation online. Data and audio transmission is usually one-way unless a dial-up communication bridge is used for two-way audio communication between the instructor and the participants. Webcasts generally provide some means for electronic interaction, including online question and answer forums. **Video conferencing** is a media rich, synchronous training approach and has the capability of linking the instructor with participants from various remote sites. Video conferencing is an appropriate delivery approach but requires the organization to purchase and maintain video equipment at various locations and stream compressed video over the computer network (Simonson et al. 2003).

Training Materials Well-designed instructional materials are critical to successful information system training (Abla 1995; Filipczak 1996; Henry & Swartz 1995). **Learning aids** are materials intended to supplement or reinforce lecture- or computer-based training. Learning aids may include outlines, diagrams, charts, or conceptual maps. **Job aids** are written instructions designed to be used as a reference in both the training and work settings. Materials supplied by the software vendor needs to be evaluated for quality and consistency and usually require edits due to information system customization. Some organizations may decide to develop training materials and not purchase them. The development can start once the detailed implementation plan is complete and clinical design of the system is under way. The development and revision of training materials may continue throughout implementation. Operational owners should review training materials and content for ease of use, accuracy, and clarity and to ensure that materials reflect workflow processes.

Proficiency Assessments

Some organizations require proficiency assessments. Instruction that is technology based and testing that is done online can be monitored electronically and provide immediate feedback and test scores that measure the acquisition of skills (Vaillancourt 2000). Proficiency assessments are designed to measure learner knowledge retention and ensure that learners can perform the required new job skills. Any instructional approach can accommodate proficiency testing (Sittig et al. 1995). Proficiency assessments can be a criterion-referenced measure to evaluate predetermined competencies, or norm-referenced tools can be used to assess performance relative to peers or other participants. Norm-referenced testing is useful in competitive hiring situations where there are more applicants than positions available. However, this type of testing is not typically used for information system training. If proficiency assessments are administered, procedures need to be in place to score and store paper-based tests, analyze training needs and prescribe remediation from the results, and report findings to administration, as required. Human resources may participate in developing policies and procedures for storing the tests and results. Whenever possible, proficiency assessments should be administered electronically to facilitate scoring, storing, and retrieving individual examination results (White & Weight 2000).

Information System Trainers Administrators decide who will conduct the information system training. Decisions are made based upon available resources, cost factors, recommendations from the information systems project team, stakeholders, and the system selection committee. Training resources may include internal training staff, employees selected who will learn how to deliver training, external and vendor-supplied trainers, and consultants. Organizations must weigh the advantages and disadvantages of each group. Internal training staff are familiar with the culture, operation, and procedures of the organization but may know little about the information system. The choice to use internal trainers

---

BOX 9–4 Selecting a Trainer: Factors to Consider

- **Teaching skills and experience.** Previous training and content development experience is helpful, as well as experience using an information system
- **Ability to interact with groups and individuals.** Most information system training occurs in a classroom with several trainees. The ability to communicate clearly and manage the training needs of the group requires patience and skill. Experienced trainers are adept at keeping the group focused and on schedule. One-on-one communication and occasional individualized training may be needed during implementation.
- **Understanding end users and their responsibilities.** Trainers must have an understanding of the various user classes and their job needs and information system requirements.
- **Training approach.** Trainers should be knowledgeable and comfortable with the selected approach. For example, if computer-based training is used, instructors must be familiar with access, content, and navigational features of the software.
- **Centralized versus departmental training.** Centralized training provides the general principles and overall functionality of the information system. Departmental training is workflow oriented, customized, and focused on individual user class responsibilities in a given area.

---

can be a positive decision and seen as a reward, an incentive, or promotion. External, vendor-supplied trainers, and consultants are knowledgeable about the information system but know little about the organization and may not be able to support a flexible training schedule, ongoing content changes, and long-term training evaluation. External, vendor-supplied trainers, and consultants may leave after the initial implementation training is complete, allowing the organization to select internal staff to take over the responsibility of training new employees and new system functionality. Box 9–4 lists factors to consider when selecting trainers.

Organizations frequently develop a core set of instructors chosen from their own personnel ranks. These individuals receive their initial system training from the vendor and are then responsible for teaching the system to employees. Instructors often come from the following areas:

- *Hospital-wide or staff development educators.* Educators may know the basic principles of adult education but may lack familiarity with specific day-to-day unit routines and workflows.
- *Clinicians.* Clinicians have expertise within their clinical practice areas and can add value by providing departmental training.
- *Department supervisors.* Supervisors are knowlegeable about their clinical area and workflow but may be unable to leave their supervisory responsibilities.
- *Information system personnel.* These individuals may include systems analysts who understand the software application and functionality, but lack a clinical perspective and have no teaching or instructional design experience.

An ideal training team would consist of a combination of clinical and information technology staff who have good communication skills and who have knowledge and experience with classroom instruction, educational technology, and curriculum development. A dedicated core group of trainers helps to provide consistent delivery of instruction. The need for training does not end once the information system has been implemented and in use. There are ongoing demands and requests to train newly hired employees, communicate new functionality, and provide post go-live or post implementation support to end users.

Super User   Another training resource to consider is the **super user.** Super users are employees who are proficient in the use of the information system and can serve as mentors to other end users in their department. Super users may be from any user class and have specialized knowledge in both the information system and the clinical area. This knowledge and skill set enables super users to assist with implementation training and to support and troubleshoot issues after go-live. Super users may be available on all shifts to answer questions and provide assistance. Some organizations have incentive programs that encourage staff to serve as super users.

ADDITIONAL TRAINING CONSIDERATIONS

Organizations support an information systems training function in order to provide employees with the knowledge required to understand and utilize workplace technology. There are several issues related to training that should be addressed in every setting. These include but are not limited to the following:

- *Responsibility for training costs.* Institutions handle training costs differently. Some organizations may charge back training fees to each department or clinical unit. This requires an attendance tracking mechanism and a standard process for monitoring departmental training budgets. Other organizations absorb the cost of training through the information systems departmental budget.
- *Responsibility for trainers.* Internal trainers are frequently recruited from several departments and training assignments may run a course of several months. Organizations need to consider transferring these employees temporarily to the information systems department. This alleviates confusion about reporting structures and relieves the trainer of clinical duties.
- *Workflow training.* Most end users benefit from training that simulates their own workflow. Training is effective when the approach incorporates realistic, job-related scenarios and examples that are seen in day-to-day practice.
- *Confidentiality.* A well planned and designed computer training environment complies with the confidentiality policies of the organization. The training client database must not contain the names of actual clients or cases nor should they be discussed in the training session.
- *System updates.* System updates and enhancements are an integral part of an information system. A communication and in-service strategy must be in place so that end users are informed of new functionality, such as new forms and documentation, changes to the electronic medication administration

record, nursing care plans, or critical pathway management. Any regulatory changes related to the use of the electronic medical record must be reviewed against current system functionality and relayed to the end users that are affected by the change.

- *The employee who fails to demonstrate system competence.* Some employees need extra training time, practice, and remediation regarding the acquisition of computer skills. Learning styles should be respected and difficult situations handled on a case-by-case basis. It is appropriate to seek the advice of Human Resources when an employee cannot or will not develop new job skills.
- *Training personnel from other institutions.* As hospitals and organizations merge and computer applications expand, information systems trainers may be asked to teach end users from other hospitals who are in various stages of an implementation. A review of the acquired hospital's initial needs assessment data, training strategy, and project scope and plan may help identify the information system training needs of the newly acquired hospital.
- *Training students.* Disciplines within the organization need to take responsibility for ensuring that students have a quality clinical experience. Training plans and content for students should be developed in conjunction with coordinators from each discipline; examples include medical, nursing, physical therapy, and pharmacy students.

Training Students

Training plans for students are reevaluated periodically to ensure that the needs of the student and the quality of the clinical experience are met. The training of students takes the same amount of time and resources as employee training, since students need to be able to review a client chart, view test results, complete assessments, and document findings in the information system. Organizations do not benefit from training students unless they seek employment with them after graduation. Organizations may consider a few options regarding student training. One option is to include students in existing end user classes, thus eliminating the need to create a separate curriculum track and instructional materials. For example, nursing students may benefit from the experience of attending a class with registered nurses, and medical students may learn from an opportunity to attend class with providers and medical staff.

Other options include the use of technology-based learning, utilizing faculty to instruct students, and integrating an informatics course into the curriculum. Any information system educational opportunity will enhance the student's clinical experience and his or her marketability upon graduation. Students should receive some degree of training so that they have the experience and responsibility of using an information system. Faculty can then act as mentors in the learning process instead of entering all documentation for their students during clinical rotations.

FUTURE DIRECTIONS

Skilled use of information systems is an expectation of today's healthcare workforce. That expectation makes effective information system training critical. As the realization of that criticality grows, additional attention will be accorded to the development and implementation of a training strategy that includes the use of proven training methods and measures of competency. Movement in this direction will accord training the respect, and subsequently the resources, that it deserves. Until that time, millions of dollars will be spent on the purchase and implementation of systems without realizing many of the benefits that they can provide because employees and providers do not use systems according to their intended design.

CASE STUDY EXERCISES

9.1　Kevin Gallagher, RN, has access to all client records on his medical-surgical unit. Consider each of the following situations:
- Kevin's mother is admitted to the unit. Is it appropriate for him to view his mother's electronic medical record? Why or why not?
- Kevin's unit clerk also has access to Mrs. Gallagher's record. Is it appropriate for her to view Mrs. Gallagher's record? Why or why not?
- Kevin's co-worker, Kaneesha, is a client on the unit assigned to another staff nurse's care. Is it appropriate for Kevin to review her chart or laboratory results? Why or why not?

9.2　Nancy Whitehorse, RN, routinely accesses client records on her medical unit. Does she violate her confidentiality statement if she performs the following actions?
- She reviews the information and does not discuss it with anyone else.
- She discusses information obtained from client records with other healthcare workers on the unit.
- She discusses clinical cases, omitting names, in social situations.

9.3　Grace Elizaga has been given the charge of training the RNs and unit clerks from the first three client care units slated to start automated order entry at Potter's Medical Center (PMC). The target implementation date is in two months. A total of 93 RNs and 11 unit clerks must receive training before that time. Based on information from other agencies that have the same information system as PMC, 8 hours of training time is projected for each individual. As the nurse manager responsible for those units, you have been asked to work with Grace to develop a detailed plan to accomplish this task and submit this plan to your vice president of Client Care Services. Include the following in your plan and provide your rationale:
- Staffing
- Costs for your personnel
- Training start and completion dates
- Length and number of training sessions

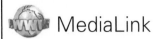 **MediaLink**

Additional resources for this content can be found on the Companion Website at www.prenhall.com/hebda. Click on "Chapter 9" to select the activities for this chapter.

- Glossary
- Multiple Choice
- Discussion Points
- Case Studies
- MediaLink Application
- MediaLink

SUMMARY

- Education is key to the successful use of an information system. Education should be guided by a training strategy and plan that identifies end user needs and includes a teaching philosophy, learning objectives, and training approach. A timetable and training schedule are essential to meeting the implementation plan time line.
- Once users are identified, a needs assessment is completed so that training content can be developed according to user class and job responsibilities. The examples of user classes include physicians, nurses, and administrative support staff. User classes are assigned different levels of access privileges needed to perform their job duties within the information system.
- The transition from manual work to automation is considered a cultural change in the work setting. End users who experience difficulty with change, use of technology, or training may affect the learning experience for both the trainer and other participants in the classroom.
- The training needs of students and replacement staff need to be evaluated to determine if these individuals are required to retrieve and document client information.
- Ideally, training sessions are conducted in classroom settings and not in the clinical areas. Classrooms provide a setting free of work-related distractions. In-services and one-on-one support sessions may be held in client areas on an as-needed basis. Information systems trainers need to ensure client confidentiality. A training environment is created that is a close parallel to the production system and simulates the features and functionality that the end users will be using once the information system is in use.
- Training is time consuming and labor-intensive and should be considered an investment in enhancing workforce knowledge and as a measurement in the successful implementation of an information system.
- Information systems training may be delivered by internal resources, such as staff development educators, clinicians, information systems analysts, the software vendor, or external consultants. Internal training resources are preferable because of their familiarity with the organization and ability to maintain a flexible training schedule.
- Super users are clinical and departmental employees with additional information system training who have an above-average mastery of the

software applications. They serve as resources in their departments and are capable of providing support, troubleshooting assistance, and collaboration with others to solve problems. Super users may come from any user class and should be able to help most end users.

- Proficiency assessments and review of classroom exercises and assignments may be included in the training activity to ensure that learners can demonstrate the expected job skills and demonstrate knowledge transfer.
- End users of an information system require technical, operational, and training support. Some training considerations include system upgrades to the computer training environment, training responsibility for updates regarding regulatory changes, training budget and costs, trainer selection and supervision, realism in training, confidentiality, end user competency, and meeting the training needs of all end users.

REFERENCES

Abla, S. (1995). The who, what, where, when, and how of computer education. *Computers in Nursing, 13*(3), 114–117.

Aldrich, C. (2000). The justification of IT training. *Gartner Research.* Note DF-11–3614.

Barritt, C. & Alderman, F. L. (2004). *Creating a learning objects strategy. Leveraging information in a knowledge economy.* San Francisco, CA: Pfeiffer.

Boisvert, L. (2000). Web-based learning. *Information Systems Management, 17*(1), 35–36.

Bush, A. M. P. (1993). Computer-based training: Training approach of choice. *Computers in Nursing, 11*(4), 163–164.

Combs, W. L. & Falletta, S. V. (2000). *The targeted evaluation process. A performance consultants guide to asking the right questions and getting the results you trust.* Alexandria, VA; American Society for Training and Development.

Craig, J. (2002). The life cycle of a health care information system. In S. Englebardt and R. Nelson (Eds.), *Health care informatics* (pp. 181–208). St. Louis, MO: Mosby.

Duggan, C. M. (2005). Designing effective training. *Journal of American Health Information Management Association, 76*(6), 28–32.

Driscoll, M. P. (2000). *Psychology of learning for instruction* (2nd ed.). Needham Heights, MA: Allyn and Bacon.

Driscoll, M. (1998). *Web-based training. Using technology to design adult learning experiences.* San Francisco, CA: Jossey-Bass Pfeiffer.

Fender, M. & Jennerich, B. (1997). The real key to success with new technology: Understanding people. *Enterprise Systems Journal, 12*(4), 38, 40, 42, 44, 46.

Filipczak, B. (1996). Training on the cheap. *Training, 33*(5), 28–34.

Fleming, M. & Levie, W. H. (1993). *Instructional message design principles from the behavioral and cognitive sciences* (2nd ed.). Englewood Cliffs, NJ: Educational Technology Publications.

Garcia, L. (2002). Squeezing the most from your training dollars. *ADVANCE for Health Information Executives, 6*(8), 55–56.

Glydura, A. J., Michelman, J. E., & Wilson, C. N. (1995). Multimedia training in nursing education. *Computers in Nursing, 13*(4), 169–175.

Guite, J., Lang, M., & McCartan, P. (2006). Nursing admissions process redesigned to leverage EHR. *Journal of Healthcare Information Management, 20*(2), 55–64.

Harvard Business School. (2003). *Guide to managing change and transition.* Boston, MA: Harvard Business School Publishing Company.

244 SECTION 2 • Healthcare Information Systems

Henry, S. A. & Swartz, R. G. (1995). Enhancing healthcare education with accelerated learning techniques. *Journal of Nursing Staff Development, 11*(1), 21–24.

Hillestand, R., Bigelow, J., Bower, A., Girosi, F., Meilli, R., Scoville, R., et al. (2006). Can electronic medical record systems transform health care? Potential health benefits, savings, and costs. *Health Affairs, 24*(5), 1103–1117.

Horton, W. (2001). *Leading e-learning.* Alexandria, VA: American Society for Training and Development.

Meister, J. C. (1998). *Corporate universities: Lessons in building a world-class workforce.* New York: McGraw-Hill, Inc.

Newbold, S. K. (1996). Maximizing technology for cost-effective staff education and training. In M. C. Mills, C. A. Romano, and B. R. Heller (Eds.), *Information management in nursing and health care* (pp. 216–221). Springhouse, PA: Springhouse Corporation.

Phillips, P. P. & Phillips, J. J. (2005). *Return on Investment (ROI) Basics.* Alexandria, VA: American Society for Training and Development.

Regan, E. A. & O'Connor, B. N. (2002). *End-user information systems: Implementing individual and work group technologies* (2nd ed.). Saddle River, NJ: Prentice-Hall.

Rossett, A. & Sheldon, K. (2001). *Beyond the podium, delivering training and performance in the digital world.* San Francisco, CA: Jossey-Bass Pfeiffer.

Simonson, M., Smaldino, S., Albright, M., & Zvacek, S. (2003). *Teaching and learning at a distance: Foundations of distance education* (2nd ed.). Upper Saddle River, NJ: Merrill Prentice-Hall.

Sittig, D. F., Jiang, Z., Manfre, S., Sinkfeld, K., Ginn, R., Smith, L., et al. (1995). Evaluating a computer-based experiential learning simulation: A case study using criterion-referenced testing. *Computers in Nursing, 13*(1), 17–24.

Slater, D. (1998). The Hidden Costs of Enterprise Software. *CIO Magazine,* January 15, 123–129.

Thielst, C. B. (2007). Effective management of technology implementation. *Journal of Healthcare Management, 52*(4), 216–219.

Troha, F. J. (2002). The right mix: A bullet proof mode for designing blended learning. *e-learning, 3*(6), 34–37.

Vaillancourt, S. (May 4, 2000). *Technology delivered learning.* Presented at Tri-State Nursing Computer Network, Pittsburgh, PA.

White, K. W. & Weight, B. H. (2000). *The online teaching guide: A handbook of attitudes, strategies, and techniques for the virtual classroom.* Needham Heights, MA: Allyn & Bacon.

Woodward, J. D., Orlans, N. M., & Higgins, P. T. (2002). *Biometics: Identity assurance in the information age.* Berkeley, CA: McGraw-Hill Osborne.

Zielstorff, R. (1996). Training issues in system implementation. In M. C. Mills, C. A. Romano, and B. R. Heller (Eds.), *Information management in nursing and health care* (pp. 128–138). Springhouse, PA: Springhouse Corporation.

CHAPTER 10

Information Security and Confidentiality

After completing this chapter, you should be able to:

1 Differentiate between privacy, confidentiality, information privacy, and information security.

2 Discuss how information systems affect privacy, confidentiality, and security.

3 Relate the significance of security for information integrity.

4 Recognize threats to system security and information.

5 Review several security measures designed to protect information and discuss how they work.

6 Compare and contrast available means of authentication in terms of levels of security, costs, and ease of use.

7 Distinguish between appropriate and inappropriate password selection and handling.

8 State common examples of confidential forms and communication seen in healthcare settings and identify proper disposal techniques for each.

9 Discuss the impact that Internet technology has on health information security.

10 Discuss the implications of the HIPAA privacy and security rules for the protection of information security.

I nformation security and confidentiality of personal information are major concerns in today's society amidst growing reports of stolen and compromised financial information and medical records. Healthcare information systems must provide rapid access to accurate and complete client information to legitimate users, while safeguarding client privacy and confidentiality. Electronic healthcare applications facilitate efficient and effective sharing of information, but the ease with which they can be accessed creates concerns over the security of the information that they house (Sax, Kohane, & Mandl 2005). At the same time, healthcare administrators must demonstrate measures that protect information to comply with Health Insurance Portability and Accountability Act (HIPAA) requirements and must meet accreditation criteria set forth by the Joint Commission (1996). These criteria continue to evolve. The HIPAA security rule does not specify the utilization of particular technologies; instead it calls for organizations to determine threats and appropriate protective measures for information in all formats. Protection of client privacy and confidentiality requires an understanding of the concepts of privacy, confidentiality, information privacy, and security as well as potential threats within an organization. Even so, breaches still occur. This fact highlights the need for constant vigilance on the part of administrators, organizations, and all employees to determine threats and implement protective measures for information in all formats. Recent events make it clear that electronic records are particularly susceptible to compromise on a large scale via loss, theft, or penetration of system safeguards. In the absence of a single, large-scale national authentication infrastructure, information must be protected through a combination of methods.

PRIVACY, CONFIDENTIALITY, AND SECURITY

While the terms *privacy* and *confidentiality* are often used interchangeably, they are not the same. **Privacy** is a state of mind, a specific place, freedom from intrusion, or control over the exposure of self or of personal information (Blair 2003; Kelly & McKenzie 2002; Kmentt 1987; Reagan 2003; Windslade 1982). Privacy includes the right to determine what information is collected, how it is used, and the ability to access collected information to review its security and accuracy. Anonymity may be requested by an individual because he or she holds public office or is a celebrity. HIPAA regulations require that clients be given clear written explanations of how facilities and providers may use and disclose their health information (Calloway & Venegas 2002). The movement to protect privacy is consistent with an international trend. The European Union established the European Network and Information Security Agency (ENISA) to address potential risks associated with the widespread use of information technology (Mitrakas 2006). Canada established its Office of the Privacy Commissioner, and Australia and South Africa also have privacy legislation (Australia's Privacy Legislation 2002; Olinger, Britz, & Olivier 2007). Ethiopia's work to establish an e-health program and attendant legislation to address access, privacy, and liability issues represents a focus on health information.

Confidentiality refers to a situation in which a relationship has been established and private information is shared (Romano 1987). Confidentiality is essential for the accurate assessment, diagnosis, and treatment of health problems. Once a client discloses confidential information, control over the release of this information lies with the persons who access it. Private information should only be shared with parties who require it for client treatment (Hill 2003). The ethical duty of confidentiality entails keeping information shared during the course of a professional relationship secure and secret from others. This obligation involves making appropriate security arrangements for the storage and transmission of private information, and ensuring that the equipment used for storage and transmission is secure and that measures are used to prevent the interception of e-mail, instant messages, Faxes, and other correspondence containing private information. Nurses are obligated by the American Nurses' Association Code of Ethics and state practice laws to protect patient privacy (Blair 2003). Inappropriate redisclosure can be extremely damaging. For example, insurance companies may deny coverage based on information revealed to them without the client's knowledge or consent. Inappropriate disclosure can also damage reputations and personal relationships or result in loss of employment. Most breaches of confidentiality occur as a result of carelessness and can be avoided through tight control of client records and by not discussing clients in public areas or with persons who do not have a "need-to-know."

Information privacy is the right to choose the conditions and extent to which information and beliefs are shared (Murdock 1980). Informed consent for the release of specific information illustrates information privacy in practice. Information privacy includes the right to ensure accuracy of information collected by an organization (Murdock 1980). **Information security,** on the other hand, is the protection of information against threats to its integrity, inadvertent disclosure, or availability (Griffiths 2003). Information systems can improve protection for client information in some ways and endanger it in others. Unlike the paper record that can be read by anyone, the automated record cannot easily be viewed without an access code. Poorly secured information systems, however, can threaten record confidentiality because records may be accessed from multiple sites with immediate dissemination of information, making clients vulnerable to the redisclosure of sensitive information. The HIPAA Privacy Rule was written to protect the privacy of people who seek care (Blair 2003).

Consent is the process by which an individual authorizes healthcare personnel to process his or her information based on an informed understanding of how this information will be used (Kelly & McKenzie 2002). Obtaining consent should include making the individual aware of any risks that may exist to privacy as well as measures in place to protect privacy.

INFORMATION SYSTEM SECURITY

Information system security is the ongoing protection of both information housed on the system and the system itself from threats or disruption (Ramanathan 2006; Vidalis & Kazmi 2007). The primary goals of healthcare information system security are the protection of client confidentiality and information integrity and ready availability of information when it is needed. Availability is necessary in today's information-driven world yet is constantly challenged as emerging technologies expand traditional security perimeters. Availability is dependent upon **survivability.** Survivability is "the capability of a system as a whole to fulfill its mission, in a timely manner, in the presence of attacks, failures, or accidents" (Ramanathan 2006, p. 50). The goals of healthcare information system security are best met when security is planned rather than applied to an existing system after problems occur. Planning for security saves time and money and should be regarded as a form of insurance against downtime, breaches in confidentiality, loss of consumer confidence, cyber-crime, liability, and lost productivity. Good security practices also help to ensure compliance with HIPAA legislation. Effective security starts with a thorough assessment of assets and risks as well as necessary resources, a well-crafted security plan and policy, and a supportive organizational culture and structure. Administrative support is essential to this effort. In addition to being secure, the system must still be easily accessible for legitimate users.

Risks

Every component in a network is constantly under attack to some degree at any one time (Ramanathan 2006). Potential threats to information and system security come from a variety of sources. These can include thieves, hackers, crackers, denial of service attacks, terrorists, viruses, snatched Web sites, flooding sites with fictitious data, power fluctuations that damage systems or data, revenge attacks, fires and natural disasters, and human error. These threats may result in jammed networks, violations to confidentiality, identity theft, interruption in information integrity, disruption in the delivery of services, monetary losses, and violation of privacy regulations. Confidential client information may also be exposed through file sharing applications on employee work stations as well as unauthorized access via e-mail, instant messaging, and Internet chat sites. Professionals may be hired to test the system for vulnerabilities. For this reason it is essential to have a real-time threat management system in place at all times. This system entails automatic intrusion detection and audit software and security training for all employees. One aspect of security training is the identification of risks and ways that these risks can be minimized.

Viruses, Worms, and Other Malicious Programs Viruses are deliberately written programs that use a host computer to spread and reproduce themselves without the knowledge of the person(s) operating the computer. Viruses need normal computer operations to spread. Originally, viruses attached themselves to other computer programs. They may, or may not, damage data or disrupt system operation. Some viruses are likened to electronic graffiti in that the writer leaves his or her mark by displaying a message. Infected e-mail and IM attachments are common means to spread malware. Executing, or opening, the attached file spreads the virus to the host computer, which then infects the hard drive. Viruses are frequently widespread at the time of detection.

Viruses may also be spread when downloading files from the Internet, visiting some Web pages, and transferring infected CDs, DVDs, and flash drives from one computer or network to another. This is a particular concern with personal use of the Internet and e-mail, which can end up compromising a single computer or the entire network to which it is connected. The infectious period for viruses varies. Infection may occur during any time that the infected program is run, or the virus may remain active in the computer memory until the computer is turned off.

Viruses are not the only program types that can damage data or disrupt computing. Other malicious programs include worms, Trojan horses, logic bombs, and bacteria. See Table 10–1 for definitions and characteristics associated with each program type.

Although antivirus software can locate and eradicate viruses and other destructive programs, the best defense against malicious programs is knowledge obtained from talking with computer users and experts about problems experienced. Some people are experts in viral detection and eradication. Box 10–1 provides tips for how to avoid malicious programs.

If a virus is contained on one machine, it must be isolated and disinfected with antivirus software. Suspect files should be deleted. All backup materials

TABLE 10–1	Characteristics of Malicious Programs
Program Type	**Characteristics**
Viruses	Require normal computer operations to spread
	May or may not disrupt operation or damage data
Worms	Named for pattern of damage left behind
	Often use local area and wide network communication practices as a means to spread and reproduce
	Usually affect memory and/or hard disk space
Trojan horses	Appear to do (or actually do) one function while performing another, undesired action
	One common example resembles a regular system log-in but records user names and passwords to another program for illicit use
	Do not self-replicate
	Are easily confined once discovered
Logic bombs	Are triggered by a specific piece of data such as a date, user name, account name, or identification or another event
	May be part of a regular program or contained in a separate program
	May not activate on the first program run
	May be included in virus-infected programs and with Trojan horses
Bacteria	Are a class of viral programs
	Do not affix themselves to existing programs

> **BOX 10–1   How to Avoid Malicious Programs**
>
> - Use only licensed software.
> - Use the latest version of virus detection software routinely. Upload updates on a regular basis.
> - Never open any file attachment from an unfamiliar source.
> - Use designated machines to check portable drives, storage media, and software for viruses before use.
> - Maintain a list of all program files, their size, and date of creation, and review these periodically for change. The complexity of today's software and computers makes this difficult.
> - Retain backup copies of original software, work files, and directory structure for each PC. Backup can quickly restore system setup and work. However, since most software is now available on CD-ROM and can be reinstalled quickly, backup may not be necessary. Keep a record of all CD product keys and the number on the package to facilitate reinstallation.
> - Have lists of vendor, purchase date, and serial number for all hardware and software items to facilitate virus tracking.
> - If a virus is found, send a copy to an expert for tracking purposes.
> - Watch for and download software patches that eliminate security problems.
> - Ensure that system safeguards have been put into place by information technology staff. Safeguards may include programming e-mail servers to reject mail containing viruses, setting up policies related to e-mail and IM use, and educating the workforce.

should be considered suspect. It should not be necessary to reformat the hard drive to eliminate the virus(es). Viruses, worms, and other malicious viruses are detrimental to the economy because of the loss of productivity and resources required to restore functionality.

Phishing Phishing refers to an attempt to get consumers to divulge personal information such as financial data and credit card and bank account numbers through social engineering and technical subterfuge (McMillan 2007). Social-engineering schemes use fraudulent e-mails to lead consumers to counterfeit Web sites, which then ask them to supply private information. Technical subterfuge schemes plant software onto computers that steals credentials directly, often by recording keystrokes. The number of phishing sites continues to increase. The Anti-Phishing Working Group is an industry association focused on eliminating the identity theft and fraud that result from the growing problem of phishing; the Group provides information on attacks, resources, and consumer advice.

Spam Spam is unwanted, or "junk" e-mail. Spam threatens security when it serves as a vehicle for the introduction of malware and when it threatens ready access to information by overloading networks and consuming valuable resources.

System Penetration Even the most secure systems can be penetrated. The best that can be hoped for is that security strategies will minimize instances of system penetration and minimize damages. A 2003 survey (Tuesday 2003) found that retail, financial services, healthcare, and federal and local government were among the top industry sectors targeted by attackers. Significant financial losses occur annually as a result of compromised systems. A 2006 Computer Security Institute survey, conducted in conjunction with the FBI, found the average cost of a computer attack was $203,606 (Gordon, Loeb, Lucyshyn, & Richardson 2006). Barriers to effective security include inadequate resources, money, time, and attention from management; the complexity of training; and the increasing sophistication of users.

Cybercrime is now a larger threat than other physical security problems. **Cybercrime** commonly refers to the ability to steal personal information such as Social Security numbers stored on computers. Cyberattackers use widely available hacker tools to find network weaknesses and gain undetected access. Inconsistent and inadequate approaches to security risks allow entry. The following types of individuals may become involved in system penetration and computer crime:

- *Opportunists.* Opportunists take advantage of the situation and their access to information for uses not associated with their jobs.
- *Hackers.* Hackers are individuals who have an average, or above average, knowledge of computer technology and who dislike rules and restrictions. Hackers penetrate systems as a challenge, and many do not regard their acts as criminal. Others, however, break into systems with the intent of obtaining information, creating mischief, destroying files, or making a profit. Members of this group are sometimes referred to as *crackers* or *black hats*.
- *Computer or information specialists.* These individuals are knowledgeable about how computers work and are in the best position to commit computer crime and disable systems while avoiding detection.

Unauthorized Users Although the most common fear is that of system penetration from outsiders, the greatest threat actually comes from inside threats, namely employees, contractors, consultants, outsourced services, and vendors who view information inappropriately, disrupt information availability, or corrupt data integrity (Steele & Wargo 2007). Such access constitutes unauthorized use and may occur at any level within an organization. Consideration must be given to the access rights accorded to all employees, including system administrators.

Even though healthcare professionals have codes of ethics to maintain client confidentiality, not all professionals act ethically. System safeguards are needed for this reason. As healthcare alliances grow and client records become more accessible, the likelihood of unauthorized system access increases. For the individual client, legal protection was limited in the United States until HIPAA compliance became mandatory. The Data Protection Act provides protection for confidentiality in the United Kingdom (Kelly & McKenzie 2002). Australia has taken action to protect health information as well. Other nations are also working on this issue. Consumer groups and healthcare professionals need to serve as advocates for healthcare consumers in the protection of privacy and confidentiality.

Concern for client confidentiality is not limited to the period of active treatment. Record access may occur later through loopholes that exist in automated systems (Hebda, Sakerka, & Czar 1994). These loopholes will be found by curious users and must be corrected as soon as information system (IS) personnel and administrators become aware of them. One example may be illustrated by the automated system that restricts access to client records during treatment but allows retrieval of any record or laboratory value after client discharge. Healthcare alliance physicians and office staff often need to see test results after the client's admission but should be able to view the results only for their clients. This type of problem represents an oversight in the design process that must be corrected. Commercial software vendors are now under greater pressure to improve the security of their products as customers use their purchasing power to exert demands. The U.S. government has started to stipulate security provisions that vendors must meet to win contracts with the government.

Sabotage The destruction of computer equipment or records or the disruption of normal system operation is known as **sabotage.** IS staff have system privileges that would permit this type of destruction, but in fact any worker may commit sabotage. Employees who are satisfied, well informed, and feel a vested interest in maintaining information and system security are less likely to wreak havoc on the system. A positive environment, a well-defined institutional ethics policy, and intact security mechanisms help to deter intentional information, or system, misuse or destruction. Consideration should be given to having background checks performed on employees and all other persons who manage and maintain computer systems or are in a position to misuse information, as a means to avert this threat. Insider threat management is an emerging focus area in information security and operational risk management (Steele & Wargo 2007).

Errors and Other Disasters Errors may result from poor design, system changes that permit users more access than they require, failure to follow policy, or absent or poorly written policies. One example of poor design is seen when information restricted during inpatient treatment is available to all users after the patient is discharged whether the users have a need-to-know or not. Errors may also arise from incorrect user entries such as inadvertent selection of the wrong client for data retrieval or documentation. A 2006 Computing Technology Industry Association survey found that nearly 60% of the surveyed organizations reported that their last security breach was due to human error (McCarthy 2006a, 2006b). This same survey found that only about one-third of their IT staffs and users received security training. Lack of adherence to established policies have resulted in several high-profile data losses when laptops and portable drives were lost or stolen.

During disasters, manual backup procedures may compromise information because the primary focus is on maintaining services. One example of this is seen when paper reports of laboratory findings are not enclosed in envelopes for delivery to client care units.

Poor Password Management Additional threats to information and system security come from poor password management, sharing passwords, posting log-on IDs and passwords on workstations, leaving logged-on devices unattended, and compromised handheld devices. Poor password management is exacerbated when users have multiple passwords to manage and it becomes difficult to remember them all.

Compromised Devices Handheld devices can transmit viruses and worms to the hospital network, threatening application, device, and network security. Given the increased risk factor associated with these devices experts recommend that handheld devices connect to the rest of the network through a firewall to optimize security (Malin 2007). Another security related concern is that handheld devices can be easily stolen because of their size and portability. Theft of information may occur once the devices are in the hands of an unauthorized user or when wireless transmissions are heard or received by unauthorized users.

SECURITY MECHANISMS

Protection of information and computer systems should receive top priority. Typically, security mechanisms use a combination of logical and physical restrictions to provide a greater level of protection than is possible with either approach alone. This includes measures such as firewalls and the installation of antivirus and spyware detection software. These measures should also be reevaluated periodically to determine what modifications need to be made. An example of a logical restriction is automatic sign-off. **Automatic sign-off** is a mechanism that logs a user off the system after a specified period of inactivity on his or her computer. This procedure is recommended in all client care areas, as well as any other area in which sensitive data exist. The level of security provided should reflect the value of the information. Some levels of information may have no particular value and do not need protection from theft, only from unauthorized change.

Physical Security

Physical security measures include placement of computers, file servers, or computers in restricted areas. When this is not possible, equipment may be removed or locked. Physical security is a challenge for remote access. **Remote access** is the ability to use the health enterprise's information system from outside locations, such as a physician's office. Secure modems and encryption are particularly useful in conjunction with remote access.

Physical security is also challenged with the growing popularity of mobile wireless devices such as notebooks, tablet PCs, and personal digital assistants (PDAs) as well as portable storage devices. These items may fall into unauthorized hands. Security cables, motion detectors, or alarms used with these devices help ward off theft. Secure, lockable briefcases should be considered for the storage of devices not in use. In the event that mobile devices are stolen, some measure of protection can be provided by making the boot-up process password protected; setting passwords on individual files; storing files in zipped, password-protected folders; or encrypting the hard drive. These actions are not foolproof because hard drives can be removed and copied. Daily backups and portable storage devices such as an external drive help to prevent data loss. It is essential to include wireless devices into organizational standards and policies to ensure that these measures are taken.

Another facet of physical security is introduced when healthcare enterprises provide Internet access within the facility for visitors and patients. Increasingly this is an expected amenity as it is in hotels, public areas, and coffeehouses (Stern 2007). Individuals who opt to use free wireless connections in public places should employ the following precautions:

- *Look for posted signs that provide the exact name of the hotspot.* This will help to steer clear of fake networks that are designed to collect passwords, credit card information, and other personal data.
- *Change settings so that permission is required before connecting to a new network.* This measure helps to avoid fake networks.
- *Avoid networks that are computer-to-computer.* Free wireless networks should be noted as such. Computer-to-computer networks are generally fake networks set up for spurious purposes.
- *Turn off file sharing.* This will keep passersby from accessing stored data.
- *Refrain from online banking or shopping.* These activities should be avoided unless network security can be guaranteed
- *Do not store passwords on your computer or other mobile devices.* These may be accessed through suspect connections or compromised when the physical device is stolen.

Public Internet access cannot be via the same network that is used to transmit secure health data unless extensive measures are used to maintain the security of that data.

Authentication

Authentication is the process of determining whether someone is who he or she professes to be. Several methods of authentication exist, ranging from log-on passwords, digital certificates, and public or private keys used for encryption and biometric measures. Authentication is one component of identity management (ID management). **ID management** is a broad administrative area that deals with identifying individuals in a system and controlling their access to resources within that system by associating user rights and restrictions with the established identity.

Passwords Access codes and passwords are a common means to authenticate access to automated records, largely because they represent a familiar, available, and inexpensive technology (Campbell, Kleeman, & Ma 2007; Lemos 2006). A **password** is a collection of alphanumeric characters that the user types into the computer. This may be required after the entry and acceptance of an access code, sometimes referred to as the *user name.* IS administrators sometimes require this information to problem-solve or reissue passwords. The password does not appear on the screen when it is typed, nor should it be known to anyone but the user and IS administrators. Recommendations for password selection and use are given in Box 10–2. Obvious passwords such as the user's name, house number, or dictionary words are easily compromised. Strong passwords use combinations of letters, numbers, and symbols that are not easily guessed. Software is available to test and eliminate easily compromised passwords before use.

Individuals should not share passwords or leave computers logged on and unattended. System administrators must keep files that contain password lists safe from view or copying by unauthorized individuals. One compromised password can jeopardize information and the system that contains it. For this reason, users should not use the same password for access to more than one site or system. Using the same password at various sites reduces security. System administrators need to allow legitimate users the opportunity to access the system while refusing entry to others. One means to accomplish this is to shut down a workstation after a random number of unsuccessful access attempts and send security to check that area. Although passwords provide considerable system protection, other defenses are still necessary. These include measures to verify user identity. Figure 10–1 shows a screen shot of a log-on screen.

BOX 10–2   Recommendations for Password Selection and Use

- Choose passwords that are at least 8, preferably 12, characters long.
- Select stronger passwords for higher levels of security.
- Avoid using the same password for more than one application.
- Do not use the browser "password save" feature.
- Use combinations of uppercase and lowercase letters, numbers, punctuation marks, and symbols.
- Do not use proper names, initials, words taken from the dictionary, or account names.
- Do not use words that are spelled backwards or with reversed syllables.
- Do not use dates or telephone, license plate, or Social Security numbers.
- Do not store or automate passwords in the computer.
- Avoid repeated numbers or letters.
- Keep passwords private.
- Change passwords frequently, with no reuse of passwords for a specified period.

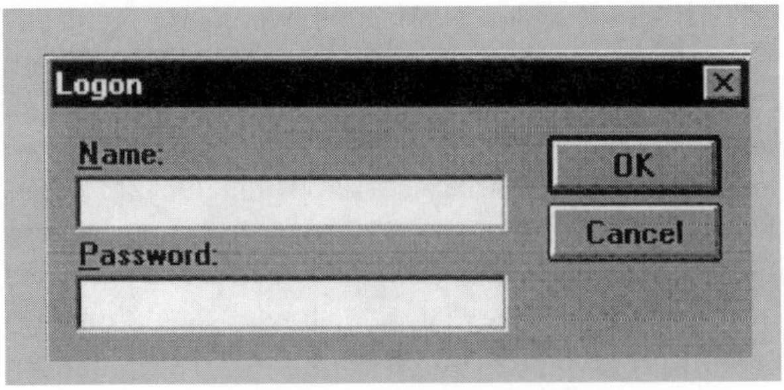

FIGURE 10–1 • Screen shot of a logon screen

Sign-on access codes and passwords are generally assigned on successful completion of system training. Passwords may be difficult for the user to recall. This leads some people to write passwords down and post them in conspicuous places. This practice should be prohibited. Users who find it necessary to record the dozens of passwords used to access various sites and systems must store them in an area away from the computer and out of casual view. Storing passwords in a file on the computer is a problem if the device is shared by others or if the hard drive crashes or is replaced. A file-wipe utility should be used to permanently erase the drive so that password files cannot be restored. When a file is used to store passwords, it should be encrypted and password protected. Passwords must be regarded as an electronic signature.

Frequent and random password change is recommended as a routine security mechanism. This can be an arduous and unpleasant task because it is difficult for users to remember new passwords. There are, however, situations that mandate immediate change or deletion of access codes and passwords, including suspicion of unauthorized access and termination of employees. Codes and passwords should also be deleted with status changes such as resignations, leaves of absence, and the completion of rotations for students, faculty, and residents. Because IS staff can view any information in the system, all members of the department should receive new passwords when IS personnel leave. In the event that an IS employee is terminated, department door locks should be changed as well.

Disadvantages associated with the use of passwords include the following: they are poorly managed, frequently forgotten, and often need reset by help desk staff; they can be shared or stolen; the complex rules for password generation are largely unenforceable; and the purpose of passwords is defeated when the user sets the browser to remember them.

Public Key Infrastructure (PKI) Encrypted key-based authentication is another, more secure technology. An example is **public key infrastructure (PKI).** PKI uses an encrypted passkey that can be provided to the user in various formats, including a smartcard, token, or wireless transmitter. The passkey provides a secret number that is verified against a registered digital certificate. The user submits the passkey information during the sign-on process, and the PKI system compares it against the registered digital certificate ID to verify a match. Digital certificates include information about the owner, such as systems that he or she may access, level of access, and biometric measures. Digital certificates provide assurance of the identity, rights, and privileges of the user. Security tokens that resemble key chain fobs are an example of this technology. Tokens strengthen authentication because the user must use both the token and a special PIN code to gain access. PKI can provide a common infrastructure that allows access to multiple delivery systems across an organization or organizations.

Biometrics Scanned employee identification may include a name badge but generally refers to biometric authentication, which is based on a unique biological trait, such as a fingerprint, voice or iris pattern, retinal scan, hand geometry, face recognition, ear pattern, smell, blood vessels in the palm, gait recognition, or keystroke cadence (Sturdevant 2007). Biometric technology is feasible and can be very accurate. Unlike passwords or devices that can be forgotten or stolen, biometric measures are always with the individual, barring major injury, and cannot be lost, stolen, or used without user consent.

The quality of biometric authentication varies by device and software used. There is a high rate of failure of first print readings as the number of users increases. This situation may require a second or third reading. Individuals must learn the proper method of placing their fingers into scanners. Skin moisture and temperature also affect the quality of the scan. Very moist or dry skin and cold fingers negatively affect reading. Some readers can be fooled by using tape, gelatin, or other measures. Infection control is a related concern when biometric authentication requires contact. No contact is required to scan the voice or iris pattern, retina, hand geometry, face, ear pattern, smell, blood vessels in the palm, or for gait recognition. Biometric authentication helps organizations to better comply with regulations and reduces the amount of time that help staff spend resetting passwords. The use of biometric measures for authentication is expected to replace password use in the near future.

Other authentication devices include proximity radio systems that detect user badges within a specified distance, picture authentication packages that use pictures instead of passwords, and digital certificates. Users should have different authentication requirements depending upon the sensitivity or value of the resources that they access. Authentication can be strengthened by requiring multifactor authentication. Authentication policy outlines acceptable forms of authentication depending on multiple factors, including user, resources, location, and time of day. The policy must also protect authentication systems from attack and sabotage. Building an authentication policy is one thing—implementing, managing, and enforcing it is another.

Firewalls and Other Network Devices

A **firewall** is a combination of hardware and software that forms a barrier between systems, or different parts of a single system, to protect those systems from unauthorized access. Firewalls screen traffic, allow only approved transactions to pass through them, and restrict access to other systems or sensitive areas such as client information, payroll, or personnel data. Firewalls, or a separate device behind them, may be able to inspect transmissions for anomalies that help to identify malware (Britt 2005). Multiple firewalls can increase protection. Strong security policies and practices strengthen firewall protection. Once a user has passed through the firewall, controlling access to individual applications takes place elsewhere. Firewalls are not foolproof. Specialists periodically create "patches" to counter flaws in security software. It is imperative to apply security patches as soon as they become available. Security protocols on network switches and routers also help. Another means to safeguard information is to segment a network into different levels of security each with its own level of priorities and set of policies (Malin 2007). It is also essential to train and remind employees about their role in security.

Application Security

Another area of concern is **application security,** which refers to protecting from harm a set of programs and the information that they store or create. Application security should be used with the client information system and other systems such as payroll records. Employees should sign off when they leave a workstation or computer or are finished using a particular software application, because failure to do so may allow others to use their code to access information. Automatic sign-off has been designed as a security measure when employees fail to properly exit a program or step away from the computer.

Antivirus Software

Antivirus software is a set of computer programs that can locate and eradicate viruses and other malicious programs from scanned memory sticks, storage devices, individual computers, and networks. The constant creation of new viruses makes it necessary to update antivirus software often. Antivirus software may come preloaded on new computers or be obtained in computer stores or over the Internet. The user must then frequently download updated virus definitions from the vendor's Web site. Some vendors automatically notify users as new virus definitions become available. Users can set up antivirus software to automatically run a virus check on the PC or server on a scheduled basis in addition to performing random checks. Networked computers are generally set by the administrator to include a virus scan in routine start-up, automatically scan new files, and to update antivirus files. Network administrators can also set privileges to prohibit unauthorized file downloads.

Spyware Detection Software

Spyware is a data collection mechanism that installs itself without the user's permission. This often occurs when the user is browsing the Web or downloading software. Spyware can include cookies that track Web use as well as applications that capture credit card, bank, and PIN numbers or other personal health information (PHI) stored on that computer for illicit purposes by an unauthorized person. This is a concern for all healthcare providers because it threatens PHI. No computer that is attached to the Internet is immune. Clues that spyware has infected a computer include the presence of pop-up ads, keys that do not work, random error messages, and poor system performance. Because of the security threat that this represents, spyware detection software should be utilized.

ADMINISTRATIVE AND PERSONNEL ISSUES

Ultimately, healthcare administrators are responsible for creating and managing the infrastructure to protect client privacy and confidentiality. This entails developing a plan, policies, designated structure for implementation, user access levels, and an adequate budget (Rainer, Marshall, Knapp, & Montgomery 2007). Upper management must have security awareness training and set a positive example for all stakeholders, including employees, students, consultants, and contractors, because security is a responsibility shared by everyone. Next, administration must work with IS personnel to establish the following centralized security functions:

- *A comprehensive security plan.* The plan needs to be developed with input from administration, information services personnel, and clinical staff. It should delineate security responsibilities for each level of personnel as well as a timeline for the development and implementation of policy and physical infrastructure. Incorporation of computer forensics as a plan component helps to build and maintain a strong security posture. **Computer forensics** refers to the collection of electronic evidence for purposes of formal litigation and simple internal investigations.
- *Correct, complete information security policies, procedures, and standards.* These should be published online for easy access, with e-mail notification of employees as new policies are released.
- *Information asset ownership and sensitivity classifications.* Ownership in this context refers to who is responsible for the information, including its security. Sensitivity classification is a determination of how damaging that information might be if it were disclosed inappropriately. The level of sensitivity may be used to determine what information should be encrypted.
- *Identification of a comprehensive security program.* A well-defined security plan can avert or minimize threats. A key part of the plan is the identification of responsibility for information integrity and confidentiality. A strong plan incorporates computer forensics.
- *Information security training and user support.* Education is an important component in fostering proper system use. Most problems with information system security are primarily related to the human factor, rather than the technical one.
- *An institution-wide information security awareness program.* Formal IS training and frequent suggestions are needed to remind users of the need to protect information.

In reality, responsibility for system and information security is shared by healthcare administrators, IS and healthcare professionals, and all system users. Involving users in system development fosters ownership of this responsibility and facilitates the ability to trace problems, limit damage, and make corrective changes. This involvement can occur on an individual level or through an institutional security committee. Security committees should consider routine maintenance, confidentiality clauses in vendor contracts, third-party payer needs, legal issues inclusive of monitoring, ongoing security needs as the institution and system evolve, and disaster planning. The IS department should address these functions when there is no security committee. Individual users are responsible for protecting their passwords, saving and backing up work files on a regular basis, securing removable storage media, and not leaving confidential information unattended on the computer screen or in paper form. They should also be responsible for reporting any observed unauthorized access. It may be necessary to outsource security if there are insufficient resources internally, but this decision needs to be carefully weighed.

Levels of Access

Access should be strictly limited to a need-to-know basis. This means no personnel, including IS staff, should have routine access to confidential information unless it is required by a particular event, at which time an audit trail is established. IS personnel must be held to the same confidentiality statement that applies to other personnel.

LIMITS

Access is determined by who needs the medical record and under what conditions and locations. Direct care providers require information on their clients. Access levels are decided by defining roles for every level of personnel. This process can be referred to as "user classes." Each user class has different privileges. Initial system access is contingent on successful completion of system training and demonstration of competence. User training should address appropriate uses of information and the consequences of information misuse. User roles and audits must be incorporated into the design of information systems to best ensure security, privacy, and confidentiality. Attempts to define user roles and implement audits into older hospital information systems is extremely difficult. Definition of user roles is instrumental to preventing unauthorized access to sensitive healthcare information. For example, nursing assistants are responsible for the documentation of hygiene, dietary intakes, vital signs, and fluid intake and output. They should not be able to access diagnostic and historical information.

User Authentication

Access by authorized individuals can be verified through user authentication. One common form of authentication is the appearance of the user's name on the screen. In the event that other staff note a discrepancy, they have the responsibility to report it immediately. It is important to develop authentication policies jointly with information technology personnel, business staff, and end users. It is also critical to factor in time to install and test drivers and hardware as well as to consider the time and resources required to enroll and update users. Support costs and training times increase as the complexity of the authentication process increases. Unwieldy authentication systems can reduce staff productivity.

Personnel Issues

Clear policies and procedures must be established and communicated for personnel handling information. Staff education is a key element for information and system security. Education for information handling and system use includes an orientation, system training, and a discussion of what is acceptable behavior. Staff should also be informed of the consequences for unauthorized access and information misuse, the use of audit trails, and ongoing measures to heighten security awareness. Staff need to know what constitutes an incident and how it should be handled. There should be periodic reminders that client information belongs to the client as well as what comprises professional, legal, and ethical behavior. Yearly review of the ethical computing statement is one way to emphasize the importance of ethical behavior. Figure 10–2 displays an example of this statement. Education and monitoring activities show administrative commitment to ethical information use.

Explicit policies and procedures provide the discipline to achieve information and system security. Policies and procedures should address information ethics, training, access control, system monitoring, data entry, backup procedures, responsibilities for the use of information on mobile devices and remote sites, and exchange of client information with other healthcare providers. Information ethics policies should do the following:

- *Plan for audit trails.* **Audit trails** are a record of IS activity. Users should know that their system access is monitored and that audit trail records will be kept for a period of years.
- *Establish acceptable computer uses.* This includes authorized access and using only legal software copies. One example of how this might be enforced is requiring licenses for all software used within the institution.
- *Collect only required data.* Limiting collection of information to what is needed, and no more, eliminates the danger of inappropriate disclosure of unneeded information and may lessen the workload.

ST. FRANCIS HEALTH SYSTEM
INFORMATION SYSTEM
USER SIGN-ON CODE RECEIPT

[] St. Francis Medical Center
[] St. Francis Hospital of New Castle
[] St. Francis Central Hospital
[] _____

ST.
FRANCIS
HEALTH
SYSTEM

Hospital Personnel or Hospital Based Physician Sign-On codes are confidential. Disclosure of your Sign-On code, attempts to discover another person's Sign-On code, or unauthorized use of a Sign-On code are grounds for immediate dismissal.

I, the undersigned, acknowledge receipt of my User Sign-On Code and understand that:

1. My User Sign-On Code is equivalent of my signature; (Please note that the electronic signature is recognized by the Health Care Finance Administration (HCFA) and the Commonwealth of Pennsylvania).

2. Accessing the system via my Sign-On Code, is recorded permanently;

3. If assigned a User Sign-On Code, I will not disclose this code to anyone;

4. I will not attempt to learn another user's User Sign-On Code;

5. I will not attempt to access information in the system by using a User Sign-On Code other than my own;

6. I will access only that information which is necessary to perform my authorized functions;

7. If I have reason to believe that the confidentiality of my User Sign-On Code has been broken, I will contact Information Services immediately so that the suspect code can be deleted and a new code assigned to me; and

I understand that if I violate any of the above statements, it will be referred to the appropriate authority.

I further understand that my User Sign-On Code will be deleted from the system when I no longer hold an appointment or am no longer employed at St. Francis or authorization is otherwise revoked.

I have read the above statements and understand the implications if confidentiality of Sign-On code is violated.

_____ Social Security #_____-_____-_____
Name (Please print)

Dept:_____Supervisor:_____ Position:_____

System: MIS:____   MEDIPAC:____   G/L:____   A/P:____   CYBORG:____   OTHER:____

Signature of Code Recipient_____ Date:___/___/___

* Trainer Signature:_____ Date:___/___/___

* Dept. Head Authorization:_____ Date:___/___/___

Issuer Signature:_____ Date:___/___/___
     Information Services

Code will not be issued without proper identification and signature in presence of issuer.
* Signature must be present prior to issuance of code.   MIS User Class:_____

FORM H-1280 Date of Origin: 2/85   File: Personnel Department
         Revised: 10/95   Physicians: Medical Staff Office

FIGURE 10–2 • Sample ethical computing statement (reprinted by permission of St. Francis Health System, Pittsburgh, PA)

- *Encourage client review of files for accuracy and error correction.* Client inspection of records ensures information integrity.
- *Establish controls for the use of information after hours and off-site.* As many employees and physicians work at home or complete projects on their own time, it is important to develop policies related to downloading files or carrying information off premises. Both the types of information that may be carried on mobile devices and the responsibilities of the staff member to safeguard that information must be spelled out.

Information ethics policies are most credible when practiced by top administrators and IS personnel.

System Security Management

System security involves protection against deliberate attacks, errors, omissions, and disasters. Good system management is a key component of a strong framework for security because it encompasses the following tasks:

- Monitoring
- Maintenance
- Operations
- Traffic management
- Supervision
- Risk management

Monitoring entails setting and enforcing standards, tracking changes, and observing all system activity. Monitoring also alerts managers to problems such as intruders or the introduction of a virus. Maintenance encompasses all activity needed for proper operation of hardware, including preventive measures such as testing, periodic applications of patches, and replacement of select components to ensure that data are available when needed. Maintenance includes documentation of all configuration settings, server protocols, and network addresses and changes to any of the above, so that records are available in the event that the system must be restored. Operations management includes all activities needed to provide, sustain, modify, or cease telecommunications. Traffic management permits rerouting of transmissions for better system performance. Supervision requires monitoring traffic and taking measures to prevent system overload and crashes. Risk management helps to identify and curtail problem areas in a timely fashion.

Although software is available to facilitate system management tasks, the paucity of commercial packages available for management of comprehensive systems across networks forced institutions to develop in-house solutions or use outsourcing agents for customized applications. Many organizations have different staff members for network and systems management. Network staff traditionally focus on hardware and connections, whereas IS personnel track information and software use. The security officer plays a pivotal role in tracking personnel information relative to system use. It is the security officer who may assign access codes and passwords to authorized users and who deletes codes for staff no longer with the organization. Increased computing needs and limited budgets require greater staff efficiency. Wise use of system and network management tools will help to provide that efficiency, minimize the number of required support staff, reduce support costs, and improve information security.

Audit Trails

Auditing software helps to maintain security by recording unauthorized access to certain screens or records. Audits show access of records by user or by password and all access by an individual or level of employee. For this reason all individuals should sign off after each use; if they encounter an active session that belongs to another user, they should log that user off and sign in under their own access. Frequent review of audit trails for unusual activity quickly identifies inappropriate use. Poorly audited systems invite fraud and abuse. The level of control in many audit systems is not sufficient for HIPAA compliance. Optimally, audits should be able to track all access, creations, updates, and edits at the data element level for each patient record. This ability will support a consumer's right to view logs of who accessed his or her data, what they saw, and when the data were accessed.

Audit trail records must now be available for protracted periods. Before HIPAA, audit logs were usually kept for limited periods. Consideration must be given now to the retention period for audit logs. Department managers must be advised when audit trails indicate that their staff have accessed records without a need. Audit trails help but may still fail to demonstrate the full range of security issues.

In the event that an audit trail identifies unauthorized access, it is important to enforce written policy. At the very least, this is a verbal reprimand or possibly a notation on the employee's performance evaluation. In many institutions, however, employees are held to the statement they signed on receipt of their access code and password, acknowledging termination of employment as a possible consequence of inappropriate system use. When employees are terminated for this reason, they may be escorted off the premises by the security department to prevent any further opportunity for unauthorized access. Audit trails may also reveal unauthorized access from outside sources, although little legal recourse has been available to punish the guilty parties until recently. There is now an increased legislative activity to prevent and punish cybercrime.

HANDLING AND DISPOSAL OF CONFIDENTIAL INFORMATION

Although most people recognize the need to keep medical records confidential, many are less attentive to safeguarding information printed from the record or extracted from it electronically for report purposes. All client record information should be treated as confidential and kept from the view of unauthorized persons.

Computer Printouts

In the past, the primary sources of inadvertent disclosure of information were printouts of portions of client records and Faxes. All papers containing personal health information (PHI), such as prescriptions, laboratory specimen labels, identification bracelets, meal descriptions, addressograph plates, and any other items that carry a patient's name, address, Social Security number, date of birth, or age, must be destroyed. This may entail using shredders or locked receptacles for shredding and incineration later. Shredding onsite may offer better control as well as cost savings. Nurses may also be responsible for erasing from the hard drive computer files containing calendars, surgery schedules, or other daily records that include PHI. Disposal policies for records must be clear and enforced. For tracking purposes, each page of output should have a serial number or other means of identification so that an audit trail is maintained that identifies what each paper record is as well as the date and method for destruction and the identity of individuals witnessing the destruction. The person designated to oversee this destruction can vary but it may be a secretary or staff from information services. Control must be established over the materials that users print or Fax. Some institutions include a header on all printouts such as lab results that display the word "Confidential" in large letters. This reminds staff to dispose of materials appropriately.

Faxes

Institutional and departmental policies must dictate the types of information that can be sent, allowable recipients, the location to which transmissions are sent, and the verification process. Information should not exceed that requested or required for immediate clinical needs. Legal counsel should review policies for consistency with federal and state law. Clients should sign a release form before Faxing information. The following measures enhance Fax security:

- *Confirm that Fax numbers are correct before sending information.* This helps to ensure that information is appropriately directed.
- *The use of a cover sheet.* This is a particularly important practice when the Fax machine serves a number of different users. A cover sheet eliminates the need for the recipient to read the Fax transmission to determine who gets it. The cover sheet may also contain a statement to remind recipients of the presence of confidential information. Figure 10–3 displays an example of a Fax cover sheet.
- *Authentication at both ends of the transmission before data transmission.* This action verifies that the source and destination are correct. This is done through use of a Fax cover sheet listing intended recipient, the sender, both phone and Fax numbers, and the transmittal confirmation sheet that lists the Fax number.
- *Programmed speed-dial keys.* Programmed keys eliminate the chance of dialing errors and misdirected Fax transmissions.
- *Encryption.* Encoding transmissions makes it impossible to read confidential information without the encryption key. This safeguards Fax transmissions that might be sent to a wrong number.
- *Sealed envelopes for delivery.* The enclosure of confidential information in sealed envelopes provides a barrier to discourage casual viewing.
- *Fax machine placement in secure areas.* Secure areas have limited traffic and few, if any, strangers.
- *Limited machine access by designated individuals.* Restricting access to a few people makes it easier to enforce accountability for actions and to identify any transgressions.

ST. FRANCIS MEDICAL CENTER
FAX TRANSMITTAL FORM

ST.
FRANCIS
HEALTH
SYSTEM

DATE: _____   NO. OF PAGES: _____
                                   (including cover sheet)

FROM: _____

FACILITY: _____

DEPARTMENT: _____

TELEPHONE: _____   FAX: _____

TO: _____

FACILITY: _____

DEPARTMENT: _____

TELEPHONE: _____   FAX: _____

COMMENTS: _____

_____

_____

_____

_____

_____

_____

FIGURE 10-3 • Sample Fax cover sheet (reprinted by permission of St. Francis Health System, Pittsburgh, PA)

- *Inclusion of a request to return documents by mail.* Inadvertent entry of a wrong telephone number can jeopardize sensitive information. In the event that information is Faxed to a wrong number, a request to return documents may limit further disclosure.
- *A log of all Fax transmissions.* A roster of all Faxes sent and received provides a means to keep track of what information is sent and to help ensure that only appropriate information is sent.

Electronic Files

Given that virtually all documents originate in electronic format, the destruction of paper printouts is almost incidental. For this reason, measures must be taken to ensure that confidential information contained on storage media, computers, and hard drives that is no longer needed is also disposed of properly. This method must go beyond the dumpster to include destruction of the storage media or electronically writing over files to ensure that no information can be retrieved from them. This is particularly important as equipment is often moved from one area of an organization to another and may even be donated to outside entities.

E-mail, Instant Messages, and the Internet

E-mail and instant messaging (IM) are discussed at length in the chapter on electronic communication and the Internet (see chapter 4). Policy should dictate what types of information may be allowed. E-mail and IM are great means of disseminating information, such as announcements, to large numbers of people quickly and inexpensively. However, information that is potentially sensitive should not be sent via these routes unless it is encrypted. Nonencrypted messages can be read, and public e-mail password protection of mailboxes can be cracked. When looking at encryption, ask whether e-mail and IM software encrypts all messages between users, whether messages are encrypted both in transit and when stored in the mailbox, and whether messages remain encrypted when sent between different e-mail programs. Unauthorized, or dormant, mail accounts should be destroyed and firewalls used for additional protection. It is all too easy to inadvertently send out messages to the wrong party, attach the wrong document, or include persons who do not need the information. Software can be used to monitor network traffic for patterns that represent client information such as lists or Social Security numbers. This same software can detect requests for files, and monitor instant messaging and Web-based mail to determine if requests come from appropriate parties or if there are problems with information going out to unauthorized recipients.

HIPAA regulations affect e-mail use and routing infrastructures. Most e-mail networks allow messages to travel through any available simple mail transfer protocol (SMTP) relay until it reaches its destination. Messages are stored at each relay and then forwarded. These relays can be hacked; encryption helps to ensure that intercepted mail cannot be read but it does not keep it secure. Security lies with access and control of decryption keys. Central administration for encryption, key management, and disclosure should be addressed via policies and training. Another concern related to e-mail and information system security is spam. **Spam** is unsolicited e-mail that uses valuable server space and employee time and can serve as an entry for malicious programs. E-mail security software can filter out spam. The downside is that this process may result in the loss of a small percentage of legitimate mail. Monitoring e-mail is important to avoid legal liability and maintain network security, employee productivity, and confidentiality of information.

Web-Based Applications for Healthcare

There is a high level of concern over the security of health information transmitted via the World Wide Web. The debate over whether the Web is safe enough to use for health information is likely to continue for some time. Technology and good practices can provide adequate security. Economic concerns may diminish safeguards. Internet use for healthcare information over the Web continues to grow. Protection of health information can be ensured by spelling out liability for its compromise and insurance.

Electronic Storage

Increased access to information through an ever-increasing number of interconnected storage devices and networks also creates additional concerns over security. Security threats to stored information mirror those that may affect any network. Unauthorized access to information is a major threat that can be curtailed through careful management of the interfaces between systems. It is crucial to ensure that authorized users can access information when they need it but that sufficient security measures are in place to prevent unauthorized access. These measures include requirements for user identification and encrypted passwords to access the various components of the network.

Confidential information may also be copied from the system in the form of electronic records. Administrators may download these records for report purposes. Once the records are no longer needed, electronic copies of sensitive data should be deleted or subjected to shredder software. **File deletion software** overwrites files with meaningless information so that sensitive information cannot be accessed.

Special Considerations with Mobile Computing

Mobile computing has the potential to improve information access, enhance workflow, and promote evidence-based practice to make informed and effective decisions at the point of care (Lu, Xiao, Sears, & Jacko 2005; Pohjonen, Ross, Blickman, & Kamman 2007). Handheld computers, or PDAs offer portable and unobtrusive access to clinical data and relevant information at the point of care. They also prove useful in areas of documentation and medical reference. For these reasons PDAs are used widely in healthcare providers' practice, and the level of use is expected to rise. Despite these many benefits there are also problems. According to a recent survey by the *British Journal of Healthcare Computing and Information Management*, one fifth of devices used to store data in the healthcare sector had no security (Survey reveals 2006). This study was limited to 117 medical professionals and IT managers. It included laptops, PDAs, Blackberry®s, and phones, most of which were individually owned. Individual devices must be subjected to the same types of safeguards applied to healthcare information systems. No patient specific information should be placed on a device unless it is protected. For example, students can use their PDAs for reference and make notes on their patient assignments but should never input identifiable information.

Staff who use PDAs should work with the information services department to help secure those devices from unauthorized view. Other problems identified with the adoption of mobile technology include usability and lack of technical and organizational support. Point-of-care devices and the software that they use must actually serve to facilitate, not hinder, the work of the bedside caregiver in order to realize the benefits associated with point-of-care technology. The mobility that provides an advantage can also pose problems because mobile devices may be left unattended in patient care areas subject to unauthorized view or theft.

FUTURE DIRECTIONS

The necessity of uninterrupted access to information makes it imperative that the systems that house the information are adequately secured. Unfortunately security has not received the attention that it deserves, as is evident from the number of recent high profile cases of theft, loss, and accidental disclosure of personal and health information. Greater awareness, sufficient resources, and an organization-wide commitment to information security are needed, particularly as development proceeds toward the realization of a lifetime electronic health record. Healthcare institutions and providers have an obligation to consumers to secure health information. Present methods are not enough. New technologies will emerge to meet this need and existing measures such as biometric authentication will become more common.

CASE STUDY EXERCISES

10.1 In the course of conversation, your nurse manager tells you that she loaded a copy of the spreadsheet program she uses on her home office PC onto one of the unit PCs so that she can work on projects at both locations. Your institution has a well-publicized policy against the use of unauthorized, unlicensed software copies. As a staff nurse, what should you do? Explain your response.

10.2 You notice several of the new physicians playing computer games on the nursing unit. You had not seen any of these games previously. What, if any, action should you take? Explain your rationale.

10.3 To remember his computer system password, university nursing instructor Pat Pawakawicz taped his password to the back of his identification badge. When Mr. Pawakawicz lost his identification badge recently, it was turned into hospital security, and subsequently the IS department, with his password still attached. When Mr. Pawakawicz picked up his identification badge, he expressed intent to use the same password. Is this an appropriate way to treat a password? Should he use the same password again? Provide your rationale. What, if any, legal ramifications might there be for Mr. Pawakawicz regarding use of his password by unauthorized users?

10.4 The administration at St. John's Hospital takes pride in their strong policies and procedures for the protection of confidential client information. In fact, St. John's serves as a model for other institutions in this area. However, printouts discarded in the restricted access IS department are not shredded. On numerous occasions, personnel working late observed the cleaning staff reading discarded printouts. What action, if any, should these personnel take relative to the actions of the cleaning staff? What action, if any, should be taken by IS administration? Provide your rationale. If current practices are maintained, are there any additional potential risks for unauthorized disclosure of client information? If you answer yes, identify what these risks might be.

10.5 The secretary on 7 Tower Oncology receives a Fax transmission about a client consult. The Fax was intended for a physician's office in the adjacent building. She places the Fax in the out bin of her desk to be delivered later by volunteers. No in-house mailer was used. Is this action appropriate? Explain why or why not.

10.6 You notice that the new nurse practitioner for one of your major orthopedic practices has a PDA on which he keeps patient information. Today he left it in the cafeteria. What should you do?

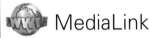 **MediaLink**

Additional resources for this content can be found on the Companion Website at www.prenhall.com/hebda. Click on "Chapter 10" to select the activities for this chapter.

- Glossary
- Multiple Choice
- Discussion Points
- Case Studies
- MediaLink Application
- MediaLink

SUMMARY

- The primary goals of healthcare information system security are the protection of client confidentiality and information availability and integrity.
- Privacy and confidentiality are important terms in healthcare information management. Privacy is a choice to disclose personal information, while confidentiality assumes a relationship in which private information has been shared for the purpose of health treatment.
- Information privacy is the right to choose the conditions under which information is shared and to ensure the accuracy of collected information.
- Threats to information and system security and confidentiality come from a variety of sources, including system penetration by thieves, hackers, unauthorized use, denial of service and terrorist attacks, cybercrime, errors and disasters, sabotage, viruses, and human error.

- Planning for security saves time and money and is a form of insurance against downtime, breaches in confidentiality, and lost productivity.
- Security mechanisms combine physical and logical restrictions. Examples include automatic sign-off, physical restriction of computer equipment, strong password protection, and firewalls.
- Ultimately, healthcare administrators are responsible for protecting client privacy and confidentiality through education, policy, and creating an ongoing awareness of security.
- One aspect of system security management includes monitoring the system for unusual record access patterns, as might be seen when a celebrity receives treatment.
- Health information on the Internet requires the same types of safeguards provided for information found in private offices and information systems.
- All chart printouts, forms, and computer files containing client information should be given the same consideration as the client record itself to safeguard confidentiality.
- More secure methods of authentication are needed as even the best passwords can be compromised.

REFERENCES

Australia's privacy legislation: A guide for nurses (2002). *Australian Nursing Journal, 10*(2), 24.

Blair, P. D. (2003). Make room for patient privacy. *Nursing Management, 34*(6), 28.

Britt, P. (2005). Protecting private information. *Information Today, 22*(5), 1–38.

Calloway, S. D. & Venegas, L. M. (2002). The new HIPAA law on privacy and confidentiality. *Nursing Administration Quarterly, 26*(4), 40.

Campbell, J., Kleeman, D., & Ma, Wi. (2007). The good and not so good of enforcing password composition rules. *Information Systems Security, 16*(1), 2–8.

Gordon, L. A., Loeb, M. P., Lucyshyn, W., & Richardson, R. (2006). 2006 CSI/FBI Computer crime and security survey. Computer Security Institute. Retrieved July 24, 2006, from http://i.cmpnet.com/gocsi/db_area/pdfs/fbi/FBI2006.pdf.

Griffiths, D. (April 22, 2003). Treat IT security as if the law required it. *Computer Weekly,* 44.

Hebda, T., Sakerka, L., & Czar, P. (1994). Educating nurses to maintain patient confidentiality on automated information systems. In S. J. Grobe and E. S. P. Pluyter-Wenting (Eds.), *Nursing informatics: An international overview for nursing in a technological era, The Proceedings of the Fifth IMIA International Conference on Nursing Use of Computers and Information Science.* New York: Elsevier Science.

Hill, J. (March 29, 2003). Speak no evil. *Lancet, 361*(9363), 1140.

Joint Commission on Accreditation of Healthcare Organizations (1996). *Medical records process.* Chicago: Accreditation Manual for Hospitals.

Kelly, G. & McKenzie, B. (2002). Security, privacy, and confidentiality issues on the Internet. *Journal of Medical Internet Research, 4*(2), e12. Retrieved November 2, 2003, from http://www.jmir.org/2002/2/e12/.

Kmentt, K. A. (Winter 1987). Private medical records: Are they public property? *Medical Trial Technique Quarterly, 33,* 274–307.

Lemos, R. (2006, May 9). Password policies. *PC Magazine, 25*(9), 116.

Lu, Y. C., Xiao, Y., Sears, A., & Jacko, J. A. (2005). A review and a framework of handheld computer adoption in healthcare. *International Journal of Medical Informatics, 74*(5), 409–422.

Malin, A. (2007). Designing networks that enforce information security policies. *Information Systems Security, 16*(1), 47–53.

McCarthy, B. (2006a). Close the security disconnect between awareness and practice. *Electronic Design, 54*(19), 20.

McCarthy, B. (2006b). Security efforts still falling short. *eWeek, 23*(46), E4.

McMillan, R. (2007). *Phishing* sites explode on the Web. *PC World,* 25(4), 22.

Mitrakas, A. (March 2006). Information security and law in Europe: Risks checked? *Information & Communications Technology Law, 15*(1), 33–53.

Murdock, L. E. (1980). The use and abuse of computerized information: Striking a balance between personal privacy interests and organizational information needs. *Albany Law Review, 44*(3), 589–619.

Olinger, H. N., Britz, J. J., & Olivier, M. S. (2007). Western privacy and/or Ubuntu? Some critical comments on the influences in the forthcoming data privacy bill in South Africa. *International Information & Library Review, 39*(1), 31–43.

Pohjonen, H., Ross, P., Blickman, J. G., & Kamman, R. (2007). Pervasive access to images and data—the use of computing grids and mobile/wireless devices across healthcare enterprises. *IEEE Transactions on Information Technology in Biomedicine, 11*(1), 81–86.

Rainer, R. K., Marshall, T. E., Knapp, K. J., & Montgomery, G. H. (2007). Do information security professionals and business managers view information security issues differently? *Information Systems Security, 16*(2), 100–108.

Ramanathan, R. (2006). Thinking beyond security. *Security Management, 15*(2), 49–54.

Reagan, M. (2003). Electronic eye can protect your health information. Retrieved June 4, 2003, from http://www.advanceforhie.com/common/Editorial/Editorial. aspx?CC-15124.

Romano, C. (1987). Confidentiality, and security of computerized systems: The nursing responsibility. *Computers in Nursing, 5*(3), 99–104.

Sax, U., Kohane, I., & Mandl, K. D. (2005). Wireless technology infrastructures for authentication of patients: PKI that rings. *Journal of the American Medical Informatics Association, 12*(3), 263–268.

Steele, S. & Wargo, C. (2007) An introduction to insider threat management. *Information Systems Security, 16*(1), 23–33.

Stern, L. (October 29, 2007). When to be wary of 'free wi-fi.' *Newsweek,* 62–63.

Sturdevant, C. (May 7, 2007). Keystrokes are us. *eWeek,* 32.

Survey reveals NHS failing to secure data on mobile devices (June 27, 2006). Retrieved July 23, 2007, from http://www.bjhc.co.uk/news/1/2006/n606012.htm.

Tuesday, V. (April 21, 2003). Security log. *Computerworld, 37*(16), 35.

Vidalis, S. & Kazmi, Z. (2007). Security through deception. *Information Systems Security, 16*(1,) 34–41.

Windslade, W. J. (1982). Confidentiality of medical records: An overview of concepts and legal policies. *Journal of Legal Medicine, 3*(4), 497–533.

CHAPTER 11

System Integration and Interoperability

After completing this chapter, you should be able to:

1 Recognize the importance of *system integration* and *interoperability* for healthcare delivery.

2 Explain what an *interface engine* is and how it works.

3 Identify several integration issues, including factors that impede the process.

4 Discuss the relevance to system integration efforts of the data dictionary, master patient index, uniform language efforts, and clinical data repository.

5 Consider how standards for the exchange of clinical data affect integration efforts.

6 Review the benefits of successful information system integration for healthcare providers and healthcare professionals.

7 Define the role of the nurse in system integration efforts.

8 Understand how Web-based tools can provide an alternative method for obtaining patient information from diverse information systems.

Most hospitals and healthcare providers have computer information systems in some, if not all, of their major departments. Historically, financial systems were computerized first, followed by registration, laboratory, order entry, pharmacy, radiology, and monitoring systems (not necessarily in that order). Some of these computer information systems were first implemented as stand-alone systems. Most departments select the information system that best meets their needs or that hospital administrators approve because of cost reasons, promises to vendors, or the preexistence of other products by the same vendor in the institution. It is rare for all departments in a given healthcare institution to agree that one vendor's product meets their information system needs. As a consequence, most institutions have several different systems that do not readily communicate or share data. Each of these systems may be highly customized to meet individual department and institutional specifications. This customization, however, complicates integration. Integration needs have increased dramatically as single institutions and providers use more systems internally and as they join with other institutions to form enterprises, alliances, and networks. In addition, integration must be achieved before the electronic health record (EHR) can be realized.

Integration is the process by which different information systems are able to exchange data in a fashion that is seamless to the end user. The physical aspects of joining networks together are not nearly as complicated as getting unlike systems to exchange information in a seamless manner. Traditionally, communication between and among most disparate systems has been the result of costly, time-consuming efforts to build interfaces. In other words, interface programs are the tools used to achieve integration. An **interface** is a computer program that tells two different systems how to exchange data.

Without integration, providers cannot realize the full advantages of automation, since sharing data across multiple systems is limited and redundant data entry by various personnel takes place. When this occurs, the likelihood of errors is increased. This situation is unacceptable in a time when managed care forces institutions to realize the benefits of automation to compete in today's healthcare delivery system. Box 11–1 lists some benefits associated with integration.

BOX 11–1 The Benefits of Integration

- Allows instant access to applications and data
- Improves data integrity with single entry of data
- Decreases labor costs with single entry of data
- Facilitates the formulation of a more accurate, complete client record
- Facilitates information tracking for accurate cost determinations

INTERFACES

Interfaces between different information systems should be invisible to the user. Many vendors claim their products are based on open systems technology, which is the ability to communicate with other systems. The reality is that there has been little incentive for vendors to market products that readily work with their competitors' products. Another problem is that the customization of vendor products by individual providers precludes off-the-shelf interface solutions. This necessitates costly and time-consuming design of custom interfaces. Another problem with customized interfaces is pinpointing the responsibility for any problems that occur. Each vendor responsible for developing an interface tends to blame the other for any difficulties encountered. Without a determination of responsibility, problem resolution is delayed and no one can be held accountable for the cost of solving the problem. All too often the institution must absorb the costs for this process; yet competition in a managed care environment does not permit this luxury. In addition, the timely flow of information is critical to cost-cutting measures and institutional survival.

There are two general types of interfaces: point-to-point and those using integration engine software. A **point-to-point interface** is an interface that directly connects two information systems. Communication and transfer of data take place only between these systems. Historically these were the first types of interfaces used in healthcare. This type of interface is achieved through customized programming and for this reason is expensive and labor-intensive to build and maintain.

More recent technology uses **interface engine** software to create and manage interfaces. This provides the ability to transfer information from the sending system to one or many receiving systems and allows users of different information systems to access and exchange information both in real-time and batch processing. **Real-time processing** occurs immediately, or with only a slight delay, whereas **batch processing** typically occurs once daily. In this situation, data are often not processed until the end of the day and therefore are not available to users until that time. Although batch processing was very common in the past, current use is primarily limited to transactions that are less time critical, such as processing charges for procedures, supplies, and special equipment.

The interface engine provides seamless integration and presentation of information results. Interface engines work in the background and are not seen by the user. This technology allows applications to interact with hardware and other applications. Interface engines allow different systems that use unlike terminology to exchange information without the need to build expensive point-to-point interfaces (Freedman 2007). This is done through the use of translation tables to move data from each system to the **clinical data repository,** a database where collective data from all information systems are stored and managed. The clinical data repository provides data definition consistency through mapping. The clinical data repository may also be referred to as the clinical data warehouse (CDW). Over time the CDW has evolved to support financial as well as clinical applications. The CDW was once developed within individual facilities but is increasingly now available commercially through vendors (Akhtar et al. 2005). **Mapping** is the process in which terms defined in one system are associated with comparable terms in another system. The major impact of using interface engines is that mappings for multiple receiving systems can be built for each sending system. For example, a client registration system can send registration transactions to the interface engine, which then forwards them on to any number of ancillary systems such as laboratory, radiology, and pharmacy. Each of these systems is able to receive updated client healthcare and demographic information, eliminating the need to manually register the client in the ancillary system. Box 11–2 discusses some of the benefits associated with the use of interface engines.

Interfacing of laboratory orders and results provides another example of how the interface engine is used in a hospital setting. On admission, the client's demographic information is entered in the hospital registration system, and portions of these data are transmitted to the clinical data repository via the interface engine. When a laboratory order is entered into the order entry system, the appropriate client demographic information is retrieved from the clinical data repository and used by the order entry system. After the order is entered, the order information may be transmitted via the interface engine to the clinical data repository and the laboratory system. When testing is complete, the results are transferred via the interface engine from the laboratory system to the clinical data repository. At this point, they are available for retrieval using the order entry system or another clinical information system.

Interface engines require new skills in the information services department. Staff may now include an integration analyst who identifies initial and ongoing interface specifications, coordinates any changes that will impact interfaces, and maintains a database for translation tables. This analyst must ascertain that data integrity is intact for all data to be sent correctly through the interface engine.

Most discussions that involve the large-scale electronic exchange of healthcare information across enterprises for the purpose of accessing and maintaining

---

BOX 11–2 Interface Engine Benefits

- Improves timeliness and availability of critical administrative and clinical data
- Decreases integration costs by providing an alternative to customized point-to-point interface application programming
- Improves data quality because of data mapping and consistent use of terms
- Allows clients to select the best system for their needs
- Preserves institutional investment in existing systems
- Simplifies the administration of healthcare data processing
- Simplifies systems integration efforts
- Shortens the time required for integration
- Improves management of care, the financial tracking of care rendered, and efficacy of treatment

longitudinal health records speak of interoperability. **Interoperability** is the ability of two entities, whether those are human or machine, to exchange and predictably use data or information while retaining the original meaning of that data (Freedman 2007; Mead 2006; Schwend 2007). While the terms *interface* and *interoperability* are sometimes used interchangeably the interface engine routes information from one system to another but stops short of enabling the second system to understand and use that information. There are two types of interoperability: syntactic and semantic. Syntactic interoperability is the ability to exchange the structure of the data, but not necessarily the meaning of the data. It is also referred to as functional interoperability. Web pages built with HTML illustrate this type of interoperability. Semantic interoperability guarantees that the meaning of the exchanged data remains the same on both ends of the transaction. This is critical for clinical data. There have been several standardization efforts to achieve interoperability for EHRs. These include: the Health Level Seven (HL7) Clinical Document Architecture (CDA); the European Committee for Standardization (CEN) EN 13606-1, also known as EHRcom; and the openEHR. All provide specifications for how information should be exchanged (Kilic 2007). HL7 relies upon XML markup language for the storage and movement of clinical documents between systems. The International Organization for Standardization (ISO) (2007) considers EN 13606-1 to be a communications standard in development. The primary focus of EN 13606-1 is to support direct care given to individuals, or to support population monitoring systems such as disease registries and public health surveillance, although EN 13606-1 may also allow the use of health records for secondary purposes such as disease registries, teaching, audits, reports, and anonymous aggregation of individual records for epidemiology or research.

The openEHR initiative is an international effort to provide semantic interoperability through the creation of specifications, open source software, and tools (Kalra 2007; Kilic & Dogac 2007; openEHR Foundation 2007). It builds upon more than 15 years of international research on the EHR. In the clinical arena, it strives to create high-quality, reusable clinical models of content and process that are defined by clinicians and known as **archetypes,** as well as formal interfaces to terminology. Each archetype contains a header, definition, and ontology section. The header has a unique code identifying the clinical concept defined as well as descriptive information such as author, version, and status. The definition includes restrictions obtained from the information model. The ontology section contains codes representing the meanings of nodes and constraints on text or terms, as well as linkages to terminologies such as SNOMED or LOINC. The Archetype Definition Language (ADL) is a formal language for the expression of archetypes.

On a second level the openEHR initiative supports the use of archetypes to model and share knowledge (Garde, Knaup, & Hovenga 2005). The development and maintenance of archetypes must be coordinated at an international level with input from health professionals for success (Garde et al. 2007). Archetypes must be consistent, link to terminology systems in an appropriate way, and meet quality standards for the capture, processing, and communication of clinical data (Kalra 2007). The EuroRec Institute has partnered with the openEHR Foundation to address quality criteria. Despite these and other efforts there is no single standard in place at present that provides complete interoperability for electronic health records despite vendor claims (Jian et al. 2007). Integrating Healthcare Enterprise (IHE®) is a global initiative dedicated to improving patient care by promoting the way that computer systems in healthcare share information by promoting the adoption of standards such as DICOM and HL7 and interoperability (HIMSS 2007). IHE®, which was conceived in the late 1990s, recently adopted principles of governance. There have been other projects for interoperability in the United States, Canada, and the European Union over the years.

Recent literature focuses upon yet another potential solution to interoperability, namely service-oriented architecture (SOA) (Bridges 2007; Cohen, Amatayakul, & Zeng 2007). SOA calls for placing key functions into modules that, along with new capabilities, may be re-used, similar to object-oriented programming. SOA defines a service as a self-contained unit of work that has well defined and understood capabilities. A service may be an entire process, a function supporting a process, or a step of a business process. Services may be built into a library that can be used to address enterprise needs. SOA does not require re-engineering of existing systems. SOA goes beyond other technologies in that it is vendor and technology neutral and does not require specific equipment or standards for operation. SOA can support information exchange among systems that use different programming languages. Its other characteristics hold promise for streamlining health information exchange. These include the ability to maintain a registry of services at the enterprise level that can be invoked after lookup, and the ability to provide quality service that includes security requirements such as authentication, authorization, and reliable messaging and policies.

INTEGRATION AND INTEROPERABILITY ISSUES

Integration is a massive project within institutions and enterprises. It generally requires more time and effort than originally projected. Several factors contribute to this situation. First, vendors frequently make promises about their products to make a sale; often these promises cannot be delivered. Second, merged institutions may prefer to keep their own systems rather than accept a uniform standard that would be easier to implement. The strategy adopted in this situation may require further negotiation and additional programming. Third, as each department and institution tries to retain its own identity and political power, it is difficult to come to an agreement on a common data dictionary, data mapping, and clinical data repository issues. Another issue is that integration brings a number of concerns for individuals, including changes in job description, learning new skills, the fear of job loss, and the general fear of change. Box 11–3 identifies several factors that may impede the integration process.

BOX 11–3 Factors That Slow Integration

- **Unrealistic vendor promises.** Vendors often promise that their information systems are interoperable with other systems. Many customers find, however, they face difficult, lengthy, and costly integration efforts after they have already purchased the system.
- **Unrealistic institutional timetable.** This is often based on a lack of understanding of the complexity of the integration process.
- **Changing user specifications.** As the integration process proceeds, users frequently request additional capabilities or change their minds regarding initial specifications.
- **Lack of vendor support.** Vendors may not provide enough support and assistance to facilitate the integration efforts.
- **Insufficient documentation.** Information regarding existing systems and related programming is imperative for achieving successful integration.
- **Lack of agreement among merged institutions.** Individual facilities within a merged enterprise may wish to continue use of their existing systems. This means there are more systems to integrate.
- **All components of a vendor's products may not work together.** Although difficulties are expected in attempts to integrate competing vendors' products, there may also be problems in integrating products developed by the same vendor.

Freedman (2007) notes that progress toward attaining true large-scale interoperability has been impeded by a lack of consensus as to how it should be achieved. Some experts feel that perfect harmonization of standards between technology systems must occur first, while others oversimplify the issue by stating that interoperability can be attained merely by mapping codes from one system to another. Rather than waiting until the issue is fully resolved, Freedman advocates using extant technology that can provide some level of semantic interoperability, and then building upon that foundation. Bridges (2007) calls SOA the next step in system evolution because it will allow enterprises to shift their efforts from maintaining a complex interface strategy to creating service-oriented applications that support interoperability while focusing more closely on the business of healthcare delivery. With the additional adoption and use of SOA within the healthcare industry, collections of services will be available for purchase or subscription serving with the end result that providers can focus on their primary business rather than duplicating the efforts of those who went before them. Other interoperability issues include:

- The need to select interoperability solutions that work with present and evolving standards
- Need for consensus on archetypes for broad clinical application
- Safe use of processes such as decision support across sites, which requires a consistent approach for naming and organizing EHR entries so that all needed information can be obtained (Kalra 2007).

NATIONAL HEALTHCARE INFORMATION NETWORK (NHIN)

Several developments led to the creation of the National Healthcare Information Network (NHIN). These include the Institute of Medicine's 2001 report *Crossing the Quality Chasm: A New Health System for the 21st Century*, which called for the development of a national health information network as a means to advance healthcare information technology and realize the benefits that a health information exchange (HIE) could offer. There are also benefits associated with interoperability, including improved physician workflow, productivity and patient care, improved safety, fully standardized healthcare information exchange, and an estimated annual savings equivalent to approximately 5% of annual U.S. healthcare expenditures (Conn 2006; FORE 2006; Kaushal 2005; Schwend 2007). The Markle Foundation started the Connecting for Health project in 2001 to promote the interconnection of healthcare information systems, then announced a contribution of $1.9 million to launch a Regional Health Information Organization (RHIO) interconnectivity project in 2005. The Robert Wood Johnson Foundation also provided financial support to this effort. In 2004 President Bush issued a directive for interoperable electronic health records by 2014. In late 2007 Mike Leavitt, secretary of the Department of Health and Human Services, announced the award of contracts totaling $22.5 million to nine HIEs to begin trial implementations of the NHIN (HHS 2007). The lessons learned and the technological gains from both projects will be available for public use. These efforts represent a start but the road to the NHIN will be an expensive one. In 2005 a study published by Kaushal (2005) in the *Annals of Internal Medicine* estimated the cost to implement the NHIN at $103 billion in total capital with another $27 billion annually for operating costs. Enrado (2007) and Larsen (2005) suggest the focus should instead be the incentives for establishing the NHIN, namely the benefits such as improved quality of care, safety, and decreased costs related to redundant services. Larsen also notes the need to establish a roadmap to establishing the NHIN, one that will allow the cost to be broken down into steps as well as a re-examination of what is meant by interoperability. In the interim, work continues on developing the framework to support NHIN. In late 2007 the Healthcare Information Technology Standards Panel (HITSP), a multi-stakeholder group working with the U.S. Department of Health and Human Services to assure the interoperability of electronic health records in the United States, approved recommendations designed to facilitate the secure exchange of information. These recommendations were sent to the American Health Information Community (AHIC), which will make further recommendations to Secretary Leavitt for his acceptance (ANSI 2007). Many other organizations are involved in the effort as well. Some of these include:

- Office of Interoperability and Standards for the Office of the National Coordinator for Health Information Technology, or ONCHIT
- The Certification Commission on Healthcare Information Technology (CCHIT)

- Commission on Systemic Interoperability
- National Committee on Vital and Health Statistics
- The Center for Information Technology Leadership (CITL).

The Centers for Disease Control are working to build their own structure for disseminating and collecting information about health issues in the United States with the hope that it will lead to sharing data with providers on an ongoing basis, shortening the time needed to spot trends and respond accordingly (Bazzoli 2004).

THE NEED FOR INTEGRATION STANDARDS

The need to exchange client data is rapidly increasing in response to the demands placed by managed care as well as consumer demands for improved levels of healthcare. To derive the utmost benefit from data, it must have a consistent or standard meaning across institution, enterprise, and alliance boundaries, facilitating the exchange of client data. This is the basis for developing a data dictionary within an enterprise and a uniform language for use on a national and global scale. It is becoming increasingly important for hospitals and information system vendors to adopt and use uniform standards for the electronic exchange of clinical information (Ball & Farish-Hunt 2003). Use of uniform standards will provide safer and more efficient healthcare delivery systems and also play a critical role in compliance with government healthcare regulations.

So many standards exist now that it adds to the difficulty of standardization. Multinational vendors are reluctant to commit to the adoption of standards that are not universal (Nusbaum 2007). In some cases only local interoperability is available. Recent initiatives such as Integrating Healthcare Enterprise (IHE) and national harmonization initiatives in the United States and abroad may help to solve that problem as they strive to create a "plug and play" solution by eliminating the optional features individual vendors supply with their version of standards such as DICOM and HL7.

Data Dictionary

The **data dictionary** defines terminology to ensure consistent understanding and use across the enterprise. Terms defined in the data dictionary should include synonyms found in the various systems used within the enterprise. This may be achieved, in some cases, through the use of the interface engine. For example, a term or data element may be a diagnosis or a laboratory test, such as "potassium." Potassium may be known in the nursing order entry system as "potassium" but be called "K" in the laboratory system. The use of the data dictionary and interface engine facilitates integration and allows for the collection of aggregate data.

Master Patient Index

The integration process may require enhancements to the data dictionary, the clinical data repository, and the master patient index. The **master patient index** (MPI) is a database that lists all identifiers assigned to one client in all the information systems used within an enterprise. It assigns a global identification number for each client and allows clients to be identified by demographic information provided at the point of care. The MPI may use first and last names, birthdates, Social Security numbers, and driver's license numbers. It cannot rely on a single type of number such as the Social Security number, because of duplicates and the fact that some people, such as noncitizens, may not have one. When the MPI cannot match records based on demographic data, all possible matches are provided for the user to view and select. The MPI is a critical component in supporting successful integration. Not all healthcare enterprises have a data dictionary, a clinical data repository, or MPI, or these components may be in various stages of development. The move toward creating a lifetime patient record creates the need to access client encounters across time. This is particularly important in a multi-institutional enterprise. The MPI, data dictionary, and clinical data repository are tools that support this effort.

The MPI saves work because vital information can be obtained from the database rather than rekeyed with each client visit. This decreases the possibility of making a mistake and eliminates the inadvertent creation of duplicate records. As a result, the registration clerk now plays a greater role in the maintenance of data integrity.

Some of the key features of an effective MPI include the following:

- It locates records in real time for timely retrieval of information.
- It is flexible enough to allow inclusion of additional identification.
- It is easily reconfigured to accommodate network changes.
- It can grow to fit an organization of any size.

It is possible to exchange information without first creating a master patient index (Getting started 2007). A research group of the American Health Information Management Association recommended starting with clinical messaging for the exchange of clinical information, such as lab results, and then adding additional information and services such as medication history, clinical summaries, quality measurement, reporting services, and administrative data.

Uniform Language

One step in the integration process is the development of a uniform definition of terms, or language. This is essential for the easy location and manipulation of data. Many efforts to develop uniform languages are under way in the healthcare arena. For example, the National Library of Medicine developed the Unified Medical Language System (UMLS), which includes the Uniform Nursing Language. In addition, the American Nurses Association sponsors the Congress of Nursing Practice Steering Committee on Databases (ANA revises criteria 1996). This group addresses issues including nursing classification schemes, uniform data sets, data elements, and national databases. One of its primary goals is to develop a mapping system to link various classification schemes. This would allow the development of national data sets for use by nursing.

There are several nursing classification systems currently in place, with the most prominent being the following three (Butcher 2004). The North American Nursing Diagnosis Association (NANDA)—now NANDA-International—is an organization that has developed a system for classifying nursing diagnoses or statements that identify those client care problems that nurses are licensed to treat independently (Thede 1999). The Nursing Intervention Classification (NIC) is a classification system developed at the University of Iowa to categorize interventions based on clinical judgment and knowledge that nurses perform to improve client outcome (Butcher 2004). And the Nursing Outcome Classification (NOC) allows nurses to measure client outcome status at any point in the continuum of care. This information can be used as input for revising the plan of care. NANDA, NIC, and NOC are designed to be used together as one large system for classifying nursing care (Thede 1999). Another classification system is the International Classification for Nursing Practice (ICNP®) which encompasses NANDA, NIC, and NOC as well as several other languages. They allow the collection of data related to nursing care, providing many benefits, such as the following:

- Collection and analysis of nursing care data for documentation in the client record
- Support of the development of an EHR by classifying and categorizing nursing data
- Facilitation of the evaluation of client care

In addition to nursing, coding systems are used in other areas of healthcare to communicate information about medical diagnoses and procedures performed. This information is most commonly captured using the **ICD-9/ICD-10** and **CPT-4** systems. *ICD-9 (International Classification of Disease—Ninth Revision)* provides a classification for surgical, diagnostic, and therapeutic procedures (Thede 1999). This information is used for hospital billing and third-party payment throughout the United States. *ICD-10* is an enlarged version of *ICD-9* that is generally used in Europe at this time. The *ICD-9/ICD-10* systems are published by the National Center for Health Statistics. Another commonly used classification is *CPT-4 (Current Procedural Terminology—Fourth Revision)*, which is published annually by the American Medical Association. This system lists medical services and procedures performed by physicians and is used for physician billing and payer reimbursement.

SNOMED (Systemized Nomenclature of Human and Veterinary Medicine) is a classification system created by the College of American Pathologists (Thede 1999). This system includes signs and symptoms of disease, diagnoses, and procedures and is meant to represent the full integration of all medical information in an electronic medical record.

Data Exchange Standards

In addition to the uniform definition of terms, integration standards facilitate the exchange of client data by providing a set of rules and structure for formatting the data.

HL7 A major standard for the exchange of clinical data for integration is Health Level 7 (HL7). HL7 refers to both an organization and its standards for the exchange of clinical data. The mission of the organization is to provide standards for the management and integration of healthcare data (Health Level Seven 2007). In particular, these standards address definitions of data to be exchanged, the timing of the exchanges, and communication of certain errors between applications. HL7 provides a structure that defines data and elements and specifies how the data are coded. The structure of the data element must follow HL7 rules, such as those specifying the length of the fields and the code nomenclature. Use of HL7 standards in individual applications improves the integration of these applications with other applications or systems using an interface engine. Benefits include easier and less costly integration within an organization and more accurate and useful data integration nationally and globally. Integration efforts and the development and use of integration standards, including HL7, are taking place at many levels. For example, integration is seen beyond the hospital setting in the form of integrated delivery systems (IDS). Although efforts are under way to develop both national and international health data networks, competition has not yet facilitated this type of information sharing. Sometimes HL7 standards have been modified by information system vendors to support various applications, creating integration issues. HL7 Version 3 was developed in response to a growing awareness that Version 2 did not guarantee meaningful exchange of data across enterprise boundaries in a cost-effective manner (Mead 2006).

HL7 standards are not the only standards that have been evolving to fit the changing healthcare model. Other organizations instrumental in supporting the development of standards and in helping to define data exchange include the Institute of Medicine, National Institute of Standards and Technology, the National Science Foundation, the National Library of Medicine, the National Committee for Health Statistics, the Centers for Medicare and Medicare Services, the National Coordinator for Health Information Technology, the American Health Information Management Association, the American Medical Informatics Association, and the Healthcare Information and Management Systems Society.

DICOM DICOM (Digital Imaging and Communications in Medicine) is a global Information technology standard first developed for the transmission of medical images and their associated information. It is now used in nearly all hospitals worldwide for the production, display, storage, retrieval, and printing of medical images and derived structured documents, as well as to manage related workflow (DICOM 2007). DICOM's goals are to achieve compatibility and improve workflow efficiency between imaging systems and other information systems. DICOM also addresses the integration of information produced by specialty imaging applications into the electronic health system, defining the network and media interchange services that allow storage and access to these DICOM objects for EHR systems. Proprietary features from some vendors limit interoperability (Broda 2007).

BENEFITS OF INTEGRATION AND INTEROPERABILITY

One major benefit of integration and the ability to exchange client data is the development of the electronic health record. In this case, integration allows data from many disparate information systems to be accessed from one point by the user, providing a complete record for each client. The clinical data repository is a key element of the EHR. It provides a storage facility for clinical data over time. The data in the clinical data repository may be generated from various systems and locations. For example, laboratory data may be generated by a laboratory system and may be collected in an acute, ambulatory, or long-term care setting. Other data may be included from clinical systems such as radiology, pharmacy, and order entry. Decision-support applications that use clinical repository data benefit other facilities if data from all facilities can be mapped to the data dictionary. One of the stumbling blocks to the creation and maintenance of the clinical data repository is poor documentation regarding term definitions in the individual systems collecting the data. Figure 11–1 depicts an example of mapping with laboratory test terms.

Hospitals and healthcare enterprises also benefit from integration. Integration strategies permit data exchange within each hospital and across healthcare networks or enterprises, allowing them to find trends in financial and clinical data. Integration opens up a realm of possibilities to trend data, such as by provider, by diagnosis, or by cost. In this way, healthcare providers obtain improved information, making them better able to react to market changes and maintain a competitive edge.

Integration of related systems such as Radiology Information System (RIS), Picture Archiving Communication System (PACS), and the EHR provides clinicians with a greatly enhanced view of diagnostic radiology information that can be accessed from many points within the hospital, or remotely. This integration provides the ability to view an electronic text report related to a radiology examination from the EHR and then seamlessly view the associated electronic images from the PACS systems. A standard client identifier

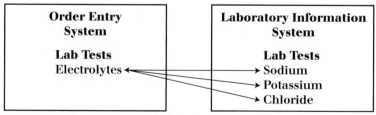

The order entry system lists a test called Electrolytes. The laboratory information system does not list a test called Electrolytes but lists its individual component tests. Before the interface engine can allow exchange of data, the relationships between the tests listed in both systems must be established by mapping.

FIGURE 11–1 • Mapping of laboratory test terms

used by all the organizations' information systems is key to creating this type of integration.

The lack of data integration is a barrier to effective data reporting and analysis. For example, executive information needs may require data regarding all aspects of an obstetric client's care, including prenatal care, risk factors, complications before admission, length of hospital stay, and cost of the entire episode of care. Some of this information may be stored in an independent information system in the physician's office. Other data may be found in the hospital clinical information system and in the financial system. Without effective integration of clinical, financial, and administrative data, it is difficult to provide a complete system information base for management and decision support.

Another benefit of integration is that it facilitates data collection for accreditation processes. For example, the Joint Commission requirements call for the ability to provide aggregate data. These requirements include the following:

- Uniform definition of data
- Uniform methods for data capture
- Ability to provide client-specific as well as aggregate data

These information standards allow the Joint Commission to compare data within and among healthcare enterprises.

IMPLICATIONS FOR NURSING

There are also particular concerns for nursing in relation to system integration and interoperability. A primary consideration is that nursing involvement is essential in the design of interfaces and interoperability solutions (While & Thomas 2007). Nurses must be involved in identifying and defining data elements that an interface may be able to supply. One way to ensure this is to recruit staff nurses to provide input during the interface design.

Another concern is ensuring that data will be collected in only one system and shared via the interface engine and clinical data repository with all other systems requiring it. This eliminates redundant effort while ensuring data integrity. For example, a client's allergies should be identified and documented by a nurse and entered into a clinical information system. These data are then transmitted to the clinical data repository via the interface engine, where they are available for retrieval by other systems that may require them, such as a pharmacy system.

Nursing must also be involved in determining measures to assure the quality of the data that are exchanged among individual information systems and in the formation and maintenance of the electronic health record. If data quality cannot be assured then clinical decision support and other important features will be suspect.

Nursing can benefit from integration and data exchange. For example, trends in client care data and cost analysis can be used to justify nursing staffing levels in the hospital setting. In addition, integration provides a tool to build nursing knowledge.

FUTURE DIRECTIONS

Several years ago Web-based tools and Internet technology were seen as a means to provide access to data from disparate information systems (Turisco 1999). This was largely a local solution that improved access to clinical information for the providers at a single hospital or healthcare system, but did nothing to advance exchange of data on a larger scale or ensure that data could be used in the same manner in both sending and receiving systems. Since that time data exchange standards have been refined, national priorities set, and work has started on building the framework needed to make interoperability of electronic health data a reality. Interoperability will become increasingly vital for the optimal management of patient care and financial success of individual institutions (Brova 2007).What remains unclear is the exact means by which this will be accomplished, or whether it will build on one of several existing models or architectures. Much work lies ahead. The road will not be easy, quick, or cheap but the promised benefits will be immeasurable.

CASE STUDY EXERCISES

11.1 You have been selected as a member of the Integration Project Team, which is charged with identifying ways that system integration could improve information flow. You work on an inpatient unit that uses a stand-alone nursing documentation system that is not interfaced or integrated with any other hospital information system. Identify the implications of this situation, and suggest integration options that could improve information flow.

11.2 You are working to identify elements in your healthcare enterprise that could be used for a master patient index (MPI). List five basic elements and describe how each could be used for an MPI.

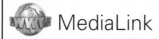 MediaLink

Additional resources for this content can be found on the Companion Website at www.prenhall.com/hebda. Click on "Chapter 11" to select the activities for this chapter.

- Glossary
- Multiple Choice
- Discussion Points
- Case Studies
- MediaLink Application
- MediaLink

SUMMARY

- An interface is a computer program that tells two different systems how to exchange data.
- Most healthcare providers have a variety of automated information systems that do not readily share data unless major efforts are made to build interfaces.
- Integration is the process by which different information systems are able to exchange data without any special effort on the part of the end user.
- The creation of networks to exchange data between systems and the process of integration are essential in today's healthcare information world, where an institution or enterprise may have multiple disparate clinical information systems.
- The interface engine is a software application designed to allow users of different information systems to exchange information without the need to build direct customized interfaces between systems.
- Other processes that facilitate the move toward and the exchange of health information include the clinical data repository, mapping, the data dictionary, the master patient index, uniform language efforts, and data exchange standards.
- The clinical data repository is a database that collects and stores data from all information systems.
- Mapping of terms establishes the relationship between terms defined in one system and those used in another.
- The data dictionary defines terms used within an enterprise to ensure consistent use.
- The master patient index lists all identifiers assigned to one client in all information systems and assigns a global identification code as a means to locate all records for a given client.
- Standardization of clinical terms through a uniform language is one means to facilitate the exchange of information across healthcare enterprises. The Congress of Nursing Practice Steering Committee on Databases and the National Library of Medicine (through its Unified Medical Language System) are working on uniform language issues.
- Three commonly used nursing classification systems are NANDA, NIC, and NOC. Efforts are underway to improve mapping of terms from one standard nursing language through the use of International Classification of Nursing Practice.
- Health Level 7 and DICOM are standards for the exchange of clinical data that provide rules and structure for how data are formatted.
- Integration improves data integrity and access for caregivers, eliminates redundant data collection, and improves data collection for staffing, for finding financial trends and client outcome trends, and for meeting requirements of regulatory and accrediting organizations.
- Integration is a necessary component for the development of the electronic health record and for integrated delivery systems.

- Interoperability is the ability of two entities, whether those are human or machine, to exchange and predictably use data or information while retaining the original meaning of that data.
- The National Healthcare Information Network (NHIN) is a proposed structure for the exchange of electronic data among individual healthcare enterprises for the purpose of supporting a longitudinal birth-to-death health record, with all of its attendant benefits, for all individuals.

REFERENCES

Akhtar, M. U., Dunn, K., & Smith, J. W. (2005). Commercial clinical data warehouses: From wave of the past to the state of the art. *Journal of Healthcare Information Management, 19*(2), 20–26.

American National Standards Institute (December 18, 2007). HITSP Delivers Next Round of Interoperability Specifications to Support U.S. Nationwide Health Information Network. Earthtimes.org. Retrieved December 25, 2007, from http://www.earthtimes.org/articles/show/news_press_release,244569.shtml.

ANA revises criteria for evaluating nursing vocabularies, classification systems. (November/December 1996). *The American Nurse, 9.*

Ball, M. & Farish-Hunt, H. (2003). Standards at center stage. *Healthcare Informatics,20*(11), 52–54.

Bazzoli, F. (1996). Providers point to index software as key element of integration plans. *Health Data Management, 4*(9), 61–65.

Bridges, M. W. (2007). SOA in healthcare, sharing system resources while enhancing interoperability within and between healthcare organizations with service-oriented architecture. *Health Management Technology, 28*(6), 6, 8, 10.

Broda, J. (2007). Going Beyond DICOM. *ADVANCE for Health Information Executives, 11*(7), 10.

Butcher, H. (2004). Nursing's distinctive knowledge. In L. Haynes, T. Boese, & H. Butcher (Eds.), *Nursing in contemporary society: Issues, trends and transition to practice* (pp. 71–103). Upper Saddle River, NJ: Pearson Prentice Hall.

Cohen, M. R., Amatayakul, R., & Zeng, X. (2007). SOA: A Potential Silver Bullet? *ADVANCE for Health Information Executives, 11*(11), 10.

Conn, J. (2006). RHIOs make it work. *Modern Healthcare, 36*(7), 22–24.

DICOM. (October 11, 2007). Strategic Document. Retrieved December 23, 2007, from http://medical.nema.org/dicom/geninfo/Strategy.pdf.

Enrado, P. (December 12, 2007). NHIN Forum: value of HIEs needs attention. Healthcare IT News. Retrieved December 25, 2007, from http://www.healthcareitnews.com/story.cms?id=8293&page=1.

Foundation of Research and Education of American Health Information Management Association. (FORE). (2006). Development of State Level Health Information Exchange Initiatives Final Report. Retrieved December 24, 2007, from http://www.staterhio.org/documents/Final_Report_HHSP23320064105EC_090106_000.pdf.

Freedman, I. (2007). What does "interoperability really mean? *Health Management Technology, 28*(10), 50–51.

Garde, S., Knaup, P., & Hovenga, E. (2005). openEHR Archetypes in Electronic Health Records: the Path to Semantic Interoperability? Retrieved December 21, 2007, from http://healthinformatics.cqu.edu.au/downloads/garde_gmds_2005.pdf.

Getting Started. (2007). *H&HN: Hospitals & Health Networks, 81*(5), 14. Retrieved December 18, 2007, from Health Source: Nursing/Academic Edition database.

Health Level Seven (2007). HL7 Mission Statement. Retrieved December 23, 2007, from http://www.hl7.org.

Healthcare Information and Management Systems Society (HIMSS). (2007a). News: Extending International Efforts, Integrating the Healthcare Enterprise Adopts Enhanced Principles of Governance. Retrieved December 24, 2007, from http://www.himss.org/ASP/topics_News_item.asp?cid=67497&tid=3.

Healthcare Information and Management Systems Society (HIMSS). (2007b). IHE. Retrieved December 23, 2007, from http://www.himss.org/ASP/topics_ihe.asp.

Garde, S., Knaup, P., Hovenga, E., & Heard, S. (2007). Towards semantic interoperability for electronic health records. *Methods of information in medicine, 46*(3), 332–343

Getting Started. (2007, May). *Hospitals & Health Networks,* Retrieved December 18, 2007, from Health Source: Nursing/Academic Edition database.

Institute of Medicine. (2001). *Crossing the Quality Chasm: A New Health System for the 2lst Century.* Washington, DC: National Academy Press.

International Organization for Standardization (ISO). (2007). ISO/FDIS 13606–1. Retrieved December 23, 2007, from http://www.iso.org/iso/iso_catalogue/catalogue_tc/catalogue_detail.htm?csnumber=40784.

Jian, W., Hsu, C., Hao, T., Wen, H., Hsu, M., Lee, Y., et al. (2007). Building a portable data and information interoperability infrastructure-framework for a standard Taiwan Electronic Medical Record Template, *Computer Methods and Programs in Biomedicine, 88*(2), 102–111.

Kalra, D. (2007). Trustworthy decision support: Is the Electronic Health Record dependable? Retrieved December 24, 2007, from http://www.haifa.il.ibm.com/Workshops/hcls2007/papers/trustworthy_decision_support.pdf.

Kaushal, R., Blumenthal, D., Poon, E. G., Jha, A. K., Franz, C., Middleton, B., et al. (2005). The costs of a national health information network. *Annals of Internal Medicine, 143*(3),165–173.

Kilic, O. & Dogac, A. (Accepted for future publication). Achieving Clinical Statement Interoperability using R-MIM and Archetype-based Semantic Transformations. *IEEE Transactions on Information Technology in Biomedicine.* Retrieved December 21, 2007, from http://www.srdc.metu.edu.tr/webpage/projects/ride/publications/KilicDogac.pdf.

Larsen, E. (October 2005). Estimating the Costs of NHIN Functions and Interoperability. HIMSS Standards Insight Summary. Retrieved December 25, 2007, from http://www.himss.org/content/files/standardsinsight/summaries/2005-10.pdf.

Mead, C. N. (2006). Data interchange standards in healthcare IT—computable semantic interoperability: Now possible but still difficult, do we really need a better mousetrap? *Journal of Healthcare Information Management, 20*(1), 71–78.

Nusbaum, M. H. (December 2007). Global interoperability now within reach. *Healthcare IT News,* 9.

Open EHR Foundation. (2007). Welcome to openEHR. Retrieved December 21, 2007, from http://www.openehr.org/home.html.

Schwend, G. T. (2007). Searching for Oz. *ADVANCE for Health Information Executives, 11*(2), 79.

Thede, L. Q. (1999). *Computers in nursing: Bridges to the future.* Philadelphia: Lippincott.

Turisco, F. (1999). Using internet technology to extend access to legacy systems. *Healthcare Financial Management, 53*(5), 86.

U.S. Department of Health & Human Services (HHS). (October 5, 2007). News release: HHS Awards Contracts for Trial Implementations of the Nationwide Health Information Network. Retrieved December 23, 2007, from http://www.hhs.gov/news/press/2007pres/10/pr20071005a.html.

While, A. & Thomas, P. (2007). Should nurses be leaders of integrated health care? *Journal of Nursing Management 15*(6), 643–648.

CHAPTER 12

The Electronic Health Record

After completing this chapter, you should be able to:

1 Define the term *electronic medical record (EMR)*.

2 Define the term *electronic health record (EHR)*.

3 Define the term *computer-based patient record (CPR)*.

4 Discuss the similarities and differences between the EHR and the CPR.

5 Understand the 12 characteristics of the CPR, as defined by the Institute of Medicine.

6 Discuss the benefits associated with the EHR.

7 Review the current status of the EHR, including impediments.

8 List several concerns that must be resolved before implementation of the EHR.

9 Discuss the *personal health record (PHR)*.

10 Compare and contrast the relationship between the PHR and EHR.

Requirements for the management of healthcare information are evolving— transforming the ways that healthcare providers store, access, and use information. The traditional paper medical record that reports client status and test results no longer meets the needs of today's healthcare industry. Paper records are episode-oriented with a separate record for each client visit. Key information, such as allergies, may be lost from one episode to the next, jeopardizing patient safety. Another drawback to paper records is that only one person can access the record at any given time. As a consequence of this fact, healthcare providers waste time looking for paper records, and treatment may be delayed. Different versions of the same information may be stored in several places. Paper records cannot incorporate diagnostic studies that include images and sound, nor do they make use of decision-support systems. The electronic health record (EHR) has the potential to integrate all pertinent patient information into one record, which will help to improve the quality of health information, patient safety, and productivity; contain costs; support research; decrease wait time for treatment; and contribute to the body of healthcare knowledge (Gearing et al. 2006; IOM 2003; Puffer et al. 2007). The Bush administration has called for the adoption of the EHR by 2014 as a means to help transform U.S. healthcare. In a letter to the U.S. House Committee on Ways and Means dated June 28, 2004, Glenn R. Breed, Chief Executive Officer and President of Medistore, a software vendor, wrote, "Our nation's goal of every man, woman and child in the U.S. having a life-long electronic health record (EHR) by 2014 is achievable if the right approach is taken" (Breed 2004).

DEFINITIONS

Numerous terms have been used over the years to describe the concept of an electronic health record. This situation continues to create confusion about the terminology and definitions related to the EHR. Government officials, vendors, and consultants have added to the confusion (Garets & Davis 2006). While there is no standard term to refer to an electronic medical file, *EHR* has been used as a generic term for all electronic healthcare systems (NCQHC 2006). It has since become the favored term for the lifetime computerized record. Some of the other frequently used terms include *electronic medical record (EMR), electronic patient record (EPR), computer-based patient record (CPR),* and *CPR system and Shared Electronic Health Record (SEHR).*

The Healthcare Information and Management Systems Society (HIMSS) (2006) outlined the differences between the terms *electronic medical record* and *electronic health record,* defining the **electronic medical record (EMR)** as the "legal record created in hospitals and ambulatory environments that is the source of data for the EHR." For many years the EMR applied to a single encounter with no, or very limited, ability to carry information from one visit to another within a care delivery system. That situation has changed so that it is now possible to bring information forward from prior visits within the organization or delivery system. The basic components of the EMR system are:

- Clinical messaging and e-mail
- Results reporting
- Data repository
- Decision support
- Clinical documentation
- Order entry

EMR result reporting and data repository components include unstructured data, which are data that do not follow any particular format and often are provided as a text report. Examples are reports produced by transcription services, including history and physical assessments, consultation findings, operative reports, and discharge summaries. The EMR also includes structured data, which are data that follow a predefined format and are often presented as discrete data elements. Structured data are often obtained from automated ancillary reporting systems; a primary example is laboratory results from an automated laboratory information system. Another type of data that may be included in the EMR is electronic imaging produced by diagnostic studies, including tomography, ultrasonography, and magnetic resonance imaging. The data in the EMR is the legal record of patient care during an encounter at the healthcare delivery system and is owned by that system (Garets & Davis 2006).

While most hospitals have some level of automation, few have attained a fully electronic environment, and many physician offices, ambulatory care areas, and long-term care settings still maintain manual processes. HIMSS Analytics (Garets & Davis 2006) created an EMR Adoption Model that identifies the levels of EMR capabilities. The stages of the model range from minimal automation at stage 0 to full automation at stage 7. Each subsequent stage presumes the existence of the functionalities listed for the preceding stage.

Stage 0: Some clinical automation exists but the laboratory, pharmacy, and radiology systems are not all operational.

Stage 1: The major ancillary clinical systems—the laboratory, pharmacy, and radiology systems—are all installed.

Stage 2: Major ancillary clinical systems send data to a clinical data repository (CDR) that allows physicians to retrieve and review results. The CDR also contains a controlled medical vocabulary and clinical decision rules engine that checks for conflict. Document imaging systems may also be linked to the CDR.

Stage 3: Basic clinical documentation (vital signs, flow sheets) is required. Nurses' notes, care plans, and/or electronic medical administration records may be present and are integrated with the CDR for at least one hospital service. Basic clinical decision support is available for error checking with order entry. Some availability is present for the retrieval and storage of diagnostic imaging. Typically this refers to the Picture Archiving Communications Systems (PACS) used for x-rays and other diagnostic images.

Stage 4: Computerized Provider Order Entry (CPOE) and a second level of clinical decision support for evidence-based practice is added to the previous stages.

Stage 5: At least one service area has the closed loop medication administration process where barcode medication administration (BCMA), Radio Frequency Identification (RFID), or other identification technology is in place and integrated with CPOE and the pharmacy to maximize patient safety.

Stage 6: At least one service area has full physician documentation, third-level clinical decision support for all clinicians for protocols and outcomes with variance and compliance alerts, and a full PACS system.

Stage 7: This is a paperless environment where all information is shared electronically.

The electronic patient record (EPR) is an electronic client record, but not necessarily a lifetime record, that focuses on relevant information for the current episode of care.

 The CPR is a comprehensive lifetime record that includes all information from all specialties. The classic definition and attributes of the CPR, as identified by the Institute of Medicine (IOM), provide the basis for today's understanding of the EHR and still apply, for the most part, to current systems (Andrew, Bruegel, & Gasch 2007).

The U.S. Department of Health and Human Services said that the electronic health record (EHR) is a "digital collection of patient's medical history and could include items like diagnosed medical conditions, prescribed medications, vital signs, immunizations, lab results, and personnel characteristics like age and weight" (HHS news release 2005). HIMSS (2007) defines the **electronic health record (EHR)** as

> "a longitudinal electronic record of patient health information generated by one or more encounters in any care delivery setting. Included in this information are patient demographics, progress notes, problems, medications, vital signs, past medical history, immunizations, laboratory data and radiology reports. The EHR automates and streamlines the clinician's workflow. The EHR has the ability to generate a complete record of a clinical patient encounter—as well as supporting other care-related activities directly or indirectly via interface—including evidence-based decision support, quality management, and outcomes reporting."

 Information in the EHR may be owned by the patient or stakeholder (Garets & Davis 2006). Unlike the EMR it provides interactive patient access as well as the ability for the patient to append information. The Department of Defense (DOD) has added dental records to the list of EHR components

(Anderson 2007). The development of the EHR relies upon the presence of fully operational EMRs and a national health information network (NHIN). HIMSS (2003) identified the following attributes of the EHR:

1. Provides secure, reliable real-time access to client health record information where and when it is needed to support care
2. Records and manages episodic and longitudinal EHR information
3. Functions as clinicians' primary information resources during the provision of client care
4. Assists with the work of planning and delivery of evidence-based care to individual and groups of clients
5. Captures data used for continuous quality improvement, utilization review, risk management, resource planning, and performance management
6. Captures the patient health-related information needed for medical record and reimbursement
7. Provides longitudinal, appropriately masked information to support clinical research, public health reporting, and population health initiatives
8. Supports clinical trials and evidence-based research

The EHR must provide secure, real-time, point-of-care, patient-centric information for clinicians at the time and place that clinicians need it. The EHR must also provide evidence-based decision support, automate and streamline the clinician's workflow, and support the collection of data for uses other than direct client care. These indirect uses include billing, quality management, outcomes reporting, resource planning, and public health disease surveillance and reporting (HIMSS 2003, p. 2).

In July 2003, the Department of Health and Human Services announced the formation of the EHR Collaborative. This group of founding stakeholder organizations was charged with the task of facilitating rapid input from the healthcare community to support the adoption of standards for the EHR. Member organizations included the following:

- American Health Information Management Association (AHIMA)
- American Medical Association (AMA)
- American Medical Informatics Association (AMIA)
- American Nurses Association (ANA)
- College of Healthcare Information Management Executives (CHIME)
- eHealth Initiative (eHI)
- Healthcare Information and Management Systems Society (HIMSS)
- National Alliance for Health Information Technology (NAHIT)

The EHR Collaborative sponsored a series of open forum meetings to solicit input, which was published as the "Final Report: Public Response to HL7 EHR Ballot 1." In 2005 the American Health Information Community (AHIC) was chartered as a federal advisory body to make recommendations to the Secretary of the U.S. Department of Health and Human Services (HHS) on how to accelerate the development and adoption of health information technology. Despite the value of this body, its charter required that its responsibilities be transferred to a successor (HHS July 2007).

The healthcare industry has been working to develop a functional model and agreed-on standards. The EHR requires both technical and clinical standards. Once completed, the nationally agreed-on standards for the EHR will affect the entire healthcare community. For example, the following entities will be affected:

- Hospitals
- Physicians
- Payers
- Researchers
- Pharmacies
- Public health agencies
- Consumers

The International Organization for Standards (ISO) Technical Committee 215 recommended definitions of electronic medical and health records that are used throughout most of the world but have not been adopted by the United States (Walton 2007). In another effort the United States is a charter member of the International Health Terminology Standards Development Organization (IHTSDO), which has acquired Systemized Nomenclature of Medicine (SNOMED) Clinical Terms as a means to foster the rapid development and adoption of standard clinical terminology for electronic health records (SNOMED CT) (HHS 2007). EHR vendors demonstrate a great deal of variation in their implementation of standards, resulting in systems that have not been interoperable (NCRR 2006).

Another concept with electronic records is the **continuity of care record (CCD).** This record is intended to improve continuity of care when clients move between various points of care. The CCD is comprised of contributions from many types of caregivers, including physicians, nurses, physical therapists, and social workers with each providing a summary of care provided (Conn 2007). The record supports the patient's safety and has a positive impact on the quality and continuity of care. The Health Level 7 and ASTM International standards groups recently reached a compromise that incorporates work done by earlier groups. The CCD is a snapshot of patient status, rather than a comprehensive record.

HISTORICAL DEVELOPMENTS

The IOM identified the following 12 major components of the CPR, which they considered the "gold standard" attributes (Andrew & Bruegel 2003):

1. Provides a problem list that indicates the client's current clinical problems for each encounter. A problem list should also denote the number of occurrences associated with all past and current problems, as well as the current status of the problem.

2. Evaluates and records health status and functional levels using accepted measures. In the current competitive healthcare market, increased attention to measuring outcomes and quality of care are imperative, and must begin to be addressed by information system departments and vendors.

3. Documents the clinical reasoning/rationale for diagnoses and conclusions. Allows sharing of clinical reasoning with other caregivers and automates and tracks decision making.

4. Provides a longitudinal or lifetime client record by linking all of the client's data from previous encounters.

5. Supports confidentiality, privacy, and audit trails. System developers must supply multiple levels of security to ensure appropriate access to confidential client information.

6. Provides continuous access to authorized users. Users must be able to access the client record at any time.

7. Allows simultaneous and customized views of the client data for individuals, departments, or enterprises. This ability improves efficiency for the specific users by allowing the data to be presented in a format that is most useful to them. The flexibility to support multiple, different, and simultaneous views of client data is a feature that many vendors find difficult to achieve.

8. Supports links to local or remote information resources, such as various databases using the Internet or organization-based intranet resources. Access to pertinent information from various external sources will provide the caregiver with needed information in a timely and effective format that can be used to support client care. Examples include access to literature searches and drug information databases.

9. Facilitates clinical problem solving by providing decision analysis tools. Examples include simple support, such as timely reminders regarding health maintenance activities, and rules-based alerts that supply decision-making support for the physician.

10. Supports direct entry of client data by physicians. The question of how to provide a simple and acceptable mechanism for direct entry of data by physicians without relying on dictation continues to be a problem for vendors.

11. Includes mechanisms for measuring the cost and quality of care. This area is vitally important in providing a significant competitive edge in today's healthcare market.

12. Supports existing and evolving clinical needs by being flexible and expandable. Many information systems address specific areas of specialty such as emergency or ambulatory care. These systems may be difficult to customize and expand to meet the specific needs of the healthcare enterprise.

Most of the data included in the CPR are structured data. Other data formats may also be linked to the CPR, including dictation and transcription, images, video, and text. These data, and collective data from all systems, are stored and managed in the clinical data repository. This database allows retrieval of

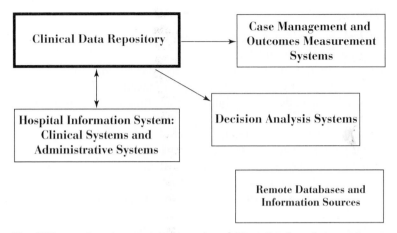

The CPR comprises the systems shown above. Client data flows between the systems as indicated by the arrows. External databases and information sources may also be accessed by the CPR, even though no client data flow to them.

FIGURE 12–1 • A Sample of EHR components

multiple elements of client data regardless of their system of origin. For example, the user may retrieve a lab result from the clinical data repository that was originally produced by the laboratory information system (LIS), along with a radiology report that was generated in the radiology information system (RIS) from a transcribed dictation. Collectively, these various systems and the clinical data repository make up the CPR.

The development of data exchange standards is instrumental for the implementation of the CPR. These standards will allow the uniform capture of data that is required to build a longitudinal record comprised of integrated information systems from multiple vendors. Figure 12–1 shows some sample components of the CPR.

 BENEFITS OF THE EHR

The driving forces for the development of the EHR are client safety and the need to restructure the healthcare delivery system to improve the quality of care delivered while containing soaring costs (NCQHC 2006). A well-developed EHR facilitates the provision of quality care and management of costs. The powerful framework of the CPR optimizes the collection, presentation, and communication of client data resulting in time and money savings for anyone who participates in the healthcare delivery process, including clients, physicians, hospitals, and insurers.

The benefits of the EHR can be best understood when considering the needs of various groups of users. Some of the benefits are general, but others relate to nurses, physicians, and other care providers, as well as the healthcare enterprise.

General Benefits

- *Improved data integrity.* Information is more readable, better organized, and more accurate and complete.
- *Increased productivity.* Caregivers are able to access client information whenever it is needed and at multiple convenient locations. This can result in improved client care due to the ability to make timely decisions based on appropriate data.
- *Improved quality of care.* The EHR supports clinical decision-making processes for physicians and nurses. For example the clinician can tailor a view of patient information that shows the most recent labs, vital signs, and current medications on one screen or select another view that graphs lab values and vital signs over time. This can be especially helpful to show renal response to ordered medications.
- *Increased satisfaction for caregivers.* Caregivers are able to take advantage of easy access to client data as well as other services, including drug information sources, rules-based decision support, and literature searches.

Nursing Benefits

- Facilitates comparisons of current data and data from previous events.
- Supports an ongoing record of the client's education and learning response across encounters or visits.
- Eliminates the need to repeat collection of baseline demographic data with each encounter.
- Provides universal data access to all who have access to the EHR.
- Improves data access and quality for research.
- Provides prompts to ensure administration and documentation of medications and treatments.
- Improves documentation and quality of care (Nelson 2007).
- Facilitates automation of critical and clinical pathways.
- Supports the development of a database that facilitates research, provides information useful to administrators and clinicians, and allows recognition of nursing work in measurable units when used with a common unified structure for nursing language (Simpson 2007).

Benefits for Healthcare Providers

- Simultaneous record access by multiple users.
- Previous encounters may be accessed easily.
- Faster chart access because the need to wait for old records to be delivered from the medical records department is eliminated.
- More comprehensive information is available.
- Fewer lost records.
- Improved efficiency of billing.
- Better reporting tools. Trends and clinical graphics are available on demand.

- Reduced liability through better decision making and documentation.
- Improved reimbursement rates.
- Enhanced compliance through system generated prompts with preventive care protocols (Martin 2007; Mitchell 2007).
- Supports pay-for-performance bonuses (NCQHC 2006).
- Early warnings of changes in patient status.
- Supports benchmarking for how well physicians manage patients with chronic disease conditions (Novogoratz 2007).

Healthcare Enterprise Benefits

- Improved client record security.
- Instant notice of authorization for procedures with integration with payer-based health records.
- Strengthened communications.
- Fewer lost records.
- Decreased need for record storage.
- Reduced medical record department costs because pulling, filing, and copying of charts is decreased.
- Improved verification of client eligibility for coverage in managed care settings.
- Faster turnaround for outstanding accounts with electronic coding and claim submission.
- Decreased need for x-ray film and physical filing, storage, and transport of films.
- Improved cost evaluation based on clinical outcomes and resource utilization data.
- Decreased length of stay (NCQHC 2006)
- Enhanced compliance with regulatory requirements.

Consumer Benefits

- Decreased wait time for treatment.
- Improved access and control over health information.
- Increased use of best practices with incorporation of decision support.
- Improved ability to ask informed questions.
- Greater responsibility for one's own care.
- Alerts and reminders for upcoming appointments and scheduled tests.
- Increased satisfaction (NCQHC 2006).
- Improved understanding of treatment choices (Martin 2007; Mitchell 2007).

Payer Benefits

- Supports pay for performance as quality measures are gathered (Martin 2007).
- Supports disease management, lowering costs for expensive diagnoses.

Despite the many cited benefits associated with the EHR, little scientific evidence now exists on the level and benefits actually delivered. HIMSS has created a Clinical Information Systems (CIS) Benefits Task Force to create a database of actual provider experiences. This lack of evidence makes it difficult to evaluate the costs, benefits, and risks of a commercial EMR purchase and for healthcare executives to make necessary organizational changes (Thompson, Osheroff, Classen, & Sittig 2007). Puffer (2007) cautioned that the mere implementation of an EMR does not guarantee that benefits will be achieved.

CURRENT STATUS OF THE EHR

No country has implemented an operational national EHR to date (Simpson 2007). There are many efforts under way to accelerate the adoption of the EHR. President Bush called for the widespread adoption of the EHR by 2014, creating the Office of the National Coordinator for health information technology. This Office has helped to provide leadership for the development and implementation of an interoperable health information technology infrastructure to improve quality and efficiency of care (NCQHC 2006). The Healthcare Information Technology Standards Panel (HITSP) (IHS Engineering 2007) is an organization that is actively working to harmonize the data standards that will allow the exchange of healthcare information needed for the EHR to occur.

The Department of Defense, the Department of Health and Human Services, the Veterans Administration, and the Centers for Medicare and Medicaid Services have all mandated the EHR for their facilities and operations (Andrew, Bruegel, & Gasch 2007). Recent legislative changes support the provision of health information technology to physician practices by healthcare organizations (Conn 2007). The Certification Commission for Healthcare Information Technology, a voluntary, private-sector initiative designed to certify healthcare IT products and service, announced plans to require interoperability EHR systems for certification. The National Health Information Exchange initiative, funded by the Markle Foundation's Connecting for Health and Robert Wood Johnson Foundation, represents one private effort supporting the move to EHRs (NCQHC 2006).

Many experts suggest that the first step toward developing an EHR is the implementation of e-prescribing. The recommendation is partly based on the fact that the Medicare Prescription Drug, Improvement and Modernization Act of 2003 required plans participating in Medicare Part D to support electronic prescription programs. Also, CMS awarded monies to fund pilot e-prescribing programs (NCQHC 2006). A recent survey showed that more than 90% of pharmacies are already equipped to handle e-prescribing (Glaser 2007). E-prescribing requires a smaller initial cost than EMR but still saves money and lives, improves efficiencies, and eliminates problems with illegible handwriting. E-prescribing does require access to patient history, allergy information, and a drug formulary. Other surveys indicated that few healthcare systems have progressed beyond stage 3 of EMR implementation (Garets & Davis 2006; Walton 2007).

BOX 12–1 Qualities of a Successful EHR	
1. Fast	The user is able to quickly enter and retrieve data.
2. Familiar	The EHR follows familiar Graphical User Interface (GUI) conventions.
3. Flexible	The EHR allows personalization of documentation style, enabling it to meet the information needs of many types and categories of users.
4. Enhances Workflow	The EHR improves work efficiency and effectiveness.
5. Improves Documentation	The user sees the EHR improving the process of documentation.
6. Meets Regulatory Requirements	The EHR supports the regulatory requirements related to data content and security measures.

Box 12–1 lists six qualities of a successful EHR. While many organizations struggle with the slow piecemeal conversion to electronic medical records, unintended negative outcomes may be seen. These include increased workloads and delayed information retrieval as clinicians search multiple data sources for client information.

 ## Considerations When Implementing the EHR

Information system vendors as well as healthcare providers are, for the most part, aware of the pressing need to develop the EHR and are continuously working toward its evolvement. Development of an electronic infrastructure and cost are the two major impediments to the creation of a fully functioning EHR. The principal requirement is that the major participants in the healthcare arena, including healthcare facilities, payers, and physicians, must be linked electronically. This is a costly undertaking in many cases. Other impediments include the lack of a common vocabulary, security and confidentiality issues, resistance among caregivers, and a lack of IT staff to create and support the necessary infrastructure (Rowland 2007).

Electronic Infrastructure The healthcare facilities, payers, physicians, and nurses all need the ability to access and update the client's longitudinal record. This ability requires linkage of the various information systems that support these stakeholders via a network infrastructure. Agreement must be reached regarding the nature and format of client data to be stored, as well as the mechanisms for data exchange, storage, and retrieval. This means that all participants use common data communication standards. The lack of standards has been a key barrier to establishing this type of electronic connectivity. First and most important is the decision regarding the recognition of a universal client identifier or MPI (master patient index) number, so that all client data can be associated with the correct client. The social security number has been widely used for this purpose but it is unreliable because it may be stolen or inaccurately provided; in addition, some individuals have used more than one number while others do not have one. Improvements in connectivity alone are not enough to support the EHR. It is also important to include components such as interoperability, comparability, decision support, and point-of-care data capture to achieve a longitudinal electronic record.

Cost Another impediment to the EHR is cost. Initial and ongoing costs for deploying and maintaining IT systems were cited as the greatest barrier to IT (Mitchell 2007). The development of the electronic links forming the infrastructure is costly, and the allocation of fiscal responsibilities is difficult. Currently each healthcare enterprise or system is paying for its own EHR development. Links to other facilities and agencies are rare and for the most part limited to provider–payer arrangements. Further progress is likely to be minimal until decisions regarding cost allocation are reached. Simpson (2007) noted one estimate that the creation of an operational EHR in the United States within the next five years would require a capital investment of $156 billion with another $48 billion in annual operating costs.

Vocabulary Standardization There is little standardization in healthcare settings regarding the medical vocabulary or language used in client records. This lack of standards prevents the integration of discrete and disparate data from multiple sources into one complete record. Additional progress in the development of a universal medical and nursing language is essential to the development of the EHR (Lunney 2006). The American Nurses' Association (ANA) recognized several standardized languages that both support the documentation of the nursing process and the aggregation of nursing data (Goossen et al. 2006). A standardized nursing language allows accurate communication among nurses and other health-care providers. Standardization also allows terms to be measured and coded (Rutherford 1998). Werley identified the need for a nursing minimum data set (NMDS) in the 1970s. The **nursing minimum data set** represents the collection of data that allows comparison of care across like settings, practice models, and other factors. The NMDS relies upon uniform definitions and categories. In the United States it includes nursing diagnoses, interventions, outcomes, and an indicator of nursing intensity. The NMDS was accepted by the ANA in 1999. Work is in process on an international NMDS; the international version goes beyond the U.S. version to include the start and end dates of episodes of care; demographic information on age, gender, year of birth, and residence; reason for admission; and data about the setting.

A conference brought together the leaders of NANDA (an international organization that began as the North American Nursing Diagnosis Association) and the Center for Nursing Classification and Clinical Effectiveness to create a common unifying structure across NANDA, the Nursing Interventions Classification (NIC), and the Nursing Outcomes Classification (NOC). The goal of this alliance was to advance the development, testing, and refinement of nursing language. The NANDA membership accepted the NANDA definition of a nursing diagnosis in 1988 (Gordon 1998). Nursing diagnoses are formulated on a nursing judgment of the individual, family, or community responses to an actual or potential health problem or life process. Determination of a nursing diagnosis determines appropriate nursing interventions. NANDA has been integrated into SNOMED. Additional work is still needed but this is a significant development in the vocabulary standardization. NANDA is comprised of a group of approved nursing diagnoses and a taxonomic structure for their classification. Work on NIC dates back to the early 1990s. A nursing intervention is a direct care treatment that a nurse performs on behalf of a patient. NIC attempts to depict the range of activities that nurses carry out during their daily work. Each individual intervention in NIC is comprised of a label, a definition, a set of activities, and background readings. Each intervention is further classified into a domain and class (Bowker, Star, & Spasser 1998). NOC provides a means to measure nursing practices across facilities, regions, and countries.

Other ANA recognized languages include the Home Health Care Classification (HHCC), the Omaha System, the Perioperative Nursing Dataset, the ABC codes, the Systematic Nomenclature of Medicine Clinical Terms (SNOMED CT), and the International Classification for Nursing Practice (ICNP®) (ANA 2007). SNOMED and ICNP® are the two most widely accepted standards in nursing. ICNP® encompasses diagnosis, interventions, and outcomes. In a 2006 interview Amy Coenen noted that it was used in 80 countries in 2006 (Ryan 2006). ICNP® includes all nursing specialties and can be used to bring together other standardized nursing languages. Hyun and Park (2002) found in their cross-mapping of ICNP® terms with NANDA, the Omaha system, the Home Health Care Classification (HHC), and the Nursing Interventions Classification (NIC) that ICNP® described the bulk of each of these diagnoses or interventions, concluding that it provided a sound foundation for a unified nursing language system.

Security and Confidentiality Security and confidentiality concerns are critical considerations in EHR development. The EHR system must be configured to allow access only to those who have been identified as authorized users. The system must authenticate the user's identity with user IDs and passwords and possibly biometrics. HIPAA considerations include the need to be able to provide the client, upon request, with a log of caregivers who have accessed his or her chart. In addition, client information should not be available to anyone without the client's approval. Data that are communicated via the Internet must be encrypted. Firewalls must be in place when data are sent and received via the Internet to safeguard data integrity.

Caregiver Resistance Resistance on the part of caregivers such as physicians and nurses also acts as an impediment to the development and use of the EHR. The fully developed EHR necessitates mandatory use of computers by caregivers as part of their daily routine. Some individuals are unable or unwilling to use computers; this may be related to various factors such as the complexity of software, the availability of workstations, and resistance to change in the work patterns. Some physicians believe that data entry is demeaning and a waste of time and interferes with their ability to provide client care on a timely basis. In addition, they may resist perceived changes to the way they practice medicine that will be required by the EHR system. Actual practice reveals that nearly all physicians will do some data entry, but only a few will do a lot.

Data Integrity

Data integrity can be compromised in three ways: incorrect entry, data tampering, and system failure. In general, data integrity can be improved by implementing security measures, including the use of audit trails, as well as the development of detailed procedures and policies.

Incorrect Data Entry The client data found in the EHR are only as accurate as the person who enters them and the systems that transfer them. Therefore, critical information, such as allergies and code status, should be verified for accuracy at each encounter. This will allow the correction of data entry errors and screen for changes that have occurred in client status. This is especially crucial because data may be entered or modified from many different encounters in the healthcare arena, such as hospitals, clinics, and home care visits. Data integrity is also compromised if an interface is not receiving or sending data correctly. When corrections to the data in the electronic record must be made, data must be corrected in multiple areas. The data in the initial system must be corrected, as well as any receiving systems. For example, if information is incorrect in the hospital information system, it must be corrected there. Any other systems that derive information from this, such as physician office systems and ancillary systems, must also be updated. This may involve correction using interface transactions or manual intervention. Some systems may not allow automated correction, which means that a person must make changes.

Data Correction In addition to accidental data entry errors, it is possible for an individual to make malicious data modifications. An effective audit trail procedure permits the tracking of who entered or modified each data element, allowing appropriate follow-up measures.

Master File Maintenance The development and maintenance of master files and data dictionaries is critical to building and maintaining an information system and data integrity. Careful attention to initial development of the files, including documentation, will ensure that data are accurate and communicate valid information. Periodic review and validation of master files, at least annually, is necessary to maintain current and accurate data.

System Failure Hardware and software malfunctions, such as a system crash, may result in incomplete or lost data. Once the problem has been resolved, it may be necessary to verify the client data that could have been affected. It may then be necessary to append paper records or manually enter data once the system is restored.

Ownership of the Patient Record

Currently, paper medical records are the property of the institution at which they are created. This institution is responsible for ensuring the accuracy and completeness of the record. With the development of the EHR, however, ownership issues become more complex. Because many providers use the same data, it is unclear who actually owns them and is responsible for maintaining their accuracy. Because the data are shared and updated from many sites, decisions must be made regarding who can access the data and how the data will be used. In addition, it must be determined where the data will actually be stored.

Privacy and Confidentiality

Preservation of the client's privacy is one of the most basic and important duties of the healthcare provider. Because one of the key attributes of the EHR is the ease of data sharing, the client's privacy rights may not be guarded by all who have access to the record. Legislation such as HIPAA has been initiated that addresses electronic access to client records. In addition, healthcare providers must address client privacy rights when developing the electronic record. In a recent survey consumers indicated that they were ready to accept electronic records if they could be assured that their health information would be kept private and secure (Chhanabhai & Holt 2007).

Electronic Signature

The healthcare provider has always been required to authenticate entries into the paper medical record with a handwritten signature. This cannot be done with the EHR because all entries are electronic. An electronic signature must be used to authenticate electronic data entries. A user's computer access code and/or password recognizes that individual by name and credentials and allows access to the system. The user should be required to sign a confidentiality statement before obtaining an access code, stating that no other person will be permitted to use the code. Other technologies, such as private encryption keys and biometric authentication, should also be used when developing an electronic signature mechanism to guarantee the source of the document.

Systems typically affix a date and time log to each entry, as well as the identity of the user in the form of an audit trail. The electronic signature is automatically and permanently attached to the document when it is created. This electronic signature cannot be forged or transferred to any other transaction and provides authentication of the healthcare provider. In the United States the Food and Drug Administration and the e-sign bill address the importance of digital signatures. The European Union has its own set of guidelines (Aharoni & Schlerf 2007).

SMART CARDS

One of the technologies associated with the EHR is the smart card. The smart card is used to store client information such as demographics, allergies, blood type, current medications, current health problems (including recent findings), and payer or insurance provider. Some cards may also include the client's photograph. The smart card is similar in appearance to a plastic credit card. The smart cards that contain a microprocessor chip are able to store thousands more bits than a magnetic strip card. Smart cards allow client information and medical history to be accessed quickly, which may be important during an emergency. In non-emergency situations, the smart card allows the client to provide his or her history easily and accurately. The Smart Card Alliance, a consortium of companies and government entities, issued best practice guidelines to address concerns surrounding citizen protection and potential rights violations with card use (Ferguson 2007).

At the present time, smart cards are widely used in Europe. A person carrying a smart card presents it to the healthcare provider at the time of treatment, and it is processed through an electronic card reader. The card provides detailed client information that is not part of an electronic network, thus ensuring accuracy and making information readily available. One of the major barriers to widespread use of the smart card is the cost. In addition to the cost of the actual smart card, there is a cost associated with card readers. Each facility must have one or more card readers to access the information on the card. The operating system and software used by one facility's card and card reader may not be compatible with those used by other facilities, so the cards may not be able to be used by more than one organization.

THE PERSONAL HEALTH RECORD (PHR)

Consumers are the primary source of information about their health history and medications. Some can provide an accurate account while others cannot. The patient-carried record (PCR) and personal health record (PHR) emerged to address this. The PCR is the client's health record on a portable card that is carried by the patient. A variation of this is the PHR (personal health record), which may be on paper, accessible via the Internet, or on a portable device. The Personal Health Record (PHR) encourages involvement and responsibility for one's own care. In China, patients are responsible for the safekeeping of their own ambulatory care record. Providers make handwritten notes on the presenting complaint, including test results, diagnosis, and prescribed medications. At the conclusion of the visit, the patient, or other responsible party, gets the book back. The book must be presented prior to each episode of care. Neither the hospital nor physician keeps a copy of these records (Cohen & Amatayakul 2007). This solution provides a comprehensive record of all episodes of care and stays with the patient. This is more than can be said for the state of healthcare records in the United States at this time. The Chinese example is portable and cost-effective but potential problems include privacy, confidentiality, liability, legibility, and loss of the record itself, which would not make it suitable here. Technology offers solutions that can be accessed from multiple points as well as by multiple authorized persons. HIMSS (2007) defines an ePHR as follows:

> An electronic Personal Health Record ("ePHR") is a universally accessible, layperson comprehensible, lifelong tool for managing relevant health informa-tion, promoting health maintenance and assisting with chronic disease man-agement via an interactive, common data set of electronic health information and e-health tools. The ePHR is owned, managed, and shared by the individual or his or her legal proxy(s) and must be secure to protect the privacy and confi-dentiality of the health information it contains. It is not a legal record unless so defined and is subject to various legal limitations.

The HIMSS definition is meant to address the immediate and future develop-mental direction of ePHRs, with the understanding that any ePHR definition is not static and will evolve with future technology advances and further adop-tion of electronic health records (EHRs), electronic medical records (EMRs), and ePHRs, which will create shifts in the culture surrounding the utilization and demand of ePHR constituents.

Distinguishing Features

Unlike other health records the PHR is patient-centered, presenting a more balanced view of an individual's health history. The portability of information helps consumers to manage their own health, which has been complicated until now with information dispersed among multiple providers, hospitals, labs, pharmacies, insurers, and related healthcare entities (Fox & Sheridan 2006; Krohn 2007; Wright & Sittig 2007). One aspect of this management includes benchmarking, or the ability to compare one's own health status against other individuals with the same conditions or age group. Considerable variation exists in format. There are four basic models in the electronic format:

1. *Independent Web sites.* This version requires the consumer to complete all fields. Partly for this reason it is not especially popular.
2. *Health plan patient portals.* These use claims-based clinical and financial information to populate fields. They often contain alerts, educational con-tent, health risk assessments, messaging, and other benefits. They may also capture medical lists, allergies, and individual and family medical history

information, and may include educational materials, interactive features such as alerts and reminders, prescription refills, and scheduling options.
3. *EMR portals.* The PHR is an adjunct to the EMR. These sites often provide educational materials, allow consumers to make appointments, request refills, and communicate directly with provider via secure messaging.
4. *Consumer-centric PHRs.* These secure sites capture information from different sources and formats, allow the viewing of pre-populating fields, and are accessible to authorized providers.

Unlike traditional health records PHRs may also include health status parameters such as exercise, nutrition and spiritual well-being, periodic risk assessment survey results, medical lists and herbal supplements, and exposure and monitoring information, as well as key contact information and living will and organ donation preferences (Ball, Smith, & Bakalar 2007; Simpson 2007). The Markle Foundation Personal Health Technology Council has developed patient and consumer principles to guide PHR design. The Markle Foundation is a group that seeks to use technology to improve the quality of life. The American Health Information Community sees the PHR as a vital steppingstone to the development of a national IT infrastructure that will eventually be integrated into physician practice–management systems for quick and easy access (Romano 2006).

At present many different groups are beginning to collect data to manage costs and quality, including pay-for-performance programs, and for predictive modeling, medication management, and member and provider portals. Most of the resulting information exists in silos with no single stakeholder seeing, let alone realizing, the benefit of the whole picture. Some proponents advocate that payers leverage their position as information brokers through the development of a payer-based health record (PBHR), which could help to further decrease costs and improve quality and safety (Rizk 2007). Rizk suggested that claims data could be sanitized and available to clinicians in a format useful to them, but the potential benefits require an agreement among competitors to share information. Employers see the potential to improve employee health and lower healthcare costs. Employees benefit through the ability to view pre-populated fields, which can be augmented as necessary.

Advantages

The PHR is patient-centered, portable, and provides a life-long record that fosters continuity of care; it should therefore improve the overall quality of healthcare (Ball, Smith, & Bakalar 2007). The value of its shared information will facilitate decision making, changing the relationship between healthcare consumer and provider. Integration of the PHR and EHR is essential to the vision of an electronic health info environment that empowers individual patients, consumers, and caregivers.

Disadvantages

It is a challenge to create easy-to-use PHRs rich in features. There are a number of unresolved issues associated with PHRs, including a lack of awareness on the part of the general consumer, security, privacy, data access and ownership, the presence of sensitive data, regulatory compliance, language used, possible secondary use of data, standards, and interoperability with EHR systems (Krohn 2007). Many consumers remain unaware of the existence of PHRs. Security issues relate to HIPAA and physical security of data. HIPAA only covers PHRs provided by covered entities such as health plans, healthcare clearinghouses, and providers. No federal coverage exists for other sites unless coverage is at the state level. PHRs can allow consumers to restrict sensitive data, such as prior psychiatric illnesses, cancer, or drug use from providers. Some portable USB-based devices can be compromised if they fall into the hands of an unauthorized user who either has access to the manufacturer's password or who finds the user password that is stored as a string in the database (Wright & Sittig 2007). The consumer empowerment working group of the American Health Information Community recommends a certification process for PHRs to avoid these types of breaches. The question of data ownership occurs particularly when it is maintained on a health or provider site. As information is shared from providers it is not generally in a form easily understood by consumers, and may be misunderstood. The fact that there is no standard language used by all providers complicates this issue.

Halamka, Mandl, and Tang (2008) suggested that control of healthcare information exchange lies with the patient because it solves the majority of privacy and consent issues faced by organizations seeking to exchange data. With the patient acting as steward of his or her own information, responsibility for the protection of patient confidentiality is largely shifted to the individual.

FUTURE DIRECTIONS

Much must be done before the benefits associated with the EHR can be realized. No country has yet realized an operational EHR, although some are closer than others. Few healthcare organizations have achieved a level of automation capable of supporting the EHR. Some experts call for stronger action on the part of the government, noting that competing software vendors and healthcare systems have little incentive to exchange information that might cause them to lose their competitive edge. Once the EHR is achieved additional changes in the way that healthcare professionals work will be visible. Not all changes will occur quickly or easily, however. The way that care is provided will evolve in ways that are barely imaginable today. Interoperability and the national health information network will afford consumers access to telemedicine services at home, work, and across the globe (Ball, Smith, & Bakalar 2007). The balance between consumers and providers will be very different than it is today as consumers will choose providers based upon their outcomes as well as their use of health information technology (HIT). The transformation of the present healthcare system requires the power of HIT as a tool, but it will take longer for some consumers and practitioners to make the transition since changes must also be seen in attitudes. Individual consumers will have greater responsibility for managing their own health with tracking and benchmarking information at their fingertips.

CASE STUDY EXERCISES

12.1 As a new student, identify advantages for when you are gathering information about your assigned patients with an electronic health record.

12.2 You are a member of the committee charged with designing the EHR at your facility. Identify which components of nursing documentation should be retained in the clinical data repository. For example, would you want to include all client vital signs from the current hospital admission? Explain why you would include or exclude the various components.

12.3 Identify several external sources of information that would be useful as part of the EHR for access by a home health nurse.

12.4 Discuss the implications of providing nurses in a hospital setting with access to all electronic client information. Identify which types of information are appropriate for access by nurses.

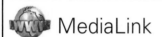 MediaLink

Additional resources for this content can be found on the Companion Website at www.prenhall.com/hebda. Click on "Chapter 12" to select the activities for this chapter.

- Glossary
- Multiple Choice
- Discussion Points
- Case Studies
- MediaLink Application
- MediaLink

SUMMARY

- The electronic health record (EHR) is an electronic client record that includes client data, medical knowledge, and other essential healthcare information.
- The Institute of Medicine identified 12 major components or characteristics of the CPR, which continue to provide the standard for current EHR systems with only slight refinement.
- The EHR offers benefits to nurses, physicians, and other healthcare providers, the healthcare enterprise, and, most importantly, the consumer.
- As of early 2008, the EHR is still being defined and developed.

- Infrastructure, cost, vocabulary standardization, and caregiver resistance are the major impediments to the development of an EHR.
- Issues that must be considered when developing the EHR include data integrity, ownership of the patient record, privacy, and electronic signature.
- An emerging technology related to EHR progress is the use of personal health records (PHR) to store client information, which will contribute to the development of a comprehensive, longitudinal record.

REFERENCES

Aharoni, G. & Schlerf, R. (June 1, 2007). The value of digital signatures in e-clinical applications. *Applied Clinical Trials.* Retrieved August 3, 2007, from http://www.actmagazine.com/appliedclinicaltrials/article/articleDetail.jsp?id=43192.

American Nurses' Association. (June 5, 2007). Relationships among ANA recognized data element sets and terminologies. Retrieved January 14, 2008, from http://nursingworld.org/npii/relationship.htm.

Anderson, H. J. (2007). EHR pioneers try to stay out front. *Health Data Management, 15*(5), 26–34.

Andrew, W. & Bruegel, R. (2003). 2003 CPR systems. *ADVANCE for Health Information Executives, 7*(9), 59–64.

Andrew, W. F., Bruegel, R. B., & Gasch, A. E. (2007). 2K6 EHR systems market summary. *ADVANCE for Health Information Executives, 11*(1), 41–44, 46, 56.

Ball, M. J., Smith, C., & Bakalar, R. S. (2007). Personal Health Records: Empowering consumers. *Journal of Healthcare Information Management, 21*(1), 76–86.

Bowker, G. C., Star, S. L., & Spasser, M. A. (1998). Classifying nursing work. *The Online Journal of Issues in Nursing, 3*(2). Retrieved January 21, 2008, from http://www.nursingworld.org/MainMenuCategories/ANAMarketplace/ANAPeriodicals/OJIN/TableofContents/Vol31998/Vol3No21998/ClassifyingNursingWork.aspx.

Breed, G. R. (June 28, 2004). Letter submitted to the Health Care Information Technology hearing before the Subcommittee on Health of the Committee on Ways and Means, U.S. House Of Representatives One Hundred Eighth Congress Second Session, June 17, 2004. Retrieved January 13, 2007, from http://waysandmeans.house.gov/hearings.asp?formmode=view&id=2239.

Chhanabhai, P., & Holt, A. (2007). Consumers are ready to accept the transition to online and electronic records if they can be assured of the security measures. *Medscape General Medicine, 9*(1), 8. Retrieved July 31, 2007, http://www.pubmedcentral.nih.gov/articlerender.fcgi?tool=pubmed&pubmedid=17435617.

Cohen, M. R., & Amatayakul, M. (2007). PHR: Is there an easier way? *ADVANCE for Health Information Executives, 11*(3), 12.

Conn, J. (2007). Agreement could put EHRs on fast track. *Modern Healthcare, 37*(9), 22.

Department of Health and Human Services (HHS). (June 6, 2005). HHS news release "Secretary Leavitt Takes New Steps to Advance Health IT National Collaboration and RFPs Will Pave the Way for Interoperability." Retrieved March 31, 2008, from http://www.hhs.gov/news/press/2005pres/20050606.html.

Department of Health and Human Services (HHS). (April 26, 2007). HHS news release "HHS Joins International Partners to Promote Electronic Health Records Standards." Retrieved August 2, 2007, from http://www.hhs.gov/news/press/2007pres/04/pr20070426a.html.

Department of Health and Human Services (HHS). (July 2007). White Paper Draft American Health Information Community Successor. Retrieved August 2, 2007, from http://www.hhs.gov/healthit/documents/m20070731/7a_whitepaper.html.

Ferguson, R. B. (January 30, 2007). Smart card alliance releases security, privacy guidelines. *PCMag.com*. Retrieved February 1, 2007, from http://www.pcmag.com/print_article2/0, 1217,a-199837,00asp.

Fox, L. A. & Sheridan, P. T. (2006). Hands-on help: The challenge and the promise of personal health records. *ADVANCE for Health Information Professionals*, *16*(17), 16.

Garets, D. & Davis, M. (2006). Electronic medical records vs. electronic health records: Yes, there is a difference. HIMSS Analytics. Retrieved August 3, 2007, from http://www.himssanalytics.org/docs/wp_emr_ehr.pdf.

Gearing, P., Olney, C. M., Davis, K., Lozano, D., Smith, L. G., & Friedman, B. (2006). Enhancing patient safety through electronic medical record documentation of vital signs. *Journal of Healthcare Information Management*, *20*(4), 40–45.

Glaser, J. (2007). Electronic prescribing. *ADVANCE for Health Information Executives*, *11*(7), 24–32.

Goossen, W. T. F., Delaney, C. W., Coenen, A., Saba, V. K., Sermeus, W., Warren, J. J., et al. (2006). In C. A. Weaver, C. W. Delaney, P. Weber, and R. L. Carr (Eds.). *Nursing and Informatics for the 21st Century: An international look at practice, trends and the future.* (pp. 305–320) Chicago: Healthcare Information and Management Systems Society.

Gordon, M. (1998). Nursing nomenclature and classification system development. *The Online Journal of Issues in Nursing, 3*(2), Retrieved January 21, 2008, from http://www.nursingworld.org/MainMenuCategories/ANAMarketplace/ANAPeriodicals/OJIN/TableofContents/Vol31998/Vol3No21998/NomenclatureandClassification.aspx.

Halamka, J. D., Mandl, K. D., & Tang, P. C. (2008). Early experiences with Personal Health Records. *Journal of the American Medical Informatics Association, 15*(1), 1–7.

Healthcare Information and Management Systems Society (HIMSS). (2003). *Electronic Health Record Definitional Model*, Version 1.1. Retrieved March 24, 2004, from http://www.himss.org/content/files/ehrattributes070703.pdf.

Healthcare Information and Management Systems Society (HIMSS). (2007). HIMSS' PHR, ePHR definition. Retrieved July 30, 2007, from http://www.himss.org/asp/topics_FocusDynamic.asp?faid=228.

Hyun, S. & Park, H. A. (2002). Cross-mapping the ICNP with NANDA, HHCC, Omaha System and NIC for unified nursing language system development. *International Nursing Review, 49*(2), 99–110.

IHS Engineering. (July 27, 2007). Health IT experts invited to contribute to standards harmonization effort, published as a news service by HIS. Retrieved September 10, 2007, from http://engineers.ihs.com/news/health-it-harmonization.htm.

Institute of Medicine. (IOM) (2003). *Key capabilities of an electronic health record system.* A letter report Committee on Data Standards for Patient Safety and Board on Health Care Services. Washington, DC: The National Academies Press. Retrieved March 24, 2004, from http://books.nap.edu/catalog/10781.html.

Krohn, R. (2007). The consumer-centric personal health record—it's time. *Journal of Healthcare Information Management, 21*(1), 20–23.

Lunney M. (2006). Helping nurses use NANDA, NOC, and NIC: Novice to expert. *Nurse Educator. 31*(1),40–46.

Martin, A. (2007). Payers get personal with online records. *Health Data Management, 15*(2), 88, 90, 92, 94, 96.

Mitchell, R. N. (2007). News Monitor. *ADVANCE for Health Information Executives*, *11*(4), 12.

National Committee for Quality Health Care (NCQHC) (2006). CEO Survival Guide Electronic Health Record Systems. Retrieved August 2, 2007, from http:\\nqfexecutiveinstitute\EHRbooksfinal.pdf.

National Institutes of Health National Center for Research Resources (NCRR). (April 2006). Electronic Health Records Overview. Retrieved August 2, 2007, from http://www.ncrr.nih.gov/publications/informatics/EHR.pdf.

Nelson, R. (2007). Electronic health records: Useful tools or high-tech headache? *AJN*, *107*(3), 25–26.

Novogoratz, S. (2007). Using EMRs to improve quality of care. *ADVANCE for Health Information Executives*, *11*(1), 51–55.

Puffer, M. J., Ferguson, J. A., Wright, B. C., Osborn, J., Anshus, A. L., Cahill, P., et al. (2007). Partnering with clinical providers to enhance the efficiency of an EMR. *Journal of Healthcare Information Management*, *21*(1), 24–32.

Rizk, E. (2007). Data Hub. *ADVANCE for Health Information Executives*, *11*(5), 43.

Romano, M. (2006). Moving IT forward. Government advances plans for electronic records. *Modern Healthcare*, *36*(6), 7.

Rowland, C. (May 14, 2007). Hospitals' move to e-files spurs a labor shortage. *The Boston Globe*. Retrieved August 2, 2007, from http://www.boston.com/business/technology/articles/2007/05/14/hospitals_move_to_e_files_spurs_a_labor_shortage/.

Rutherford, M. A. (1998). Standardized nursing language: What does it mean for nursing practice? *The Online Journal of Issues in Nursing*, *3*(2). Retrieved January 21, 2008, from http://nursingworld.org/MainMenuCategories/ANAMarketplace/ANAPeriodicals/OJIN/TableofContents/Vol31998/Vol3No21998/StandardizedNursingLanguage.aspx.

Ryan, S. (2006). AddedInterview. Multidisciplinary terminology: the International Classification for Nursing Practice (ICNP)... Amy Coenen. *Online Journal of Nursing Informatics*, *10*(3), 2.

Simpson, R. (2007). Easing the way for the electronic health record. *American Nurse Today*, *2*(2), 48–50.

Thompson, D. I., Osheroff, J., Classen, D., & Sittig, D. F. (2007). A review of methods to estimate the benefits of electronic medical records in hospitals and the need for a national benefits database. *Journal of Healthcare Information Management*, *21*(1), 62–68.

Walton, G. (2007). The Status of Acute Care EMRs. *ADVANCE for Health Information Executives*, *11*(5), 59.

Wright, A. & Sittig, D.F. (2007). Encryption characteristics of two USB-based personal health record devices. *Journal of the American Medical Informatics Association*, *14*(4), 397–399.

CHAPTER 13

Regional Health Information Organizations (RHIOs)

After completing this chapter, you should be able to:

1 Define the term *Regional Health Information Organization (RHIO)*.

2 Discuss key factors in the RHIO movement.

3 Compare and contrast different RHIO models for their respective advantages and disadvantages.

4 Identify obstacles to RHIO development and ongoing operation.

5 Describe the current status of RHIOs in the United States.

6 Differentiate between a *Clinical Data Network (CDN)* and an RHIO.

7 Envision ways in which RHIOs might impact healthcare delivery.

In today's mobile society achieving a comprehensive, longitudinal electronic health record for one individual is unlikely without the ability to exchange information among different providers and care delivery systems. Healthcare Information Exchange initiatives address this issue. A **Healthcare Information Exchange (HIE)** is the sharing of patient information, such as demographic data, allergies, presenting complaint, diagnostic test values, and other relevant data, between providers such as primary physicians, specialists, hospitals, and ambulatory care settings. This sharing should be bi-directional. For example, Mr. Smith has positive results on a urine culture for a urinary tract infection. His physician determined this fact when he accessed his office computer system, which is linked to the hospital information system. Before the physician orders an antibiotic, he needs to check allergies. Mr. Smith is a new patient who has never been seen by a physician except at a local urgent care center. Mr. Smith's doctor is still able to retrieve allergy information because these information systems exchange data. HIE has long been an essential part of the healthcare delivery system. Until recently it was entirely a manual process, one that was often inefficient with key pieces of information lost in the process. As mentioned above, electronic information exchange is presumed to occur bi-directionally. An HIE requires a focus on the areas of technology, interoperability, and standards utilization. **Regional Health Information Organizations (RHIOs)** exemplify an effort to attain this type of exchange (Thielst 2007). RHIOs represent the initiative in which physicians, healthcare systems, payers, and businesses exchange information for the collective good. While the term *RHIO* is now used with greater frequency it is not universally accepted and may be simply referred to as a Health Information Exchange (HIE) (A primer 2006).

The following must be in place to achieve HIE:

- *Patient identifier.* This is the foundation of any successful HIE because it ensures that the correct patient record is selected, which is essential for patient safety. Inaccurate data may lead to linking unrelated records or may indicate that no records are available when they do exist, (Fernandes & O'Connor 2006). No national identifier exists, which forces exchange partners to agree upon identifiers or to rely upon a mapping process (National network keeps debate 2006).
- *Technology infrastructure.* This includes interoperability as well as security measures such as encryption and authentication, shared terminology, and network connections (Glaser 2007; Grabscheid 2006).
- *A model.* Participants need to identify a business model. RHIOs need an ongoing source of revenue, but most RHIOs have not identified a business model. This may be due to the fact that there seem to be two schools of thought about RHIOs (A primer 2006; Dillehunt 2007). The first school focuses primarily upon the exchange of healthcare information, while the second group's focus is the potential cost savings associated with a RHIO. The development and operation of a RHIO requires a substantial financial investment initially as well as an ongoing source of income to remain sustainable. This is best illustrated by the fact that the

information exchange provides a service, namely information. When the information exchange can provide that service at a lower cost than other providers, such as physician offices, then the health information exchange operates at a profit and the arrangement is beneficial for all parties involved. This is an example of a for-profit business model. Lack of attention to the creation of a business model contributes to a nonsustainable effort. The Santa Barbara RHIO, for example, collapsed largely because there was no provision for income to meet operating expenses once grant monies were spent.

- *Participants.* All parties that require patient information for treatment purposes should be involved in HIE. Hospitals, physicians, pharmacies, and independent laboratories are among the primary participants. It is important to provide linkages to ambulatory care settings, long-term care facilities and public health agencies.
- *Funding.* The benefits of HIE have the potential to outweigh the costs to establish the infrastructure. Some RHIOs establish fees for certain services. Types of fees include enrollment, transaction, and access fees.
- *Policies.* Policies need to include access restrictions. Participating RHIO providers may only access their patient records. This limited access will help to ensure record privacy and confidentiality (Leviss 2006; Martin 2007a).
- *Consent management.* Consumers have the option to share their information across the HIE system. Consent information is then housed where it can readily be accessed to determine what, if any, information can be released to HIE participants. Consumers who elect not to share information need to understand the risks associated with incomplete health information (Grabscheid 2006).
- *Community buy-in.* The majority of stakeholders see the potential benefits of HIE, but there are often lingering concerns over security of health information. It is important to obtain the support of the community.
- *Scalability.* The size of the exchange effort must be defined to make it manageable. Ease of use is also important to participants. Web-based access has become popular in recent years.

DRIVING FORCES

The forces supporting HIE include a combination of governmental and private initiatives. The National Committee on Vital and Health Statistics (NCVHS) called for the creation of a national health information infrastructure in 2001 (Overhage, Evans, & Marchibroda 2005). The Medicare Modernization Act (MMA) of 2003 included some provisions to support HIE, namely electronic prescribing. In 2004 President Bush escalated federal health information technology (HIT) activities when he signed Executive Order 13335. This order recognized the need to develop and implement a national HIT infrastructure and established the Office of the National Coordinator for Health Information Technology (ONCHIT) in the

Department of Health and Human Services. The HHS report titled *The Decade of Health Information Technology: Delivering Consumer-centric and Information-rich Health Care* provided a 10-year plan to accomplish the following: build a national health information infrastructure or network; bring EHR systems to providers; use technology to give consumers more access and involvement in health decisions; and improve population health. Support for regional collaborations to exchange health information comprised one strategy identified to meet the goals of this plan (Coleman, May, Bennett, Dorr, & Harvell 2007; HHS 2004; Glaser 2007). The national health information network (NHIN) provides the technology, standards, and management to integrate the exchange of data across the country. In subsequent years ONCHIT convened the Secretary's Health Information Technology Leadership Panel, a group of nine CEOs from major companies outside of healthcare, and concluded that the federal government should provide the leadership for HIT.

The Agency for Healthcare Research and Quality (AHRQ) is another federal agency that staunchly supports HIE and RHIO development (Clancy 2006; Coleman et al. 2007). Among notable nonprofit agencies providing financial support are the Markle Foundation's Connecting for Health program, which actively promotes the interconnection of healthcare information systems, and the Robert Wood Johnson Foundation (Conn 2006). Box 13–1 lists examples of information and services available to participants.

BOX 13–1   Information Available to RHIO Participants

- E-prescribing
- Laboratory results
- Pathology results
- Radiology results
- Diagnostic images
- Physician's dictation, including history and physical, progress notes, and discharge summaries
- Inpatient medication treatments
- Nursing care documentation
- Client demographic information
- Client healthcare insurance information
- Names of primary and consulting physicians
- Long-term health records
- Ambulatory care/clinic visits
- Public health records
- Home health information
- Decision support
- Quality measurement and reporting services
- Telehealth consults
- Immunization records
- Prescribed medications, vitamins and supplements, and homeopathic remedies

The following include some of the purported benefits associated with HIE:

- *Saves money.* Electronic health information exchange is projected to save the U.S. economy $78 billion (Beneftis of RHIOs 2006). HIE eliminates problems associated with paper record management and expedites authorization and claims processing.
- *Improves outcomes.* Shared access to records allows providers to spot warning signs faster and initiate treatment earlier.
- *Improves provider-patient relationships.* Shared information eliminates the need to ask the same questions multiple times, saving time and improving credibility.
- *Streamlines workflow.* Less paper management allows providers to spend more time with patients, resulting in greater satisfaction for clinicians and consumers.
- *Provides a positive perception.* Hospitals and other participants in information exchange are viewed as working to improve the health of individuals and the community.

RHIO Models

There is a wide variation in the objectives, governance, and financial structures for RHIOs (A primer 2006). No dominant RHIO form has emerged, nor has the federal government expressed any preferences for a particular model (Scalise 2006; Thielst 2007). Some terms for the different models include community-based, proprietary, federation, and co-op. A brief description of each follows:

- *Community-based.* This type is comprised of multiple, unrelated stakeholders.
- *Proprietary.* All stakeholders are either owned by, or affiliated with, a single corporate entity.
- *Federation.* Multiple independent enterprises in a region agree to allow access to information that they maintain, often developing a system to index or locate data. This arrangement affords more direct control over security but with the challenge of dealing with multiple systems.
- *Co-op.* Multiple enterprises agree to share technology, a common data repository, and administrative overhead to create a central utility. This choice is generally favored by smaller enterprises.
- *Hybrid.* This combines federation and co-op networks to allow exchange within and across organizations.

RHIOs typically work in one of two ways: as a centralized database that serves as an information exchange, clearinghouse, or locator service; or as a facilitator that brings together competitors who then build a consensus on policies and rely upon the use of open standards rather than proprietary software. The first approach offers quick retrieval of information because it relies upon a single server and consistent format. It is usually faster to put into operation but leads to more difficulty in keeping records up-to-date. The second approach, however, permits records to be updated quicker.

RHIOs derive income in several ways. Most charge individual participants a fee for information services that reduce administrative burden (deBrantes, Emery, Overhage, Glaser, & Marchibroda 2007; Martin 2007b). Typically physicians do not pay to access patient data such as lab results but may pay to access a physician practice management system, on-line prescribing, and electronic charting systems. Additional sources of revenue may come from the sale of secondary data useful to medical device and pharmaceutical manufacturers and the inclusion of third-party payers that could also provide incentives for participating providers through quicker reimbursement and payment for performance. Secondary use of data for profit presents an ethical issue. This issue must be weighted carefully to avoid HIPAA violations. A study conducted on behalf of ONCHIT by the American Health Information Management Association (AHIMA) identified clinical messaging and medication histories as services that offer the best chance for immediate revenue generation (FORE 2007). Other services included e-prescribing, shared patient summaries, quality measurement and reporting services, and credentialing. One HIE generated extra revenue for providers by asking emergency room patients without a primary care provider to sign a release to have their information sent to clinics and practices to determine acceptance for follow-up care (Experienced networks 2006). Patients received almost instant notice and the accepting provider benefited via additional revenue.

Current Status

The technology to support HIE exists now and is within financial reach (Smaling 2005). The **community health information network (CHIN)** concept of the 1990s was similar to that of a RHIO but failed to achieve widespread acceptance, partly because the costs and technology of that time made it unfeasible (Bazzoli 2007; Benefits of RHIOs). A CHIN was an organization that offered electronic connections that enabled all providers, payers, and purchasers of care to exchange financial, clinical, and administrative information in a defined geographic location, eliminating redundant data collection and reducing paperwork (Tabar 2000). Regulatory agencies could receive information directly from CHINs. Only a few communities created CHINs. Primary features of a CHIN included:

1. *Open communications.* An interface engine connected the computer-based patient record, various data repositories, and payer information, making all data available to the various participants.
2. *Clinical data repository.* The CHIN clinical data repository combined clinical data from all individual data repositories.
3. *Mechanisms for cost, outcome, and utilization analysis.* Information provided by the payers, as well as the outcomes recorded by the healthcare providers, was used and analyzed by decision support software (Bir & Zerrenner 1995).

The key factors that doomed CHINs were a lack of clear agreed-on objectives at the beginning and the focus on administrative transactions instead of safety and quality (Marietti 2004). The CHIN concept made an important contribution to the expectation for the EHR in terms of the ability to share information across systems. A few surviving CHINs are working toward achieving RHIO status (Experienced networks 2006).

The maturation of several RHIOs has led to a growing acceptance of the concept. Of the providers who responded to a recent survey, 70% expect HIE to start with RHIOs even though the majority of those same respondents are not yet involved in an RHIO (The provider's perspective 2006).

There have been more than 200 regional HIEs, many of which have been funded by the federal government (Coleman, Benent, Dorr, & Harvell 2007; Conn 2005; Experienced networks 2006; FORE 2006; Smaling 2005). More than 40 states have some phase of RHIO planning, implementation, or projects. Only a portion of these are expected to achieve a sustainable business model once public and private grant monies allocated for start-up and initial operating costs are depleted. One notable failure was the Santa Barbara County Care Data Exchange, one of the first and most prominent RHIOs. For this reason the Center for Health Transformation advocates ongoing federal support. There have also been legislative efforts to provide ongoing funds. The federal government is in the process of developing best practices to address governance and sustainability for RHIOs, practices that include a requirement for funded organizations to show viability. Many healthcare providers have taken a wait-and-see attitude before committing limited resources on RHIO development until viability is proven (Roop 2007).

RHIOs need to be responsive to what stakeholders need and want. Financial return on investment has not been a primary factor in the decision to participate although it is critical to sustainability. Successful RHIOs need to deliver:

- *Relevant information to clinicians where and when they need it.* Relevant information includes medication history, test results, pharmacy data, diagnostic images, prior treatment locales, discharge summaries, and home health reports (Strating 2007). Individual clinicians should then be able to pick the view that enhances their workflow.
- *Decision support to help process the huge volumes of information* (Thielst 2007). RHIOs impact both clinical operations and business functions including customer service, medical record management, information security, facilities management, patient outreach, and various back-office functions. Decision support can be used to facilitate safe, as well as cost-effective, interventions. For example, decision support can be used to suggest the most cost-effective antibiotic for a particular patient.

Obstacles

Several obstacles have been identified to the formation and long-term success of RHIOs (dbMotion 2006; Glaser 2007; Leviss 2006; The provider's perspective 2006; Smaling 2005; Stats Snapshot 2007; Thielst 2007). These include:

- *Governance.* This is the largest obstacle, along with funding. It is difficult to reach agreement on information exchange, economic factors, and incentives among multiple entities particularly when they have competing interests. The ever-changing, dynamic nature of member institutions contributes to the complexities. Strong leadership is needed to set balanced, attainable goals.
- *Funding.* Although the majority of HIEs received start-up funds, few began with a comprehensive business plan.
- *Competition.* Potential stakeholders are often in competition for the same patients.
- *Internal policies.* Individual organizations vary widely in access to information policies.
- *Consumer privacy concern.* The added complexity of a RHIO makes this a very real issue. The need for information versus a need-to-know limitation must be balanced. Close, frequent dialogue with all members and the public is needed to address the issues of privacy and security.
- *Trust.* RHIOs offer greater trust for the healthcare consumer when there is local control rather than a national framework for HIE.
- *Legal and regulatory issues.* There are uncertainties regarding liability for security breaches, concerns over anti-kickback restrictions with for-profit business models, and unanswered questions as to who owns data housed in RHIOs. Healthcare consumers must be informed of how information is shared and may be offered an option to restrict information access. HIPAA regulations are now seen as an enabler of RHIOs because they provide a baseline of standards.
- *Technology.* The number of technical challenges has decreased in recent years so that business and legal concerns create more issues. Interoperability, security testing, authentication, and the ability to conduct audits fall within this realm. Rarely do participants share the same type of information systems or share the same approach.
- *Scarce human resources.* There are few people who have the experience and expertise needed to establish and maintain a RHIO (Conn 2006). Clinicians may not be eager to participate if they see the cost of time, equipment, and other scare resources outweighing perceived benefits.

Clinical Data Networks

A **Clinical Data Network (CDN)** is a community based group of providers, clinicians, and organizations that share health information using a common information technology framework in order to improve the quality of patient care and safety (Lang 2007). CDNs are a smaller variant of RHIOs. CDNs share most of the same issues faced by RHIOs but technology is generally a lesser issue because it is sponsored by the dominant provider organization in the community.

FUTURE DIRECTIONS

As we move toward a longitudinal health record for all citizens, it is important to pull in records from all sources, including long-term healthcare and public health records, such as immunizations and monitoring efforts. Patients are particularly vulnerable at points of transition such as during transfers between different levels of care and care settings. Full HIE will improve both safety and quality of care. Inclusion of public health records is especially important in the case of an outbreak of a contagious disease.

As HIE gains momentum at the community level the next step is to link to a National Health Information Network (NHIN), enabling information sharing across the country and eventually across the globe to meet the needs of a mobile population (Glaser 2007; Theilst 2007). In the interim, RHIOs must remain responsive to what stakeholders need and want while taking care to keep patient care, privacy, and security of health information as top priorities. Findlay and Rein (2007) indicated that this may not be enough: government intervention is needed to address healthcare privacy and confidentiality policy; to make specific recommendations on medical privacy in the electronic age; and to draft legislation to address gaps in HIPAA for privacy protection. RHIOs must also anticipate and deal with challenges early. This includes the selection of the most appropriate legal structure for the present and future, allowances for growth, changes in requirements and technology, and a long-term financial plan (Bazzoli 2007; dbMotion 2006). Glaser (2007) noted that many RHIOs will fall victim to market forces and ineffective approaches to data exchange over the next few years until more is known about what models are most viable.

CASE STUDY EXERCISES

13.1   What benefits do you, as a clinician, perceive associated with HIE?

13.2   You work in a prominent surgeon's office. You have noticed that the office manager has accessed the RHIO for information on another employee in the practice who is not currently being treated by the surgeon. How should this situation be handled?

13.3   You work in the medical ambulatory clinic. When reviewing your list of patients for the day you notice that one, John Pauvlik, has not had the pneumonia vaccine according to data pulled from the RHIO. What measures should be in place to determine that you have information on the correct patient?

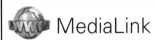

MediaLink	• Glossary
	• Multiple Choice
Additional resources for this content can	• Discussion Points
be found on the Companion Website at	• Case Studies
www.prenhall.com/hebda. Click on	• MediaLink Application
"Chapter 13" to select the activities for	• MediaLink
this chapter.	

SUMMARY

- The ability to exchange information among different providers and care delivery systems, frequent known as healthcare information exchange (HIE), is an essential step toward the EHR.
- A Regional Health Information Organization (RHIO) is a network of stakeholders within a region who are committed to improving the quality, safety, access, and efficiency of healthcare through the use of health information technology.
- HIE requires agreement upon how patient information will be found from one system to the next, technology, finances, access policies, funding, consent management, "buy-in" by participants, and trust that information privacy will be maintained.
- Healthcare consumers must be informed as to who will be able to access their information, and consumers may be given the opportunity not to fully disclose all information to all RHIO participants.
- Several forces are behind the push toward HIE. These include a presidential executive order, support by several government agencies, the move toward the EHR, and the need to reform healthcare.
- Purported RHIO benefits include cost savings, improved outcomes, better provider-patient relationships, and improved work efficiencies.
- No one RHIO model for structure is dominant.
- RHIOs are the building blocks of the proposed National Health Information Network (NHIN).
- A Clinical Data Networks (CDN) is a community based group of providers, clinicians, and organizations that share health information using a common information technology framework in order to improve the quality of patient care and safety. It is a smaller variant of a RHIO that generally avoids the issue of information exchange across different systems.

REFERENCES

A primer for building RHIOs. (February 2006). *Hospitals & Health Networks, 80*(2).

Bazzoli, F. (February 1, 2007). RHIOs make a renewed push for profitablity. *Healthcare Finance News*. Retrieved August 8, 2007, from http:www,healthcarefinancenews. com/story.cms?id=5998.

Benefits of RHIOs. (2006). *Hospitals & Health Networks, 80*(2), 55.

Bir, N. & Zerrenner, W. (1995). Network design and implementation of a CHIN from a hospital's perspective. Toward an electronic patient record '95. *Proceedings, 2,* 50–58.

Brailer, D., Q & A. (2005). Policy: Brailer Q & A. *Hospitals & Health Networks, 79*(12), 20–22.

Clancy, C. (February 13, 2006). Health Care IT: The foundation for improving care. Remarks for HIMSS 2006 Conference. Delivered by Scott Young, M. D. Retrieved August 8, 2007, from http://www.ahrq.gov/news/sp021306.htm.

Coleman, E. A., May, K., Bennett, R. E., Dorr, D., & Harvell, J. (February 2007). Report on health information exchange in post-acute and long-term care. Prepared for Office of Disability, Aging and Long-Term Care Policy, Office of the Assistant Secretary for Planning and Evaluation, U.S. Department of Health and Human Services. Retrieved August 8, 2007, from http://aspe.hhs.gov/daltcp/reports/2007/HIErpt.pdf.

Conn, J. (2005). Destination RHIO: As regional data networks continue to grow in number, some find financial strength. *Modern Healthcare, 35*(42), 28, 32.

Conn, J. (2006). RHIOs make it work. *Modern Healthcare, 36*(7), 22–24.

Department of Health and Human Services (HHS). (July 21, 2004). News release Thompson Launches "Decade of Health Information Technology." Retrieved August 9, 2007, from http://www.hhs.gov/news/press/2004pres/20040721a.html.

dbMotion. (January 2006). White Paper: A practical approach to RHIO formation. Retrieved August 8, 2007, from http://www.himss.org/HIEForums/d/whitepapers/dbMotionRHIOWhitePaper.pdf.

deBrantes, F., Emery, D. W., Overhage, M., Glaser, J., & Marchibroda, J. (2007). The potential of HIEs as infomediaries. *Journal of Healthcare Information Management, 21*(1), 69–75.

Dillehunt, D. B. (2007). RHIOs: An alternative approach. *ADVANCE for Health Information Executives, 11*(9), 47.

Executive Order 13335: Incentives for the Use of Health Information Technology and Establishing the Position of the National Health Information Technology Coordinator. (2004). *Federal Register, 70*(236), 76287–76288.

Experienced networks offer business model. (2006). *Health Data Management, 14*(2), 50, 52, 56, 58, 60, 62.

Fernandes, L. & O'Connor, M. (2006). What's in a RHIO? *ADVANCE for Health Information Executives. 10*(6), 43–46.

Findlay, S. & Rein, A. (2007). On IT, privacy is the priority. Retrieved August 8, 2007, from http://modernhealthcare.com/apps/pbcs.dll/article?AID=/20070116/FREE/70116001&SearchID=7328965563818137(3).

Foundation of Research and Education of the American Health Information Management Association (FORE). (2007). *Development of State Level Health Information Exchange Initiatives Final Report: Extension Tasks.* Retrieved August 15, 2007, from http://www.staterhio.org/documents/Final_Report_HHSP23320064105EC_090106_000.pdf.

Glaser, J. (2007). The advent of RHIO 2.0. *Journal of Healthcare Information Management, 21*(3), 7–9.

Grabscheid, P. (2006). RHIOs and reality. *ADVANCE for Health Information Executives, 10*(10), 10.

Lang, R. D. (2007). Provider-sponsored clinical data networks. *Journal of Healthcare Information Management, 21*(3), 2–3, 5.

Leviss, J. (2006). Identity and access management: The starting point for a RHIO. *Health Management Technology, 27*(1), 64, 63

Marietti, C. (2004). Healthcare transformation via infrastructure. *Healthcare Informatics, 21*(2), 44–50.

Martin, Z. (2007a). Building a RHIO, Bit by bit. *Health Data Management, 15*(6), 58, 60.

Martin, Z. (2007b). Virginia RHIO: Taking baby steps. *Health Data Management, 15*(2), 120, 122.

Mitchell, R. N. (2007). Tackling RHIO initiatives. *ADVANCE for Health Information Executives, 11*(2), 43–44, 46, 48, 50, 52–54.

National network keeps debate over patient identifier alive. (2006). *Health Data Management, 14*(2), 54.

Overhage, J. M., Evans, L., & Marchibroda, J. (2005). Communities' readiness for health information exchange: The national landscape in 2004. *Journal of the American Medical Informatics Association, 12*(2), 107–112.

A primer for building RHIOs. (2006). *Hospitals & Health Networks, 80*(2), 51.

The provider's perspective of RHIO participation. A CGI White paper. (2006). Retrieved August 8, 2007, from http://www.cgi.com/cgi/pdf/cgi_whpr_65_rhio_e.pdf.

Roop, E. S. (2007). Hospitals leery of funding information exchanges, seek assurances. *Hospitals & Health Networks, 81*(5), 14, 16.

Scalise, D. (2006). Which way RHIO? *Hospitals & Health Networks, 80*(6), 2–22.

Steen, R. S. (January 26, 2007). IBM approach to health information network service provider business model. Retrieved August 8, 2007, from http://www.hhs.gov/healthit/healthnetwork/presentations/Steen.pdf.

Smaling J. (2005). A dose of RHIOlity: The toughest RHIO integration challenges are not technology-based. *Health Management Technology, 26*(12), 34–36.

Stats Snapshot. (2007). *Health Data Management, 15*(8), 55.

Strating, D. (2007). Regional data exchange to the north. *ADVANCE for Health Information Executives, 11*(2), 46.

Tabar, P. (2000). The latest work: A glossary of healthcare information technology terms. *Healthcare Informatics, 17*(3), 75–133.

Thielst, C. B. (2007). Regional Health Information Networks and the Emerging Organizational Structures. *Journal of Healthcare Management, 52*(3), 146–150.

CHAPTER 14

Regulatory and Accreditation Issues

After completing this chapter, you should be able to:

1 Review legislation that impacts the protection of healthcare information, including HIPAA and the Patriot Act.

2 Discuss issues related to the implementation of HIPAA administrative simplification requirements.

3 Analyze the impact of HIPAA security and privacy requirements on the healthcare delivery system.

4 Consider the issues related to identity theft.

5 Discuss the influence of major accrediting agencies and reimbursement issues on the design and use of information systems.

6 Review design and implementation considerations for automated documentation systems in specialized facilities in light of legal and regulatory requirements.

SIGNIFICANT LEGISLATION FOR HEALTH INFORMATION TECHNOLOGY USE

Healthcare institutions deal with an increasing number of legislative and regulatory issues daily. There are local, state, and federal laws as well as watchdog agencies that safeguard private health information and monitor the quality of care delivered. Some of the organizations that perform accreditation and establish standards for healthcare delivery in the United States include:

- The Joint Commission
- Commission for Accreditation of Rehabilitation Facilities (CARF)
- National Committee for Quality Assurance (NCQA)
- American Medical Accreditation Program (AMAP)
- American Accreditation Healthcare Commission/Utilization Review Accreditation Commission (AAHC/URAC)
- Accreditation Association for Ambulatory Healthcare (AAAHC)
- American Association for the Accreditation of Ambulatory Surgical Facilities (AAAASF)
- Accreditation Commission for Health Care (ACHC)
- Utilization Review Accreditation Commission (URAC)
- Community Health Accreditation Program (CHAP)

In addition, the Agency for Healthcare Research and Quality (AHRQ) plays an important role in ensuring the quality of healthcare. Accreditation entails an extensive review process that monitors performance against predetermined standards. The accreditation process certifies to the public that the facilities involved meet nationally accepted standards through a recognized program. The amount of documentation required for compliance with these various laws, regulations, and performance standards is voluminous. There is a growing recognition that information systems can and must be used to improve client safety and quality of care as well as enhance regulatory compliance through improved data capture and system prompts, thereby relieving demands on already overburdened healthcare providers. This capture should occur as a by-product of daily documentation activities.

PRIVACY AND CONFIDENTIALITY LEGISLATION

The ability to access sensitive health information in electronic patient records by many different parties generates growing concerns over privacy and confidentiality (Robezniek 2005; Win & Fulcher 2007). A 2005 California HealthCare Foundation survey revealed consumer concern over the possible misuse of private health information. These results were mirrored by a recent Harris poll that found that 70% of adults surveyed expressed worry about possible compromise of sensitive health information due to weak data security (Amatayakul & Cohen 2007). Several large-scale breaches of client privacy have occurred when personal health information (PHI) was accidentally posted to the Web or stolen. These breaches highlighted the need to safeguard client privacy. The incorporation of consent mechanisms into EHRs has the potential to help protect confidentiality but fails to provide legal protection. Until the 1996 passage of the Health Insurance Portability and Accountability Act (HIPAA), legal protection for PHI had been poor. HIPAA, also known as the Kennedy-Kassebaum Bill, represented the first federal legislation to protect automated client records and to provide uniform protection nationwide. This legislation called for the establishment of an electronic patient records system and privacy rules (Frank-Stromborg & Ganschow 2002; Information Policy Committee 1997). PHI refers to individually identifiable health information such as demographic data; facts that relate to an individual's past, present, or future physical or mental health condition; provision of care; and payment for the provision of care that identifies the individual. Examples include name, address, birth date, Social Security number, allergies, claims data, lab results and other diagnostic history, prescription history, past visits to physicians, emergency rooms and other healthcare encounters, vaccination records, and prior in- and outpatient procedures.

Previous attempts to legislate medical records privacy included the Individual Privacy Act, the Fair Health Information Practices Act of 1995, and the Medical Records Confidentiality Act of 1995. However, none of these bills were passed into law. Table 14–1 provides a synopsis of each of these proposed bills.

TABLE 14–1	Important Legislative Efforts to Protect the Privacy of Medical Records
Title	**Synopsis**
Individual Privacy Protection Act of 1991	Designed to amend the Privacy Act of 1974, increasing the minimum amount of civil damages when records are not properly maintained
	Provided penalties for violations of privacy rights
	Established an individual privacy protection board
	Not enacted into law
The Fair Health Information Practices Act of 1995	Required healthcare providers, information service organizations, benefit plan sponsors, and health researchers to allow individuals to examine their own records
	Set forth provisions concerning the use and disclosure of protected information
	Established penalties for violations of the Act
	Not enacted into law
Medical Records Confidentiality Act of 1995	Designed to ensure medical record privacy
	Defined *health information trustee*
	Established circumstances for disclosure
	Required trustees to establish safeguards and to maintain records of disclosures not related to treatment

Title	Synopsis
	Established penalties for failure to comply with the Act
	Not enacted into law
The Health Insurance Portability and Accountability Act (HIPAA) of 1996	Established minimal level of legal protection for privacy and personal health information
	Ensured portability of health insurance for individuals
	Sought to reduce paperwork associated with processing claims
	Enacted into law
Medical Privacy in the Age of New Technologies Act of 1997	Established safeguards for health information
	Restricted the use and disclosure of information
	Proposed civil and criminal sanctions for failure to comply with the Act
	Not enacted into law; referred back to committee
Fair Health Information Practices Act of 1997	Required healthcare providers to allow individuals to examine their records
	Restricted the use of protected information to the purpose for which it was collected or for which disclosure authorization has been obtained
	Mandated the establishment of standards for electronic document transmission, receipt, and maintenance
	Established civil and criminal penalties for violations of the Act
	Authorized research on protecting health information
	Not enacted into law

Source: Adapted from "Legislative information on the Internet," Thomas, 2003. On the Internet at: http://thomas.loc.gov/home/thomas.html.

The Medical Records Confidentiality Act, otherwise known as the Bennett Bill, was notable because it contained the following points (Braithwaite 1996):

- A definition of *health information trustee* as a person or entity that creates, receives, obtains, maintains, or transmits protected health information and any employee, agent, or contractor of same
- Conditions for the inspection and copying of protected information
- Provisions for the correction or amendment of protected health information
- Time limits and additional constraints over disclosure of information

- Authorization and accountability for disclosure of information, including electronic disclosure
- Stiff sanctions for inappropriate access or use of health-related information

Although the Bennett Bill did propose safeguards for healthcare information, the American Civil Liberties Union (ACLU) and several consumer rights groups opposed the bill because they thought it did not adequately address client control over the use and dissemination of health information. Other critics thought that its wording would prevent legitimate exchange of client information between institutions (Barrows & Clayton 1996; Braithwaite 1996). Box 14–1 lists some principles identified by the ACLU for the formulation of a health information privacy policy.

The Privacy Act of 1974 protected federally managed records, such as those of Medicare and Medicaid, and mandated that federal agencies develop, implement, and disclose their plans for maintaining the security of stored data (Frawley 1995; Hebda, Sakerka, & Czar 1994; Robinson 1994; Rothfeder 1995). Veteran Affairs and Administration hospitals published their plans. There were no similar federal mandates for private institutions and providers at that time. As a result, European agencies refused to transmit medical information to the United States.

It is important to note that the Privacy Act of 1974 was enacted before widespread computer use. As a result, protection of medical records varied, from state to state, necessitating that practitioners be familiar with the regulations of the states in which they practiced. Some states had regulations, statutes, and case laws that recognized the confidentiality of medical records and limited access.

BOX 14–1   American Civil Liberties Union (ACLU) Principles for Formulating a Health Information Privacy Policy

- Strict limits on access and disclosure of all personally identifiable health data
- Individual control of all personally identifiable health records, with no disclosure without informed consent
- Security measures that protect against unauthorized access or misuse by authorized persons
- No access to personally identifiable health information for employers or potential employers
- The right of all individuals to access, copy, and/or correct any information contained in their own medical records
- Full notification of clients of all uses of their health information
- Establishment of a private right of action and government enforcement to prevent or correct wrongful disclosures or information misuse
- Establishment of a federal system to ensure compliance with privacy laws and regulations

Source: Adapted from "Privacy, confidentiality, and electronic medical records" by R. C. Barrows and P. D. Clayton, 1996, *Journal of the American Medical Informatics Association, 3*(2), 139–148; and *Toward a new health care system: The civil liberties issues,* an ACLU Public Policy Report, 1994.

Breach of confidence might lead to disciplinary action for healthcare professionals by their state boards for licensure. Other states had criminal sanctions against violations of client confidentiality, but enforcement and quantification of damage were difficult.

Several groups besides the ACLU have a strong interest in privacy issues for medical records; these include the Center for Democracy and Technology, the Electronic Privacy Information Center (EPIC), and the Center for Patient Advocacy, among other professional organizations and regulatory bodies. Each group maintains its own Web site.

The Health Insurance Portability and Accountability Act (HIPAA)

HIPAA (Public Law 104–191) was passed into law by Congress in 1996. This Act had the following objectives (Haramboure 1999; Hellerstein 2000):

- To ensure the portability of health insurance
- To prevent healthcare fraud and abuse
- To ensure the security and privacy of health information
- To enforce health information standards that will improve the efficiency of healthcare delivery, simplify the exchange of data between healthcare entities, and reduce cost
- To reduce the paperwork associated with processing healthcare transactions

HIPAA Standards HIPAA affects all aspects of health information management, including privacy and security of patient records, coding, and reimbursement. The broad scope and complex nature of HIPAA resulted in an extensive definition of its rules since its enactment in 1996. The Clinton Health Security Act provided the framework for the national standards created by HIPAA (Annas 2003). The Department of Health and Human Services (DHHS) developed the privacy rule after Congress failed to do so within the timeframe prescribed by HIPAA. It was released in final form in 2002. The deadline for compliance was 2003 but some small health plans were given until 2004 to achieve compliance. The Office of Civil Rights in the Department of Health and Human Services is responsible for implementing and enforcing the privacy rule with respect to voluntary compliance and civil monetary penalties. The privacy rule attempts to ensure that PHI is properly protected while allowing the flow of data needed to promote high-quality care and protect the public's health and well-being. HIPAA sets a minimum level of protection (Annas 2003). It does not override state laws that are more stringent in their provisions.

The HIPAA privacy rule affects all organizations and individuals involved in the delivery of healthcare. Organizations, including hospitals, physician offices, home health agencies, nursing homes, and all individual clinicians, instructors, students, and volunteers, now have additional responsibilities and must examine current policies and practices to comply with the provisions of this legislation. Also affected are payers, employers, data services, clearinghouses, regulatory agencies, information system vendors, Medicare, and Medicaid. HIPAA affects individual care providers, including physicians, nurses, and other clinicians. Others who have direct or indirect access to client information are also affected. Examples include utilization review staff as well as housekeeping and maintenance personnel.

HIPAA affects daily clinical practice in several ways. Clients must receive a privacy notice that includes a clear written explanation of the allowable uses and disclosures of their PHI and they must be notified of their rights to see and amend health data and learn who has seen their healthcare records. Providers, in turn, must make a good faith effort to obtain written acknowledgment that each client has received a copy of the provider's privacy notice and maintain an audit log of all parties who have requested access to a client record or PHI. Authorization, rather than consent, is requested for the disclosure of information for nonclinical and reimbursement issues. Authorization differs from consent because it is specific to the release of PHI for a specific purpose and expires on a particular date. Individual clinicians must take reasonable precautions to avoid disclosure during care and to protect written, spoken, and recorded information (Anderson 2007). One example to protect PHI is the use of a password selected by the client in order for information to be given out for inquiries. Clients can then disclose the password to individuals who may secure information concerning their condition. Other protective measures include the elimination or modification of sign-in sheets, locking up medical records when cleaning crews and other workers come in, exercising care when sending Faxes and mail, not sharing log-ons and passwords, reconfiguring offices and nurses stations to remove charts and x-rays from casual view, not posting client names outside rooms or on assignment boards that can be viewed by the public, turning monitor screens so they cannot be viewed by outsiders, and respecting the rights of individuals who opt out of the hospital directory. Employees should not take medical records home, and when remote access is used special precautions should be taken to avoid unauthorized view.

HIPAA allows the use or disclosure of PHI without authorization or permission when required by law and for public health activities such as controlling disease, abuse, violence, Food and Drug Administration tracking, and for work-related illnesses. PHI may also be shared in the following instances:

- Audits or investigations by health oversight agencies
- Judicial and administrative proceedings
- For law enforcement purposes
- As needed by funeral directors and coroners
- Donation/transplantation of tissues
- Research
- Essential government functions such as combat
- Worker's Compensation

The use or disclosure of PHI for any of the reasons listed above removes it from HIPAA's privacy requirements (Frank-Stromborg & Ganschow 2002; DHHS 2003).

HIPAA Privacy Rule Compliance HIPAA mandates administrative and technical procedures to protect privacy. Administrative procedures include information access controls, contingency plans, formal mechanisms for processing records, security configuration and management, security incident procedures, security management processes, security training, certification of compliance, chain-of-trust partner agreements, and termination procedures. Certification of compliance is implicit with the act of filing a claim, as this indicates that the organization has met Medicare and Medicaid statutes and regulations (Nowicki & Summers 2001). The certification process confirms the ability of software products and users to submit readable transactions but does not guarantee payment of claims. Chain-of-trust partner agreements are required when a provider exchanges individually identifiable client information. These agreements must include language that certifies HIPAA compliance (Maddox 2003). Organizations may self-certify and audit every business partner in its chain of trust. Business partners in this chain can include all payers, providers, employers, and clinical service vendors such as independent laboratories and radiology or therapy departments. Certification may also be obtained through third-party reviewers.

Technical measures include audit controls, authorization controls, data authentication, communication and network controls, encryption, and various types of authentication for event reporting, integrity controls, message authentication, message integrity, and user authentication. Compliance requires incorporation of HIPAA into the strategic plan for the entire system, starting with a review and revision of policies and procedures, designation of a privacy officer, and implementation of a security plan with specific safeguards (Buppert 2002; Welker & Podleski 2003; Wilson 2003). The chief nurse executive, informatics nurse, and representative clinicians all share a responsibility for health information privacy and confidentiality and should be actively involved in the development of strategies to achieve compliance. As an advanced practice clinician, the informatics nurse understands clinical processes, information systems, and the significance of relevant legislation. This makes the informatics nurse ideally suited to serve as a member of the HIPAA team. There must also be representatives from medical records, information systems, accounting, client intake and registration, risk management, public relations, ancillary services, human resources, and the compliance office. Designation of a chief privacy officer assigns accountability for HIPAA compliance. The privacy officer is responsible for the following areas:

- Periodic risk analysis to review current systems, procedures, personnel, and overall compliance. Risk assessments should be conducted every 12 to 18 months (Davis 2007)
- Identification of changes that must be made, including system changes, to improve compliance
- Formulation of a plan to carry out needed revisions
- HIPAA training

- Communication and education of all staff regarding system revisions and updates to policies and procedures
- Implementation of a mechanism to track requests to view PHI and maintain that documentation
- Means to archive privacy policies and procedures, privacy notices, disposition of complaints, and other documentation required by the privacy rule for 6 years after their creation or last effective date

Gard (2002) noted that with proper security systems in place, including encryption, passwords, and unique client identifiers, electronic records may be more secure than paper records. Box 14–2 lists examples of security measures that should be evaluated for HIPAA compliance.

One highly visible requirement of the privacy rule is the privacy notice sent to all healthcare consumers. The content of this notice must address the following:

- Ways in which PHI may be used or disclosed
- Responsibility of providers to protect privacy, provide a notice of privacy practices, and abide by the terms of the notice
- Description of individual's rights, including the right to complain to the Department of Health and Human Services and the provider in the event that the individual believes that his or her rights have been violated
- Point of contact for further information and complaints

BOX 14–2   Evaluation of Current Security Measures for HIPAA Compliance Examples of Security Measures That Should Be Evaluated

- **Determine what types of data are stored on PCs and storage media such as memory sticks.** Do they hold individual patient data?
- **Secure workstations.** Do workstations require a unique sign-on for each user? Are workstations and point-of-care devices protected from theft?
- **System security.** Is there an automatic log-off procedure in place?
- **Review of user accounts, privileges, and permissions.** Is there a policy for regular review?
- **Personnel policies.** Are there procedures in place, such as background checks, to scrutinize personnel responsible for PHI, including those individuals who had access to restricted areas but who have left or changed job responsibilities, and those who play a key role in incident response, business continuity or emergency mode operations?
- **Review of business parties.** Is there a plan to review business partners at least twice annually?
- **Evaluate network security.** Is the network protected from unauthorized access?
- **Update hardware and software inventories.**
- **Examine physical features in accordance with security requirements.** Identify location of backup media and workstations in relation to public access.
- **Printout security.** How are paper reports containing patient information disposed of?
- **Monitor environment for unusual activity.** Is there a review of tools used to monitor the environment for unusual activity, such as intrusion detection, help desk tickets, visitor logs, and work logs from facility maintenance and housekeeping?

HIPAA also includes requirements for electronic signature standards if an organization chooses to use them. The electronic signature standard is applicable only with respect to use with the specifics defined in the Health Insurance Portability and Accountability Act of 1996.

Electronic or digital signatures include an encrypted digital tag added to an electronic document. This technology has the following features:

- User authentication that guarantees the user's identity
- Evidence that supports the validity of the signature
- Assurance of the integrity of the message

HIPAA Security Rule Compliance The final security rule was published in 2003. This rule mandates safeguards for the physical storage, maintenance, transmission, and access to PHI to ensure its confidentiality, data integrity, and availability when required for treatment. Like the privacy rule, the security rule specifies administrative, technical, and physical procedures to keep personal health information secure. The security rule does not apply to all individually identifiable information. The security rule requires covered entities to appoint a security officer, just as the privacy rule requires the appointment of a privacy officer. Security readiness involves people and processes, as well as information technology. Covered entities must conduct a risk analysis and then determine the security measures that best meet their needs. These may vary by the size of the office and the transactions that take place there. Physician offices may elect different disaster recovery measures than large healthcare systems. Critical gaps should be addressed first. These may include simple solutions such as locking storage areas or emptying confidential trash more frequently. Compliance with HIPAA security and privacy rules is closely linked. The final security rule requires encryption of PHI transmitted via open networks (Goedert 2003a). Organizations and providers should exercise ongoing measures to comply with both the privacy and security rules. A 2006 HIPAA survey conducted by HIMSS & the Phoenix health systems found only 55% compliance with the security standards (Albright 2007). The Office of Inspector General now has plans to conduct a systematic examination of security compliance (Amatayakul & Cohen 2007).

The HIPAA legislation includes descriptions of the various penalties for non-compliance, which can be severe. For example, the penalty for violating transaction standards may range from $100 per person per violation to $25,000 per person per violation of a single standard per calendar year. Penalties for wrongful disclosure of client information include large fines as well as possible imprisonment.

HIPAA Issues There are many issues surrounding HIPAA. They include:

- *A weakened final privacy rule.* The removal of the requirement for written client consent before the circulation of PHI by hospitals or other providers involved in routine uses of information for treatment, payment, or other healthcare constitutes one of the greatest issues. This action leaves consumers unaware of how their data are being used and creates concern over possible abuse of information by business partners or via data mining (Cohen & Amatayakul 2007). One noted area of weakness is the lack of protection for identifiable prescription information (Capizzi, Blenkinsop, & Glaser 2006). The Patriot Act, officially known as the Uniting and Strengthening America by Providing Appropriate Tools Required to Intercept and Obstruct Terrorism Act of 2001, and developing case law have considerably altered expectations of privacy (Brous 2007; Horowitz 2006; Kluge 2006). The Patriot Act allows federal authorities to collect personal information on citizens for the sake of national security without notification of the involved parties. The Patriot Act was amended in 2006 to protect privacy rights and minimize random searches.

- *Offshore outsourced services.* Foreign countries are not bound by HIPAA regulations. A significant amount of data processing of personal information and medical transcription occurs outside of the United States. Many states have drafted laws seeking to limit overseas outsourcing of personal data (Capizzi, Blenkinsop, & Glaser 2006). Healthcare providers are not responsible if service providers release information without proper authorization, but they must take appropriate steps to correct the situation or terminate the contract (Wilson 2006). The cost of negative publicity associated with such a breach in trust is difficult to measure.
- *Incomplete compliance.* This may be due to several reasons including the relatively small number of total complaints filed, apathy, virtually no legal consequences for security violations, and that it may seem less expensive to settle rather than comply (Amatayakul & Cohen 2007; Davis 2007). Privacy complaints are more visible with resultant legal action, while there are several hundred security complaints each month with an increased number of security breaches (Amatayakul 2007). An increasing number of threats and data breaches necessitate ongoing efforts to safeguard data security, particularly since healthcare data typically contain social security numbers, insurance account numbers, payment and financial information, and treatment data.
- *A growing market for data mining.* Some advocates of privacy express concern that the Department of Health and Human Services promotes a national health information technology (HIT) infrastructure that supports the financial interests of a few commercial interests over individual privacy. Courts have determined that data mining companies have a right to free speech that supersedes patient rights (Conn 2007a). Data that have been de-identified and aggregated have potential economic value to companies buying and selling data. Data kept in hospital or medical practice electronic records may be resold without consumer knowledge (Cohen & Amatayakul 2007).
- *Costs.* Enactment of HIPAA was supposed to help reduce healthcare costs by simplifying the claims submission process. No savings have yet been realized given the additional costs associated with training and the implementation of privacy and security rules and standard identifiers (Edlin & Johns 2006).

- *Lingering confusion.* Many clinicians remain unclear on HIPAA requirements despite the finalization of its rules and extensive training programs (Levine 2006; Wilson 2006). HIPAA has been used inappropriately as a means to either withhold information or make it more difficult to obtain information. HIPAA permits disclosure of healthcare information to other individuals. This requires a written statement naming the person who can receive this information.
- *Varying levels of legal protection.* A patchwork of widely varied, stricter state privacy laws contributes to the perplexity, particularly for individuals and organizations that cross state lines. Multiple jurisdictions complicate the ability to know, understand, and track changes in laws (Anderson 2007; Brous 2007; Capizzi, Blenkinsop, & Glaser 2006). More stringent state laws must be met. Most state laws are similar to the privacy rule's requirements but some have special provisions that address HIV/AIDS status, genetic testing, and mental health. Others have a broader definition of covered entities that extend to marketing communications or require written authorization to permit contact for promotional purposes. Federal legislative efforts to create a single privacy standard have not been successful to date (Broder 2006).
- *Limited protection.* The National Committee on Vital and Health Statistics recently asked the Secretary of Health and Human Services to extend HIPAA privacy protections to entities not presently covered but deemed essential to the operation of a national health network. These include community access services, health information exchanges (HIEs), medical record banks, system integrators, record locator services, and entities not yet named (Government Advisory Group 2007). While not specifically named, personal health records housed on some commercial sites are exempt from HIPAA protection. The Department of Health and Human Services has been criticized for its failure to develop a national privacy policy for healthcare information technology (Conn 2007b). International standards and enforcement have been lacking as well (Kluge 2006).
- *Vendor contracts.* Vendor contracts for electronic health record systems and possibly other services must be reviewed carefully to ensure compliance with privacy rules (Conn 2007c).
- *Need-to-know access.* It has been suggested that third-party payers may have access to far more information than they actually need (Wilder 2007).
- *Implications for researchers.* Adherence to the Privacy Rule has increased the cost of performing research, primarily by changing the way that subjects are recruited (Erlen 2005; Wilson 2006). There are now added privacy protections for research subjects, which make it more difficult to recruit subjects and track populations such as cancer survivors. Researchers cannot approach potential subjects or ask providers to supply a list of names without authorization from the patient or family. Instead other recruitment means must be used such as brochures and

advertisements that enable possible participants to contact the researchers. Providers and organizations can only supply protected health information to researchers if the study has obtained consent from patients, HIPAA authorization, or waivers of authorization from institutional review boards. Study recruitment information must disclose how information will be used and who will have access.

- *Storage of patient information on medical devices.* Patient information is stored on an increasing number of devices that include infusion pumps, glucometers, and various monitoring devices (Klein & Keller 2006). Some of these devices transmit data across hospital networks. Plans to protect patient information must include these devices. These plans must address responsibility for purchasing and implementing security upgrades, physical security of the equipment, encryption of data transmissions from devices to the information system, and measures to prevent inappropriate access to patient data by vendors or service personnel.

Other Privacy Legislation

There have been many efforts in recent years to draft legislation to protect privacy and strengthen patient consent rules (Sloane 2007). Many of these bills have been sent back to committee, and some have elicited criticism that they would create too much regulation. The Veterans Benefits Health Care and Information Technology Act of 2006 took effect immediately. It was drafted in response to the theft of a computer from the home of a programmer that compromised personal data of more than 26 million veterans (Conn 2007d). The aim of this legislation was to prevent further data security breaches at the Department of Veterans Affairs. The VA is to follow with regulations that will govern medical record data-mining, notification of persons potentially affected by breach, fraud alerts, credit monitoring, identity theft insurance and credit-protection services, and data processing and maintenance contracts that require vendors to promptly report any data breaches and establish liability for damages.

Identity Theft Identity theft now represents a growing concern in the health-care arena (Foust 2007). Several variations exist. In the first type, persons impersonating the unsuspecting victim use his or her insurance information to receive costly healthcare. Providers are defrauded. The victim's credit history is tarnished, and there is a real danger that information from the imperson-ator will be mixed with that of the victim, endangering him or her with future treatment episodes. In another variation, established providers submit fraudulent claims. In a third approach, organized crime rings either offer free screenings as a means to obtain information or just steal it outright. Electronic records may actually worsen this type of fraud because information is so readily available. Consumers should protect themselves by reading the "explanation of benefits" letters sent to them by their payers to ascertain that no unauthorized treatments were performed and that frequent checks are made to their credit reports.

Other Important Legislation for Health Information Technology Health information technology has been the focus of many bills introduced in recent years with dominant themes that center on improving healthcare quality, creating a national health information network, making healthcare more affordable, developing funding for technology, and establishing electronic records. The majority of these bills have been referred back to committee. The Department of Health and Human Services, the Centers for Medicare and Medicaid Services, and the Internal Revenue Service all published exceptions to anti-kickback statutes in an attempt to bolster the adoption of technology in physician offices (Conn 2007e). These rulings allow affiliated hospitals to provide information technology to nonemployed physicians without allegations of kickbacks for referrals.

ACCREDITATION AND REIMBURSEMENT

Several agencies have a major effect on healthcare providers. Accreditation determines whether providers receive funding. It also serves to enhance provider image, instills confidence in the quality of services rendered, and attracts qualified professionals. This process has direct implications for how documentation and information systems are structured. These agencies may be subdivided into accrediting bodies and agencies that dictate reimbursement criteria. Several accrediting bodies exist. The Joint Commission and the Commission on Accreditation of Rehabilitation Facilities fall into the first group, with Medicare and Medicaid and other third-party payers in the second group, as well as ambulatory payment classifications (APCs).

The Joint Commission

The mission of the Joint Commission is "To continuously improve the safety and quality of care provided to the public through the provision of healthcare accreditation and related services that support performance improvement in healthcare organizations" (The Joint Commission 2007). The Joint Commission has focused on client safety and the safe administration of medications for several years. One example of this is the attempt to ensure consistent interpretation of medication dosages that fall within a range that is subject to nursing judgment (Manworren 2006). Once limited to acute care facilities, The Joint Commission standards now exist for ambulatory, long-term, home health, mental health, and hospice care, as well as managed care. The Joint Commission accreditation benefits providers by helping them to meet all, or portions of, state and/or federal licensure and certification requirements. Accreditation also expedites third-party payment and provides guidelines for the improvement of care, services, and programs. Other benefits include community confidence in the organization and improved staff recruitment and retention.

The Joint Commission standards and goals shape organization practice and documentation, thereby affecting information system documentation design (Ridge 2006). Each year specific target areas are selected, or refined, as safety goals. When accreditation standards change, documentation must reflect additional requirements. The Joint Commission introduced information management standards for healthcare organizations in 1994. Those standards addressed the following areas:

1. Measures to protect information confidentiality, security, and integrity, inclusive of:
   - Determination of user need for information and level of security
   - Retrieval of information with ease in a timely fashion without compromising security or confidentiality
   - Written and enforced policies restricting removal of client records for legal reasons
   - Protection of records and information against loss, destruction, tampering, and/or unauthorized use
2. Uniform definitions and methods for data capture as a means to facilitate data comparison within and among healthcare institutions
3. Education on the principles of information management and training for system use. This may include education about the transformation of data into information for subsequent use in decision support and statistical analysis
4. Accurate, timely transmission of information as evidenced by the following characteristics:
   - 24-hour availability in a form that meets user needs
   - Minimal delay of order implementation
   - Quick turnaround of test results
   - Pharmacy system designed to minimize errors
   - Efficient communication system
5. *Integration of clinical systems* (i.e., pharmacy, nursing, laboratory, and radiology systems) and nonclinical systems for ready availability of information
6. *Client-specific data/information.* The system collects, analyzes, transmits, and reports individual client-specific data and information related to client outcomes that can be used to facilitate care, provide a financial and legal record, aid research, and support decision making
7. *Aggregate data/information.* The system generates reports that support operations and research and improve performance and care. For example, information may be provided by practitioner, client outcomes, diagnosis, or drug effectiveness
8. *Knowledge-based information.* The system is capable of providing literature in print or electronic form
9. *Comparative data.* The system can extract information useful to compare the institution against other agencies. Deviations from expected patterns, trends, length of stay, or numbers of procedures performed may be noted

In 2006 the Joint Commission expanded information standards to include business continuity and disaster recovery planning, data and information retention, decision support, and specific documentation areas and formats.

Information standards may be demonstrated through the presence of the following: planning documents, institutional and departmental policy and procedures, data element definitions and abbreviations, observations, continuing education outlines and records, interviews with administrators and staff, and meeting minutes. A scoring system notes the degree to which each standard is met. Scoring criteria can be found in the Joint Commission's accreditation manual.

Commission on Accreditation of Rehabilitation Facilities

The Commission on Accreditation of Rehabilitation Facilities (CARF) is another healthcare accrediting body (CARF 2007). In addition to its focus on the improvement of rehabilitative services to people with disabilities, CARF provides accreditation in the following areas: aging services; behavioral health; child and youth services; durable medical equipment, prosthetics, orthotics, and supplies (DMEPOS); employment; and community services. CARF provides a template for operations as well as a tool for evaluation. CARF is a private, nonprofit organization that uses input from consumers, rehabilitation professionals, state and national organizations, and third-party payers to develop standards for accreditation. Although similar in purpose and structure to the Joint Commission, CARF places a greater emphasis on the following factors:

• Accessible services
• Comprehensiveness and continuity in individual treatment plan
• Input from consumers about CARF and its decision making
• Safety of persons with disabilities and their evacuation in the event of an emergency
• Post-discharge outcomes

CARF standards also shape institutional practices and documentation requirements. This may necessitate changes in automated documentation systems to comply with standards.

Reimbursement Issues

Medicare, Medicaid, and other third-party payers dictate reimbursement criteria to healthcare organizations. Health maintenance organizations (HMOs) also have numerous criteria that must be met for the reimbursement of services. Failure to demonstrate client need for a service may result in denial of that service or reimbursement for that service. For example, Medicare will pay for a client's care in a transitional or subacute care unit only if the client has a preceding hospital stay. Medicare also requires a demonstrated daily need for skilled services. Documentation plays an essential role in this process. Missing or insufficient documentation leads to denial of payment from insurance companies. Automated documentation systems should support entry of information about client need through initial screen design and the use of prompts to elicit needed information. Automated systems can also remind providers of remaining days of coverage for each client, as well as services not covered by Medicare, Medicaid, or their third-party payers. And last, information systems can be used to help track claims and report denials. These features can be incorporated into clinical information systems to encourage use and improve documentation and ultimately reimbursement.

Recent reimbursement rulings from the Centers for Medicare and Medicaid Services require more educational and preventive services as well as evidence-based treatment protocols. These requirements will likely be extended to other government-funded programs (Levine 2006). Additional rulings are expected that will stipulate remote security requirements to reduce the likelihood of unauthorized use and disclosure of sensitive health information and set standards for electronic prescribing under Medicare Part D (Security update 2007).

Standardized coding systems help to ensure consistent processing of claims. The Healthcare Common Procedure Coding System (HCPCS) is one of the standard code sets used for Medicare claims and by many other payers (Himiak 2006; Isenberg 2007). HCPCS consists of two levels. Level I is comprised of Current Procedural Terminology (CPT), a numeric coding system maintained by the American Medical Association (AMA) to identify medical services and procedures furnished by physicians and other healthcare professionals. The AMA determines when to add, delete, or revise CPT codes. Level II was developed in the 1980s to identify products, supplies, and services not included in the CPT codes, such as products, supplies, services and durable medical equipment, prosthetics, orthotics, and supplies (DMEPOS), used outside a physician's office and covered by Medicare and other insurers. The Centers for Medicare and Medicaid Services are responsible for the maintenance and distribution of HCPCS Level II Codes.

Ambulatory Payment Classification (APC) describes reimbursement criteria for ambulatory procedures for Medicare patients, criteria that became effective in August 2000 (CMS 2007). Similar to diagnosis-related groups (DRGs) used for inpatients, APCs were designed to promote efficiency in the delivery of services and to save money. There are specific coding guidelines for ambulatory reimbursement and guidelines for managing APC compliance. APC compliance requires verification of the integrity of the charge description master (CDM) to address issues of overlapping charges and duplication of charges for services and to develop appropriate management reports to facilitate reimbursement. The CDM is a master list of charges for all procedures, tests, and visits to the provider. Failure to code and bill properly can lead to lost revenue and noncompliance. Revenue may be lost with double coding, missed coding, charge-capture problems, missing modifiers, and denials. This is particularly problematic because APC coding is primarily done by clinicians rather than by coders who have had extensive training in the process. The information services staff must work closely with the clinicians and coders to maintain an updated CDM in the information system.

The Centers for Medicare and Medicaid Services (CMS) assumes responsibility for the review, revision, addition, and deletion of International Statistical Classification of Diseases and Related Health Problems codes (ICD-9-CM) (Bryant 2006; National Center for Health Statistics 2007). ICD-9-CM is based on the World Health Organization's International Classification of Diseases

Ninth Revision (ICD-9). ICD-9-CM is the official system of assigning codes to diagnoses and procedures associated with hospital utilization in the United States. The CM stands for Clinical Modification. Work is under way on ICD-10, which will replace ICD-9. Use of ICD-9 codes is an essential part of the coding and billing process. This has relevance for nurses in outpatient services because reimbursement is secured by services provided. For example when the flu vaccine is administered, there is a code attached to the vaccine and a second code attached to the actual injection. Both are reimbursable. Nurses need to be aware of this fact to secure payment for all services.

Electronic Data Interchange (EDI)

The CMS published regulations in August 2000 mandating all providers, insurers, and middlemen involved in healthcare claims submission, referrals, eligibility verification, and the transmission of other client-related information to use a common format to send and receive electronic information by October 2002. An act of Congress extended that deadline to October 2003. CMS extended that deadline again when it announced that it would continue to process nonstandard claims for an unspecified period of time, as many providers petitioned for an extension. Paper claims are exempt from this requirement. While many providers have submitted claims electronically for several years, others have delayed making changes in their computer systems. It may take several more years before this standard is fully met. Providers also have the option to buy and maintain a HIPAA-compliant practice management system (PMS) or use a claims clearinghouse to meet this standard. Either of these options may prove to be cost effective.

HIPAA Administrative Simplification provisions mandated the adoption of National Provider Identifier (NPI) guidelines by spring 2007. These guidelines require each covered provider to obtain a unique 10-digit identifier that allows the provider to use just one number when submitting claims, whether the claims are sent electronically or not. For the purposes of the NPI providers include individual physicians, dentists, chiropractors, podiatrists, psychologists, pharmacists, physician assistants, nurse practitioners, and other healthcare practitioners. Implementation of the NPI impacts billing, reporting, and **claim payment.** Software vendors, health plans, and clearinghouses are responsible for supporting the use of NPI within their respective systems.

QUALITY INITIATIVES

The federal government is moving forward in its efforts to link reimbursement to quality and performance (Cohen & Cooper 2007). The Deficit Reduction Act (DRA), enacted into law in 2006, requires all general acute care hospitals to report secondary diagnoses present on admission (POA) for Medicare beneficiaries effective October 2007, although reimbursement is not affected until October 2008. The Deficit Reduction Act also demands more accountability from providers for complications that occur during a patient stay. This is an important step in tracking and assessing a hospital's performance. These requirements come at a time when oversight organizations, such as the Leapfrog Group, are questioning reimbursement for treatment of certain hospital-acquired conditions identified by the National Quality Forum as serious, largely preventable events in the healthcare setting. The Leapfrog Group is a consortium of Fortune 500 companies and other large private and public healthcare purchasers that uses its purchasing leverage to reward entities that meet or demonstrate progress toward meeting standards that enhance safety practices and reduce preventable medical errors. Several states require collection of the POA indicator to all payers, not just Medicare, and to outpatient services as well as inpatient services. Consistent with the Government Performance and Results Act (GPRA), CMS is now focusing on identifying outcome-oriented performance goals (Zimmet & Rosenfield 2007).

The U.S. Agency for Healthcare Research and Quality (AHRQ) funds studies that identify preventable injuries and complications and demonstrate how technologies such as decision-support systems, electronic medical records and data warehouses, and computer models can improve care. Electronic data warehouses can be used to track quality indicators for best practices of care based on client outcomes. AHRQ maintains the National Quality Measures Clearinghouse (NQMC) (www.qualitymeasures.ahrq.gov). NQMC is a Web-based resource that allows users to search for measures that target a particular disease/condition, treatment/intervention, age range, gender, vulnerable population, setting of care, or contributing organization and to compare quality measures to determine which best suit their needs. The intent is to provide information on the most up-to-date, clinically proven measures (AHRQ 2007). For example, studies have shown that pneumonia patients who receive their first antibiotic within four hours after their arrival at the hospital demonstrate a significantly lower mortality rate. These findings led the Infectious Diseases Society of America/American Thoracic Society (IDSA/ATS) to make the recommendation that antibiotics be administered as soon as the diagnosis of pneumonia is suspected. NQMC is accessible to the public as well as healthcare professionals. It is clearly written and could be understood by lay individuals.

The National Committee for Quality Assurance (NCQA) is a private, non-profit organization dedicated to improving healthcare quality (NCQA 2007). NCQA accredits and certifies healthcare organizations and manages the evolution of the Health Plan Employer Data and Information Set (HEDIS), a set of standardized performance measures that health plans use to measure and report on their performance. NCQA introduced a Web-based Interactive Survey System (ISS) that is expected to change the way in which healthcare organizations are reviewed, making the process faster and more efficient while providing organizations with more immediate feedback.

The Institute of Medicine (IOM) is an advisory body to the national academies. The IOM launched a concerted, ongoing effort focused on assessing and improving the nation's quality of care in 1996. This effort remains part of the IOM's strategic purpose (IOM 2007).

SPECIAL FACILITY ISSUES

Specialized facilities have unique needs with implications for automated documentation systems. Not all of these needs are covered by the Joint Commission accreditation. State regulations, including mental health legislation, play an important role in dictating standards for information systems. No attempt is made here to address each type of facility, but pertinent considerations are noted.

Geriatric and Long-Term Facilities

Because of long stays and high client ratios for each nurse, documentation in nursing homes and long-term facilities must be concise, while addressing specific problems for this client population. Many institutions have developed their own forms to expedite this process and address required areas in accord with the mandated frequency of charting for reimbursement. For example, monthly comprehensive summaries on each resident are required. Box 14–3 identifies areas that a monthly summary might include. Figure 14–1 displays a sample documentation screen from an automated summary. When long-term or skilled beds (beds occupied by clients who require specialized nursing care) are located within an institution with automated documentation, additional screens are needed to meet the special needs of this population. Automation can speed updates, provide prompts to ensure appropriate response, decrease entry errors on ICD–9 reimbursement codes, and generate automated plans of care. Screen design of documentation

---

BOX 14–3 Minimum Data Set for Nursing Home Resident Assessment and Care

- Identification and background information
- Cognitive patterns
- Communication/hearing
- Vision patterns
- Physical functioning and structural problems
- Continence in last 14 days
- Psychosocial well-being
- Mood and behavior patterns
- Activity pursuit patterns
- Disease diagnoses
- Health conditions
- Oral/nutritional status
- Oral/dental status
- Skin condition
- Medication use
- Special treatment and procedures
- Identification information
- Resident information
- Discharge information

Section B. Cognitive Patterns

1 Comatose   ❑   Yes (skip to Section E)
                                  ❑   No

2 Memory   Short-term—recall after 5 minutes
                                  ❑   OK
                                  ❑   Problem
                                  Long-term
                                  ❑   OK
                                  ❑   Problem

3 Memory/recall ability   ❑   Current season
                                  ❑   Location of own room
                                  ❑   Staff names/faces
                                  ❑   That he/she is in a nursing home
                                  ❑   None of the above

4 Cognitive skills   ❑   Independent
    for daily decision   ❑   Modified independence—some difficulty with new situations
    making   ❑   Moderately impaired—poor decisions, requires supervision
                                  ❑   Severely impaired—never makes decisions

5 Indicators of delirium/   ❑   Less alert, easily distracted
    disordered thinking   ❑   Changing awareness of environment
                                  ❑   Episodes of incoherent speech
                                  ❑   Periods of motor restlessness or lethargy
                                  ❑   Cognitive ability varies over course of day
                                  ❑   None of the above

6 Change in cognitive status   ❑   None
                                  ❑   Improved
                                  ❑   Deteriorated

FIGURE 14–1 • Sample screen shot from an automated summary for a nursing home resident

requires an increased emphasis on psychosocial functioning and several other areas. The requirements of the Joint Commission, Medicare, and Medicaid are driving forces in documentation design. The Minimum Data Set (MDS) is the primary driver of Medicare Part A reimbursement for skilled nursing facilities (SNFs) via the Resource Utilization Group (RUG) system (Zimmet & Rosenfield 2007). Accurate completion of the MDS is necessary for compliance and reimbursement. The RUG and other assessment information transfers to another document known as the UB-92 for billing. Coding for too few services, also known as **downcoding,** results in lost reimbursement. Overbilling is referred to as **upcoding**.

Psychiatric Facilities

Each state has its own public health and mental health legislation and regulations that affect information system design. For example, regulations relative to the use of restraints vary from state to state. Documentation must comply with state law as well as the Joint Commission requirements. Essential information for charting on the application of restraints, for example, includes date and time applied, reason for use, type of restraint applied, length of time the client remains in restraints, neurovascular status distal to the restraint, and frequency of assessments done on the client in restraints. Policy must be established that includes these areas and identifies a maximum length of time that a client may remain in restraints without a renewal order from a physician. This policy should be reflected in time limits on documentation screens. Seclusion policies should be basically the same. Figure 14–2 shows a suggested documentation screen for restraint use and seclusion.

There also is a greater tendency for interdisciplinary documentation in psychiatric care, due to the need to provide adequate system and record access to many different personnel. Nursing staff, psychiatrists, psychologists, social workers, art therapists, music therapists, and play therapists require access to psychiatric client records regardless of the unit to which the client is admitted.

Documentation of Restraint Application/Assessment

Time applied: __:__ (Maximum time policy identifies for removal automatically shown)
Time scheduled for release: __:__
Reasons for use: (indicate all that apply)
❏ Behavior harmful to self/to others
❏ Necessary to prevent injury
❏ Assaultive behavior
❏ Increased agitation
❏ Impulsive behavior
❏ Other (Specify): _____

Type of restraint applied:
❏ Soft wrist
❏ Waist
❏ Jacket posey
❏ Geriatric chair
❏ Locked leather wrist
✓ One
✓ Two
❏ Locked leather ankle
✓ One
✓ Two
Time restraints removed: __:__
Neurovascular status distal to restraints:
-Pulses: may select from predetermined responses or indicate "other" and describe
-Color: may select from predetermined responses or indicate "other" and describe
-Sensation: may select from predetermined responses or indicate "other" and describe
Frequency of nursing assessments: __:__

FIGURE 14–2 • Suggested screen design for restraint use in an automated documentation system

Assisted Living Facilities (ALFs)

Assisted Living Facilities now come under various state regulations as the general population ages and there is a concerted effort to try to allow residents to age "in place" as they decline in health (Kissam, Gifford, Mor, & Patry 2003; Williams 2007). The scope of services provided has increased according to what is allowed by state laws and community philosophies, blurring the distinction between ALFs and skilled care. These additional services can result in additional reimbursement but at the cost of greater liability. As the number of persons residing in these facilities continues to increase, a commensurate number of new regulations are expected.

FUTURE DIRECTIONS

As the number of threats to PHI continues to grow, additional legislation and regulation is expected. This will require additional awareness and education for all healthcare professionals, coders and billers, and various business partners and vendors, as well as for informatics professionals who are responsible for its safekeeping. Consumers will also become more wary. Hopefully these actions will prove sufficient to prevent large-scale problems with identity theft and hardship.

Pay for performance initiatives will replace the existing claims reimbursement process through the healthcare industry. Proposed cuts to reimbursement will force providers to increase their efficiency at a time when additional legislation and regulation impose additional demands on an already scaled back workforce.

CASE STUDY EXERCISES

14.1 You are teaching an undergraduate course titled Nursing Informatics. One class session is scheduled for a discussion on the protection of client record information. How would you summarize the current status of legislative safeguards in the United States? What, if anything, would you suggest that students might personally consider to improve this situation?

14.2 You have been appointed to the Clinical Information Systems Committee, which is charged with looking at ways that automation can facilitate data collection for the next accreditation visit by the Joint Commission. List examples of how your community hospital demonstrates adherence to the Joint Commission information standards, and state your rationale for why you feel these examples display compliance.

14.3 You are the general nursing information systems liaison person at Wilson Rehabilitation Institute. CARF accreditation is coming up. What would you do to ensure that your automated documentation is in compliance with CARF standards? Explain your rationale.

14.4 You are instructing new healthcare employees during orientation regarding HIPAA. A question is asked regarding how family members receive information on a delusional client. Discuss how you would deal with the issue and how you would provide additional safeguards over the disclosure of healthcare information.

14.5 You are part of a research team studying CVA treatments. Discuss how you use patient data and how data is de-identified.

14.6 You serve on the Medication Administration Process Committee to improve safety and efficiency. Patient complaints have surfaced that identification bands reveal too much information. How would you proceed?

14.7 Your mother has proudly announced that she now has a PHR. When she proudly displays it to you online you note that it is available through the Web page of a large drugstore chain located in another state. What, if any, issues might this raise in terms of protection of PHI?

14.8 You are in the midst of a clinical rotation at the local community hospital as part of your baccalaureate nursing education. Please list examples of how your practice demonstrates compliance to the Joint Commission standards.

 MediaLink

Additional resources for this content can be found on the Companion Website at www.prenhall.com/hebda. Click on "Chapter 14" to select the activities for this chapter.

- Glossary
- Multiple Choice
- Discussion Points
- Case Studies
- MediaLink Application
- MediaLink

SUMMARY

- Legislative, regulatory, and accreditation issues and quality initiatives place increased demands on healthcare providers to safeguard, track, provide, and manage information. Information systems can and must facilitate this process.
- Several pieces of legislation address health record privacy and confidentiality. HIPAA represents one of the best known examples.
- HIPAA affects all aspects of information management, including reimbursement, coding, security, and client records.
- HIPAA compliance requires a broad approach that incorporates administrative and technical procedures on an ongoing basis. Education, the development and enforcement of policies, and process changes are key factors.
- Accrediting agencies such as the Joint Commission and CARF, Medicare and Medicaid regulations, third-party payer demands, state and federal laws, and ambulatory payment classifications dictate documentation requirements.

- Electronic claims submission must meet standards set forth by HIPAA. These standards were established to streamline the claims submission process and now require all providers to use a unique 10-digit identification number.
- Information systems and the design of automated documentation must incorporate safeguards for information privacy as well as standards for quality of care imposed by accrediting agencies.
- Automated documentation can facilitate the collection of data for accrediting bodies, third-party payers, and state and federal requirements.
- Special care facilities have documentation requirements that require additional automated screen design.
- There are several bodies that focus on quality and safety in the delivery of healthcare. These include, but are not limited to, AHRQ, NCQA, the Leapfrog Group, and the IOM. All recognize the potential of information technology to help ensure client safety.

REFERENCES

AHRQ. (2007). Mission & Budget. Retrieved September 17, 2007, from http://www.ahrq.gov/about/budgtix.htm#background.

Albright, B. (2007). Guarding the perimeter. *Healthcare Informatics, 24*(3), 42–44.

Amatayakul, M. & Cohen, M. R. (2007). Is HIPAA spelled apathy? *ADVANCE for Health Information Executives, 11*(5), 10.

American Civil Liberties Union. (1994). *Toward a new health care system: The civil liberties issues.* An ACLU Public Policy Report. New York: American Civil Liberties Union.

Anderson, F. (2007). Finding HIPAA in your soup: Decoding the privacy rule. *AJN, 107*(2), 66–72.

Annas, G. (2003, April 10). HIPAA regulations—A new era of medical-record privacy. *The New England Journal of Medicine, 348*(15), 1486–1490.

Barrows, R. C. & Clayton, P. D. (1996). Privacy, confidentiality, and electronic medical records. *Journal of the American Medical Informatics Association, 3*(2), 139–148.

Braithwaite, W. R. (1996). National health information privacy bill generates heat at SCAMC. *Journal of the American Medical Informatics Association, 3*(1), 95–96.

Broder, C. (2006, March 16). Congress tackles HIT, privacy issues. www.healthcareitNews.com/story.cms?id=4665.

Brous, E. A. (2007). HIPAA vs. Law Enforcement. *AJN, 107*(8), 60–63.

Bryant, G. (2006). ICD-9-CM changes make a big impact. *ADVANCE for Health Information Professionals, 16*(21), 28.

Buppert, C. (2002). Safeguarding patient privacy. *Nursing Management, 33*(12), 31–36.

Capizzi, M. D., Blenkinsop, P., & Glaser, R. E. (2006). The complexities of privacy law. *ADVANCE for Health Information Executives, 10*(5), 63–64, 66, 68, 70.

CARF. (2007). Who we are. Retrieved September 17, 2007, from http://www.carf.org/consumer.aspx?content=content/About/News/boilerplate.htm.

CMS. (June 21, 2007). OCE Background. Retrieved September 17, 2007, from http://www.cms.hhs.gov/OutpatientCodeEdit/30_Background.asp.

Cohen, C. & Cooper, L. (2007). Merging quality with reimbursement coding for present on admission. *ADVANCE for Health Information Professionals, 17*(1), 15.

Cohen, M. R. & Amatayakul, M. (2007). Who's using your data? *ADVANCE for Health Information Executives, 11*(8), 10.

Conn, J. (2007a). In the interest of privacy. *Modern Healthcare, 37*(20), 30–32.

Conn, J. (2007b). GAO rebukes HHS on milestones. *Modern Healthcare, 27*(26), 46.

Conn, J. (2007c). Invasion of privacy? *Modern Healthcare, 37*(29), 20.

Conn, J. (2007d). Giving vendors the bill. *Modern Healthcare, 37*(1), 12.

Conn, J. (2007e). IT might be, IT could be, IT isn't. *Modern Healthcare, 27*(18), 18–19.

Davis, C. (2007). Diagnosis: HIPAA apathy. *ADVANCE for Health Information Executives, 11*(6), 43–46.

Department of Health and Human Services. (May 2003). *OCR privacy brief: Summary of the HIPAA privacy rule.* Retrieved December 7, 2003, from http://www.hhs.gov/ocr/privacysummary.pdf.

Edlin, M. & Johns, S. (2006). High standards. A decade after the law went into effect there is still debate about the pros and cons of the HIPAA privacy and electronic transaction regulations. *AHIP Cover, 47*(6), 26–29.

Erlen, J. A. (2005). HIPAA—implications for research. *Orthopaedic Nursing, 24*(2), 139–142.

Feds clarify HIPAA compliance plans. (2003). *Health Data Management, 11*(10), 26.

Foust, D. (2007, January 8). Diagnosis: Identity theft. *BusinessWeek, 30, 32, 33.*

Frank-Stromborg, M. & Ganschow, J. R. (2002). How HIPAA will change your practice. *Nursing, 32*(9), 54–57.

Frawley, K. (1995). Achieving the CPR while keeping an ancient oath. *Healthcare Informatics, 12*(4), 28–30.

Gard, C. (2002). How private are your medical records? *Current Health 2, 29*(3), 30–31.

Government advisory group urges expansion of HIPAA rules. (2007, July 12). iHealthBeat. Retrieved July 16, 2007, from http://www.ihealthbeat.org/Articles/2007/7/12/Government-Advisory-Group-Urges-Expansion-of-HIPAA-Rules.aspx#.

Haramboure, D. (1999). An industry unready for HIPAA's proposed privacy legislation. *Health Management Technology, 20*(8), 16–17.

Hebda, T., Sakerka, L., & Czar, P. (1994). Educating nurses to maintain patient confidentiality on automated information systems. In S. J. Grobe & E. S. P. Pluyter-Wenting (Eds.). *Nursing informatics: An international overview for nursing in a technological era.* The Proceedings of the Fifth IMIA International Conference on Nursing Use of Computers and Information Science. New York: Elsevier Science.

Hellerstein, D. (2000). HIPAA and health information privacy rules: Almost there. *Health Management Technology, 21*(4), 26–31.

Himiak, L. (2006). AMA and CMS establish clearinghouse. *ADVANCE for Health Information Professionals, 16*(13), 17.

Horowitz, I. L. (2006). Privacy, publicity and security: The American context. *EMBO Reports, 7* (Special Issue), 540–544.

Information Policy Committee National Information Infrastructure Task Force (April 1997). Options for promoting privacy on the National Information Infrastructure. Retrieved January 20, 2008, from http://aspe.hhs.gov/datacncl/privacy/PromotingPrivacy.shtml.

Institute of Medicine (IOM). (2007). About. Retrieved September 17, 2007, http://www.iom.edu/CMS/AboutIOM.aspx.

Isenberg, S. F. (2007). HCPCS codes. *ENT: Ear, Nose & Throat Journal, 86*(6), 337.

Joint Commission on Accreditation of Healthcare Organizations (1996). *Medical records process.* Chicago: Accreditation Manual for Hospitals.

The Joint Commission. (2006). Critical Access Hospital 2006 Management of Information. Retrieved September 11, 2007, from http://www.jointcommission.org/NR/rdonlyres/DD06404B-66AE-4C7F-9D67-6419734651D7/0/06_cah_im.pdf.

The Joint Commission. (2007). About us. Retrieved September 11, 2007, from http://www.jointcommission.org/AboutUs/joint_commission_facts.htm.

Kissam, S., Gifford, D. R., Mor, V., & Patry, G. (2003). Admission and continued-stay criteria for assisted living facilities. *Journal of the American Geriatrics Society*, *51*(11), 1651–1654.

Klein, S. R. & Keller, J. P. (2006). A new paradign for medical technology procurement. *Journal of Healthcare Information Management, 20*(4), 14–16.

Kluge, E. W. (2006). E-health, the USA Patriot Act and other hurdles: The black lining on the silver cloud. *The British Journal of Healthcare Computing and Information Management 23*(9), 16–23.

Levine, C. (2006). HIPAA and talking with family caregivers: What does the law really say? *AJN, 106*(8), 51–53.

Manworren, R. (2006). A call to action to protect range orders. *AJN, 106*(7), 65–68.

National Center for Health Statistics. (Reviewed January 11, 2007). Classifications of Diseases and Functioning and Disability. Retrieved September 17, 2007, from http://www.cdc.gov/nchs/about/otheract/icd9/abticd9.htm.

National Committee for Quality Assurance (NCQA). (2007). About NCQA. Retrieved September 17, 2007, from http://web.ncqa.org/tabid/65/Default.aspx.

NCQA shifts to Web-based survey. (July 31, 2003). *US Newswire*, p1008212n4868.

Nowicki, M. & Summers, J. (2001). Managing impossible missions: Ethical quandaries and ethical solutions. *Healthcare Financial Management, 55*(6), 62.

Ridge, R. A. (2006). Focusing on JCAHO National Patient Safety Goals. *Nursing 2006, 36*(11), 14–15.

Robeznieks, A. (2005). Privacy fear factor arises. *Modern Healthcare, 35*(46), 6–16.

Robinson, E. N. (1994). The computerized patient record: Privacy and security. *M.D. Computing, 11*(2), 69–73.

Rothfeder, J. (1995). Invasion of privacy. *PC World, 13*(11), 52+.

Security update part of Fed agenda. (2007). *Health Data Management, 15*(6), 12.

Sloane, T. (2007). D.C. (not) confidential. *Modern Healthcare, 37*(10), 24.

Thomas, Legislative information on the Internet. (2003). Retrieved from http://thomas.loc.gov/home/thomas.html.

Welker, J. & Podleski, J. M. (2003). Preparing the front office staff to carry out HIPAA privacy procedures. *The Journal of Medical Practice Management, 19*(2), 67–70.

Wilder, B. L. (2007). Getting beyond economics. *ADVANCE for Health Information Executives, 11*(8), 49–50.

Williams, L. (2007). Be careful what your assisted living facility offers. *Nursing Homes: Long Term Care Management, 56*(8), 40–42.

Wilson, J. F. (2006). Health Insurance Portability and Accountability Act Privacy Rule causes ongoing concerns among clinicians and researchers. *Annals of Internal Medicine, 145*(4), 313–316.

Win, K. & Fulcher, J. (2007). Consent mechanisms for electronic health record systems: A simple yet unresolved issue. *Journal of Medical Systems, 31*(2), 91–96.

Wilson, M. (2003). Mobilizing the right resources to achieve HIPAA compliance. *Journal of Healthcare Information Management, 16*(2), 5–7.

Zimmet, M. N. & Rosenfield, S. B. (2007). Make the MDS Work for You. *ADVANCE for Health Information Professionals, 17*(9), 14.

CHAPTER 15

Continuity Planning and Disaster Recovery

After completing this chapter, you should be able to:

1 Discuss the relationship between continuity planning and disaster recovery.

2 Outline the steps of the continuity planning process.

3 Review the advantages associated with continuity planning.

4 Identify events that can threaten business operation and information systems (IS).

5 Discuss how information obtained from a mock or an actual disaster can be used to improve response and revise continuity plans.

6 Discuss legal and accreditation requirements for continuity plans.

Until recently, disaster planning focused primarily on the recovery and restoration of data. However, as reliance on timely access to data grows, so does the importance of continuity planning for all organizations that rely on timely access to and processing of information for continued operation. This is true for healthcare agency information systems, networks, and freestanding personal computers (PCs). Lost or damaged data have a negative impact on business processes, impede the delivery of safe care, reduce productivity, and undermine public confidence. Lost data are costly to re-create and threaten the survival of a business or healthcare delivery system in a highly competitive environment. It is estimated that somewhere between 40% to 90% of organizations that have incurred a significant downtime with data loss will go out of business within five years (Kirschenbaum 2006; Lawton 2007). Since it is obvious that the primary focus of healthcare delivery is the well-being of the clients, it is essential to protect the technology and data that support client care. At the same time information technology must be seen for what it is, a resource to support daily operations. Healthcare providers must determine how a disaster may affect the delivery of services, and identify strategies to ensure availability of information and continuity of care on a 24-hours-a-day, 7-days-a-week basis.

WHAT IS CONTINUITY PLANNING?

Continuity planning is the process of ensuring uninterrupted operation of critical services regardless of any event that may occur. This includes all critical applications, resident data, and Web, database, and file servers for the business. A continuity plan is a critical aspect of an organization's risk management strategy and is instrumental to its survival should a disaster occur (Wainwright 2007). Tolerance for information technology (IT) downtime is rapidly declining, with a recent survey setting the figure at five hours or less (Lindeman 2007; Witty 2006). Continuity planning historically began as disaster recovery, but increased dependence on automation for daily operations created a shift toward more detailed planning to maintain daily functions. Continuity planning is sometimes referred to as business continuity planning (BCP) or contingency planning. BCP now encompasses disaster recovery planning for information technology and data as a component (Glenn 2006; G'Sell 2007; Wainwright 2007). Disaster planning and recovery is focused primarily on risks to information systems and the data that they house. Information services staff are primarily responsible for this area. Data recovery and protection are required for healthcare providers but rapid access to usable data is essential. BCP has evolved into its own specialty, resulting in the formation of the Disaster Recovery Institute International and a certification process for its experts. The development of a continuity plan is the most difficult aspect of business continuity. The broader scope of continuity planning now requires the expertise of many different disciplines. Consultants may be brought in to help develop a plan, but its ultimate success requires consultation with persons across the organization who ultimately know it best (Glenn 2007). Building continuity into the design of the infrastructure helps to prevent local events from disrupting an entire organization.

A disaster is an occurrence that disrupts or disables necessary organizational functions and has the potential to destroy an organization by wiping out financial, administrative, and—in the case of healthcare institutions—clinical data needed for ongoing operations (Martin 2007). Disasters necessitate immediate action. Disasters strike without warning. For this reason, every institution needs to develop a plan that anticipates potential problems, implements measures to avoid problems whenever possible, and institutes measures to maintain the availability and security of client information under adverse or unexpected conditions. Continuity plans also address alternative means to support the retrieval and processing of information in the event that information systems fail. Disaster recovery plans enable the retrieval of critical business records from storage, restore lost data, and allow organizations to resume system operations, but this process may take 48 hours or longer to accomplish. This timeframe is unacceptable in today's information-driven society. There also is another difference between restoration and business continuity (McCormick 2003; Price 2003): restored data do not typically show the relationship between how information is created and used. One example may be seen in a physician's office when the daily backup does not occur, and the system loses pieces of information that are key to the patient's treatment.

Plans should ensure uninterrupted operation or expedite resumption of operation after a disaster while maintaining data access, integrity, and security. Plans must identify scope and objectives, including the multiple vendor platforms found in most organizations, and address the implications for other agencies of an inoperable system (Price 2007). For example, if a healthcare information system is down for a lengthy period of time, treatment may be slowed and information will not be available to third-party payers and suppliers. A comprehensive plan consists of separate plans for each of the following areas:

- *The emergency plan.* Provides direction during and immediately after an incident. This may include a provision to switch to duplicate hardware as a means to minimize disruption of services (Wainwright 2007).
- *The backup plan.* Outlines steps to ensure the availability of key employees, vital records, and alternative backup facilities for ongoing business and data processing operations.
- *The recovery plan.* Restores full operational capabilities.
- *The test plan.* Uncovers and corrects defects in the plan before a real disaster occurs.
- *The maintenance plan.* Provides guidelines ensuring that the entire plan is kept up to date.

Consideration of each of these areas as separate plans may provide for better division of responsibility and increased awareness of significance.

The security officer should have a key role in disaster planning, starting with a basic understanding of the plan development process to help direct the effort. Part of the security role is the protection of information. Data security is particularly important with federal mandates and accreditation requirements.

STEPS OF THE CONTINUITY PLANNING PROCESS

The **first step** in continuity planning is a **business impact assessment or analysis (BIA).** This is the process of determining the critical functions of the organization and the information vital to maintain these operations as well as the applications and databases, hardware, and communication facilities that use, house, or support this information (G'Sell 2007). This is critical in healthcare delivery because patient care requires timely access to accurate information. Interviews with employees in each area establish the following:

- Description, purpose, and origin of the information
- Information flows
- Recipients, or users, of the information
- Requirements for timeliness
- Implications of information unavailability

The importance of information dictates the priority given to maintaining its continuity. The BIA identifies threats and risks and includes a workflow analysis to determine interdependencies. General policy and procedures, hardware and software, troubleshooting, backup, training, testing, and overall costs must be weighed. Interviews with department heads help to identify the most appropriate strategies to be used to maintain or recover business functionality and sequencing for restoration. Data flowcharts help to ensure that all critical processes are documented. Each company must select its criteria for business recovery timeframes based on its own perspective (Croy 2007). Typically the faster that a business or department needs to recover, the more the recovery will cost (Lawrence 2007).

Even after information critical to system users has been identified, it is important to realize that critical information is more than the information required for direct client care. Individual areas within the institution have vendor contracts, personnel files, financial or claim documentation, important e-mails, permits, building blueprints, regulatory compliance documentation, equipment manuals, and reporting data in a variety of formats and places. Approximately 60% of an organization's valuable information is not protected because it resides on PCs, laptop computers, and personal digital assistants (PDAs); on remote sites that are not backed up regularly; or solely in paper format (Moore 2006). Much of this information would be difficult or time consuming to replace. For this reason, each area should develop a disaster plan and complete a physical vital records inventory, such as the one depicted in Figure 15–1. This inventory should specify:

- Volume and description of information
- Format; for example, whether information is maintained on paper, CDs, DVD's, tapes, or removable drives
- When the information was created, its use, and how it relates to other records
- When the information is transferred to storage or destroyed
- Equipment used to store critical information
- Consequences for the loss of this information

Make one copy of this page for each record listed. When parentheses appear, select one response from within them.

Record name:
Scheduled and Unscheduled Meds Due lists/Parenteral Therapy lists

Purpose of record:
Used to administer medications to patients

Who is responsible for this record:
HIS*-generated document based on MD orders

Media (paper, fiche, mainframe, etc.):
HIS paper document

Where is the record stored:
HIS system, on nursing units for 24 hours

Volume/frequency of change:
Many times/day

Retention requirement:
24 Hours

Originating office:
Nursing units

Location of any copies:
Nursing units/outdated copies

The record is: (irreplaceable, unique/difficult to replace/not hard to replace)

The record is: (essential for business/not essential but important/not important)

How would you obtain this record if your copy were destroyed?
If HIS system available, reprint; if not, go through each patient's chart

How would you re-create the information on this record?
Through patient's chart and current hard copy of Patient Care Plans

How long after a disaster could you work without this record?
Few hours—would use documents available

How is this record protected from destruction? (not protected, sprinklered office area, fireproof cabinet, duplicates kept in other locations, sprinklered warehouse, mainframe computer files, easily re-created, etc.)
HIS backups—paper documents not protected

Duplication and off-site storage is: (already being done/should be done/is not necessary)
Already being done—HIS

Are you prepared to supply input data, or work in progress, to allow the rerun of your critical applications from the last off-site backup?

Who is in charge of removing/restoring this record if it is damaged? What provisions have been made to restore/remove damaged records? What is the relocation destination? Who will transport damaged records and what is this person's 24-hour telephone number and security clearance?

* HIS, hospital or healthcare information service.

FIGURE 15–1 • Example of a physical vital records inventory sheet

The **second step** is the planning process. This is broken down into several phases:

1. *Secure top management support and commitment resources.* This is critical because administrative support is essential to the development of a viable plan, which in turn can make the difference between an organization's demise and survival and provides a competitive advantage. Placing continuity planning within the business context of information technology makes the investment appear more palatable (G'Sell 2007). Administrators need to weigh actual costs against the potential cost and damage to the institution for failure to sustain operations.

2. *Select the planning committee.* Agency staff may develop a continuity plan, but consultant expertise on the team can develop a plan more quickly, objectively, and knowledgeably because no one individual can know everything needed to implement an effective plan for a large, complex system. For this reason, each section of the plan should be authored by the parties with the greatest expertise in the area. The chief information officer should play a role on the committee and in the development of the plan (Spath 2002).

3. *Risk Assessment.* During this phase, the planning committee identifies the following information:

   a) Types and probabilities of various types of disasters; risks range from low to high (Croy 2007)
   b) Potential impact of a particular disaster scenario
   c) Estimated costs of lost/damaged information/records and lost time and customer goodwill
   d) Costs to replace and restore records, equipment, and facilities, as well as to hire or replace staff, versus the costs to develop and maintain the disaster plan
   e) Risk of the worst-case scenario striking the organization

4. *Set processing and operating priorities.* During this phase, the committee determines the equipment and telecommunication links and vital records needed to perform daily business functions and viable alternatives in the event that these are not available.

5. *Data Collection.* This phase entails a determination of available resources. This includes external resources such as backup and duplication systems, recovery services, and internal resources. Internal assets include staff information; inventories of vital records, equipment, supplies, or forms; policies and procedures; contact lists for staff, vendors, and other service providers; a review of security systems; and an evaluation of facilities for potential problems.

6. *Writing the plan.* A common mistake is to assign the responsibility for writing the plan to an individual who already has a full workload or who lacks authority to confront managers about the criticality of information in their areas. If the task is tackled internally, it needs to be divided among persons

with expertise in specific areas. A successful plan must be well organized, up to date, concise, and simple to follow. Software tools are available to aid the process; these include personal software or office productivity tools, enterprise software, and Web-based tools. Office productivity tools are readily available, but plans tend to get locked away on desktops with issues of version control and contact lists, and pager and telephone numbers that are not kept up to date. Enterprise software offers a proven track record but may be expensive, difficult to install and learn, and antiquated in design. Web-based software is easy to use and provides version control and free access to extensive information and instant, interactive communication. It offers wide dissemination, the ability to incorporate questionnaires and surveys, automated contact management, and security. The plan must catalog all strategies needed to sustain delivery of services and to test the plan.

Well-documented systems and procedures are essential for the continuity of operations and disaster recovery. Although each institution and system are different, the plan should identify the following (Bermont 2007; Lindeman & Grogan 2007):

- Planning process description
- Purpose of the plan
- General system policies and procedures, including who can declare a disaster, the mechanism for calling a disaster, and the distribution and maintenance of the plan
- Persons for emergency notification (this may include a traditional calling tree/call schedule with telephone, cell phone, and pager numbers or utilize software specific for this purpose) and the length of time required for each identified person to arrive, whether the person is an employee, or any other individual key to the recovery process
- Responsibilities for each administrator and key employee
- Floor plans for water, gas, and oxygen lines and exits
- Cable, electrical, and telecommunication diagrams
- System configurations inclusive of server configurations and port connections
- Schematics for backup systems and schedules
- Outline of what users should do in the event of a disaster, including their responsibilities with manual systems and restoration efforts
- Projected timeline for system restoration
- Troubleshooting and problem resolution
- Data backup, security, and restoration procedures
- Insurance documents
- Repair procedures
- List of basic resources required to perform services, including equipment and software vendors, and restoration and storage services
- Vital record inventory that includes, but is not limited to, vendor/service provider and warranty information
- Provisions for nonclinical vital record access, backup, and, if needed, appropriate restoration techniques for each type of storage medium used

- Vendor service agreements along with identification numbers
- Mechanism to store and retrieve passwords and software from a protected site
- Locations of all operations
- Auditing procedures
- Evacuation plan

Documentation must be explicit because staff come and go. For example, instructions should provide details on responsibilities and where staff will report in an emergency (Lindeman & Grogan 2007). Key information, such as persons responsible for implementing the plan and their roles, must be kept up to date. Consideration must also be given to whether human resources are intact. Documentation should include goals for the implementation of suggested and/or required changes.

The **third step** of continuity planning is the implementation of the strategies identified to maintain business continuity, delivery of client services, and restoration of lost or damaged data. This includes the implementation of policies and procedures as well as contracts with vendors and various service providers necessary to ensure business continuity in the presence of a threat or disaster.

The **fourth step** in continuity planning is evaluation. Once developed, the plan should be carefully reviewed for weak spots. This includes consideration of the reliability, adequacy, compatibility, and appropriateness of backup systems, facilities, and procedures. The plan should be evaluated periodically and when major changes occur in system processes. Training for team members should occur at this time. An actual test of the plan should be done in sections after peak business hours and evaluated for effectiveness. Strategies and methods must then be determined to test and evaluate the plan periodically to determine if it is workable, documentation is appropriate, and staff is trained. Testing twice a year, with a 6-month period in between, is recommended (Sheth & McHugh 2007). Offsite service providers and vendors should be included in tests. Actual disaster or outage situations provide an excellent test opportunity (Kirchner & Ziegenfuss 2003). Much has been written, and many lessons learned, since Hurricane Katrina struck in 2005 and after the terrorist attacks on September 11, 2001.

ADVANTAGES OF CONTINUITY PLANNING

It is not always possible to avoid a disaster or to provide 100% protection against every threat, but a good plan can anticipate problems and minimize losses incurred by damage (Pelant 2003). A good plan is clear and concise and does the following (Miano 2003; Midgley 2002):

- Identifies strategies for correction of vulnerabilities within the organization
- Provides a reasonable amount of protection against interruption in services, downtime, and data loss
- Ensures continuity of the client record and delivery of care
- Expedites reporting of diagnostic tests

- Captures charges and supports billing and processing of reimbursement claims in a timely fashion
- Ensures open communication with employees and ensures customers of availability of services or interim arrangements
- Provides a mechanism to capture information needed for regulatory and accrediting bodies
- Helps to ensure compliance with HIPAA legislation and requirements of the Joint Commission
- Establishes backup and restoration procedures for systems, databases, and important files
- Allows time for restoration of equipment, the facility, and services

In short, an effective disaster plan saves patients from unnecessary delays in treatment and redundant procedures. It also saves money up front and over time through limiting loss of data, equipment, and services. Any agency that requires information integrity and availability cannot afford to be without a disaster plan. A good plan can make the difference between institutional survival and demise, as the likelihood of bankruptcy increases with each moment those data are unavailable.

DISASTERS VERSUS SYSTEM FAILURE

Hazards come from a variety of sources, including environmental disasters, human error, sabotage and acts of terrorism and bioterrorism, high-tech crime, operating system or application software bugs, viruses, overtaxed infrastructure, power fluctuations and outages, and equipment failure (Midgley 2002; Wiles 2004). Table 15–1 lists some information system threats. A thorough appraisal by information services personnel can minimize the risk of damage from various situations.

Environmental Disasters

Environmental disasters may be natural or man-made. Plans must anticipate the predictable and the unpredictable, inclusive of climate, location, building features, internal hazards such as fire or smoke damage, and utility service. Many hospitals and providers lack the infrastructure to accommodate and support information systems. Often key clinical services, computers, and data are housed in areas threatened by floods, potential plumbing leaks, or exposure to dangerous materials, such as oxygen, anesthetic agents, or other hazardous chemicals. Both the security of the IS power supply and the availability of backup power to sustain uninterrupted computer operation, ventilation, and cooling of the data center must be considered. Excessive heat can shut computers down and cause processing errors (Barry 2007). Power capabilities must be kept up to date as data center consumption has increased (Johnston 2007; Komoski 2007; Rizzo 2006). Enough fuel should be on hand to power generators for at least one week. Hospital utility lines may be at risk because of their location, particularly if construction is under way and if power or telephone lines have not been marked and protected from inadvertent damage.

TABLE 15–1 Threats to Normal System Operation	
Threat	**Examples**
Accidents	Brown-outs and power outages/grid failures
	File corruption
	Transportation accidents
	Chemical contamination
	Toxic fumes
Natural disasters	Avalanche
	Floods
	Earthquakes
	Tsunamis
	Hurricanes
	Tornadoes
	Blizzards
	Pandemics
Internal disasters	Hardware or software errors
	Water line breaks
	Construction accidents
	Fire
	Sabotage
	Theft
	Ex-employee violence
Malicious or violent acts	Hackers
	Bombs
	Terrorism and bioterrorism
	Electromagnetic pulse
	Civil unrest
	Armed conflict

Workforce Disruption and Bioterrorism

In the event of a major disaster—such as the terrorist attacks of September 11, Hurricane Katrina, a pandemic, or bioterrorism—there will be problems securing and maintaining sufficient resources to carry out critical operations. An unanticipated problem after Katrina was the loss of qualified healthcare professionals and knowledgeable IT staff, who chose not to return or were unable to return post-disaster (Martin 2007; Picking up 2006). A shortage of workers can also result from direct casualties, morbidity, problems getting to work sites, travel restrictions, fear, and family obligations (Epstein & Nilakantan 2007; Zirkel 2007).

A pandemic is the emergence of a new communicable disease, such as bird flu, that infects humans, creates serious illness and death, and spreads into a global outbreak (Chandler, Wallace, & Coombs 2006). In the event of a pandemic, managers must assume that at least 40% of their workers will be unavailable for a period of six to eight weeks (Myers 2006). Good planning and frequent communication take on even more importance under these circumstances to safeguard the safety of human resources and retain a sense of community. Consideration must also be given to the family and loved ones of the workforce. The implications of this type of situation call for major changes in the way that key applications are supported and the ability to run services remotely (Glenn 2007). In planning for pandemics, strategies must address the need for providing employees with laptops with extra batteries, connectivity from home, and some form of wireless communication. Planning for pandemics is a relatively new event in continuity planning. On a related note, a recent Health Information Management Systems Society (HIMSS) (2007) poll of chief information officers rated external threats such as bioterrorism low (3.1%) on their list of IT priorities. The U.S. Centers for Disease Control and Prevention (CDC) has several emergency plans posted on its Web page for an array of disasters. The Agency for Healthcare Research and Quality of the Department of Health and Human Services posted a sample disaster recovery plan on its Web site to help organizations plan for pandemics and other health emergencies (www.ahrq.gov/research/health/happk.htm).

Human Error

Human error is the largest factor contributing to data loss, followed by mechanical failure. Both account for 75% of all data loss (Margeson 2003; Sussman 2002). Examples of human error include accidental file deletion, failure to follow proper backup procedures, unintended overwriting of files, the introduction of viruses or vandalism, theft, and loading flawed programs. Flawed programs are more commonly referred to as programs having "bugs." This comes from the programmer jargon of "debugging" a software application as it is written to ensure that it works as designed. Commercial software that is distributed without being tested adequately first may include "bugs." Bermont (2007) noted that several studies cite human error as the primary cause of problems in the data center, an area routinely responsible for the completion of file backups and for the support of hardware that runs major enterprise-wide applications. Training, fully tested documented procedures, and comprehensive maintenance records are suggested strategies to protect against human error in the data center. Nurses in the clinical area should be certain to save their documentation after entry because data may not be saved to the permanent record otherwise. Nurses and other healthcare professionals in clinical settings should also avoid downloading software from the Internet to hospital computers because this may have unintended consequences, such as poor computer performance and interference with institutional software.

Sabotage, Cybercrime, and Terrorism

Both current and former employees pose the greatest risk to IS in terms of their capabilities to change data and damage systems because of their special knowledge and access. For this reason, random, unannounced background investigations of employees with access to sensitive and critical IS organizational information should be considered as a means to avert sabotage, inadvertent disclosure of PHI, and wrongful system use, such as identity theft and credit card fraud (Marcella 2004). In the clinical area personnel who note suspicious behaviors, such as changes in computer performance, deviant co-worker online behavior, and increased spam or e-mail traffic, should alert the information service department.

On a national and international level, it is essential to consider the impact of terrorism and bioterrorism on the delivery of care and the potential effects on all services, not just information services. Threats that once seemed remote are now considered high risk. These include explosions, radiation, biological warfare, and electromagnetic pulses, which can kill and damage unshielded electronic devices (Maggio & Coleman 2007). Events associated with September 11 demonstrated what happens when infrastructure is destroyed, leaving parts of a major city without power, communication, and water, and leaving the workforce for entire companies devastated (Ballman 2006). Since the September 11 attacks, efforts to improve responses to emergencies include the adoption of the Incident Command System (ICS) by the Department of Homeland Security. The ICS provides a unified approach for multiple agencies to use when responding to a disaster with the goal of improving communication and coordination of people and other resources. It has since been adopted by the healthcare industry as well and is mandated by the Joint Commission (Koch & Marks 2006). Another outcome of September 11 is the emergence of building vulnerability criteria (Kemp 2007). These criteria include visibility, criticality, significance of the site outside of its immediate location, public accessibility, presence of possible hazards, height of the edifice, type of construction, total capacity, and potential for collateral casualties. While many of these areas have no obvious connection to health information technology, there are questions as to whether IS and support personnel could sustain operations in the face of an attack.

System or Equipment Failure

System or equipment failure may occur in the absence of any of the preceding environmental disasters. System failure may result from the failure of a component part or parts. Central processing unit (CPU) crashes, cabling and software problems, and even loose plugs may cause difficulties. When feasible, spare parts such as hubs, patch cables, extra printers, PCs, and servers as well as trained support staff should be available to troubleshoot system problems, avert downtime, and initiate recovery. Redundancy in system design raises the initial system cost but increases IS reliability. A well-executed physical system prevents many problems or makes them easier to discover. A review of the facility, system, policies and procedures, and disaster plan conducted quarterly can identify vulnerable

BOX 15–1	Suggested Areas for Review to Avert System Disasters

- Organizational continuity plan
- Documentation
- Vital records
- Vendor service and maintenance agreements
- Vendor continuity plans
- Backup procedures
- Recovery procedures
- Network access controls
- Physical security
- Archived data
- Backup equipment
- Backup facility
- Network diversity
- Communications links
- Spare parts inventory
- Backup services
- LAN configurations
- Off-site storage
- Personnel availability
- Operations personnel
- Technical personnel
- Antivirus updates

areas. A review should also be done whenever major changes are introduced. Box 15–1 lists areas for consideration.

CONTINUITY AND RECOVERY OPTIONS

The 24-hour-a-day operations of healthcare providers make continuity of services essential. Although continuity planning must encompass all aspects of daily operation, the information focus should guide the selection of computer services, hardware and software for day-to-day operations, backup, and recovery. Problems are exacerbated by the fact that an estimated 60% of critical business data resides in remote sites away from IT staff with backup hampered by limited and busy staff, slow WAN connections, and exploding data storage requirements (Moore 2006). Hardware redundancy is the first line of defense in providing continuous systems; hardware redundancy allows operations to continue even when individual components fail. This redundancy may be accomplished via redundant processors and disk arrays in one location or at two separate locations of the same agency or another facility. An increasing number of organizations now split their information technology between two locations for added protection. A second data processing site requires sufficient space for equipment and staff, especially if it may double as a backup data center. Functional requirements include mainframe and/or server capacity, printers, storage devices, sufficient cabling, power, an uninterrupted power source, air conditioning and space for a help desk, and an operations center and test room. Online replication of data is an integral part of business continuity, providing data availability, averting disaster, and reducing costs and recovery time. Redundant network storage provides multiple data paths, preventing damage and loss.

Advances in technology in recent years help organizations to be better prepared in the event of a major disaster. These include improvements in data replication hardware, servers, and other equipment that require less electricity and better battery backup systems for small businesses. Improved software and equipment options for emergency notification make it easier and quicker to contact key administrators, employees, vendors, and suppliers (Ballman 2006; Veldboom 2007). Automated emergency notification applications expedite the traditional calling tree to contact personnel within the span of minutes, using methods that range from interactive voice response phone calls to e-mail, freeing personnel for other tasks in the process.

Backup and Storage

Data availability, recovery time, disaster avoidance, retention requirements, and costs determine the best backup and storage options for a given organization (Lindeman 2007). Continuous delivery of services is the goal, but solutions to achieve zero downtime are expensive and not always possible. For these reasons, organizations must determine data storage requirements and acceptable recovery time on a system-by-system basis. These decisions help to determine media choices. Common antidisaster protection methods include the following: automated backups, off-site media storage, data mirroring, server replication, remote data replication, a virtual tape library that emulates multiple tape drives (by backing up data to disks with later conversion to physical tapes for off-site vaulting), and snapshots of data at prescribed intervals (Lindeman 2007). Virtual disaster recovery pools IT resources, masking boundaries between hardware to increase capacity. Data mirroring is the creation of a duplicate online copy. This technique eliminates wait time but may also replicate corrupt data. Best practices for long-data retention include the selection of standardized file formats, good management of metadata, the selection of media intended for long-term storage and proper housing, and regular inspection and maintenance of stored media. **Metadata** is a set of data that provides information about how, when, and by whom data are collected, formatted, and stored (Morgenthal & Walmsley 2000). It is essential to the creation and use of data repositories. Backup allows restoration of data if, or when, they are lost. Losses may occur with disk or CPU crashes, file deletion, file corruption secondary to power or application problems, or overwritten files.

Fast data recovery minimizes the worst consequences of downtime, including a tarnished image and financial losses. Networked storage area networks (SANs) and electronic vaulting provide the type of protection needed to ensure business continuity. Server replication is recommended for the most widely used applications because it ensures continuity by providing a reliable secondary infrastructure. Electronic vaulting sends backups over telecommunication links to secure storage facilities. This approach eliminates labor costs and the need to physically transport tapes. It also improves data integrity and shortens recovery efforts. Electronic vaulting may be provided by commercial enterprises that provide backup services for customers. Customers receive backup software at their site and at a central, remote file server. The customer dials to the remote server to back up data. Each customer has a separate account, and file access is limited to authorized persons. Remote backup service (RBS) staff protect both data and data integrity. Data retrieval, when needed, is limited only by the speed of the communication link. RBSs also provide reports to show which files have been backed up. Tape and other older media do not support fast data recovery efforts. Recovery may require 12 to 48 hours depending on recovery location and the number of critical systems that must be rebuilt before applications and data can be loaded (Lindeman 2007).

Backup may fail because of faulty software, bad network connections, worn tapes, or poor storage conditions. For this reason, backup should be verified and periodically tested. Advancements in technology and changes in the costs of backup options and storage media provide more options to maintain business continuity and backup and storage. Newer tape drives have well-developed error correction, eliminating the need to verify backup copies but not the need to test stored media. Storage conditions must be climate controlled and free from electromagnetic interference to avoid degradation of media. Agencies may opt to outsource storage to cold sites. A **cold site** is a commercial service that provides storage for backup materials or the capacity to handle the disaster-stricken facility's computer equipment (Wold & Vick 2003). Often backup materials are found on a combination of different media. Materials are shipped from the institution to the cold site, where backups from multiple organizations are kept in protected vaults under controlled conditions. Agency personnel are responsible for backup, dating, and labeling materials for storage. Cold sites should be located in areas free from floods and tornadoes and at least five miles away from the agency to avoid disaster conditions. Commercial cold sites provide environmental controls and possibly communication links and uninterrupted power sources. They are relatively inexpensive but cannot be tested as a backup facility unless equipment is shipped there and communication links are installed.

Traditional backup dumps data to a storage medium for transfer to another site for storage and, if needed, system restoration. While tape is still used, higher-capacity forms of media and faster processes are preferred, although tape may be used in combination with other media (Taylor 2007). Tape dumps for off-site storage start off with a gap between creation and pickup/delivery time. Data may be lost in this gap and recovery from tapes can be unreliable and time consuming. Increasingly critical data are stored on disk for quick restoration. For these reasons backup reporting and analysis software is an emerging field of data protection management (MacDonald 2007).

Storage media differ but should permit permanent or semi-permanent record keeping. Magnetic tape is still used as a relatively inexpensive, storage medium.

Optical disks are another storage option with a longer shelf-life but a higher cost. Electronic transfer over high-speed telephone lines to another site is a faster, more reliable means of backup that eliminates transportation concerns. When electronic transmission is not an option, a second set of backup media should be made and transported separately to ensure against accidental loss or destruction. Archived data must be inspected regularly to ensure that they can be processed and that the medium has not deteriorated or become outdated in light of current backup systems. Backup criterion include the following four points: (1) backups must contain the requested data; (2) backups must complete within the prescribed timeframe; (3) backups must occur as scheduled—full backup on some days and incremental on others; and (4) backups must be set to expire at the correct time.

Personal and Notebook Computers Although the primary focus for IS disaster plans is on the major systems, large amounts of information important for daily operations are also found on PCs, notebook computers and PDA's. This is particularly true as mobile workers and telecommuters comprise a greater percentage of the workforce (McKilroy 2003). Mobile workers spend at least 50% of their time at a location outside of the main institution, using notebooks or PDAs. Homecare staff exemplifies one such group of mobile workers. Another population of healthcare professionals telecommute using the Internet and remote connections to access and transmit information. Telecommuters face information system threats that do not affect internal employees, such as firewall maintenance and denial of service attacks, and lost productivity when network connections are not available. For these reasons, IS disaster plans need to include notebook computers, PDAs, mobile devices, and remote users. Routine maintenance prevents many problems. Box 15–2 lists

---

BOX 15–2 Recommended PC/Notebook Maintenance

- Keep original software handy in the event that it must be reinstalled.
- Establish a secure place for backup media away from the PC, preferably in a fire-proof safe or file cabinet. Backup media stored under poor conditions or kept in the same area as the PC are vulnerable to the same threats. Another backup option is online backup. This may be accomplished through the information services department or a vendor.
- Do an incremental backup daily, a full backup weekly, and a full system backup monthly and back up/store files on network drives whenever possible. This is particularly important for remote sites not covered by IS staff.
- Test backup media to ensure that they are good. Establish a policy for routine replacement of backup media.
- Periodically delete files from the hard drive that are no longer needed.
- Defragment all hard drives monthly.
- Maintain air flow around the PC/notebook to allow cooling.
- Keep storage media away from magnetic fields, including electronic devices.
- Periodically clean PCs/notebooks.
- Run virus protection software regularly and obtain updated versions as available.

tasks suggested for maintenance. Agencies cannot assume that users know how to perform these chores or perform them regularly. Instruction and assistance should be provided. For example, computer support personnel should perform periodic backups using standardized backup procedures and media.

MANUAL VERSUS AUTOMATED ALTERNATIVES

The decision to use manual alternatives when the system is down has implications for the delivery of care, the cost of care given, record management, and employee system training. A backup alternative is a different means to accomplish a common task than what is ordinarily used. An example of a manual backup alternative is the completion of paper requests for laboratory tests that are then delivered to the laboratory, instead of selecting ordered tests from menus on computer screens. Implementation of a backup alternative may delay delivery of services for several reasons. First, personnel are less familiar with the alternative procedure and will take longer to accomplish their work. Results reporting and processing requests for services will be delayed. Manual forms may no longer exist or may not be current in listing available tests or test names. Because automation eliminated personnel who supported the manual process, there may be few people available who know the manual alternative. Automated backup alternatives may also be available. For example, staff may be able to access information through a different screen than the one they generally use. Despite these problems, implementation of backup alternatives permits ongoing delivery of care, even if it is at a slower pace.

Calculation of backup costs goes beyond initial setup costs and ongoing expenditures. Recovery costs can be high because of several reasons: the personnel costs for hiring and training staff to use backup alternatives; additional costs for dual entry of data; costs for cleanup, repair, or replacement of computer equipment; and payment for backup computing or recovery services. Another cost is the impact on the quality of services rendered during the downtime.

The expense for manual versus automated alternatives varies according to the length of time that the system is down, backup alternatives employed, and the resources they require. Because implementing a backup alternative is costly, administrators must decide if the anticipated downtime merits initiating the alternative. Extremely short down periods are usually not worth the additional time and trouble. Costs include additional labor for IS and other personnel, increased potential for error, and space requirements. Data entry into the system following a manual backup requires additional personnel and a place for them to work. For example, laboratory tests that were requested but not completed before downtime must be requested by nursing again manually. During downtime, laboratory staff must try to match manual requisitions against those that were entered but not processed before downtime. When the system goes live, laboratory tests that were ordered and completed during downtime, along with results, must be entered so that the client record is not fragmented.

Staff Training The successful implementation of a manual alternative plan hinges on the cooperation and support of everyone in the institution. One way to ensure this success is through training. Detailed instruction on every aspect of the system, the plan, and implementation of manual alternatives may be incorporated into initial computer training. However, this approach requires a longer training period, and recall of manual procedures is often poor when long periods elapse between instruction and implementation. A more effective strategy entails posting plans in conspicuous places, yearly review of continuity plans, mock disasters, and the provision of step-by-step reference guides to help staff implement manual alternatives. Other measures to increase disaster awareness and ensure successful recovery efforts are listed in Box 15–3.

When it is not possible to maintain IS continuity, recovery is the next option. It sounds simple, but it is not. Few institutions have actually reconstructed Information Systems from backups, and few information technology staff are well equipped to deal with data recovery (Margeson 2003). Recovery also requires a safe place for employees to gather and a means for them to get there in times of travel restrictions (Lindeman 2007). Even when it would appear that equipment and storage media are damaged, no assumptions should be made that data are permanently lost, nor should persons unacquainted with salvage measures attempt to restore equipment or storage media (Olson 2002). For these reasons, it is best to call in recovery specialists when significant data loss has occurred. Successful recovery requires stabilization of the affected system and good problem-solving skills, staff preparedness, and good backups. Recovery is complicated when backups are not verified, delaying the detection of problems until restoration is attempted. Also,

---

BOX 15–3   Ways to Ensure Business Continuity and Successful Recovery

- Display continuity plans in conspicuous places, and post revised versions as soon as they are available.
- List key contact people responsible for implementing continuity and recovery plans.
- Review staff responsibilities periodically.
- Provide clear step-by-step reference aids for staff to guide them through continuity and recovery options including manual alternatives.
- Emphasize the importance of disaster preparedness by incorporating mock disaster situations into training.
- Review the continuity and recovery plans at least twice each year.
- Schedule at least two mock disasters per year—one of which is community wide.
- Test backups periodically.
- Label backup materials and include explicit directions with them.
- Provide up-to-date hot and cold site information to persons responsible for recovery.
- Test the emergency notification periodically. This may include a calling tree, but more likely it will rely upon special software that provides almost instant, simultaneous notification of all key persons.
- Emphasize the need for emergency care arrangements for dependents and pets to personnel involved in disaster and recovery plan implementation.

large institutions have information located in several areas: the mainframe, networks, PCs, laptops, PDAs, and paper documents. Last, most institutions use a combination of backup formats and programs.

Restoration of system operation may result from one of several techniques. First, materials stored at a cold site can be shipped back to the institution and reloaded onto the system. Second, information may be restored from RBSs or electronic vaulting. A third option is the use of **hot sites.** Commercial hot sites are fully equipped with uninterrupted power supplies, computers, telecommunication capabilities, security, and environmental equipment. Hot sites may accept transmission of backup copies of computer data, allowing restoration of operations using backup media. This is accomplished at another location served by a different power grid and central telephone office to avoid the effects of the disaster that affected the healthcare enterprise. The organization may develop its own hot site or outsource for services. When possible, hot sites should be close enough for practical employee travel, with sufficient space, power, cabling, parking, and satellite dish accommodations to support IS function. Hot sites are expensive and it may be difficult to get employees to the hot site location (Martin 2007).

A dedicated hot site usually sits idle when not needed but is available in the event of an emergency and is compatible with agency systems for ease of system restoration and updates. The creation of redundant computer capabilities and the acquisition of a dedicated hot site are costly. At one time, it was common to share the center with other healthcare alliance partners. A tenant would have to agree to relinquish the site in the event of a disaster. Sharing a site presumes that it is unlikely that two or more partners at separate locations would have a disaster at the same time. Shared arrangements are no longer practical because most systems now have extensive online processing. Hot sites may not be adequate to process critical applications or be able to provide for special equipment needs such as unique laser printers and forms handling equipment. Mobile hot sites are also available. Another option is the creation of a backup facility on-site in another building owned by the organization. This option reduces real estate costs but still requires system redundancy. Internal hot sites can continue to provide processing for critical business functions, although typically this occurs at a reduced level of service. When not in use as a hot site, it can be used for other processing, eliminating fees.

Commercial hot site services charge monthly reservation fees in addition to restoration charges but are less costly than establishing an independent site. There is a risk of being bumped by another client who requires services at the same time, particularly during a regional disaster when several organizations are affected by the same event (Martin 2007). Commercial vendors should be able to offer the assurance of a proven track record for mainframe recovery. Unfortunately, the uniqueness of most client–server environments made commercial recovery services unprofitable and unavailable until recently, forcing institutions to develop their own internal recovery options.

Although clinical staff have no involvement in the establishment of hot and cold sites it may have relevance for them in terms of possible delays in information access.

Vendor Equipment Vendors may offer processing capability through their equipment either at their location or at the location of the disaster. This solution may work for a select few applications but does not address the needs of an entire organization. There are also issues related to costs, software versions and customizations, availability, and testing. Sending equipment in from other locations can take days before the equipment arrives, the software is loaded, and the data are recovered from backup media. This option can be problematic in a regional disaster in which several organizations need the same type of services at the same time (Martin 2007).

An alternative to system restoration is distributed processing. Distributed processing uses a group of independent processors that contain the same information, but these may be at different sites. In the event that one processor is knocked out, information is not lost because remaining processors can continue IS operation with little or no interruption. Distributed processing is more expensive upfront but eliminates downtime. Rapid replacement of equipment is yet another recovery strategy, but it is not always feasible because it is costly to maintain extra hardware.

Salvaging Damaged Equipment and Records

Once alternative arrangements have been made to maintain business options, restoration of the equipment and records needed becomes a focus. Few IS staff possess the skills necessary to salvage damaged records and equipment, but internal staff should know how to act quickly and effectively to contain damage and to obtain outside help (Spetter 2007). Quick action and a basic knowledge of recovery techniques can expedite return to full operation and minimize loss of equipment, records, and costs. Whether the computing center was without climate control or was physically damaged by an event that exposed it to heat, humidity, and/or smoke damage, there are guidelines to follow to salvage materials; Box 15–4 lists some of these. The first rule is to stabilize the site. In most scenarios, internal staff

---

BOX 15–4   General Salvage Rules

- Stabilize the site.
- Pump any standing water out of the facility.
- Decrease the temperature to minimize mold and mildew growth and damage.
- Vent the area.
- Do not restore power to wet equipment.
- Open cabinet doors, remove side panels and covers, and pull out chassis to permit water to exit equipment.
- Absorb excess water in equipment with cotton, using care not to damage pins and cables.
- Call in professional decontamination specialists when hazardous chemicals or wastes are present.
- Initiate salvage options within 48 hours.

do not participate in the actual recovery process. Many processes require the use of hazardous and dangerous chemicals or knowledge of detailed salvage methods.

Disaster recovery experts can best ensure data recovery from damaged media, particularly from magnetic media. Fires, heat, and floods leave behind residues that damage electronic equipment and storage media. Additional damage may occur when media are improperly stored and handled after the disaster and with the passage of time. Degradation of media also impedes recovery efforts. Data integrity is compromised when storage media are damaged. Recovery specialists must verify data bit by bit and reconstruct files before data can be recorded onto new media. Having written agreements with restoration companies is particularly crucial in times of widespread disasters, such as earthquakes or floods, when many organizations will be seeking help at the same time. Box 15–5 lists some recovery measures.

Recovery Costs The cost for recovery is frequently overlooked (Spetter 2007). It should not be. It can be an extremely expensive process, involving the following factors:

- Lost consumer confidence
- Lost profits
- Temporary computer services, including space rental, equipment, furniture, extra telephone lines, and temporary personnel

---

BOX 15–5 Recommended Storage Media Recovery Techniques

General efforts recovery methods for paper-based materials:

- Have record salvage professionals on retainer. Initiate recovery within 48 hours of the disaster for best results.
- Consult recovery specialists before attempting any record salvage!
- Separate coated papers such as ECG tracing and ultrasound records to prevent them from permanently fusing together.
- Remove noncoated documents from file cabinets or shelves in blocks—do not pull each page apart, as this increases mold growth.
- Store paper documents in a diesel-powered freezer trailer until proper drying arrangements can be finalized.
- Remove excess mud and dirt before freezing documents.
- Pack wet files or books in a box with a plastic trash liner and allow room for circulation of air.
- Place files with open edges facing up and books with spines down.
- Label all boxes precisely and create a master inventory.
- Freeze-dry priority documents and sterilize and use fungicide as needed.

General magnetic media recovery techniques:

- Freeze-dry tape cartridges, then use recovery software to recover and copy information to new tape cartridges.
- Dry reel-to-reel tapes on a tape-cleaning machine, using warm air to evaporate moisture. Use recovery software to recover and copy information to new storage media.

- Shipping and installation costs
- Post-disaster replacement of equipment
- Post-disaster repairs and bringing the building up to new codes
- Recovery and possible decontamination
- Overtime hours for staff during the disaster for the implementation of manual alternatives, and after the disaster for entering data into the system that was generated during system downtime
- Reconstruction of lost data

Insurance coverage is recommended as a means to help pay for IS disasters. It is imperative that a complete inventory with photographs, replacement values for equipment, and all other documentation be finalized prior to submitting a claim (Baldwin 2007). Table 15–2 lists types of available coverage. One person should be designated to interact with the insurance company and a mechanism should be identified for how disaster-related costs will be documented.

Restarting Systems

System restarts after downtime must be planned carefully. All critical data for client management and agency administration should be targeted for

TABLE 15–2 Recommended Insurance Coverage

Coverage	Purpose
Business interruption	Provides replacement of lost profits as a result of a covered loss. Must be certain that insurance covers the same period as the event.
Extra expense	Provides financial recovery for out-of-the-ordinary expenses such as a temporary office or center of operations, and additional costs for rent, staff, and rental of equipment and furniture while regular facilities cannot be used.
Code compliance	Often overlooked. Insurance will normally reimburse only for expenses associated with repair or replacement of a damaged building, but not additional costs associated with building code changes implemented since the building was built. This coverage provides for those additional costs.
Electronic data processing	Replaces damaged or lost equipment and media from a covered incident such as storm damage not covered in normal property insurance. May also include coverage for business interruption and extra expenses.

Source: Adapted from Cox, L. P. (1996). Disaster recovery: How do you pay for it? *Disaster Recovery Journal, 9*(2), 19–20; Baldwin, W. (2007). After a disaster strikes. *Disaster Recovery Journal, 20*(1). Retrieved September 28, 2007 from http://www.drj.com/articlees/winter07/2001–10.pdf.

restoration first. For example, client admission systems are needed before client-related entries can be made. Therefore, it is logical to make the admissions and discharge functions one of the first areas restored. Users can help identify critical functions. Usage tends to be heavy once the system is live again as users try to catch up on their work. Communication is critical at this point. IS personnel must provide users with a sense of confidence, prevent system overload, and bring the system back online slowly to prevent further problems. Economic factors should also be considered. For instance, if charges are calculated with the documentation of a medication, or intravenous fluid, this process must be restored as soon as possible. Nonessential functions and reports should be deferred until the system is fully operational to prevent additional downtime.

Decisions Regarding the Extent of Data Reentry Healthcare administrators must determine how they will handle late entries and documentation that occurs during system downtimes. One factor that frequently goes unconsidered is the cost for entering information gathered manually into the system once normal operations have resumed. This is a labor-intensive process. The importance of data for inclusion in the automated record and the possible legal ramifications for data stored only on paper must be weighed. For example, is it necessary to include all vital signs and intake and output in the automated record, particularly if these have been within normal limits? A mechanism must be developed that indicates the availability of additional record information in paper form. Additional considerations include whether the entry of information collected manually and entered into the automated record later might be more prone to error and how the original paper record should be dealt with.

PLANNING PITFALLS

Continuity plans are subject to the following pitfalls:

- *Few information technology budgets have sufficient funding for business continuity efforts.* Continuity plan budgets need to be spread across the organization.
- *Lack of access to the plan.* If the plan is available online, measures must be taken to ensure that the computers that house the plan are accessible. All employees responsible for implementing any part of the plan should have a copy at home, at work, and in their briefcase. These copies may be on paper, PDAs, and/or notebooks. CD-ROM or DVD may also be an acceptable distribution method. Everyone should be aware of their roles and responsibilities (Stephens 2003).
- *Failure to include all information and devices in the plan.* Businesses evolve and institute new processes. Many plans lag behind the technology in use. An increasing amount of important information is found on laptops, desktop PCs, PDAs, and even paper format. Many plans fail to consider the

importance of e-mail, enterprise resource planning (ERP) systems, and Web-based transactions to daily operations. Many healthcare providers also have separate databases for various populations. Information services may not be aware of these separate databases until problems arise. There are also applications supported by application service providers (ASPs). One such example might include a renal database for dialysis patients. Continuity plans must consider how services will be provided in the event that the vendor's database is unavailable due to failure on the vendor's end or because of an inability to access the database due to downed Internet or telephone connections (Bannan 2002). Another example might include the failure to consider the multivendor environment seen in most healthcare systems today. Data are frequently housed on several computers.

- *Failure to plan for regional disasters.* The 2005 Gartner survey (Witty 2006) showed that the majority of organizations planned for a single facility outage rather than a regional disaster. Subsequent events surrounding September 11 and Hurricane Katrina demonstrate the inadequacy of plans that focus on just one facility (Ballman 2006).
- *Failure to incorporate data growth into the plan.* Unprecedented data growth threatens recovery plans. Organizations need to focus on critical data to ensure business continuity and reduce recovery time. This can be done by separating inactive from active data as a means to keep operating databases at a manageable size and improve application availability (Lee 2003).
- *Failure to update the plan.* The continuity plan is a fluid document that is subject to change as operations and personnel change and determinations are made that some portions of the plan do not work well. The planning committee should control the change process and should print review and revision dates on each page. A change manual can be used to note changes, including the date and reason for each change. While not specific to the healthcare industry, a 2005 survey by AT&T found that one in four companies that had a continuity plan had not updated it in the past 12 months (Ballman 2006).
- *Failure to test the plan.* A significant percentage of organizations that have continuity and disaster recovery plans have either never tested them, do not know if they have been tested, or have not tested them within the past year (Ballman 2006).
- *Failure to consider the human component* (Kirschenbaum 2006; Mitchell 2007; Zirkel 2007). Preservation of human life is the top priority in any disaster, followed by preservation of critical functions. Even so, in any disaster, the loss of personnel is a distinct possibility. In times of disaster, the institution should be prepared to assist employees and their families, including communication links to check on employees and providing such amenities as transportation to work and possibly temporary housing. Restoration of peace of mind for employees and families is just as important as recovering data from a computer and maintaining business continuity. This includes reestablishing user confidence once normal operations are restored and addressing the emotional impact that the disaster had on employees.

USING POST-DISASTER FEEDBACK TO IMPROVE PLANNING

Post-disaster feedback is invaluable in revising disaster plans for future use and should be an integral part of continuity planning (Price 2007). Personnel input after mock disasters or prolonged downtime should be used to identify what worked and what did not. Systems and organizations change. Plans that looked good before a disaster may not look good after one. Recovery expenses usually exceed anticipated costs, leading to a change in recovery strategies for future use. Figure 15–2 depicts a checklist to evaluate the success of a disaster and recovery plan.

Checklist Item	Yes	No
Are backup(s) available? tested?	☐	☐
Are disaster/recovery plan copies available/accessible?	☐	☐
Are duplicate processors or storage options in place?	☐	☐
Are hot-site contract copies available/accessible?	☐	☐
Do key personnel have emergency care arrangements for dependents? pets?	☐	☐
Is home-site staffing coverage adequate?	☐	☐
Are the hot-site locations and access procedures known?	☐	☐
Are the cold-site storage sites and procedures for retrieval of backups known/arranged?	☐	☐
Is travel to the cold and hot sites feasible?	☐	☐
Has authorization for recovery-related expenses been confirmed?	☐	☐
Are contracts with record salvage services in place?	☐	☐
Is shipping information accurate for backup tapes from cold to hot sites and back again?	☐	☐
Is documentation accurate for tape restoration available with starting and ending tape numbers?	☐	☐
Are backup media labeled accurately?	☐	☐
Have network/communications persons been sent to the hot site?	☐	☐
Do restoration procedures agree with current software?	☐	☐
Have previous arrangements been made to have persons stay after hours at the remote site?	☐	☐
Are communications links for backup confirmed, appropriate, and available?	☐	☐
Are phone numbers available for all vendors and services?	☐	☐
Are stored supplies intact/usable?	☐	☐
Is a timeline for anticipated restoration of operations identified and appropriate?	☐	☐
Are packing materials and labels available to ship media from cold to hot sites and back again?	☐	☐
Is an extra container for reports among supplies?	☐	☐
Are human needs for food and rest adequately included in the plan?	☐	☐

FIGURE 15–2 • Checklist for successful implementation of an IS disaster and recovery plan

Another option for the development, revision, and management of continuity plans for resource-strapped organizations is the use of a managed service provider (Midgley 2002). Managed service providers offer continuous data backup, safeguarding against data loss while allowing for immediate recovery and restoration of services in the event of a disaster. Organizations using managed service providers retain control of data processing operations while the managed care provider provides the resources. Customers can manage their data processing through a personalized Web management interface that allows them to initiate recovery from any location.

Challenges for the future include (1) finding ways to protect the growing amount of information, no matter where it is stored or used; and (2) finding ways to make sure people can stay connected to their data, no matter what the disruption. Without addressing and linking these two elements, a plan may fall far short of its goals.

LEGAL AND ACCREDITATION REQUIREMENTS

A 2005 Gartner survey on business continuity and disaster recovery that spanned various types of industries including healthcare found that an increasing number of regulatory bodies require a documented methodology for conducting business continuity and disaster recovery activities (Witty 2007). The HIPAA security rule requires continuity planning and disaster recovery processes (Averell 2003; Bogen 2002; Miller & Lehman 2002; Zawada 2003). All healthcare organizations must have a data backup plan, a recovery plan, an emergency mode of operation plan, and testing and evaluation procedures. Although HIPAA does not specify the exact processes or procedures for compliance, it does demand safeguards for the security of protected health information while operating in both normal and emergency modes. These safeguards encompass the creation, access, storage, and destruction of manual records. The final continuity planning component of the HIPAA regulations required compliance by April 2006. The Federal Information Privacy and Security Act of 2002 established a minimum standard of performance for the protection of information and information systems managed by federal agencies, their contractors, and other agencies acting on their behalf, and required the institution of continuity plans for information systems supporting the operations of the agency (Collmann 2007). Other federal legislation also exists that requires current access to information for organizations (Lindeman 2007).

The Pandemic and All-Hazards Preparedness Act was enacted at the end of the 109th Congressional session (Goedert 2007). This law authorized development of a national, near-real-time information network to coordinate federal and state response to public health emergencies within two years of enactment. The Secretary of Health and Human Services was charged with leading the federal response to these types of emergencies, usurping the role previously accorded to the Department of Homeland Security. Similar legislation focused upon hospital readiness to deal with disasters.

The Joint Commission set disaster preparedness standards as a requirement for hospital accreditation more than 30 years ago (Cutlip 2002). Until 2000, standards focused on disasters and accidents such as power plant failures and chemical spills. In 2001, the Joint Commission introduced new emergency management standards for hospitals, long-term care facilities, and behavioral health and ambulatory care that focus on the concept of community involvement in the management process. These guidelines address information security, disaster preparedness, and recovery planning. The Joint Commission has since added bioterrorism to the list of events that organizations must consider in their plans (McGowan 2002).

The Joint Commission suggests that organizations conduct at least two emergency drills per year with one community-wide drill. Accreditation standards mandate that healthcare organizations have an emergency plan that identifies potential hazards, their impact on services, and measures to handle and recover from emergencies. Accredited organizations must demonstrate a command structure, emergency preparedness training for staff, and a mechanism to enact an emergency plan, and they must identify their role in community-wide emergencies. The 2008 emergency management standards for hospitals, critical access hospitals, and long-term care facilities call for planning and testing plans during conditions when the local community cannot support the healthcare organization. It is no longer sufficient to plan for a single, simple event (The Joint Commission 2007).

Together the Joint Commission and HIPAA require that healthcare providers perform a business impact analysis and crisis management analysis; conduct employee training; implement ongoing continuity plan reviews; plan for information technology disasters and recovery; and audit their continuity plan processes (Zawada 2003). Several other accrediting bodies require disaster plans, though their focus is personal safety rather than information safety. There are other groups that demonstrate varying levels of interest in business continuity management; these include the Food and Drug Administration (FDA), the Federal Emergency Management Agency (FEMA), the National Institute of Standards and Technology (NIST), the Disaster Recovery Institute International, the Bioterrorism Task Force of the Association for Professionals in Infection Control and Epidemiology, and the Bioterrorism Working Group of the Centers for Disease Control and Prevention. Recommendations from these other groups provide voluntary guidelines for better business continuity management that help continuity planners to achieve HIPAA and compliance with the Joint Commission.

There has been a move toward voluntary compliance with the Sarbanes-Oxley Act by not-for-profit healthcare oganizations in recent years (Giniat & Saporito 2007; Greene 2005; Peregrine & Schwartz 2002). The Sarbanes-Oxley Act of 2002 was enacted by the federal government as a means to legislate corporate responsibility. While it only applied to publicly traded corporations, Sarbanes-Oxley impacts the healthcare industry by increasing demands for fiscal responsibility and accurate financial reports and disclosure. Voluntary compliance with Sarbanes-Oxley is widely seen as a part of enterprise risk management and an opportunity to demonstrate good governance to the community. It requires the creation of audit functions and the presence of an expert in accounting on a corporate audit committee. Auditors must clearly see that a plan exists to protect and recover financial data. Voluntary compliance with Sarbanes-Oxley helps not-for-profit entities justify their not-for-profit status and maintain their reputation in the community. Compliance with Sarbanes-Oxley requires continuity of records.

FUTURE DIRECTIONS

Continuity planning will receive greater attention for a variety of reasons. Consumers have come to expect a level of service that requires immediate access to data. Wait time decreases satisfaction and can diminish quality of care. Healthcare organizations are catching up with other industries in understanding the business case for continuity of operations. Compliance will become a larger issue, particularly as more legislation and regulatory bodies require the presence of a workable continuity plan. More professional organizations are now focused upon various aspects of continuity planning and response to disasters. The creation of a national network that will allow improved monitoring of the population's health for suspicious symptoms or early onset of epidemics will make it more imperative to maintain all links in the process.

As the national monitoring of disease outbreak and bioterrorism activities improves, healthcare organizations can stockpile supplies, bring in additional staff, delay vacations, make bed space available, and put into place plans for remote and backup options to ensure continuity of overall operations (Goedert 2007). It is only a matter of time before another disaster occurs. The preparation provided by an effective business and continuity plan can minimize loss of life and data and can support ongoing operations. Healthcare organizations must be able to effectively deal with crises.

CASE STUDY EXERCISES

15.1   As the clinical representative for your unit on the Disaster Planning Committee, you are charged with identifying all forms in your area that require completion of a physical vital records inventory sheet. What forms would you list and why?

15.2   Work crews at Wilmington Hospital inadvertently cut the cable connecting all terminals at the hospital with the computer center. As the on-duty nursing supervisor, what should you tell your employees and why? Who would you contact for further information? How do you determine whether to initiate manual alternatives?

15.3   An early morning train wreck near St. Luke's Hospital derailed seven freight cars carrying chemicals that can emit toxic fumes. The accident took out power lines for the neighborhood and for St. Luke's. Emergency crews evacuated a 7-block area, stopping just outside of the hospital's main entrance. Power has already been out for 12 hours, and restoration is not expected for at least another 12 to 24 hours. You are on an executive administrative committee charged with determining what information will be brought online first and what will remain in paper form. What would you restore first? What records, if any, would you not restore? Explain your rationale. How would you document, for record management purposes, that part of the record is automated and part is manual?

15.4   As the informatics nurse, you are responsible for helping the Renal Department select a new database. One of the top vendors must cancel its Web-based demonstration because its server was stolen. This particular application is designed to run over the Internet with data housed at the vendor site. What types of questions should this situation raise for disaster planning with the use of vendor-supported applications?

15.5   You recently learned that the information services network engineer responsible for conducting backups on the server for the tumor registry database failed to ensure that regular backups occurred properly. This was discovered when the database was found to be corrupt. Approximately 20,000 entries were lost as a result. As the liaison between the tumor registry and the IS department, how would you ensure that this would not happen again?

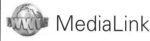 MediaLink

Additional resources for this content can be found on the Companion Website at www.prenhall.com/hebda. Click on "Chapter 15" to select the activities for this chapter.

- Glossary
- Multiple Choice
- Discussion Points
- Case Studies
- MediaLink Application
- MediaLink

SUMMARY

- Continuity planning is the process of ensuring the continuation of critical business services regardless of any event that may occur. It includes information technology disaster planning.
- Continuity planning consists of several steps. The first step requires business impact analysis and a determination of vital organization functions and information. The business impact analysis should be done as soon as possible.
- The second step in continuity planning is the development of the plan itself. This step determines the probabilities of all types of disasters, their impact on critical functions, and factors necessary for restoration of services.

- The third step in continuity planning is the implementation of the strategies identified to maintain business continuity, delivery of patient services, and restoration of lost or damaged data. This includes policies and procedures and contracts with vendors and various service providers.
- The fourth step in continuity planning is evaluation.
- Disasters that threaten information systems operation may be natural or man-made. Continuity plans help to ensure uninterrupted operation or speedy resumption of services when a catastrophic event occurs.
- The identification of information vital to daily operation is best determined through interviewing system users. The purpose, flow, recipients, need for timeliness, and implications of information unavailability must be considered in this process.
- Not all information used in daily operations is automated. A vital records inventory should be conducted to identify additional information that requires protection.
- Documentation is essential to the development and successful implementation of a disaster plan. Plans must be detailed, current, and readily available to be useful.
- Careful attention to backup and storage helps ensure that information may be retrieved, or restored, later. Backup may be handled internally or outsourced. Commercial backup services provide transport or electronic transmission of backup media and special storage conditions until materials are needed.
- Manual alternatives to information systems ensure ongoing delivery of services, although it is at a slower rate. Staff must receive instruction and support as they resort to manual methods.
- Restoration of information services post-disaster is not simple because backup media may be faulty and some information kept on other media is lost forever.
- System restoration may reload backup media stored at cold sites or resort to remote backup service or hot sites. Distributed processing and rapid replacement of equipment are other alternatives.
- Restoration is costly because it generally requires outside professional services, additional equipment, and extra hours from support staff. Expenses may be partially recouped through insurance coverage.
- Salvage of damaged records is an important aspect of recovery that is best handled by experts.
- System restarts require planning to avoid system overload as users try to catch up on work. Administrators must consider what functions should be restored first and how to integrate backup paper records with automated records.
- Post-disaster feedback is key to the design and implementation of a better plan for future use.
- Continuity planning needs to consider legal and regulatory requirements.

REFERENCES

Averell, H. (2003, June 1). Disaster recovery, HIPAA style. *ADVANCE for Health Information Executives*. Retrieved January 27, 2004, from http://www. advanceforhie.com/.

Baldwin, W. (2007). After a disaster strikes. *Disaster Recovery Journal, 20*(1). Retrieved September 28, 2007, from http://www.drj.com/articlees/winter07/2001-10.pdf.

Ballman, J. (2006). September 11—5 years later. *Disaster Recovery Journal, 19*(4). Retrieved September 17, 2007, from http://www.drj.com/articles/fall06/1904-01p.html.

Bannan, K. J. (2002, January 29). Building your safety net—Every company needs a disaster recovery plan, but e-businesses have some special needs to guarantee they're running around-the-clock. *PC Magazine, 21*(1), 2.

Barry, S. (2007). Heat—the death knell for hard drives. *Disaster Recovery Journal, 20*(2). Retrieved September 17, 2007, from http://www.drj.com/articles/spr07/2002-11.pdf.

Bermont, T. (2007). Ensuring your data center is in compliance. *Disaster Recovery Journal, 20*(2). Retrieved September 17, 2007, from http://www.drj.com/articles/spr07/2002-05.pdf.

Bogen, J. (2002). Implications of HIPAA on business continuity and disaster recovery practices in healthcare organizations. *Healthcare Review, 15*(5), 14.

Chandler, R. C., Wallace, J. D., & Coombs, W. T. (2006). Current state of pandemic disaster preparedness. *Disaster Recovery Journal, 19*(4). Retrieved September 17, 2007, from http://www.drj.com/articles/fall06-1904-10.html.

Collmann, J. (January 2007). The Federal Information Security Management Act of 2002 Title III-Information Security, Electronic Government Act, Public Law (PL) 107-347. Health Information Management and Systems Society (HIMSS). Retrieved September 27, 2007, from http://www.himss.org/content/files/CPRIToolkit/version6/v6%20pdf/D68_FISMA.pdf.

Croy, M. (2007). Enterprise, know thyself! *Disaster Recovery Journal, 20*(2). Retrieved September 17, 2007, from http://www.drj.com//articles/spr07/2002-02.pdf.

Cutlip, K. (2002). Strengthening the system: Joint commission standards and building on what we know. *Hospital Topics, 80*(1), 24.

Disaster resource guide. (2003). Business continuity planning: All the right moves. Retrieved January 7, 2004, from http://www.disaster-resource.com/articles/02p_045.shtml.

Epstein, K. & Nilakantan, C. (2007). Double jeopardy in a "slow" disaster. *Disaster Recovery Journal, 20*(2). Retrieved September 17, 2007, from http://www.drj.com/articles/spr07/2002-07.pdf.

Giniat, E. & Saporito, J. (August 2007). Sarbanes-Oxley impetus for enterprise risk management. *Healthcare Financial Management, 61*(8), 64–70.

Glenn, J. (2006). Business continuity vs. protecting data. *Disaster Recovery Journal, 19*(4). Retrieved September 17, 2007, from http://www.drj.com/articles/fall06/1904-04p.html.

Glenn, J. (2007). Planning for the pandemic. *Disaster Recovery Journal, 20*(3). Retrieved September 17, 2007, from http://www.drj.com/articles/sum07/2003-09.pdf.

Greene, J. (2005). Looking harder: Not-for-profit hospitals use Sarbanes-Oxley to strengthen their boards' financial accountability. *Hospitals and Health Networks, 79*(6), 52–54, 56, 58.

G'Sell, D. M. (2007). From the beginning. *Disaster Recovery Journal, 20*(3), Retrieved September 17, 2007, from http://www.drj.com/articles/sum07/2003-04.pdf.

Health Information Management Systems Society (HIMSS). (April 10, 2007). 18th Annual HIMSS leadership survey, CIO Results Questionnaire Index. Retrieved September 27, 2007, from http://www.himss.org/2007Survey/DOCS/2007Healthcare_CIO_questionnaire_index.pdf.

Johnston, E. (2006). Business owners are reminded of the perils of power loss. *Disaster Recovery Journal, 19*(4). Retrieved September 17, 2007, from http://www.drj.com/articles/fall06/1904-06p.html.

Joint Commission. (May 2007). Joint Commission Online. Retrieved September 28, 2007, from http://www.jointcommission.org/Library/jconline/jo_05_07.htm.

Kemp, R. L. (2007). Assessing the vulnerability of buildings. *Disaster Recovery Journal, 20*(2). Retrieved September 17, 2007, from http://www.drj.com/articles/spr07/2002-11.pdf.

Kirchner, T. A. & Ziegenfuss, D. E. (2003). Audit's role in the business continuity process. *Disaster Recovery Journal, 16*(2). Retrieved January 7, 2004, from http://www.drj.com/articles/spr03/1602-11.html.

Kirschenbaum, A. (2006). The missing link in business continuity. *Disaster Recovery Journal, 19*(4). Retrieved September 17, 2007, from http://www.drj.com/articles/fall06/1904-09p.html.

Koch, R. & Marks, C. (2006). Prepare for the next wave of BC planning. *Disaster Recovery Journal, 19*(4). Retrieved September 17, 2007, from http://www.drj.com/articles/fall06/1904-12.html.

Komoski, E. (2007). Is power your weakest link in data center flexibility? *Disaster Recovery Journal, 20*(3). Retrieved September 17, 2007, from http://www.drj.com/articles/sum07/2003-13.pdf.

Lawrence, D. (2007). Hurricanes, floods and fires, *Healthcare Informatics, 24*(8), 37–39.

Lawton, S. (2007). When protecting an SMB image is everything. *Disaster Recovery Journal, 20*(3). Retrieved September 17, 2007, from http://www.drj.com/articles/sum07/2003-17.pdf.

Lee, J. (2003). Effective strategy for meeting disaster recovery SLAs for mission-critical applications. *Disaster Recovery Journal, 16*(2). Retrieved January 20, 2004, from http://www.drj.com/articles/spr03/1602-15p.html.

Lindeman, J. (2007). The next level of disaster recovery. *Disaster Recovery Journal, 20*(3). Retrieved September 17, 2007, from http://www.drj.com/articles/sum07/2003-01.pdf.

Lindeman, J. & Grogan, J. (2007). Beyond disaster recovery. *Healthcare Informatics, 24*(8), 72, 74.

McDonald, J. (2007). Successful backups are not enough for disaster preparedness. *Disaster Recovery Journal, 20*(3). Retrieved September 17, 2007, from http://www.drj.com/articles/sum07/2003-06.pdf.

Maggio, E. J. & Coleman, K. G. (2007). A new face for an old threat. *Disaster Recovery Journal, 20*(3). Retrieved September 17, 2007, from http://www.drj.com/articles/sum07/2003-05.pdf.

Marcella, A. J. (2004). CYBERcrime: Is your company a potential target? Are you prepared? *Disaster Recovery Journal, 17*(1). Retrieved April 23, 2004, from http://www.drj.com/articles/win04/1701-04p.html.

Margeson, B. (2003). The human side of data loss. *Disaster Recovery Journal, 16*(2). Retrieved January 20, 2004, from http://www.drj.com/articles/spr03/1602-08p.html.

Martin, Z. (2007). Disaster recovery. *Health Data Management, 15*(1), 30–32, 34, 36, 38, 40.

McCormick, J. (2003). Picking up the pieces: To prepare for a disaster, whether natural or man-made, you will need both backup and recovery applications—and a plan. *Government Computer News, 22*(5), 42.

McDaniel, L. D. D. (1996). First steps to take after a fire. *Communication News, 33*(3), 26.

McGowan, B. (2002). The board's role related to disaster preparedness. *Healthcare Review, 15*(2), 15.

McKilroy, A. A. (2003). Connecting the islands: Disaster recovery planning for tele-working environments. *Disaster Recovery Journal, 16*(1). Retrieved Janaury 20, 2004, from http://www.drj.com/articles/win03/1601-07p.html.

Meyers, J. (2006). Preparing for the worst. *Healthcare Informatics, 23*(7), 44–45.

Miano, B. (Fall 2003). Key considerations for proactive planning. *Disaster Recovery Journal, 16*(4). Retrieved January 20, 2004, from http://www.drj.com/articles/fall03/1604-04p.html.

Midgley, C. (2002). Protecting your data, protecting your business. *Disaster Recovery Journal, 15*(3). Retrieved January 20, 2004, from http://www.drj.com/articles/sum02/1503-09p.html.

Mitchell, V. J. H. (2007). Take your own pulse first. *Disaster Recovery Journal, 20*(3). Retrieved September 17, 2007, from http://www.drj.com/articles/sum07/2003-07.pdf.

Miller, V. & Lehman, K. (2002). Assessment of HIPAA security requirements on disaster recovery planning. *Disaster Recovery Journal, 15*(1), 62–64.

Moore, R. (2006). Living on the edge: Remote site backup. *Disaster Recovery Journal, 19*(4). Retrieved September 17, 2007, from http://www.drj.com/articles/fall06/1904-15p.html.

Morgenthal, J. P. & Walmsley, P. (February 2000). Mining for metadata. *Software Magazine.* Retrieved January 27, 2004, from http://www.findarticles.com/cf_0/m0SMG/1_20/61298805/print.jhtml.

Olson, G. (2002). Recovering data in a snap. *Disaster Recovery Journal, 15*(4). Retrieved January 20, 2004, from http://www.drj.com/articles/fall02/1504-12p.html.

Peterka, A. (2007). Influenza pandemic presents unique challenges. *Disaster Recovery Journal, 20*(3). Retrieved September 17, 2007, from http://www.drj.com/articles/sum07/2003-08.pdf.

Pelant, B. F. (2003). Business impact analysis. *Disaster Recovery Journal, 16*(1). Retrieved January 4, 2004, from http://www.drj.com/articles/win03/1601-03p.html.

Peregrine, M. W. & Schwartz, J. R. (December 2002). What CFOs should know—and do—about corporate responsibility. *Healthcare Financial Management, 56*(12), 59–63.

Picking up the pieces. (2006). *American Journal of Nursing, 106*(9), 102.

Price, E. S. (Summer 2003). Application-aware solutions: The building blocks of business continuity. *Disaster Recovery Journal, 16*(3). Retrieved January 20, 2004, from http://www.drj.com/articles/sum03/1603-20p.html.

Price, Jr., J. O. (2007). Planning to exercise or planning to recover. *Disaster Recovery Journal, 20*(3). Retrieved September 17, 2007, from http://www.drj.com/articles/sum07/2003-11.pdf.

Rizzo, S. (2006). Aligning operational resilience to business requirements. *Disaster Recovery Journal, 19*(4). Retrieved September 17, 2007, from http://www.drj.com/articles/fall06/1904-08p.html.

Sheth, S. & McHugh, J. (2007). CIOs! How good is your disaster recovery plan? *Disaster Recovery Journal, 20*(2). Retrieved September 17, 2007, from http://www.drj.com/articles/spr07/2002-08.pdf.

Spath, P. (September 2002). Treatment is priority, but plan to safeguard info. Retrieved December 27, 2003, from http://www.findarticles.com/cf_0/m0HKF/9_2-/012-6010/print.jhtml.

Stephens, D. O. (January–February 2003). Protecting records in the face of chaos, calamity, and cataclysm: Even organizations that do not think they are prime targets for terrorists do not have the luxury of considering themselves exempt from disaster planning. *Information Management Journal, 37*(1), 33.

Sussman, S. (2002). Securing windows workstations in real time. *Disaster Recovery Journal, 15*(4). Retrieved January 21, 2004, from http://www.drj.com/articles/fall02/1504-15p.html.

Taylor, C. (2007). Is tape dead? *Disaster Recovery Journal, 20*(3). Retrieved September 17, 2007, from http://www.drj.com/articles/sum07/2003-14.pdf.

Veldboom, K. (2007). Emergency notification in a time of crisis. *Disaster Recovery Journal, 20* (2). Retrieved September 17, 2007, from http://www.drj.com/articles/spr07/2002-09.pdf

Wainwright, V. L. (2007). Business continuity by design. *Health Management Technology, 28*(3), 20–21.

Wiles, J. (2004). Auditing your disaster recovery plan: A closer look at high tech crime. Will this be your most likely disaster in the 21st century? Retrieved January 8, 2004, from http://www.disaster-resource.com/cgi-bin/article_search.cgi?id='93'.

Witty, R. J. (2006). 2005 BCM/DR survey results from Gartner, DRJ. *Disaster Recovery Journal, 19*(4). Retrieved September 17, 2007, from http://www.drj.com/articles/fall06/1904-03p.html.

Wold, G. H. & Vick, T. L. (2003). Comparing & selecting recovery strategies. *Disaster Recovery Journal, 16*(2). Retrieved January 4, 2004, from http://www.drj.com/articles/spr03/1602-05p.html.

Zalewski, S. (2003). Online data replication…provides new opportunities for business continuity. *Disaster Resource Guide.* Retrieved February 5, 2004, from http://www.disaster-resource.com/articles/03p_062.shtml.

Zawada, B. J. (2003). Regulatory pressure on technology for business continuity. *Risk Management, 50*(7), 20.

Zein, M., Cohn, S., & Broadway, T. (2002). Business continuity: Planning is a process not a project. Retrieved January 7, 2004, from http://www.disasterresource.com/articles/02p_036.shtml.

Zirkel, S. (2007). Ensuring workforce continuity during a pandemic. *Disaster Recovery Journal, 20*(3). Retrieved September 17, 2007, from http://www.drj.com/articles/sum07/2003-10.pdf.

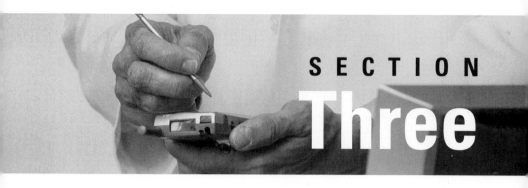

SECTION
Three

Specialty Applications

CHAPTER 16

Using the Computer to Support Healthcare and Patient Education

After completing this chapter, you should be able to:

1 Identify specific ways that computer technology may be used to support and enhance education.

2 List benefits associated with *Virtual Learning Environments (VLE), distance learning,* and *Web-based instruction (WBI).*

3 Compare and contrast *e-learning* with other educational uses of computers.

4 Provide examples of how computer technology may support education in each of the following settings: formal nursing programs, continuing education, and client or consumer education.

5 Compare and contrast various Web 2.0 applications and describe their use in education, social networking, professional collaborations, and patient care.

6 Explain to a colleague the various mobile learning technologies and demonstrate the ability to find information regarding the development of these tools for educational purposes.

Educational applications of computer technology can enhance the presentation of content, ease the burdens associated with course management for faculty, erase geographic boundaries for students, make learning opportunities available 24 hours a day, tailor instruction to individual learning needs, improve learning outcomes, provide a safe learning environment, and reduce the challenge of acquiring, maintaining, collaborating with other educators, and expanding skill sets—helping to keep the present workforce competent (Bradley 2003). Proponents see its potential to revolutionize education for healthcare professionals and consumers and promote critical thinking and problem-solving skills. The realization of this potential requires well-developed learning objectives, good planning, design, wise use, and evaluation by educators and administrators. Technology is increasingly prevalent in today's mobile society and dynamic workplaces. Technology should be a part of the education process but only when there is a match with the objectives of the curriculum, it is well used, and it facilitates the learning process. Educators must become adept in the evaluation and use of the technology that they plan to use. Today's students and healthcare consumers expect access to emerging technologies that will assist them with searching for healthcare content by category and that will allow them to actively participate in topical online groups.

INSTRUCTIONAL APPLICATIONS OF COMPUTER TECHNOLOGY

Computer-related technology may be used in a variety of ways to support, provide, and enrich learning. These often include:

- Word-processing software to prepare student handouts.
- Slide presentation software to create presentations and audio-visual aids.
- Spreadsheets or course management tools to maintain attendance records and grades.
- Course management system (CMS) tools to develop, administer, and score examinations and provide formative evaluation tools.
- Communication tools such as instant messaging, e-mail, weblogs (blogs), podcasts, threaded discussions, chats, and wikis to answer student questions and provide feedback to students on their progress.
- Online literature searches that may be used to research content prior to developing or revising a presentation. Searches can be done directly through databases available through libraries or through Websites such as Sigma Theta Tau's Virginia Henderson Library and the National Library of Medicine's portal For Healthcare Professionals (www.nlm.nih.gov/portals/healthcare.html). Abstracts and some full text articles can also be retrieved online.

Other instructional applications of computer technology include Virtual Learning Environments (VLE), competency-based training, teleconferencing, multimedia presentations, simulation, virtual reality, and distance education. Some examples of instructional applications may be found at www. Merlot.org.

Merlot.org is an online, multimedia educational resource housing various types of learning packages that can be accessed without charge. Content is submitted by the authors, evaluated by peers, and made available to the academic community at no cost. Box 16–1 lists some ways that computers may be used to facilitate education.

Virtual Learning Environment

A Virtual Learning Environment (VLE) is a system that uses the Internet to assist the educator in developing, managing, and administering educational materials for students. Other terms used for VLEs are *Course Management System (CMS)*, *Managed Learning Environment (MLE)*, and *Learning Management Systems (LMS)*. These programs facilitate electronic learning (e-learning), may track students' progress in a course, and generally run on servers (Wikipedia 2007a). Examples of VLEs are Moodle Learning Management System, CyberExtension Virtual Managed Learning, Blackboard, and WebCt. The Sakai Project (2007) is an example of a free and open-source CMS. This project is spearheaded by a group of academic institutions and volunteer organizations around the world that have developed an online collaboration and learning environment. This open-source learning platform provides generic "collaboration" tools, such as

---

BOX 16–1 Applications of Computers in Healthcare Education

Formal opportunities

- Continuing education
- Distance education
- Online journal retrieval
- Client education

Informal opportunities

- E-mail
- Listservs and Real Simple Syndication (RSS) (automatic news retrieval)
- Support groups
- Online literature searches and databases
- Chats or instant messaging
- Blogs
- Podcasts
- Wikis
- Social Networking Applications

Administrative support

- Webcasts
- Preparation of presentations, handouts, and slides
- Record keeping
- Course management tools inclusive of test administration scoring and statistical analysis
- Student services

threaded discussion boards, an announcement board, Web content, a chat room, and more. The "core" tools consist of teaching tools, such as a grade book, course syllabus, and assignments. Furthermore, there are portfolio tools that allow the student and educator to use templates, forms, and evaluations for professional electronic portfolios.

Advocates of VLE allege that it enhances computer literacy, facilitates decision-making skills, reduces computer anxiety, and positively affects student achievement. Although originally designed to promote individualized learning, VLE and Web 2.0 applications can enhance group learning as well (Calderone 1994; Maag 2006). Numerous studies have been conducted comparing the efficacy of VLE to traditional instruction. The general finding is that a VLE is at least as effective as traditional instruction although some critics find the methodology of many of these studies faulty—calling for more research (Wang & Sleeman 1993a, 1993b; Rouse 2000). It has been suggested that VLE may provide a means to introduce technology into the curriculum and even to pave the way for distance education (Greco & O'Connor 2000; Kozlowski 2002). A VLE is often used to supplement classroom instruction (Myles 2000; Second Health 2007).

VLE offers the following advantages:

- *Improved reading habits.* Learners can proceed at a pace conducive to comprehension.
- *Convenience.* VLE can be offered at any site that has computer access. Programs may be available for single users on freestanding PCs or via network connections.
- *Reduced learning time.* Because learners can proceed at their own pace, they can skim through familiar content and focus on weak areas.
- *Increased retention.* The active nature of the media facilitates learner participation, which in turn, improves retention.
- *Twenty-four-hour access.* VLE is available at any time of the day or night so that learners can use it at times convenient to them.
- *Consistent instruction in a safe environment.* VLE allows learners to practice new skills without fear of harm to themselves or others.
- *Flexibility of faculty schedules.* VLE makes it easier to teach around clinical instruction.

Three major variables influence VLE effectiveness: quality of the software, the environment of computer use, and characteristics of the learner. Some factors that can lead to negative attitudes toward VLE include the following design issues:

- *Poor design.* Many VLE applications do nothing more than automate page turning.
- *Lack of feedback on incorrect answers.* This is frustrating to learners who want to know why their selections were wrong.
- *Lack of control.* Control encompasses the ability to advance, repeat, or review portions of the program, or to quit at any point.
- *Lack of intellectual stimulation.* Programs that fail to maintain interest may cause learners to feel that they wasted their time.

Drug calculation programs are a common VLE application in many nursing schools. These programs are popular because drug calculation is a basic skill needed by all nurses, and, as such, drug calculation programs fit well into the curriculum, while programs on other content areas may not match curriculum objectives. An example of an interactive VLE that assists students and nurses with drug dosages is the "Med-Calc Tutorial" (Hansen 2007a).

Competency-Based Training

Competency-based training and testing are particularly important in the clinical setting as institutions need to demonstrate that staff are able to perform skills safely (Bradley 2003; O'Gara 2003). Simulation technology allows users to learn and then demonstrate their skills or test different scenarios without negative consequences. Initial research indicates highly positive effects of simulation on skill and knowledge acquisition (Ravert 2002). Computer-based competency training and testing have the potential to free instructor time, streamline instruction and testing, and eliminate costs associated with employee travel. An example of a high fidelity simulation and case-based learning lab is at the University of Tasmania School of Nursing and Midwifery (2007). The manikins used in the simulation lab assist students in practicing assessment skills through computer-assisted case scenarios. It is vital that the case studies be developed around well-planned learning objectives, and that the students' learning outcomes be evaluated on a continuous basis. Simulation labs are popular in healthcare education; however, caution needs to be taken so that they do not totally replace clinical education.

Multimedia

Nursing education has always used multimedia, whether that media included chalkboard diagrams, overhead transparencies, slide presentations, videos, skill demonstrations, computer-based instruction, interactive video disks (IVDs), compact discs (CDs), digital video discs (DVDs), or streaming video (Batscha 2002; Billings 1995; Calderone 1994; Gleydura et al. 1995; Simpson 2002; Smith-Stoner & Willer 2003; Sternberger & Meyer 2001). Now it is possible to add virtual reality to the list of examples. Quite simply, multimedia refers to presentations that combine text, voice or sound, images, and video, or hardware and software that can support the same. Interactive technological tools that facilitate different forms of online communication, learning, and collaboration among educators, students, and colleagues include Web 2.0 technologies. According to Wikipedia (2007b), Web 2.0 is "a second phase of development of the World Wide Web, including its architecture and its applications." (O'Reilly 2005). The concept of Web 2.0 began with a brainstorming session in which O'Reilly participated. These technologies include blogs, podcasts, vodcasts, wikis, and YouTube (see Appendix). Murray and Maag (2006) claimed these tools could enhance effective communication, manage information, and enrich professional collaboration. Currently, health informaticians are proposing an International Medical Informatics Association (IMIA) Web 2.0 exploratory task force in order to provide knowledge about these applications (Moura, Murray,

Hammond, Hansen, & Erdley, 2007). Another novel online interactive learning tool is "Second Health: The Future of Healthcare Communication" (2007). The three dimensional (3D) virtual world of Second Life is an exciting online tool that allows healthcare students and professionals to interact with other visitors in a virtual hospital and help shape future healthcare.

While interactive multimedia is an excellent approach for nurses because they are required to learn and communicate complex issues to clients, specific learning objectives need to be in place before the multimedia is presented. Research has shown that learning retention is facilitated with an approach that incorporates seeing, hearing, doing, interactivity, and repetition (Mayer 2001; Barrett, Lacey, Sekara, Linden, & Gracely 2004). Multimedia has been found to be at least as effective as traditional instruction, offers greater satisfaction, and has value as an additional learning resource (Maag 2004a; Palmer & Devitt 2007). Group-paced instruction with multimedia decreases costs associated with individual instruction, increases comfort with computers, and improves learning as long as the environment is conducive to group use. Nurse educators need to select and use multimedia well and creatively to realize its benefits (Cuellar 2002; Ross & Tuovinen 2001). Multimedia can be incorporated into formative and summative evaluation as well (Rossignol & Scollin 2001; Hansen 2007b). Virtual reality is a form of multimedia that fully envelops learners in an environment. It is already used to help medical students, surgeons, and other healthcare professionals with procedural skills such as the insertion of urinary catheters and surgical procedures (Go Virtual Medical 2007). Virtual reality offers the next best option to performing the skill on a real person but without any risks to the learner or the client. More research is being conducted in order to determine if a carefully engineered integrated simulator and an i-Pod video for male and female urinary catheter insertion will increase student confidence levels and enhance skill acquisition and retention (Doherty et al., 2007; Hansen et al., 2007c).

Changing technology now makes tailored multimedia presentations feasible via the use of CDs, DVDs, and videoclips on the Web (Calderone 1994; Gleydura et al. 1995; Goodman & Blake 1996; Smith-Stoner & Willer 2003). The tools to produce streaming video are increasingly available. Streaming video can be uploaded to Web pages or course management tools such as Blackboard and WebCT. Streaming video may also be reproduced and distributed on CDs. Video is converted to a digital format for use on the Web or CD. Quality multimedia should reduce labor costs for instructor and participant time, improve overall instructional effectiveness, and foster productivity through user satisfaction and enjoyment. DVD drives are standard equipment on PCs that support CDs as well as DVDs. Multimedia enhances VLE by using the interactivity, information management, and decision-making capabilities of computers (Billings 1994; Cambre & Castner 1993; Goodman & Blake 1996). Skiba (2007) reports that students entering higher education are digital natives who understand multimedia, prefer multimedia, and are comfortable using technology. The aforementioned author suggested that nurse educators think about using "YouTube" in order to transform nursing education. "YouTube is a place for people to engage in new ways with video by sharing, commenting on, and viewing videos" (YouTube Website, 2007).

Authoring tools allow program design to match learning objectives and foster higher cognitive development. Authoring tools are software applications designed to allow persons with little or no programming expertise to create instructional programs. These tools require time for mastery: As many as 50 to 200 hours may be needed to prepare one hour of instruction and work out the program bugs. Educators can exercise creativity in the design of multimedia. It is possible to use slide presentation software to prepare and customize programs for student learning (Batscha 2002; Smith-Stoner & Willer 2003). Slide presentation software is easily learned, is adaptable, allows the insertion of simple programming commands, and is easily revised. It can also be used to house streaming video presentations or narrate audio. Faculty who are comfortable with the various forms of multimedia usually do a better job of integrating it into their instruction for optimal student benefit. Figure 16–1 depicts an online tutorial on arterial blood gases that was developed by a faculty member.

Videoteleconferencing

Videoteleconferencing is the use of computers, audio and video equipment, and high-grade dedicated telephone lines to provide interactive communication between persons at two or more sites. Recent developments make videoteleconferencing capability possible from desktop computers. Teleconferencing

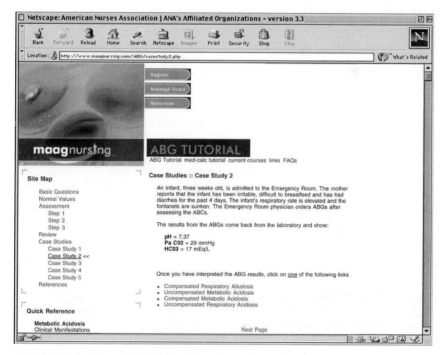

FIGURE 16–1 • An example of online educational offering (Reproduced with the permission of the author Dr. Margaret Maag.)

is particularly useful for graduate and doctoral students and staff nurses because it brings educational opportunities to areas that may not otherwise offer courses or programs. In teleconferencing, learners at one site view and interact with an instructor and other learners at separate locations. Participants can pool resources to establish collaborative programs, thus maximizing resources through shared classes and conferences. Videoteleconferencing requires start-up funds and an investment in equipment, transmission media, and adaptation in communication methods, particularly when used in conjunction with traditional on-site classes. Classes, assignments, and feedback may be offered entirely online. Content may be clinically oriented or focus on nursing informatics. Videoteleconferencing extends the reach of educational programs and continuing education courses by accommodating students who would otherwise be unable to attend programs because of their distance from offered programs. The drawbacks associated with videoteleconferencing are eye contact and appearance self-consciousness. Advanced technology is capable of addressing the problem of eye contact. As people experience more video interaction, their feelings of self-consciousness before a video camera will subside.

Another technology that is free to the public is Skype. Skype is a "peer-to-peer" Internet telephony network that allows individuals to call one another via the computer and communicate via microphone and a video camera. Its popularity is rising around the globe. According to Wikipedia (2007c) there are 240 million users. The program offers instant messaging, file transfer, short messaging, video phone, and videoteleconferencing. Nurse educators may benefit from using Skype as an educational and collaborative tool.

There are some guidelines that educators may wish to consider before embarking on videoconferencing. Broadband is requisite as well as equipment that is easy to use with a cross-platform capability. Individuals may need to collaborate on editing the video that is produced for educational purposes. Some users may be interested in viewing and intereacting with all attendees if it is a small group while others prefer collaborative editing. Still others may prefer still photos as the video portion of the production. The equipment for the videoconferencing should meet standards, and the individual making the video should decide if head or full body shots are desirable. The individual making the video needs to consider how many people are required to control the cameras (distant, local, or both). Participants should be made aware of any other information technology or software that is needed during the videoconferencing or presenation (Erdley 2008).

Distance Education

Distance education is the use of print, audio, video, computer, teleconferencing capability, or the World Wide Web to connect faculty and students who are located at a minimum of two different locations. Print media is inexpensive and low technology and can be developed quickly. Audio conferences may take place over the telephone or via Skype. Video and teleconferencing have been popular in recent years. Video signals may be one-way or two-way transmissions over telephone lines, cable, satellite, or network connections. Improved Internet capabilities, telephone use, and teleconferencing have virtually eliminated the barriers faced by nurses in remote locations who wish to further their education via formal study or through continuing education programs, or who require additional job training (Corwin 2000; Kozlowski 2002). Distance education may occur in real, or synchronous, time or via a delay. In real time, all parties participate in the activity at the same time; this may include a classroom session or chat. With the delayed, or asynchronous, approach, the learner reviews material at a convenient time, which is generally not at the same time as other participants. Asynchronous learning can be enhanced with the incorporation of ongoing electronic discussion to aid the clarification of ideas, promote retention, and aid critical thinking (Cartwright 2000; Harden 2003). Synchrony influences instructional design, delivery, and interaction. Distance education requires additional course preparation and organization by faculty and a concerted effort on the part of students to remain active participants. The transition from traditional classroom to online learning is not easy. It can, however, be an effective means of instruction.

There is a strong push among institutions of higher learning to offer distance education as a means to improve student access, meet student demands, extend geographic boundaries, remain viable, and keep students on the cutting edge of technology (Bentley, Cook, Davis, Murphy, & Berding 2003; Charp 2003; Cuellar 2002). However, good market research and planning remain key to the success of distance education courses and programs (Wong, Greenhalgh, Russell, Boynton, & Toon 2003). Careful consideration must be given to the market, course objectives, choice of software platform, staff training, design of active learning, quality, technical and administrative issues, finances, and the fit with the overall institution. Distance education has rapidly become an acceptable mode of nursing education, with more than one-half of all schools of nursing surveyed by the American Association of Colleges of Nursing demonstrating some involvement in distance education (Faison 2003; Sapnas et al. 2002). As more institutions and faculty move toward Internet-based distance education, the Institute for Higher Education Policy prepared a report sponsored by the National Education Association and Blackboard Inc., an Internet education company, that identified 24 benchmarks deemed essential to ensure excellence in Internet-based distance education (IHEP 2000). These benchmarks are broken down into seven categories and are summarized here:

Institutional Support Benchmarks
- Documented technology plan that includes security measures such as password protection, encryption, and back-up systems
- Reliable technology delivery system
- Centralized support system for building and maintaining the distance education infrastructure

Course Development Benchmarks
- Guidelines that specify minimum standards for course development, design, and delivery

- Periodic review of instructional materials for compliance with program standards
- Course and program requirements call for students to use analysis, synthesis, and evaluation

Teaching/Learning Benchmarks
- Students interact with faculty and other students as a part of instruction; communication facilitated through voice and/or e-mail
- Timely and constructive faculty feedback to students on questions and assignments
- Instruction on the methods of effective research and evaluation of resources for students

Course Structure Benchmarks
- Counseling for students on online instruction before starting a course or program to determine if they meet the technology and commitment requirements
- Supplemental course materials that address course objectives, concepts, and learning outcomes
- Access for students to sufficient library resources
- Agreement by faculty and students on course expectations

Student Support Benchmarks
- Students receive program information inclusive of admission requirements, tuition and fees, and technical and proctoring requirements
- Hands-on training is provided to help students access electronic databases, interlibrary loans, government archives, news services, and other pertinent resources
- Technical assistance is available at all times
- Student services answer questions accurately and quickly and have a mechanism to handle complaints

Faculty Support Benchmarks
- Technical assistance is available to faculty
- Assistance is available to help faculty make the transition from traditional to online teaching
- Instructor training and assistance, including peer mentoring, are available all through online courses
- Faculty have written guidelines to help students with issues related to the use of electronically accessed data

Evaluation and Assessment Benchmarks
- Evaluation processes use several methods and specific standards to determine educational effectiveness
- Enrollment data, costs, and applications of technology are used to evaluate program effectiveness

- Learning outcomes are regularly reviewed for clarity, utility, and appropriateness
- Faculty must acquire new skills and teaching methodologies for distance education (Geibert 2000; Im & Lee 2003; Kozlowski 2004; McKenna & Samarawickrema 2003)

Communication and flexibility are essential qualities. Students may feel isolated, particularly if they experience difficulties in getting online. For this reason, technical assistance should be readily available for all involved. Faculty are wise to maintain frequent communication with students in order to maintain a feeling of connection. This communication may take place through postings to the class as well as e-mail to an individual or a group of students. Students come to distance education with varying levels of technical skills. Students must be enrolled in the course and the electronic roster for access to the distance education offering. Late course registration, servers that are not working, and poor computer skills can frustrate students. Internet access is necessary for online instruction. Time spent on e-mail may seem excessive but actually frees up time otherwise spent in group meetings addressing concerns (VandeVusse & Hanson 2000). All assignments should be clearly communicated via a well-planned CMS. Course requirements need to stipulate file formats for paper submission. Faculty must realize that students may experience difficulty with firewalls, file transfer, and occasional Internet problems. A sense of community needs to be established by the instructor in order to prevent students' feelings of isolation. Online collaboration may be accomplished via the use of e-mail, videoconferences, online supported group projects, instant messaging, threaded discussions, bulletin board postings, and the use of Web 2.0 applications. Thurmond (2003) stated that interaction opportunities are a core element of online courses. Learners must engage with course content, other learners, the instructor, and technology. Learner-content interaction occurs when students examine content and participate in class activities. Print media is less likely to engage a learner than are hyperlinks, interactive software, and discussions. Reciprocal action aids learning. Learner-to-learner interactions provide an opportunity to share ideas and benefit from the experiences of others. Collaborative projects facilitate this interaction through the creation of a community. Learner-to-instructor interactions occur with prompt feedback and scheduled meetings. Frequent communication through postings, e-mail, and online discussion facilitates this process. Learner-to-interface interaction is facilitated when students are successful in getting online and accessing course materials. Today's Internet savvy student requests automatic "push technology" instead of "pull technology." This entails a change in how course materials are provided. Traditionally faculty expect students to obtain data from the course management system via downloads or "pulling" the information from the CMS. Students now request that educators set up tools that will automatically disseminate (or "push") the information out to them. An example of this "push" technology is iTunes University. Podcasting lectures has become a mainstay over the past few years (Kaplan-Leiserson 2005; Lane 2006; Maag 2006; Malan 2007; Murray & Maag 2006).

Distance education offers many advantages, but it also requires student commitment. Distance learners must assume responsibility for active learning, thus becoming more independent and self-disciplined (Theile 2003). Box 16–2 lists key points for the participant in distance education. Distance education broadens educational opportunities and eliminates long commutes. For this reason it may serve as a recruitment and retention mechanism for schools of nursing and healthcare agencies. It can provide access to experts and cut costs by paying faculty to teach at one site rather than multiple sites. Despite these advantages, distance education often faces budget constraints as well as slow planning and decision making.

The growth of distance education programs has implications for library services as well (Gandhi 2003). Academic libraries must demonstrate the ability to provide equivalent resources and services electronically or through some other means to both on-campus and distance learners to meet accreditation requirements. Some institutions have distance education librarians who work closely with faculty who teach distance education. This may be done through digitizing reserve materials and placing them on electronic reserves accessible only to students enrolled in the course. Restricted access, along with a prominent display of copyright notices on all readings, helps to ensure compliance with copyright and fair use laws. Permission should be obtained from the copyright holder for each item used. Reserve lists must be submitted in sufficient time to allow librarians time to scan materials.

As more schools of nursing move to distance education, there are concerns over the ability to socialize students to the profession. Obviously, this aspect of education requires careful attention in any setting. It is even more critical when there are no regular, face-to-face meetings between faculty and student. Studies

---

BOX 16–2   Key Points for Students Involved in Distance Learning

- Reception sites may be in students' homes, workplaces, or recreational areas.
- Increases educational opportunities by eliminating long commutes.
- Class rosters with phone numbers and addresses are generally distributed to all class members (pending individual approval) as a means to encourage interaction among students.
- Faculty may hold office hours online and provide feedback by telephone, electronic posting, Instant Messaging, e-mail, and Skype as well as during class time.
- Students may remain online after class to ask questions.
- The sponsoring agency notifies students of information pertaining to hardware and software requirements, reception sites, parking, and technical support.
- Additional effort is required from both students and faculty to maintain interactive aspects of the education process.
- Some modifications may be required in the use of audiovisual aids. Additional attention must be given to how well audiovisual aids transmit and whether they are visible to persons at other sites.
- Successful offerings are the result of a team effort that involves instructional designers, graphic artists, faculty training, and technical support.

indicate that it can take place in distance education, although additional research into this area is suggested (Faison 2003). Hirumi (2002) noted that technological advances are happening faster than research can keep up with the effectiveness of these advances. There are also issues related to faculty workload, effective class size, and intellectual property rights for electronic courses (Bentley et al. 2003).

Web-Based Instruction

Web-based instruction (WBI) uses the attributes and resources of the World Wide Web, such as hypertext links and multimedia, for educational purposes. WBI may be offered as a stand-alone course or as a complement to traditional classes. Independent WBI provides access to most or all class materials, resources, and interaction via Internet technology. This is in contrast to Web-enhanced courses that rely on physical meetings of students and teachers but integrate assignments, readings, computer-mediated communications, and/or links to sites into the course activities. Some synonyms for WBI include Web-based training (WBT), Web-assisted instruction (WAI), Internet-based training (IBT), Web-based learning (WBL), Web interactive training (WIT), and online courses.

WBI is a popular educational use of computers (Cragg, Edwards, Yue, Xin, & Hui 2003; Cragg, Humbert, & Douchette 2004; Geibert 2000). It shares many of the advantages associated with VLE, such as self-paced learning, 24-hour availability, prompt feedback, and interactivity. Web-based instruction also supports multimedia, a high level of learner interactivity, and hypertext links, which enable learner-centered control over information and learning (Vogt, Kumrow, & Kazlauskas 2001). WBI is free from geographic constraints and can be revised as needed. The Web provides a user-friendly format along with access to multimedia in a fairly consistent manner. Most WBI sites provide basic course information, such as syllabus, schedule, announcements, and reading lists. Many other sites include synchronous or asynchronous communication, online testing, discussion groups, conferences, whiteboards, streaming audio and video, and, in some cases, online help. WBI can be used as a stand-alone course for distance education or as a complement to traditional courses. Teleconferencing capability is sometimes included. There is debate as to whether WBI is actually cost effective when development and support costs are considered. In the case of course materials, printing costs are shifted from the institution to the student.

It is important to consider a number of issues before Web-based instruction is offered (Bruckley 2003; Chen 2003; Choi 2003; Gould III 2003; Rose, Frisby, Hamlin, & Jones 2000; Sakraida & Draus 2003). These include:

- *Institutional commitment of resources.* WBI requires human and material resources. It is labor intensive to develop and manage. It requires administrative support for needed equipment, technical staff, and help for faculty interested in using this medium. Good design requires input from software specialists, service technicians, learning specialists, and possibly psychologists.
- *The technology infrastructure.* Networking and technical support staff should be consulted to determine server and network specifications, technical

standards, bandwidth, and software requirements for Web-based instruction. Requirements to support and receive instruction must be identified.

- *Web course management tools and online peer collaboration tools.* This type of software provides the infrastructure, or shell, for faculty to present content, documents, and media (Kropf 2002; Mills 2000). Common features include tracking, threaded discussions, chat capability, a whiteboard, e-mail, the ability to post information, scheduling capability, templates, the ability to share files, grading components, exam and evaluation capability, and administrative and security features that limit access to authorized users. Some examples include Blackboard, FirstClass, TopClass, LearningSpace, LearnLinc I-Net, and Centra Software's Symposium. Course management tools may be used to supplement traditional instruction or to supplant it. Some course management tools are fairly intuitive while others require a higher learning curve for faculty use. Typically colleges and universities make the software available and provide instruction and support to faculty and students seeking to use it (Sakraida & Draus 2003).
- *Adaptation of course materials and delivery for online instruction.* Successful WBI makes use of the hypertext capabilities of the Web; this includes links to other sites of potential interest. It represents a deviation from traditional class structures and acknowledges that the locus of control for learning lies with the learner. For this reason, activities that require active involvement on the part of the learner such as structured or threaded discussions and group projects are recommended.
- *Faculty commitment.* Web-based instruction is time consuming to create and maintain. Students require more feedback than might be needed in a traditional setting. Faculty must learn the tools and the teaching methodologies and keep materials and links up-to-date.
- *Practice time before the actual start of instruction.* One cannot assume that faculty or students come to Web-based instruction with an intuitive grasp of the technology. For this reason, it is important to practice using the tool before the start of a course. Preparatory tutorials ensure that instructional time is not squandered on technical assistance for a few. Faculty must consider that Web-based courses generally have a slow start because Web-based learning is still a new learning environment for many students. They must exercise patience and ensure that technical support is available until all students demonstrate the basic skills required to navigate the course. Support may be available via orientation sessions, written and online materials, and telephone support.
- *Develop and communicate a contingency plan.* While the advantages of WBI include 24-hour availability from any location, there may be instances when access cannot be accomplished. This may be related to an individual's PC or Internet service provider, power outages, or problems with the organization's infrastructure. It is of particular concern when classes are synchronous. Identify alternative means of communicating assignments early in the class.

Box 16–3 includes a few suggestions for faculty who are developing Web-based instruction or considering its use.

WBI requires time for planning, implementation, and maintenance. Course design needs to incorporate learning activities that encourage collaborative efforts. Faculty and student roles shift with the move from a content-driven or teacher-centered approach to a student-centered approach. Faculty must move

---

BOX 16–3 Do's and Don'ts for Teaching a Web-Based Course

Do's

- **Communicate software standards.** Tell students what office productivity software is supported by the school and will be used for shared course files. Even with established software standards there may be instances when the institution and many of the students are in a transition phase between different operating systems and versions of productivity and browser software. Be prepared to save files in the older software version during this phase.
- **Humanize the course.** Encourage students to provide background information about themselves and their goals at the onset of the course. Providing students with a profile of yourself and a current photograph will add a personal touch that the student will appreciate.
- **Post materials prior to class and discussions.** This provides reinforcement and promotes active listening when WBI is used as an adjunct to traditional classes.
- **Provide mechanisms for student feedback.** Use threaded discussions, chats, e-mail, blogs, wikis, tagging, and whiteboard capability.
- **Keep lessons short and modular.** Long documents online do not facilitate learning.
- **Use methods to foster interaction.** Include situations and ask participants to identify how they would respond. Encourage discussion among classmates. Assign group projects suggesting that students use the collaborative work space for real-time efforts or rely on e-mail to develop their work.
- **Incorporate a mechanism to access library resources.** Provide reserve lists to the library well in advance to allow time to procure material.
- **Use formative feedback.** This will allow faculty to modify the course as needed to benefit students.
- **Provide information related to resources for technical support.**
- **Be flexible.** Not all students have the same level of computer skills; therefore, provide them with a frequently asked questions (FAQ) printout at the beginning of the course.

   Give students opportunities to check back with the faculty and other students following the completion of the course by providing an alumni event.

Don'ts

- **Don't assume preexisting knowledge.** Provide a tutorial prior to class or as part of the first class to familiarize students with the technology.
- **Don't assume that everyone has the latest versions of software or the fastest processor.** Students who cannot access all documents or portions of the class will become frustrated.
- **Avoid items that take a long time to download.** People will not wait. Large files also place a heavy demand on the server and network.
- **Avoid "plug-ins."** These programs can change the way the user's computer processes tasks as well as place additional demands on the processor.

into the role of facilitator as they help students to organize information and use critical thinking (Kozlowski 2002). WBI increases access to educational offerings but learners still need access to computers and the Internet and basic computer skills before they enter the workforce. Students will be encouraged to become self-regulated learners as they are given more opportunity to access assignments that are to be "self-learned" online and when they are provided with the necessary expert support throughout the learning experience.

E-learning

E-learning is the delivery of content and stimulation of learning primarily through the use of online telecommunication technologies such as blogs, podcasts, streamed video recorded videos, e-mail, bulletin board systems, electronic whiteboards, inter-relay chat, desktop video conferencing, and the World Wide Web (Hirumi 2002; Maag 2006). It may also occur as the result of a satellite broadcast, audio/video tape, interactive TV, YouTube, and/or CD-ROM. E-learning is often associated with advanced learning technology (ALT), which not only includes the specific technology but also the methodology involved in the learning process associated with e-learning. E-learning offers convenience, flexibility, availability anytime and anywhere there is an Internet connection, and self-paced instruction within a semi-formal environment. As cities around the world become wireless, there will be more of an opportunity for mobile learning opportunities. Imagine students riding a city bus or subway and having access to e-learning via mobile technologies, such as iPods or cellular phones. Another important aspect of e-learning is the ability to network with fellow students who may be anywhere around the globe. However, there have been reports that some students feel isolated in e-learning environments. This feeling of isolation may be ameliorated by giving assignments that foster the use of technologies, such as video-enabled Skype, message boards, whiteboards, and instant messaging that create an interactive environment.

Web 2.0 Applications in Education, Healthcare, and Social Networking

Interactive technological tools that facilitate different forms of online communication, learning, and collaboration among educators, students, and colleagues across international borders are becoming popular in healthcare education and clinical practice. Blogs, podcasts, wikis, and some other Web 2.0 applications that are evolving in healthcare education and clinical practice will be covered herein. While not all of these cutting-edge technologies are mobile per se, many of them are, and as technology advances, common items, such as the ubiquitous cell phone, will become handy learning tools. Therefore, the term *mobile learning*, or *m-learning*, is a popular term that denotes the use of mobile technologies, such as the mobile phone, personal digital assistant (PDA), and iPod. There is grant funding available for healthcare educators who wish to pursue this area of educational research (Cell Phone 2007). An extremely comprehensive explanation of Web 2.0/3.0 is available for healthcare educators who are interested in technological advances to improve, enhance, and/or stimulate learning for healthcare students, professionals, and patients (Yourdon 2007). Since Web 2.0 is now considered the "read-write-listen" Web, it provides an avenue for users to comment, annotate, create, mix, and share content that is related to health education (Boulos 2007).

Blogs

Weblogs, also known as "blogs," are innovative writing tools that are exciting and intuitive to use, Internet based, and encourage health profession students to write and publish their writing instantaneously. Lewis (2004) reported "blogs" as innovative pedagogical aids for students studying different disciplines, such as medicine, business, and journalism. The Institute of Medicine (2003) recommended that healthcare professionals be taught to use informatics in order to "communicate, manage knowledge, mitigate error, and support decision making using information technology" (p. 46). The use of blogs as social networking and professional collaborating tools is evident on the Internet (Erdley, Murray, Hansen, Oyri, Ward, & Perry 2007; Ward 2007). Blood (2000) wrote about the culture, theory, and creation of weblogs, and discussed the change of the nomenclature from "wee-blog," initially proposed by Peter Merholz. Maag (2004b) described a "blogger toolbox" as containing software programs that are free to use on the Internet and are based on Real Simple Syndication (RSS). Yensen (2005) explained RSS and how this feed to the World Wide Web fuels frequently updated content in order for individuals to access information on blogs, podcasts, and latest news headlines Some of the blogging tools include, but are not limited to, *Blogger, Moveable Type, Haloscan, Typepad, Slash,* and *now.Mac.* Maag (2004b) provided a step-by-step method of creating a blog and gave various examples of how blogs may be utilized in healthcare education and clinical settings. A blog is generally edited, organized, and published using a Content Management System (CMS), many of which are built with Linux/Apache/MySQL/PHP architecture (Murray & Maag 2006). Moreover, there are various applications available that link posts from different blogs containing similar subject matter, using either permalinks or tags, such as Technorati tags (2007).

Clinical educators may encourage healthcare students to blog about their clinical experiences. This Web 2.0 application is ideal for this aspect of education because it is convenient for students, and educators may respond online to the students' experience in a timely fashion via the "comment" component of the blog. Clinical blogs may be easily password protected in order to prevent inadvertent disclosure of a patient's identity via a blog. Educators need to keep in mind the Family Education Rights and Privacy Act (FERPA) in order to respect and protect students' privacy. An anonymous posting or a pseudonym may be used by the student blogger. Clinical cases and images may be delivered automatically via RSS and viewed on iGoogle. This free program offered by Google allows the user to create his or her own private Web page and allows for YouTube videos to be selected and viewed. The user may add RSS feeds as tabs, such as medical journals, medical podcasts, updates in hospital medicine, and healthcare informatics for daily updates. Educators could ask healthcare students to create their own iGoogle pages as an online assignment; this would provide the student and educator with a gateway to current healthcare information. It is easy to create an iGoogle page, and the user may use creativity and create "widgets" to add to his or her personal Web page. An example of a self-created widget is seen as "The hi-blogs.info krew" (http://www.differance-engine.net/krew/); widgets may be shared with colleagues and peers. All that is needed is a free Google e-mail account in order to create an iGoogle home page. Another interesting example of a healthcare blog that examines Web 2.0 applications in healthcare is the "Constructive Medicine: Bench side to Bed side 2.0" (2007). Improved patient care may be achieved through the collaboration of healthcare professionals, sharing of knowledge, and active discussion via Internet-based platforms, such as blogs, podcasts, vodcasts (video-enhanced podcasts), and dynamic wikis.

Students who blog their clinical experiences have been known to increase their writing over time, interact with the instructor and peers more readily, and share experiences as the semester progresses. Students' writing has been observed to improve over the course of the semester. In order to make the clinical assignment more interactive, students may be asked to comment on a peer's blog each week; this, in turn, enhances communication and support of the student who is blogging. Software applications, such as Blogger, have a comment button that may be activated by the reader of the blog. Furthermore, students may create an audio blog (PodBean 2007), and this may prove to be convenient for the student following a long clinical day. Moreover, a school of nursing blog may spark students' interests in posting their artwork, poetry, and other creative musings. Healthcare providers may encourage their patients to blog about their medical experiences, thereby allowing patients to share with others their challenges and experiences, and to offer support to others who are newly diagnosed with a similar disease process. Another popular use of blogs is by universities who wish to showcase students' ideas about their experiences in a specific field of study. An example of this is the University of Michigan School of Medicine blog (2007).

Podcasts

Podcasting, a portmanteau of "broadcasting" and the popular "iPod" (Apple Computer's MP3 player), is another example of an Internet-based technology that allows for an audio event, conversation, lecture, presentation, speech, group-learning occurrence, video, or a song to be distributed via RSS. The beauty of a podcast is that it may be listened to via a desktop computer or from a MP3 player via free podcasting software, such as Apple iTunes or iPodder. An enhanced podcast involves the creation of text, chapters, images, and/or video. Educators have the ability to create enhanced podcasts by using software packages, such as Podcast Maker or Apple iLife07. The audio, text, and video components provide many creative opportunities for truly "any time, anywhere" distance education. As more cities around the globe become wireless, learners will be able to access podcasts, YouTube videos, and blogs with great ease in a car, train, bus, or subway.

Jeiesiewicz (2007) reported that iPods help facilitate stethoscope skills among medical students at Temple University School of Medicine and Hospital. Listening repeatedly (400 times) to five common heart murmurs via iPods improved students' heart sound identification by 80%. Medical students studying at the University of Michigan have the opportunity to listen and view lecture and exam video podcasts (2007). These are examples of how this mobile technology may assist with education and with the healthcare of patients. Malan (2007) reported that 45% of students attending Harvard University stated that a lecture podcast was used for "review" rather than as an alternative to attendance (18%). Furthermore, Malan stated that 71% of the students in the study were more inclined to listen to or watch lectures on their desktop computers, versus 19% of the participants relying on audio-only or 10% on video iPods. Maag (2006) examined podcasting and MP3 technology in nursing education by providing portability for listening to lectures (iTunes "Maag" Podcasts 2007), training more clinicians, and using podcasts to reach the public at large. Many universities are subscribing to iTunes University, therefore, making it easier for educators to make their lectures, presentations, and students' work available on the Internet. Maag (2006) provided a step-wise instruction on how to create a podcast. The technical components and interactions of podcasting are presented by Carnegie Mellon's teaching with technology white paper (2007). The authors of the white paper set out to evidence the "creation and distribution of lecture archives for review, the delivery of supplemental educational materials and content, and assignments requiring students to produce and submit their own podcasts" (2007, p.1). Educating the Net Generation requires educators to know and understand their audience prior to developing learning objectives and the delivery of educational materials. A new wave of learning and flexibility is available to our learners; students need not be anchored to desktops in computer labs. Palmer and Devitt (2007) demonstrate how case studies and anatomical images, such as a view of a patient's retina as seen via an ophthalmoscope, may be accessed via an iPod for clinical learning. Also, from a clinical standpoint, an iPod video may be just the prescription for an anxious patient awaiting surgery. The patient may view nature scenes and listen to relaxing music, guided imagery, or meditative audio via an iPod video.

Wikis

Web pages may now be created by individual users via dynamic "wikis." The well-known Wikipedia (2007), an online editable encyclopedia, is an example of such a Web page. A wiki, which actually means "quick" in Hawaiian, allows anyone visiting the Website to create, update, or change content at one's whim. This asynchronous group socialization tool provides a place for communication, collaboration, and archiving various writings and information. Another form of a wiki is Google Docs. This enhanced wiki is a technological application that is affecting education and professional development. It allows anyone to compose online (write and edit) as an electronic word processor, allowing collaboration with others in real time. As with the iGoogle page, Google Docs is free to Google mail (Gmail) users.

Wiki software programs, such as Wiki Media, (2007), are intuitive and easy to use. However, the important question to first ask is "why" am I creating a wiki or implementing any of these other tools? A specific purpose (such as a subject matter) should be kept in mind, and the user may consider how many people will be involved in the project and use/contribute to the interactive page. Another important issue is to decide how much of the content will be made public or kept private. Free guides for installing the wiki program are available at Free Software Daily (2007). Furthermore, Wikipedia (2007b) offered a nice table comparing various wiki software programs for those interested in comparing and contrasting various programs before constructing a wiki. Oyri (2007) shares a wiki project, "Biomedical Wireless Sensor Network Project," that demonstrates a wiki created by using TikiWiki. There are concerns regarding the "piracy" of wikis, since anyone who has access can change information on the Web page and potentially corrupt the validity of the information provided to the public. Hence, some instructors do not accept students citing Wikipedia in their assigned papers. Nonetheless, Wikipedia is being referenced more often by well-known authors. The validity of the information may be double-checked with a follow-up reference and then added to the wiki for future use by others.

VIRTUAL LEARNING ENVIRONMENTS

Educational applications of computers adapt well to a diversity of settings and learners. The very flexibility of the educational application of computer technology makes it suitable for use in formal healthcare education programs, as well as continuing education and consumer education.

Formal Healthcare Education

Advocates of computer-enhanced education note that its applications in healthcare are limited only by imagination (Bloom & Hough 2003; Charp 2003; Greco & O'Connor 2000). Critics of e-learning claim that computers and the Internet only promise to revolutionize the way that nursing content is delivered not the overall methodology. As instruction moves away from the traditional classroom lecture and clinical instruction to modalities that better accommodate the learning needs of individual students, the development of critical thinking skills and skills needed in the workplace are fostered (Bentley et al. 2003; Choi 2003; Cragg et al. 2003). The activities that can accomplish this may include simulations, virtual reality, VLE as a supplement to classroom instruction, slide presentations, Internet searches, collaborative learning, computerized testing, and the availability of reference materials online and on Personal Digital Assistants (PDAs) (Bloom & Hough 2003; Myles 2000). IBM (2007) recently released a three-dimensional (3D) anatomic and symbolic mapper engine that provides physicians with the ability to interact with medical data as they would with a human being. The interactive 3D software program allows healthcare students to get under simulated skin to view the cardiovascular and muscular systems. Furthermore, a physician or student clicks on the anatomical part the patient is complaining about, such as pain in the elbow, and all of the patient's important medical records (such as lab reports, body scans, and x-ray results) regarding the body part are displayed on the screen for immediate review. This software program is like an electronic health record (EHR) with interactive 3D images of the human body. These activities may replace, or supplement, the traditional lecture format, which supports passive rather than active learning. Institutions are also responding to consumer demands for new models and methods for instructional delivery. Computer-enhanced communication and education may increase student access to experts and educational programs through the removal of geographical boundaries. The inclusion of computers in education is vital to the development of basic computer skills needed in the workplace. Many programs suggest, and some require, that students purchase and use PDAs in the classroom and clinical settings to access reference materials and take notes. Computers are used in the clinical setting to document client care on hospital information systems. As a result of this expanding use of computers, most nursing programs have institutional academic computer plans, policies, and facilities. This reflects expectations that nursing graduates possess basic computer literacy skills (AACN 1998; ANA 2001). Nursing education programs are a logical place to introduce or expand basic computer skills such as word processing, Internet access, e-mail, electronic searches, and spreadsheet and database applications. These computer literacy skills are important in the everyday workplace, as they serve to increase access to information, facilitate the teaching/learning process, decrease anxiety associated with computer use, and enhance job skills. Basic computer literacy provides a framework for the development of another skill set expected of new graduates, namely rudimentary information management. For these reasons, basic nursing programs require that students take an introductory computer course, and an increasing number require an introduction to a nursing informatics course.

While in school, many nursing students are exposed to the Health Education Systems, Incorporated (HESI) exit exams and the National Council Licensure Examination for Registered Nurses (NCLEX-RN) review programs. The HESI exams serve as a predictor of NCLEX performance. Exposure to these examinations is important because all nurses in the United States take their licensure examination via computer. The NCLEX-RN examination uses computer adaptive testing (CAT) with the goal of determining candidate ability based on the difficulty of questions answered correctly, not the number answered correctly (NCSBN 2008; Wendt 2003). When a question is missed, the candidate is given an easier item to answer. If the candidate is able to answer the easier item correctly, the next item is more difficult. The NCLEX-RN uses an established minimum number of questions that must be answered but the total number of questions will vary by candidate. CAT offers several advantages over paper-and-pencil examinations. It saves time by matching items to individual ability, examinations are tailored to the individual, results may be available immediately, and it supports a variety of different reports (Latu & Chapman 2002; Van Horn 2003). NCLEX-RN preparation programs vary in quality, ranging from simple drill and practice to those that provide rationale for answers. An example of an NCLEX-RN educational endeavor is the weekly NCLEX question that is available to students online

---

BOX 16–4   Features to Look for in NCLEX-RN Preparation Programs

- Clearly defined system requirements such as types of computer, operating system, memory requirements, and any special software needed such as a media player
- Ease of use
- Feedback for answers. For example, does it provide rationale for answers and scores?
- Screen design and keyboard use that simulates the NCLEX-RN
- High quality and clear questions
- Random generation of questions similar to the NCLEX-RN
- A match between the preparation program content and NCLEX-RN examination content
- A bookmark feature that allows students to exit the program and return to the same spot later
- Clear instructions
- Adequate technical support
- System requirements such as type of computer and memory requirements

---

(Kaplan Nursing 2007). Educators and nursing students need to be discriminating consumers. One question to consider is the approach and intended purpose of the program. For example, some provide a means to decrease anxiety over the NCLEX-RN examination through practice under similar conditions. They may also attempt to simulate the examination experience. Other programs claim to predict student success on the NCLEX-RN examination. Box 16–4 lists some criteria to consider when selecting NCLEX-RN preparation software.

The benefits associated with computer-supported learning have led to an increased availability of courses and educational software related to nursing and healthcare topics. It is important to evaluate the quality of these applications and to use them in an effective manner. The nurse educator is responsible for evaluating the merits of available tools prior to their implementation. It is not necessary to be a software expert to do this. Faculty should use the same criteria to evaluate computer uses in education that they apply to any other instructional medium. Box 16–5 lists criteria that may be used to evaluate the quality of instructional software.

Administrative computer applications improve record keeping for program attendance, performance, and evaluation and can save time for the construction,

---

BOX 16–5   Evaluation Criteria for Instructional Software

- Does it support the overall course objectives?
- Is the material presented clearly?
- Is content accurate?
- What is the quality of the design? Does it maintain learner interest and provide the ability to customize learning to individual needs?
- Is information presented in a logical order?
- Does it provide appropriate and immediate feedback?
- Does it make good use of graphics, design, and multimedia?

administration, and scoring and statistical analysis of test results. Although most evaluative tools focus on testing, computers and PDAs lend themselves nicely to notes and anecdotal accounts of clinical learning, which can be used to evaluate individuals and the quality of specific learning experiences as well as support curriculum changes (Meyer, Sedlmeyer, Carlson, & Modlin 2003). An increasing number of faculty are turning toward software applications and technology to make the clinical evaluation process less arduous. In some cases, Web-based tools accept input from both faculty and students, tabulating results and providing information for curriculum decisions.

Hospital Information Systems (HIS) Connectivity with real hospital information systems (HIS) is another important use of computers in nursing education. The incorporation of hospital and nursing information systems into nursing school curricula promotes professional socialization, helps students see the effects of their decision making with care plans or maps, and decreases orientation time for new graduates. Computer-generated care plans or maps allow students to devote more time to the analysis of data, rather than to the writing of care plans, and allow staff more time to mentor students. This use of information systems ensures that graduates have exposure to computers and that they possess marketable job skills, and helps students to see the whole clinical picture. Students may receive live training sessions in system use by faculty or by hospital-based trainers or use computer-based training (CBT). Training may occur at the school or healthcare facility. Students can retrieve information for use in preparing for client assignments, but should not be able to make changes or add information to the actual client record from remote sites.

Access to hospital information systems as a learning tool in schools of nursing offers the following benefits (Doorley, Renner, & Corron 1994; Kennedy 2003; Poirrier, Wills, Broussard, & Payne 1996):

- Provides time to analyze clinical information
- Provides the student with adequate time to compose care plans or review critical pathways
- Allows students to review their plans with faculty or hospital nursing staff prior to entry into the system
- Increases students' knowledge and proficiency when they enter the actual clinical setting

HIS connectivity may be provided at schools of nursing. This requires negotiation with the vendor for permission. Other considerations include increased demands upon the information system and concerns related to confidentiality of client information. HIS connectivity allows students to be more familiar with their assigned clients and poses fewer interruptions for staff from students requesting information. HIS connectivity provides students with the opportunity to retrieve diagnostic results, vital signs, admission assessment data, and nursing documentation for review prior to their assigned clinical hours. Incorporation of hospital and nursing information systems at schools of nursing also facilitates role transition from student to graduate nurse, makes graduates more attractive to prospective employers, and allows hospitals to cut orientation time for graduates with prior HIS training.

Continuing Education

Nationwide budget cuts caused many institutions and employers to reduce or eliminate continuing education program offerings provided by traditional classes, conferences, and workshops. There is now an increased reliance on outside agencies and technology to meet this need. The traditional approach to this problem has been home study offered through professional journals and organizations. Readers review articles, answer related questions, send in their test form and fee, and wait to find out whether they received credit. The journal approach offers little, if any, interaction with peers. Mandatory education requirements such as fire safety were often met through the review of video or paper self-learning modules. Another approach is the use of the Internet for continuing education courses. This approach offers several benefits. It is available without a subscription 24 hours a day to a large population. Furthermore, it can provide instant feedback and highly individualized instruction, since the incorporation of links allows users to skip familiar content or seek additional information as required. It allows staff to attend mandatory programs at convenient times without interruption to client services and decreases expenses for travel between sites and instructor hours (Harrington & Walker 2003). Internet continuing education programs may be found through professional publications and organizations, as well as Web searches. Unfortunately, this option requires access to a computer.

Computers can also be used for administrative support of continuing education (Cragg et al. 2004). For example, computerized records can be searched rapidly to determine if and when a particular student attended a program, such as fire safety or cardiopulmonary resuscitation (CPR). It is also possible to administer and score proficiency examinations and evaluation tools. Other tracking features can show individuals who started, but did not complete, an educational unit or the number of attempts needed to achieve successful completion. Improved records also help to determine program costs and demonstrate staff development or continuing education staff productivity.

E-learning has been suggested as an alternative delivery method for mandatory educational programs as well as other programs that provide employees with opportunities to improve or maintain skill sets (Hequet 2004; Hirumi 2002; Joch 2003). The rationale for this approach is that e-learning allows employees to learn at their own pace and skip material that they already know. There are no costs associated with travel, lodging, or meals. It also helps to meet deadlines for mandatory education programs. Training is available upon demand, and course materials and tests are online. Institutions using e-learning to meet mandatory educational programs should choose a product that easily allows customization, as regulations change and programs need to be revised. In addition, e-learning can support synchronous or asynchronous communications, but asynchronous communications are more common and are often mediated by technology. Appraisal of the effectiveness of e-learning may be done through participant evaluation as well as a review of technical support logs.

Client Education

Although many computer applications directly benefit nurses and other healthcare professionals, consumers derive much of their healthcare information from the Internet, educational software, and e-mail. Some sites allow consumers to pose questions and then provide an answer within 24 hours. Home pages on the World Wide Web provide information on a variety of topics, including preparation for diagnostic tests. They may even show video clips of medical-surgical procedures. Web-based client education materials must be designed with the following factors in mind: purpose, target population, expected clinical and learning outcomes, educational framework, design principles, and ongoing site evaluation for readability and ease of navigation (Smith, Cha, Puno, Magee, Bingham, & Van Gorp 2002). Effective instructional Websites should also incorporate different learning modalities (Vogt et al. 2001). Client education materials and discharge instructions can be generated by hospital information systems as well.

An example of this application may be seen with a client who had heart bypass surgery. Instructions should include the following: when to schedule a follow-up visit with the cardiac surgeon and the primary physician, wound care, signs or symptoms that should be reported to the physician, and discharge medications. Computer generation of discharge instructions can tailor instructions to the individual client and the physician authorizing the discharge, and offers the following advantages:

- Consistent instruction despite the fact that different nurses provide teaching
- Improved quality and detail
- Speed
- Clarity and legibility
- Eliminates repetition so nurses no longer need to write the same instructions over and over again.
- Compliance with physician recommendations.
- Provides individualized, printed discharge teaching instructions with the capability to incorporate evidence-based guidelines

ISSUES RELATED TO COMPUTER-ENHANCED EDUCATION

The mere presence and use of computers for education do not ensure successful learning. Consideration of the following factors and guidelines will enhance the effectiveness of using computers for education:

- *Institutional planning.* Computer-enhanced education must be a part of an overall plan that makes provisions for infrastructure, as well as financial and technical support.

- *Hardware and software must be accessible.* This includes technical support, servers, and all software that the learner is expected to use. Problems with access and poor service immediately set a negative tone.
- *User comfort with the technology.* Not all learners are familiar with computers or know how to use them. This lack of knowledge and skills may lead to anxiety. For this reason, computer literacy should be a prerequisite, and a basic introduction to computers should be provided to faculty and students before the introduction of any new technology. Short, highly interactive training sessions that cover small amounts of information at one time are recommended. Once the learner is comfortable with the technology, other learning needs can be met (Chen 2003; Scollin 2001).
- *Opportunities to ask about material not understood.* Although the computer is an invaluable instructional aid, the ability to question and discuss information presented must also be available.
- *Instruction is well designed and well matched to course objectives.* High-quality Web-based instruction and computer programs for education must maintain learner interest and provide the appropriate information (Bloom & Hough 2003).
- *Evaluation criteria are identified to monitor the effectiveness of the computer as a tool.* These may include increased use of e-mail, increased job satisfaction, and improved student achievement. Online course evaluations may also be used.

There are a number of issues that must be addressed for faculty who are either interested in developing online courses and other means of computer-enhanced instruction, or who feel that they are under pressure from their respective institutions to teach online courses. These issues include:

- *Faculty workload, or hours, for the development and presentation of computer-enhanced instruction.* Administrative support of faculty who develop and present online courses, computer tutorials, and other applications that support education should include release time and/or financial rewards.
- *Promotion and tenure policies.* The design, development, and ongoing support of computer-enhanced or online instruction are time-consuming and labor-intensive. However, this time-intensive work is recognized by today's students, who expect technology to be woven throughout their educational experiences. Therefore, students will evaluate faculty accordingly, and perhaps positive teaching evaluations will have a direct effect on promotion in rank and tenure. As more institutions adopt computer-enhanced instruction this area is being considered by peer-review committees.
- *Intellectual ownership.* Many faculty remain unclear on questions of intellectual ownership for computer-enhanced learning activities and online courses that they develop or materials that they post online as part of a course. Institutional policy needs to address this. Most faculty feel that they "own" a course that they developed and that no one else should be given that course to teach without their permission. Typically, however, this attitude conflicts with the policies of the organization.

EDUCATIONAL OPPORTUNITIES IN NURSING INFORMATICS

Until recent years, the opportunities for nurses and other healthcare professionals to learn more about informatics were largely limited to programs sponsored by special-interest groups. Only a handful of undergraduate and graduate nursing programs offered introductory nursing informatics courses. This situation is changing rapidly now as nursing informatics has become a popular topic. An increasing number of schools offer a graduate degree or a certificate with a nursing informatics focus. Some of these programs use distance or Web-based education, while others use the traditional classroom setting. Doctoral programs are still limited. There are also a number of programs with a focus on health information management or health informatics.

PERSONAL DIGITAL ASSISTANTS

Contributed by Dee McGonigle, PhD, RN, FACCE, FAAN

Personal digital assistants, or PDAs, have gained appeal due to their small size. Usually designed to fit in a pocket, PDAs are easily portable and have impressive performance capabilities that allow you to store, access, and organize information such as calendar entries, documents, spreadsheets, databases, notes, and to-do lists. Your capabilities and access are limited by the processing speed and memory; the faster and more robust the memory capabilities are, the bigger the price tag. If you are considering purchasing a PDA, it is important that you reflect on your current and future needs. You want to be able to expand your capabilities as needed without having to replace your PDA. Therefore, it is important to review all of the PDAs available (c|net 2008a; c|net 2008b; Softpedia 2007a; Softpedia 2007b).

Most of today's PDAs use Linux, PocketPC (Windows), or PalmOS (Palm) operating systems. Since PDAs can be used in networked environments, including wireless configurations, they can theoretically give the clinician constant access to patient information, colleagues, and other necessary resources.

The applications provide a wide range of functionality, from simple to highly complicated software tools. You can take dictation, practice telenursing, and access dosage calculators, drug and specialty databases, educational applications, and clinical forecasting tools—all from your PDA. Since the PDA is compact and you use a stylus or scroll bars to manage your information, there are many add-ons available to enhance functionality as well as ease of use in inputting, accessing, and output.

How to Use a PDA

The PDA could have the following equipment: a display/touch screen, IR (infrared) port, USB connector, SD slot (secure digital memory), clock icon, menu icon, sync icon, find icon, web browser button, navigator button or pad, calendar icon, home icon, contacts icon, scroll button/bar, headphone jack, internal

Bluetooth, internal Wi-Fi, speaker, multi-connector, reset button, stylus, microphone, and/or cell phone capabilities. Examine a PDA at a vendor or online at Softpedia (2007c). The configuration of the PDA will affect its performance and your ability to use it. The navigation buttons and scroll functions allow you to see, access, and open applications, files, and documents. Depending on the PDA you choose, how you input your data and commands will vary. There are handwriting and voice recognition capabilities available but typically you will use a blending of a plastic stylus, touch screen, and handwriting recognition software. The handwriting software that recognizes the characters you write and transfers them to letters and numbers is Graffiti on Palms and Block Recognizer for Pocket PCs. The Transcriber software used on the Pocket PC will recognize legible normal handwriting, printing, or a combination of both; thus, you do not have to remember the character codes for the letters and numbers. You can also type in your input using the soft keyboard, a small keyboard on the screen, or add-ons such as a small or full size peripheral keyboard using a Bluetooth or USB connection.

Almost all of the current PDAs come with an expansion slot enabling you to increase your memory or storage space. Secure Digital (SD) is a common type of card that provides inexpensive additional memory. If you are thinking about purchasing a PDA, an expansion slot is a must-have item in today's environment.

Most PDAs come with office applications, sync software, Bluetooth, cables, and an IR port. The office applications could include word processing, spreadsheets, database, and/or presentation software. The sync software is short for "synchronize" and functions to match and update information on both your computer and PDA. Bluetooth is a form of wireless connection that is commonly used in cell phones; although it usually does not provide Internet access, it does facilitate file transfer between your PDA and a computer. You can purchase an adaptor if you have a PDA without Bluetooth. Cables are an inexpensive way to connect to a computer. You essentially plug the PDA into your computer. The downside is that you must be near the computer in order to connect. The IR beams of light are used as a unidirectional means to wirelessly transfer select data or entire programs to other PDAs. The data and information are not exchanged or traded but rather transferred in one direction. If you had something that was needed in hard copy, you could also beam a document to an IR enabled printer. People most commonly beam their business cards. For example, if you are at a career fair or conference visiting exhibitor booths, you could beam your business card into a vendor's PDA. The quest to beam across platforms would require additional software.

As PDAs continue to evolve, so do their capabilities and connectivity. The Internet connectivity (Web browser and e-mail) provides the clinician with communication capabilities and constant access to real time online data and information. Since the PDA is portable, your connectivity must be ready whenever and wherever you need it. One way to establish connectivity is through the use of Wi-Fi. The Wi-Fi compatibility provides for use at hotspots throughout the country, such as coffee shops, hotels, restaurants, universities, and other sites. It can also use your existing wireless network in your agency or office. You can add this feature to a PDA by purchasing a Wi-Fi adaptor.

Some cell phones, called smartphones, have limited PDA capabilities, and some PDAs are phone enabled. Smartphones have limited PC functionality; they have an operating system and facilitate the use of e-mail and other applications. The addition of the phone features could be an important consideration based on your practice setting.

Applications

As nurses, there are tremendous advantages to using a PDA. They can be used to track patients, as Point of Care (POC) devices, or as calculators. The PDA could take your dictation at the bedside or on the go as you travel between patients. As reference tools, PDAs can provide ready access to clinical and/or drug databases; electronic textbooks and reference materials; online journals in real-time, such as the Online Journal of Nursing Informatics (OJNI) and MEDLINE; educational tools such as study guides; and care planning documents (Skyscape, n.d.; Dykes Library, 2008: PDA Cortex, n.d.). You can transfer information within your network even when you are in the field, such as sending a note to a case manager, updating a physician on the status of a patient you visited in her home, or sending a prescription to the pharmacy. The PDA allows you to maintain your calendar or schedule and receive reminder alarms. You can even use your PDA for professional development such as continuing education offerings or furthering your academic education online. Get involved and participate in the online group that discusses PDA use in nursing at http://www.rnpalm.com/nursing_pdas_listserv.htm.

As a nursing student, the reference materials and podcasts available for your coursework could be stored on your PDA for easy access. You could upload and download clinical documents and information with your instructor and clinical setting staff.

The PDA can enhance the healthcare for patients as well. We can monitor our patients and send surveys and questionnaires; patients can submit their responses to us as their healthcare provider or to the healthcare institution. The PDA can enhance their access to their clinicians, especially if the patient is mobile; the PDA can go where the patients go and they can keep in touch via e-mail, phone, Fax, and instant or text messaging. Patients can maintain their appointment and medication schedule as well as receive patient education materials and access clinician-recommended Websites/Listservs.

We have certainly not included an exhaustive list of PDA applications or equipment, and the current will be the past by the time this is in print. PDAs continue to evolve and become smaller and more robust (About.com n.d.; Seko 2005; Softpedia 2007a; Softpedia 2007b). As this future continues to unfold, so will our uses for PDAs in nursing.

FUTURE DIRECTIONS

All forms of education will continue to evolve as more is understood about individual learners, their learning styles, and desired outcome behaviors. Technology will continue to support and enhance learning in ways that can scarcely be imagined at the present time, making learning more convenient anywhere, anytime. Simulation provides the means to foster learning in an environment that is safe for the student as well as the healthcare consumer. It is particularly useful for experiences that are difficult to provide for all students. As technology continues to become more pervasive throughout society it will also become more available and easier to use, affording yet more educational opportunities.

CASE STUDY EXERCISES

16.1   Locate and evaluate at least one online continuing education offering.

16.2   You are on the education committee at your small community hospital. Your staff development department was eliminated several years ago. You and your colleagues are charged with developing strategies to meet the educational needs of agency registered and licensed practical nurses. Limited capital and the isolated location of your community make this a difficult assignment. Your institution does have Internet and World Wide Web access in the medical library, as well as teleconferencing capability. Develop a proposal to meet your charge using available resources. Be prepared to defend your proposal to an administration loathe to part with monies beyond those already budgeted.

16.3   You are the client educator at a medical center in the Pacific Northwest. Your clientele are drawn from a 150-mile radius and beyond. It is difficult to have clients complete diabetic education or other classes. You have been told to improve client completion of classes or face elimination of your department. The medical center has both teleconferencing capability, presently used for consults, and an established Web page that provides basic information about the institution. How might you use these resources to develop alternative strategies for client education? Address budget considerations, necessary resources, target populations that might be better served, and how you propose to link distant clients with instructional offerings.

16.4   You recently joined the faculty at a small, private rural college. Because you express an interest in computers and are slightly more knowledgeable about computers than are your faculty colleagues, you have been asked to establish online sites for all of the traditionally taught courses to post the course syllabi, announcements, handouts, and other relevant course materials as a mechanism to facilitate learning. Your institution already owns a course management system. How would you proceed? What, if any, additional applications might you consider when working on this project?

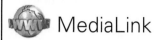 MediaLink

Additional resources for this content can be found on the Companion Website at www.prenhall.com/hebda. Click on "Chapter 16" to select the activities for this chapter.

- Glossary
- Multiple Choice
- Discussion Points
- Case Studies
- MediaLink Application
- MediaLink

SUMMARY

- Computer technology can help revolutionize education in formal healthcare programs, continuing education, and consumer education. It also provides informal opportunities for networking among professionals via e-mail, and social networking systems, such as wikis, blogs, and podcasts.
- Successful use of computers for education requires careful planning, specific learning objectives, orientation to the technology, convenient access, opportunities to question what is not understood, instructional design, and sound evaluation of learning outcomes.
- Formal nursing education is a logical place to introduce or expand basic computer skills, such as word processing, Internet access, e-mail, online literature searches, and use of Web 2.0 applications.
- Educational software should be subject to the same review criteria applied to other instructional materials before their adoption and following student use.
- Computer instruction should clearly match curriculum level and objectives.
- NCLEX-RN preparation programs and HESI exit exams are a popular use of computerized test programs in basic nursing programs.
- Connectivity to hospital information systems from schools of nursing allows students more opportunity to analyze client information before scheduled clinical experiences and facilitates professional socialization.
- Computers provide invaluable assistance in the preparation of educational materials and presentations, the delivery of instruction, examinations and evaluations, and the maintenance of educational records.
- Virtual Learning Environments are examples of the use of a computer to teach a subject other than computing. A VLE offers the following advantages: convenience, decreased learning time, and increased retention.
- Teleconferencing is the use of computers, audio and video equipment, and high-grade dedicated telephone lines, cable, or satellite connections to provide interactive communication between two or more persons at two or more sites. It may occur via desktop computers or via larger systems with multiple persons participating at one time.

- Distance education is the use of print, audio, video, computer, or tele-conference capability to connect faculty and students located at a minimum of two different sites. Distance education may take place in real time or on a delayed basis. It expands educational opportunities without the need for a long commute.
- Web-based instruction uses the attributes and resources of the Internet to deliver and support education. It may be used as a stand-alone course or to supplement traditional classes.
- E-learning uses electronic media to present instruction. It is often suggested for corporate training because it is considered to be efficient. It allows users to skip material that they already know.
- Multimedia refers to the ability to deliver presentations that combine text, voice or sound, images, and video. Multimedia presentations tend to improve learning by actively engaging the senses.
- Educational opportunities in nursing informatics range from the informal to the formal. There are numerous introductory courses on undergraduate and graduate levels. Some institutions offer areas of specialization within a degree on the graduate level or certificate programs. Opportunities for doctoral work in nursing informatics are limited.

REFERENCES

American Association of Colleges of Nursing (AACN). (1998). *Essentials of baccalaureate education for professional nursing practice.* Washington, DC: AACN.

American Nurses Association (ANA). (2001). *Scope and standards of nursing informatics practice.* Washington, DC: American Nurses Publishing.

Barrett, M. J., Lacey, C. S., Sekara, A. E., Linden, E. A., & Gracely, E. J. (2004). Mastering cardiac murmurs. *Chest, 126,* 470–475.

Batscha, C. (2002). The pharmacology game. *CIN Plus, 5*(3), 1, 3–6.

Bentley, G. W., Cook, P. P., Davis, K., Murphy, M. J., & Berding, C. B. (2003). RN to BSN program: Transition from traditional to online delivery. *Nurse Educator, 28*(3), 121–126.

Billings, D. M. (1994). Effects of BSN student preferences for studying alone or in groups on performance and attitude when using interactive videodisc instruction. *Journal of Nursing Education, 33*(7), 322–324.

Billings, D. M. (1995). Preparing nursing faculty for information age teaching and learning. *Computers in Nursing, 13*(6), 264, 268–270.

Blood, R. (September 7, 2000). Weblogs: A history and perspective. [*Rebecca's Pocket* Website]. Retrieved September 27, 2007, from http://www.rebeccablood.net/essays/weblog_history.html.

Bloom, K. C. & Hough, M. C. (2003). Student satisfaction with technology-enhanced learning. *CIN: Computers, Informatics, Nursing, 21*(5), 241–246.

Boulos, M. N. K. (2007). e-Health and Web 2.0: Looking to the future with sociable technologies and social software. Retrieved January 14, 2008, from http://www.slideshare.net/sl.medic/ehealth-and-web-20the-3d-web-looking-to-the-future-with-sociable-technologies-and-social-software-121698

Bradley, C. (2003). Technology as a catalyst to transforming nursing care. *Nursing Outlook, 51*(3), S14–S15.

Bruckley, K. M. (2003). Evaluation of classroom-based, web-enhanced, and web-based distance learning nutrition courses for undergraduate nursing. *Journal of Nursing Education, 42*(8), 367–370.

Calderone, A. B. (1994). Computer-assisted instruction: Learning, attitude, and modes of instruction. *Computers in Nursing, 12*(3), 164–170.

Cambre, M. & Castner, L. J. (March 1993). The status of interactive video in nursing education environments. Presented at FITNE: Get in Touch with Multimedia, Atlanta, GA.

Carnegie Mellon (2007). Podcasting: A teaching with technology white paper. Retrieved January 16, 2008, from http://www.cmu.edu/teaching/technology/research/index.html#podcasting.

Cartwright, J. (2000). Lessons learned: Using asynchronous computer-mediated conferencing to facilitate group discussion. *Journal of Nursing Education, 39*(2), 87–90.

Cell Phone as a Platform for Healthcare Request for Proposals 2007. (2007). Microsoft Research. Retrieved October 11, 2007, from http://research.microsoft.com/ur/us/fundingopps/RFPs/CellPhoneAsPlatformForHealthcare_RFP.aspx.

Charp, S. (2003). Technology for all students. *T.H.E. Journal, 30*(9), 8.

Chen, T. (2003). Recommendations for creating and maintaining effective networked learning communities. *International Journal of Instructional Media, 30*(1), 35.

Choi, H. (2003). A problem-based learning trail on the Internet involving undergraduate nursing students. *Journal of Nursing Education, 42*(8), 359–363.

Constructive Medicine: Benchside to Bedside 2.0. (2007). Retrieved January 14, 2008, from http://www.medicine20.org/wiki/index.php/Main_Page.

Corwin, E. J. (2000). Distance education: An ongoing initiative to reach rural family nurse practitioner students. *Nurse Educator, 25*(3), 114–115.

Cragg, C. E., Edwards, N., Yue, Z., Xin, S. L., & Hui, Z. D. (2003). Integrating web-based technology into distance education for nurses in China. *CIN: Computers, Informatics, Nursing, 21*(5), 265–274.

Cragg, C. E., Humbert, J., & Douchette, S. (2004). A toolbox of technical supports for nurses new to web learning. *CIN: Computers, Informatics, Nursing, 22*(1), 19–23.

Cuellar, N. (2002). Tips to increase success for teaching online: Communication! *CIN Plus, 5*(1), 1, 3–6.

Doorley, J. E., Renner, A. L., & Corron, J. (1994). Creating care plans via modems: Using a hospital information system in nursing education. *Computers in Nursing, 12*(3), 160–163.

Doherty, I., Hansen, M., McCann, L., Oosthuizen, G., Hardy, K., Greig, S., et al. (2007). Simulated learning for clinical skill acquisition and retention: Report on a research project with trainee medical interns. Paper is accepted for EdMedia 2008 Conference, Vienna, Austria.

Erdley, S. (2008). Videoconferencing. Personal communication. January 14, 2008.

Erdley, W. S., Murray, P. J., Hansen, M. M., Oyri, K., Ward, R., & Perry, W. F. (July 19, 2007). Connections, collaboration, and creativity: Exploring Web 2.0 applications in health informatics and professional development. Panel presentation at MedInfo2007, Brisbane, Australia

Faison, K. A. (2003). Professionalization in a distance learning setting. *The ABNF Journal: Official Journal of the Association of Black Nursing Faculty in Higher Education, 14*(4), 83–85.

Free Software Daily (2007). Retrieved September 17, 2007, from http://www.fsdaily.
  com/Business/New_InstallationWiki-org_Website_Launches_with_Free_
  Guides_for_Installing_Software/.
Gandhi, S. (2003). Academic librarians and distance education: Challenges and
  opportunities. *Reference & User Services Quarterly, 43*(2), 138.
Geibert, R. C. (2000). Integrating web-based instruction into a graduate nursing
  program taught via videoconferencing: Challenges and solutions. *Computers
  in Nursing, 18*(1), 26–34.
Gleydura, A. J., Michelman, J. E., & Wilson, C. N. (1995). Multimedia training in
  nursing education. *Computers in Nursing, 13*(4), 169–175.
Glover, S. M. & Kruse, M. (1995). Making the most of computer-assisted instruction.
  Nursing 95, 25(9), 32N.
Goodman, J. & Blake, J. (1996). Multimedia courseware: Transforming the classroom.
  Computers in Nursing, 14(5), 287–296.
Go Virtual Medical Ltd. (2007). Retrieved September 12, 2007, from http://www.
  govirtualmedical.com/.
Gould, J. W. III. (2003). Program planning of asynchronous online courses design
  complexities and ethics. *Acquisition Review Quarterly, 10*(1), 63.
Greco, J. F. & O'Connor, D. J. (2000). A role for computer-assisted instruction in the
  beginning undergraduate course. *Financial Practice & Education, 10*(1), 239–244.
Hansen, M. (2007a). Med-Calc Tutorial. Retrieved September 7, 2007, from
  http://www.m2hnursing.com.
Hansen, M. (2007b). m2hnursing.com ECG activity. Retrieved September 9, 2007,
  from http://www.m2hnursing.com/flash/ecg_activity.html.
Hansen, M., Doherty, I., McCann, L., Oosthuizen, G., Hardy, K., Greig, S., et al.
  (2007). Medical interns' clinical skills acquisition and self-confidence levels:
  Enhanced via iPods? Paper accepted for EdMedia 2008 Conference,
  Vienna, Austria.
Harden, J. K. (2003). Faculty and student experiences with web-based discussion
  groups in a large lecture setting. *Nurse Educator, 28*(1), 26–30.
Harrington, S. S. & Walker, B. L. (2003). Is computer-based instruction an effective
  way to present fire safety training to long-term care staff? *Journal for Nurses in
  Staff Development, 19*(3), 147–154.
Hequet, M. (2004). Training no one wants: Restive, rebellious, reluctant—Sometimes
  you're faced with employees who just don't want to be trained. What should you
  do? *Training, 41*(1), 22 (6p).
Hirumi, A. (2002). The design and sequencing of e-learning interactions: A grounded
  approach. *International Journal on E-Learning, 1*(1), 19–27.
IBM (2007). IBM (2007). Anatomic and symbolic mapper engine provides an interactive 3D model of the human body that displays health information at a glance.
  Retrieved September 27, 2007, from http://www-03.ibm.com/press/us/en/
  pressrelease/22375.wss.
Im, Y. & Lee, O. (2003). Pedagogical implications of online discussion for preservice
  teacher training. *Journal of Research on Technology in Education, 36*(2), 155.
Institute for Higher Education Policy (IHEP). (2000). *Quality on the line: Benchmarks
  for success in Internet-based distance education.* Retrieved February 19, 2004,
  from http://www.ihep.com/Pubs/PDF/Quality.pdf.
Institute of Medicine (2003). *Health Professions Education: A Bridge to Quality.*
  Washington, DC: The National Academies Press.
Jeiesiewicz, E. (2007, March 14). iPods help docs improve stethoscope skills. *Temple
  Times.* Retrieved September 27, 2007, from https://develop.temple.edu/
  temple_times/march07/DociPod.html.

Joch, A. (2003). Sites for sore eyes. *Healthcare Informatics, 20*(4), 31–33.

Kaplan Nursing (2007). Retrieved January 16, 2008, from http://www.kaplanmedical. com/Kaplan/Article/Nursing_Domestic/NCLEX-RN/Practice-the-NCLEX-RN/ question-of-the-week.html;jsessionid=PSWEV0EP24FAZLA3AQJHB NVMDUCBG2HB.

Kaplan-Leiserson, E. (2005). Trend: Podcasting in academic and corporate learning. *Learning Circuits.* Retrieved September 12, 2007, from http://www. learningcircuits.org/.

Kennedy, R. (2003). The nursing shortage and the role of technology. *Nursing Outlook, 51*(3), S33–S34.

Khoiny, F. E. (1995). Factors that contribute to computer-assisted instruction effectiveness. *Computers in Nursing, 13*(4), 165–168.

Kozlowski, D. (2002). Using online learning in a traditional face-to-face environment. *Computers in Nursing, 20*(1), 23–30.

Kozlowski, D. (2004). Factors for consideration in the development and implementation of an online RN-BSN course: Faculty and student perceptions, *CIN: Computers, Informatics, Nursing, 22*(1), 34–43.

Kropf, R. (2002). How shall we meet online? Choosing between videoconferencing and online meetings. *Journal of Healthcare Information Management, 16*(4), 68–72.

Latu, E. & Chapman, E. (2002). Computerised adaptive testing. *British Journal of Educational Technology, 33*(5), 619.

Lane, C. (2006). Podcasting at the UW: An evaluation of current use. Retrieved September 12, 2007, from catalyst.washington.edu/research_development/ papers/2006/podcasting_report.pdf.

Maag, M. (2004a). The effectiveness of an interactive multimedial learning tool on nursing students' math knowledge and self-efficacy. *CIN: Computers, Informatics, Nursing, 22*(1), 26–33.

Maag, M. (2004b). The potential use of *blogs* in nursing education. *Computers Informatics Nursing, 23*(1), 16–24.

Maag, M. (2006). Podcasting and MP3 players: Emerging education technologies. *Computers Informatics Nursing, 24*(1), 9–13.

Maag, M. (2007). iTunes lectures.

Malan, D. J. (2007). Podcasting computer science E-1. *SIGCSE'07.* 389–393.

Mayer, R. E. (2001). Multimedia Learning. New York: Cambridge University Press.

McKenna, L. G. & Samarawickrema, R. G. (2003). Crossing cultural boundaries: Flexible approaches and nurse education. *CIN: Computers, Informatics, Nursing, 21*(5), 259–264.

Meyer, L., Sedlmeyer, R., Carlson, C., & Modlin, S. (2003). A web application for recording and analyzing the clinical experiences of nursing students. *CIN: Computers, Informatics, Nursing, 21*(4), 186–195.

Mills, A. C. (2000). Creating web-based, multimedia, and interactive courses for distance learning. *Computers in Nursing, 18*(3), 125–131.

Moura, J. R., Murray, P., Hammond W. E., Hansen, M., & Erdley, S. (2007). IMIA Web 2.0 Exploratory Task Force: A Proposal. Retrieved April 7, 2008, from http://www.AMINA.org

Murray, P. J. & Maag, M. (2006). Towards health informatics 2.0: Blogs, podcasts and web 2.0 applications in nursing and health informatics education and professional collaboration. A discussion paper.

Myles, J. (2000). The Internet advances nursing education. *Healthcare Review, 13*(10), 4. Available at http://www.findarticles.com/cf–0/m-HSV/10_ 13/82393991/print.jhtml. Accessed January 21, 2004.

NCSBN (2008). NCLEX Examinations. Retrieved January 16, 2008, from https://www.ncsbn.org/nclex.htm.

O'Gara, N. & American Academy of Nursing. (2003). Recommendations of the American Academy of Nursing Conference participants. *Nursing Outlook, 51*(3), S39–S41.

O'Reilly, T. (2005). What is Web 2.0? Design patterns and business models for the next generation of software. Retrieved January 14, 2008, from http://www.oreillynet.com/pub/a/oreilly/tim/news/2005/09/30/what-is-web-20.html.

Oyri, K. (2007). Biomedical wireless sensor network project. Retrieved January 16, 2008, from http://www.bwsn.net/tiki-index.php.

Palmer, E. J. & McDevitt, P. G. (2007). A method of creating interactive content for the iPod, and its potential use as a learning tool: Technical advances. *BMC Medical Education, 7*(32). Retrieved January 14, 2008, from http://www.biomedcentral.com/1472–6920/7/32.

PodBean (2007). Podcast hosting. Retrieved January 14, 2008, from http://www.podbean.com/.

Poirrier, G. P., Wills, E. M., Broussard, P. C., & Payne, R. L. (1996). Nursing information systems: Applications in nursing curricula. *Nurse Educator, 21*(1), 18–22.

Ravert, P. (2002). An integrative review of computer-based simulation in the education process. *CIN: Computers, Informatics, Nursing, 20*(5), 203–208.

Rose, M. A., Frisby, A. J., Hamlin, M. D., & Jones, S. S. (2000). Evaluation of the effectiveness of a web-based graduate epidemiology course. *Computers in Nursing, 18(4),* 162–167.

Ross, G. D. & Tuovinen, J. E. (2001). Deep versus surface learning with multimedia in nursing education. *Computers in Nursing, 19*(5), 213–223.

Rossignol, M. & Scollin, P. (2001). Piloting use of computerized practice tests. *Computers in Nursing, 19*(5), 206–212.

Rouse, D. P. (2000). The effectiveness of computer-assisted instruction in teaching nursing students about congenital heart disease. *Computers in Nursing, 18*(6), 282–287.

Sakai Project (2007). Retrieved September 26, 2007, from http://sakaiproject.org/.

Second Health (2007). Retrieved September 27, 2007, from http://commons.wikimedia.org/wiki/Image:Web_2.0_Map.svg.

Sakraida, T. J. & Draus, P. J. (2003). Transition to a web-supported curriculum. *CIN: Computers, Informatics, Nursing, 21*(6), 309–315.

Sapnas, K. G., Walsh, S. M., Vilberg, W., Livingstone, P., Asher, M. E., Dlugasch, et al. (2002). Using web technology in graduate and undergraduate nursing education. *CIN Plus, 5*(2), 1, 33–37.

Scollin, P. (2001). A study of factors related to the use of online resources by nurse educators. *Computers in Nursing, 19*(6), 249–256.

Simpson, R. L. (2002). Virtual reality revolution: Technology changes nursing education. *Nursing Management, 33*(9), 14–15.

Skiba, D. (2007). Nursing education 2.0:YouTube. *Nursing Education Perspectives, 28*(2), 100–102.

Smith, C. E., Cha, J., Puno, F., Magee, J. D., Bingham, J., & Van Gorp, M. (2002). Quality assurance processes for designing patient education web sites. *CIN: Computers, Informatics, Nursing, 20*(5), 191–200.

Smith-Stoner, M. & Willer, A. (2003). Video streaming in nursing education. *Nurse Educator, 28*(2), 66–70.

Sternberger, C. & Meyer, L. (2001). Hypermedia-assisted instruction: Authoring with learning guidelines. *Computers in Nursing, 19*(2), 69–74.

Technorati Tags (2007). Retrieved September 16, 2007, from http://www.technorati.com.

Theile, J. E. (2003). Learning patterns of online students. *Journal of Nursing Education, 42*(8), 364–366.

Thurmond, V. A. (2003). Defining interaction and strategies to enhance interactions in web-based courses. *Nurse Educator, 28*(5), 237–241.

University of Tasmania School of Nursing and Midwifery (2007). Retrieved September 7, 2007, from http://www.m2hnursing.com.

University of Michigan Blog (2007). Retrieved September 16, 2007, from http://www2. med.umich.edu/medschool/reality/.http://www.med.umich.edu/medstudents/ curRes/streamingVids/podcast/index.html.

VandeVusse, L. & Hanson, L. (2000). Evaluation of online course discussions: Faculty facilitation of active student learning. *Computers in Nursing, 18*(4), 181–188.

Van Horn, R. (2003). Technology: Computer adaptive tests and computer-based tests. *Phi Delta Kappan, 84*(8), 567.

Vogt, C., Kumrow, D., & Kazlauskas, E. (2001). The design elements in developing effective learning and instructional web-sites. *Academic Exchange Quarterly, 5*(4), 40.

Wang, S. & Sleeman, P. J. (1993a). A comparison of the relative effectiveness of computer-assisted instruction and conventional methods for teaching an operations management course in a school of business. *International Journal of Instructional Media, 20*(3), 225–235.

Wang, S. & Sleeman, P. J. (1993b). Computer-assisted instruction effectiveness: A brief review of the research. *International Journal of Instructional Media, 20*(4), 333–348.

Ward, R. (2007). Informaticopia. Retrieved September 17, 2007, from http://www. rodspace.co.uk/blog/blogger.html.

Wendt, A. (2003). Frequently asked questions about computer-adaptive testing. *Computers, Informatics, Nursing: CIN Plus, 21*(1), 46–48.

Wikipedia (2007). Retrieved January 16, 2008, from http://www.wikipedia.com.

Wikipedia (2007a). Virtual Learning Environment. Retrieved September 17, 2007, from http://en.wikipedia.org/wiki/Virtual_learning_environment.

Wikipedia (2007b). Web 2.0. Retrieved September 17, 2007, from http://en.wikipedia. org/wiki/Web_2.

Wikipedia (2007c). Skype. Retrieved September 12, 2007, from http://en.wikipedia. org/wiki/Skype.

Wikimedia (2007). A multilingual free encyclopedia. Retrieved January 18, 2008, from http://www.wikimedia.com.

Wong, G., Greenhalgh, T., Russell, J., Boynton, P., & Toon, P. (2003). Putting your course on the web: Lessons from a case study and systematic literature review. *Medical Education, 37*(11), 1020–1023.

Yensen, J. A. P. (2005). Leveraging RSS feeds to support current awareness. *Computers, Informatics, Nursing: CIN Plus, 23*(3), 164–167.

YouTube Website (2007). Retrieved September 9, 2007, from http://www.youtube. comhttp://docs.google.com/TeamPresent?docid=dd2trp3s_0tj8txc&pli=1.

PDA REFERENCES

About.com (n.d.). Palmtops/PDAs: Fossil Wrist PDA FX2008 with Palm OS Review. Retrieved on January 12, 2008, from http://palmtops.about.com/od/ palmhardware/fr/FossilWristPDA.htm.

c|net. (2008a). c|net Reviews: Compare PDAs. Retrieved on January 12, 2008, from http://reviews.cnet.com/4244-5_7–0.html?query=PDA&tag=srch&target=.

c|net. (2008b). c|net Reviews: What to look for in handhelds. Retrieved on January 12, 2008, from http://reviews.cnet.com/4520-3127_7-5021319-1.html?tag=wtlf%5C%22%3Ehttp://computers.cnet.com/hardware/0-1087-8-20549052-1.html?tag=wtlf.

Dykes Library. (2008). Popular freeware for PDAs. Retrieved on January 12, 2008, from http://library.kumc.edu/resources/PDAFreebies.htm.

PDA Cortex. (n.d.). The Journal of Mobile Informatics and PDA Resources for Healthcare Professionals. Retrieved on January 12, 2008, from http://www.rnpalm.com/.

Seko, S. (2005). Ir Watch Ver 0.3 The version only for WristPDA. Retrieved on January 12, 2008, from http://www.pamupamu.com/soft/irmoniw/irw.htm.

Skyscape. (n.d.). Nursing. Retrieved on January 12, 2008, from http://www.skyscape.com/estore/store.aspx?category=36.

Softpedia. (2007a). Handhelds area and latest handheld devices (RSS). Retrieved on January 12, 2008, from http://handheld.softpedia.com/#devices.

Softpedia. (2007b). Headline News: Handhelds news and latest handhelds news. Retrieved on January 12, 2008, from http://news.softpedia.com/cat/Telecoms/Handhelds/.

Softpedia. (2007c). Handhelds area and PDA Manual 1.0 Download (for the PocketPC). Retrieved on January 13, 2008, from http://handheld.softpedia.com/get/Documents-E-Books/Pda-Manual-36435.shtml.

CHAPTER 17

Telehealth

After completing this chapter, you should be able to:

1 Define the term *telehealth*.

2 List the advantages of telehealth.

3 Identify equipment and technology needed to sustain telehealth.

4 Discuss present and proposed telehealth applications.

5 Describe legal and practice issues that affect telehealth.

6 Review the implications of telehealth for nursing and other health professions.

7 Identify several telenursing applications.

8 Discuss some issues pertaining to the practice of telenursing.

Telehealth is the use of telecommunication technologies and computers to exchange healthcare information and to provide services to clients at another location. This was once known as *telemedicine*, but applications are now widely used by other members of the healthcare community. The American Nurses Association (1996) prefers the term *telehealth* as a more inclusive and accurate description of the services provided. Telehealth services include health promotion, disease prevention, diagnosis, consultation, education, and therapy. Teleconferences and videoconferences are tools used to deliver these services. Electronic, visual, and audio signals sent during these conferences provide information to consultants from remote sites. Many common medical devices have been adapted for use with telemedicine technology. Distant practitioners and clients benefit from the skills and knowledge of the consultants without the need to travel to regional referral centers. Telehealth is a tool that allows healthcare professionals to do the following (Coyle, Duffy, & Martin 2007; Cross 2007; Demiris, Edison, & Vijaykumar 2005; Liaw & Humphreys 2006; Merrill 2007; Yun & Park 2007):

- Consult with colleagues
- Conduct interviews
- Assess and monitor clients
- View diagnostic images
- Review slides and laboratory reports
- Extend scarce healthcare resources
- Decrease the number of hospital visits for patients with chronic conditions
- Decrease healthcare costs
- Tackle isolation and loneliness
- Provide health education
- Improve the coordination of care
- Improve the equity of access to services
- Improve the quality of client care
- Improve the overall quality of the client's record

Numerous terms have been coined to describe these capabilities (see Box 17–1 for a partial listing).

TERMS RELATED TO TELEHEALTH

Initially *telemedicine* was the predominant term for the delivery of healthcare education and services via the use of telecommunication technologies and computers. It has since largely been replaced by the term *telehealth*. Telehealth encompasses telemedicine but is a broader term that emphasizes both the delivery of services and the provision of information and education to healthcare providers and consumers. For example, federal agencies use the Internet to provide healthcare professionals, consumers, and their families with medical information. The Public Health Service's Agency for Health Care Policy and Research (AHCPR) places clinical practice guidelines online. The U.S. National Library of Medicine provides information on health, various medical

BOX 17–1   Some Common Telehealth Terms

- **E-care.** The provision of health information, products, and services online as well as the automation of administrative and clinical aspects of care delivery.
- **E-health.** A broad term often used interchangeably with the term *telehealth* to refer to the provision of health information, products, and services online.
- **E-medicine.** The use of telecommunication and computer technology for the delivery of medical care.
- **Telecardiology.** Transmission of cardiac catheterization studies, echocardiograms, and other diagnostic tests in conjunction with electronic stethoscope examinations for second opinions by cardiologists at another site.
- **Telecare.** The remote delivery of healthcare services into the home via information and communication technology that include the use of monitoring devices.
- **Teleconsultation.** Videoconferencing between two healthcare professionals or a healthcare professional and a client.
- **Telehomecare.** The use of telecommunication and computer technologies to monitor and render services and support to home care clients.
- **Telementoring.** Real-time advice offered during a procedure to a practitioner in a remote site via a telecommunication system.
- **Telenursing.** The use of telecommunication and computer technology for the delivery of nursing care.
- **Telepathology.** Transmission of high-resolution still images, often via a robotic microscope, for interpretation by a pathologist at a remote site.
- **Teleprevention.** The use of telecommunication technology to provide opportunities to promote health.
- **Telepsychiatry.** Variant of teleconsultation that allows observation and interviews of clients at one site by a psychiatrist at another site.
- **Telerehabilitation.** The use of interactive technology to facilitate exercise and rehabilitation activities.
- **Teleradiology.** Transmission of high-resolution still images for interpretation by a radiologist at a distant location.
- **Telesurgery.** Technology that allows surgeons at a remote site to collaborate with experts at a referral center on techniques.
- **Teletherapy.** The use of interactive videoconferencing to provide therapy and counseling.
- **Teleultrasound.** Transmission of ultrasound images for interpretation at a remote site.

conditions and procedures, clinical trials, and the capability to conduct searches of several databases on its Website. There also are a number of professional journals and articles available online. Some require subscription; some do not. One example of an online journal is the National Cancer Institute's *JNCI Cancer Spectrum*. This publication incorporates a wide range of cancer information from respected sources. It allows readers to browse by topic, and does require a subscription. As a consequence of the information explosion, healthcare professionals and clients gain access to the most current treatment options at essentially the same time. No matter what term is used, the basic premise of telehealth is that it can provide services to underserved communities. Another frequently used term is *e-health*, which is often used interchangeably with the term *telehealth*. **Telenursing** is the use of telecommunications and computer technology for the delivery of nursing care.

Teleconferencing

Teleconferencing implies that people at different locations have audio, and possibly video, contact, which is used to carry out telehealth applications. The terms *teleconference* and *videoconference* may be used synonymously, because both use telecommunications and computer technology.

Videoconferencing

Videoconferencing implies that people meet face-to-face and view the same images through the use of telecommunications and computer technology even though they are not in the same location. It saves travel time and costs, which actually encourages people to meet more frequently. Videoconferencing is an appealing concept that can be used for many applications, especially distance learning and telehealth (although some applications may require high resolution and audio quality and high-speed transmission). For example, videoconferences provide a means to improve quality and access to care in Alaska, where clinics are connected. Live conferences are used to view critically ill clients, and specially adapted medical equipment is used to collect and send assessment data digitally. Communities benefit by saving travel time and costs for this arrangement, and appropriate care can be initiated in a timely fashion (Smith 2004).

Desktop Videoconferencing

Desktop videoconferencing (DTV) is a synchronous, or real-time, encounter that uses a specially equipped personal computer with telephone line hookup, DSL or cable connections to allow people to meet face-to-face and/or view papers and images simultaneously. DTV is less expensive than custom-designed videoconference systems, but it may not be acceptable for telehealth applications that require high-resolution or high-speed transmission, such as interpretation of diagnostic images where slower frame rates produce a jerky image or lengthy transmission times.

HISTORICAL BACKGROUND

Telehealth began with the use of telephone consults and has become more sophisticated with each advance in technology. During the past four decades the U.S. government played a major role in the development and promotion of telehealth through various agencies. Interest waned as funding slowed to a trickle in the 1980s but subsequent technological advancements made telehealth attractive again. Federal monies and the Agriculture Department's 1991 Rural Development Act laid the groundwork to bring the information superhighway to rural areas for education and telehealth purposes.

The most aggressive development of telehealth in the United States has been by NASA and the military (Brown 2002). NASA provided international telehealth consults for Armenian earthquake victims in 1989. The military has also had several projects to feed medical images from the battlefield to physicians in hospitals and on robotics equipment for telesurgery for improved treatment of casualties.

Another large U.S. telehealth application has been the provision of care to state inmates by the medical branch of the University of Texas at Galveston (Brown 2002). Other states also use telehealth to treat prisoners, avoiding the costs and danger of transporting prisoners. New York piloted a telepsychiatric project that was well received (Manfredi, Shupe, & Batki 2005).

One major barrier to telehealth was removed with the passage of the Telecommunications Act of 1996, which allowed vendors of cable and telephone services to compete in each others' markets (Schneider 1996). This event helped to open the door to create the information superhighway needed to provide the framework to support telehealth. The Snowe–Rockefeller Amendment required telecommunications carriers to offer services to rural health providers at rates comparable to those charged in urban areas so that affordable healthcare may be available to rural residents.

Grant monies to fund the development of telehealth applications and studies have been provided by several federal and state agencies including the U.S. Departments of Defense, Commerce, Agriculture, Education, Justice, Health and Human Services, Veterans Affairs, and the Department of Homeland Defense. There are also private, nonprofit groups such as the Center of Excellence for Remote and Medically-Underserved Areas (CERMUSA) and the Acumen Fund. The majority of private parties providing funds focus on specific applications, often to promote a particular product. Additional research is needed before there will be widespread acceptance of telehealth applications (Bonneville & Pare 2006; Gagnon, Lamothe, Hebert, Chanliau, & Fortin 2006). Questions remain about the evidence of the efficacy, cost-benefits, and quality of telehealth applications. These questions arise not so much because of a lack of projects but rather because of a lack of a coordinated approach to the development, research, testing, and evaluation of applications. The Lewin Group (2000) noted that despite an earlier call by the Institute of Medicine (IOM) (1996) to evaluate telemedicine applications in terms of quality of care, outcomes, access to care, healthcare costs, and the perceptions of clients and clinicians, methodology problems remained. These included small sample sizes and a lack of control groups Agency for Healthcare Research and Quality, (AHRQ 2001). There was also a lack of long-term data (Waldo 2003). AHRQ recommended that projects involving chronic conditions that use the bulk of resources or have the greatest barriers to care receive the highest priority for telemedicine research. The National Institute of Nursing Research solicited grant applications to study telehealth technologies that can improve clinical outcomes. The National Cancer Institute's Center to Reduce Cancer Health Disparities has been looking for technology and telehealth applications that can facilitate early detection and screening. Despite the emphasis in this text on U.S. development of telehealth, it is an international phenomenon.

The United States may lead in the development of technologies that enable telehealth, but Australia, Canada, Norway, and Sweden are among the current world leaders in the use of telehealth. Work has been done in Canada on policies and procedures for allied health professionals (AHPs) who provide telehealth services as a means to enhance and expand successes already achieved with telehealth delivery of services and for use by accreditation criteria (Hailey, Foerster, Nakagawa, Wapshall, Murtagh, Smitten, Steblecki, & Wong 2005; Hogenbirk, Brockway, Finley, Jennett, Yeo, Parker-Taillon, Pong, Szpilfogel, Reid, MacDonald-Rencz, & Cradduck 2006). Topics covered by these policies include the scope and limitations of services, staff responsibilities, training, reporting, professional standards, and cultural considerations.

DRIVING FORCES

Recent attention to patient safety, cost containment, managed care, disease management, shortages of healthcare providers, uneven access to healthcare services, and an emphasis upon keeping an aging population functional in their own homes makes telehealth an attractive tool to improve the quality of healthcare and save money (Brantley, Laney-Cummings, & Spivack 2004; Introducing: telehealth and telecare 2007; Smith 2004; Stronge, Rogers, & Fisk 2007).

Savings may be realized via the following measures:

- Improved access to care, which allows clients to be treated earlier when fewer interventions are required.
- The ability of clients to receive treatment in their own community where services cost less.
- Improved quality of care; expert advice that is more easily available.
- Extending the services of nurse practitioners and physician assistants through ready accessibility to physician services.
- Improved continuity of care through convenient follow-up care.
- Improved quality of client records; the addition of digital information such as monitored vital signs and wound images, which provide better information for treatment decisions and help to decrease errors.
- Time savings; the ability of healthcare professionals to cut down on the amount of time spent in travel and instead spend it in direct client care.

Telehealth is also a marketing tool. Many institutions post health promotion or quality benchmark information on their Web pages with the hope that it will attract new customers. Large institutions offer links with the understanding that additional services will be rendered at their facilities. For example, imagine that a client with symptoms of coronary artery disease is seen at a community hospital that has no facilities for cardiac surgery. The client is more likely to follow up at the larger institution that has established links to the community hospital, because a rapport has been established with the consulting physician. Telehealth services can eliminate the need for visas for international clients. Some facilities provide scheduling and online claim authorization as convenient services. Telehealth services deemed valuable by physicians can also attract

---

BOX 17–2   Telehealth Benefits

- **Continuity of care.** Clients can stay in the community and use their regular healthcare providers.
- **Centralized health records.** Clients remain in the same healthcare system.
- **Incorporation of the healthcare consumer as an active member of the health team.** The client is an active participant in videoconferences.
- **Collaboration among healthcare professionals.** Cooperation is fostered among interdisciplinary members of the healthcare team.
- **Improved decision making.** Experts are readily available.
- **Education of healthcare consumers and professionals.** Offerings are readily available.
- **Higher quality of care.** Access to care and access to specialists is improved.
- **Removes geographic barriers to care.** Clients living away from major population centers or in economically disadvantaged areas can access care more readily.
- **May lower costs for healthcare.** Eliminates travel costs. Clients are seen earlier when they are not as ill. Treatment may take place in local hospitals, which are less costly.
- **Improved quality of health record.** The record contains digitalized records of diagnostic tests, biometric measures, photographs, and communication.

---

new medical staff. As a result of the above factors, many agencies offer telehealth or plan to do so in the near future. Telehealth services need to be addressed in enterprise-wide strategic plans. Box 17–2 lists some additional benefits associated with telehealth.

APPLICATIONS

Telehealth applications vary greatly. Examples include monitoring activities, diagnostic evaluations, decision-support systems, storage and dissemination of records for diagnostic purposes, image compression for efficient storage and retrieval, research, electronic prescriptions, voice recognition for dictation, education of healthcare professionals and consumers, and support of caregivers. Sophisticated equipment is not always necessary. Some applications are "high tech," whereas others are relatively "low tech." Real-time videoconferencing between physicians or healthcare professionals and clients and the transmission of diagnostic images and biometric data are examples of high-tech applications. An example of a low-tech application is a home glucose-monitoring program that uses a touch-tone telephone to report glucose results. Desktop PCs outfitted with video cameras can provide telehealth opportunities for applications that do not require high resolution. Current telehealth technologies can be grouped into at least nine broad categories, although for general discussion purposes, there are two types: store-and-forward and interactive conferencing. Store-and-forward is used to transfer digital images and data from one location to another. It is appropriate for nonemergent situations. It is commonly used for teleradiology and telepathology. Interactive conferencing primarily refers to video conferencing and is used in place of face-to-face consultation. Telehealth is not a technology so much as it is a technique for the delivery of services. Increasingly it is perceived as a framework for a comprehensive health system integrating various applications, as well as the management of information, education, and administrative services. Box 17–3 lists some other actual and proposed applications.

BOX 17–3 Current and Proposed Telehealth Applications

- **Cardiology.** ECG strips can be transmitted for interpretation by experts at a regional referral center, and pacemakers can be reset from a remote location.
- **Counselling.** Clients may be seen at home or in outpatient settings by a counselor at another site.
- **Data mining.** Research may be conducted on large databases for educational, diagnostic, cost/benefit analysis, and evidence based practice.
- **Dermatology.** Primary physicians may ask specialists to see a client without the client waiting for an appointment with the specialist and travelling to a distant site.
- **Diabetes management.** Clients may report blood glucose readings by using the touch-tone telephone.
- **Mobile unit post-disaster care.** Emergency medical technicians (EMTs) and nurses at the site of a disaster can consult with physicians about the health needs of victims.
- **Education.** Healthcare professionals in geographically remote areas can attend seminars to update their knowledge without extensive travel, expense, or time away from home.
- **Emergency care.** Community hospitals can share information with trauma centers so that the centers can better care for clients and prepare them for transport.
- **Fetal monitoring.** Some high-risk antepartum clients can be monitored from home with greater comfort and decreased expense.
- **Geriatrics.** Videoconference equipment in the home permits home monitoring of medication administration for a client who has memory deficits but who is otherwise able to stay at home.
- **Home care.** Once equipment is in the client's home, nurses and physicians may evaluate the client at home without leaving their offices.
- **Hospice.** Palliative and end-of-life services via technology can increase access to services in remote areas or supplement traditional care.
- **Military.** Physicians at remote sites can evaluate injured soldiers in the field via the medic's equipment.
- **Pharmacy.** Data can be accessed at a centralized location.
- **Pathology.** The transmission of slide and tissue samples to other sites makes it easier to obtain a second opinion on biopsy findings.
- **Psychiatry.** Specialists at major medical centers can evaluate clients in outlying emergency departments, hospitals, and clinics via teleconferences.
- **Radiology.** Radiologists can take calls from home and receive images from the hospital on equipment they have in place. Rural hospitals do not need to have a radiologist onsite.
- **School clinics.** School nurses, particularly in remote areas, can quickly consult with other professionals about problems observed.
- **Social work.** Social workers can augment services with telehealth home visits.
- **Speech–language pathology.** More efficient use can be made of scarce speech–language pathologists.

- **Virtual intensive care units.** Remote monitoring capabilities and teleconferencing allow experts at medical centers to monitor patients in distant, rural hospitals, particularly when weather conditions or other factors do not allow transport.
- **Extended emergency services.** Remote monitoring and teleconferencing support allow emergency care physicians to view and monitor ambulance patients, supervise emergency medical technicians, and initiate treatments early and re-direct patients to the most appropriate facilities, such as burn centers or trauma units, without being seen first in the emergency department.

Online Databases and Tools

Online resources can include the following:

- *Standards of care.* These may include recommended guidelines for care for a particular diagnosis.
- *Evidence-based practice guidelines.* Best practices based upon research findings are increasingly available online for reference and use.
- *Computerized medical diagnosis.* This database assists the physician to match symptoms against suspected diagnoses.
- *Drug information.* One important application is the determination of the most effective, least expensive antibiotic for a particular infection.
- *Electronic prescriptions.* This permits the physician to "write" a prescription that is sent automatically to the pharmacy. It decreases errors associated with poor handwriting and sound-alike drugs. When integration exists among healthcare systems, physicians, and pharmacies, there is no need to enter patient history, allergies, demographic, and insurance information more than once. Electronic prescribing is being adopted in more systems as part of patient safety initiatives.
- *Abstracts and full-text retrieval of literature.* These can be retrieved easily at any time of the day.
- *Research data.* This information is available via literature searches and Web access.
- *Bulletin boards, reference files, and discussion groups on various specialty subjects.* Ready access to information improves care delivery and decreases related costs. For example, the incorporation of national standards of care and drug information eliminates redundant efforts by individual institutions to prepare their own standards and formularies. It also decreases malpractice claims through adherence to standards of care. Standards of care reflect best practices based on research findings. Online research databases facilitate research through the systematic collection of information on large populations, with potential for data mining at a later time. Further benefits from online resources will be accrued as more projects are implemented to develop common terms to facilitate sharing of data, such as the National Library of Medicine's Unified Medical Language System.

Education

Telehealth affords opportunities to educate healthcare consumers and professionals through increased information accessibility via online resources, including the World Wide Web, distance learning, and clinical instruction. Grand rounds and continuing education are two of the most touted applications for education.

Grand rounds are a traditional teaching tool for health professionals in training (Ellis & Mayrose 2003; Sargeant, Allen, O'Brien, & MacDougall 2003). As the name indicates, a group of practitioners review a client's case history and his or her present condition, at which time they mutually determine the best treatment options. Grand rounds help to maintain clinical knowledge and expertise but are not always available in smaller institutions. Telehealth facilities allow the incorporation of diagnostic images, client interviews, and biometric measurements from outlying hospitals into medical center grand rounds, thereby allowing practitioners from two or more sites to participate. Videoconferencing allows more practitioners to attend this educational offering than might otherwise be possible. In like fashion, consultations and images from major teaching centers may be made available to remote facilities to enhance the practice of professionals in outlying areas.

Continuing Education

Telehealth offers direct access to traditional continuing education and extemporaneous teaching opportunities with every teleconsultation and distance education offering. Training costs for continuing education may be decreased by bringing people together from many distant sites without travel or lodging expenses or extended time away from their responsibilities.

Home Healthcare

Telecommunication technology can reduce costs and increase choices and the availability of services that can keep people in their own homes longer (Garrett & Martini 2007; Hi-tech home help 2007; Brennan 1996). This is particularly important as the population over age 65 explodes without a concomitant increase in funds for healthcare services (Demiris, Oliver, & Courtney 2006). Telecommunication technology also supports automatic collection of data and allows clinicians to handle more clients than via traditional care models. For example, use of a home monitoring system in Japan provides 24-hour contact and medical response for clients as needed in addition to regularly scheduled visits. Biometric measurements such as heart rate and pattern, blood pressure, respiratory rate, and fetal heart rate can be monitored at another site, with electronic or actual house calls provided as needed. Women with high-risk pregnancies, diabetics, and cardiac and postoperative clients can be monitored at home. Clients who require wound care comprise another population that can be managed well at home through telehealth applications. Nurses can also transmit digital photographs of wounds to certified wound ostomy continence nurses (WCONs). Photographs are stored in the database. The WCON can make recommendations and follow more clients through the use of telehealth than would otherwise be possible. Internet access for home health clients and their families also provides convenient access to support groups, treatment information, and electronic communication with their healthcare providers, while decreasing feelings of isolation. The REACH (Resources for Enhancing Alzheimer's Caregiver Health) initiative sponsored by the National Institutes for Health exemplifies a support program for caregivers that encourages them to engage in relaxation exercises. As the number of elderly grows, televisits eliminate the discomfort and inconvenience of travel and long waits to be seen by physicians. Equipment needs are dictated by the nature of the monitoring. For example, telemetry requires continuous monitoring, necessitating a dedicated telephone line as well as the monitoring devices supplied by the home healthcare agency. Other clients may require less expensive, low-technology monitoring, while another group requires equipment with videoconference and monitoring capability. A Web-based solution for care coordination can integrate information from biometric measures and diagnostic tests and automatically alert the clinician of panic values. The benefits of telehealth technology allow clinicians to cut travel time without decreasing client contact and help to improve the organization of the health record with automatic collection of data and better coordination of care among clinicians. Figure 17–1 depicts a teleconference that connects a home healthcare client, a nurse, and a physician.

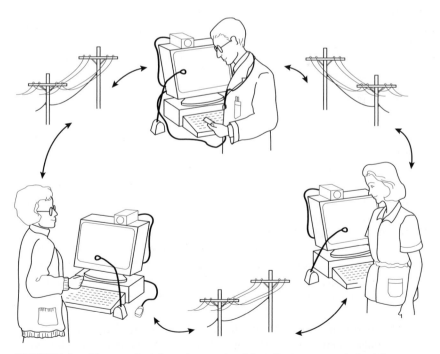

FIGURE 17–1 • Diagram of a teleconference involving client, nurse, and physician at separate sites

The use of sensors can also detect falls and whether the refrigerator has been opened and closed as a means to alert nurses to problems in the homes of elderly and frail individuals. Coming trends include the integration of wireless sensors, wearable monitoring technology into telehealth systems, smart homes, and helper robots (Karunanithi 2007; Koch 2006; Lamprinos, Prentza, & Koutsouris 2006).

Some providers of advanced home telemonitoring services have formed partnerships with home care companies that make the technology available to providers. This arrangement eliminates the need for home healthcare companies to invest in the equipment needed to support telehealth (Strategic Partnership 2003).

The American Telemedicine Association developed clinical guidelines for the use of telemedicine for home care that include criteria for patients, care providers, and technology (ATA adopts telehomecare clinical guidelines 2007). These are listed on their Website (www.atmeda.org/news/guidelines.htm).

Disease Management

The bulk of U.S. healthcare costs result from chronic conditions. For this reason it is essential to find better ways to manage the health of individuals with chronic medical conditions. Telehealth applications can help. The U.S. Department of Veteran Affairs has several telemedicine initiatives nationally monitoring over 20,000 chronically ill veterans with heart disease, depression, diabetes, post-traumatic stress disorder, pulmonary problems, and other chronic illnesses in their own homes and coordinating regional programs that reduce travel and wait time (Department of Veteran Affairs 2006; Kline & Schofield 2006; Midwest VA Service 2007; Riverside County 2006; Wertenberger, Yerardi, Drake, & Parlier 2006). Technology ranges from automated reminders to take medications and handheld vital sign monitors to two-way video computers that are equipped with everything from a stethoscope to an electrocardiograph, and a personal health record (PHR) for veterans. Monitoring devices load results into the veteran's PHR. While technology costs may be substantial, they are significantly less than the cost of an inpatient admission. Similar initiatives are under way at home care agencies and through private medical centers throughout the country. Examples of other programs include Resource Link of Iowa (RLI), the Diabetes Education and Telemedicine Project (IDEATel), and the use of Health Buddy.

The RLI uses two-way interactive video to manage the care of chronically ill patients in their homes throughout Iowa (Coen Buckwalter et al. 2002). Criteria for enrollment included a high utilization of care, clinical indications that more aggressive monitoring could reduce use of services, and a willingness to use technology. The technology has been well received and has led to a reduction in the number of face-to-face visits.

IDEATel began in February of 2000 as a 4-year clinical trial to maximize clients' control of their diabetes by providing them with a computer link to their caregivers for input of glucose and vital signs. Eligibility requirements included a high utilization of care, clinical indications that aggressive monitoring could reduce the use of services, and an expressed willingness to use technology. Caregivers received alerts with critical values.

Health Buddy is an in-home communication device that has been used to provide heart failure disease management (Rosenberg 2007). It prompts patients to take their medicine, keep their legs elevated when sitting, and monitors subjective reports of difficulty breathing or increased edema. On the other end of the connection nurses receive alerts when patients gain weight or indicate other problems.

The U.S. federally funded Jewish Home and Hospital Services Lifecare Plus study showed that telehealth patients decreased their overall utilization of healthcare resources significantly with fewer office visits, ER visits, and readmissions (Lehmann et al. 2006). In a newer twist cell phones are now used to provide programmed reminders to check blood sugars, take medications, or accept downloads from blood sugar monitors, which can then be transmitted to caregivers (Goedert 2007).

In Great Britain several pilot programs are using telecare systems in an attempt to help the elderly maintain a safe environment and manage their chronic conditions at home (Hi-tech home help 2007).

LEGAL AND PRIVACY ISSUES

Reimbursement and licensure issues remain two of the major barriers to the growth and practice of telehealth (Cwiek, Rafiq, Qamar, Tobey, & Merrell 2007; Dickens & Cook 2006; Kennedy 2005; Starren et al. 2005). The Centers for Medicare & Medicaid Services (CMS) have not formally defined telemedicine for the Medicaid program, and Medicaid does not recognize telemedicine as a distinct service. Medicaid reimbursement for telehealth services is available at the discretion of individual states as a cost-effective alternative to traditional services or as a means to improve access for rural residents (CMS 2007; Cross 2007; Gray, Stamm, Toevs, Reischl, & Yarrington 2006). Advocates are struggling to increase state Medicaid reimbursement. Several states have passed legislation mandating private insurance coverage of telehealth services (States require reimbursement 2004). There are also concerns about the impact of telehealth on record privacy, particularly with the implementation of the Health Insurance Portability and Accountability Act (HIPAA).

HIPAA, Referral, and Payment

Brantley et al. (2004) concluded that federal, state, and private sector policies have impeded the advance of telehealth and that an entirely new framework is necessary to determine reimbursement for telehealth services. The Balanced Budget Act of 1997 first authorized Medicare reimbursement for some services that did not traditionally require a face-to-face meeting between client and practitioner, such as radiology or electrocardiogram interpretation. Almost two years passed before any reimbursement occurred. There were limitations on who could receive services, what services were covered, who got paid, and how services were reimbursed. Only clients in federally designated rural areas deemed as having a shortage of health professionals were eligible. Store-and-forward technologies were not covered in some cases. And there were issues related to which practitioners were eligible for reimbursement and how they were paid. Reimbursement rules were loosened with the Medicare, Medicaid, and SCHIP Benefits Improvement and Protection Act of 2000 but not enough to make a significant difference in Medicaid reimbursement or to encourage other third-party payers in the United States to pay for telehealth services. As a result, some physicians and other providers who did teleconsultation did not receive payment for their services. A temporary procedural (CPT) code for billing developed by the American Medical Association may help to increase physician interest in performing online consultations (Dannenfeldt 2004). Up until now, increased client volume at referral centers has been regarded as a means to make up for lost revenue.

Support Personnel

While the technology behind telehealth should be easy to use, technical support may be required as new and different skills are required. Support staff should be capable, flexible, and preferably experienced. At the present, questions have not been fully resolved as to who will train healthcare professionals to participate in telehealth and how compensation will be derived for the additional hours associated with installation, training, and use of telehealth technology. There is also an issue of confidentiality. Technical support staff who are present during the exchange of client information need to be aware of institutional policies as well as laws such as HIPAA that are designed to protect client privacy. These individuals should sign the same sort of statement that clinical personnel sign on the receipt of their information system access codes. In the case of home monitoring, support is crucial to help participants feel comfortable with the technology, particularly when using Internet access and Web applications (Cudney, Weinert, & Phillips 2007).

Liability

Telehealth is plagued by a number of liability concerns (ANA 1996; Dickens & Cook 2006). First, there is the possibility that the client may perceive it as inferior because the consulting professional does not perform a hands-on examination. The American Nurses Association (ANA) cautions that telehealth shows great promise as long as it is used to augment, not replace, existing services. Second, professionals who practice across state lines deal with different practice provisions in each state and may be subject to malpractice lawsuits in multiple jurisdictions, raising questions about how that liability might be distributed or which state's practice standards would apply. Theoretically, clients could choose to file suit in the jurisdiction most likely to award damages. The basic question here is, where did the service occur? Third, how might liability be spread among physicians, other healthcare professionals, and technical support persons? And fourth, HIPAA legislation added new concerns to the mix. These issues remain concerns today.

Telehealth has the potential to raise or lower malpractice costs. For example, Pennsylvania's HealthNet recorded teleconferences to provide a complete transcript of the session. Clients were given a videotape for later review and as a means to clarify their comprehension, and the original videotape was kept as part of the client record. The American Nurses Association (1999) called for the development of documentation requirements for telehealth services that addressed treatment recommendations as well as any communication that occurs with other healthcare providers. This strategy should decrease malpractice claims through better documentation and improved client understanding. On the other hand, liability costs may increase if healthcare professionals can be sued in more than one jurisdiction.

Major issues for nurses include questions of liability when information provided over the telephone is misinterpreted, when advice is given across state lines without a license in the state where the client resides, or, particularly, when an unintentional diagnosis comes from the use of an Internet chat room. Liability is unclear in these areas. Regulation of telenursing practice by boards of nursing is difficult when practice crosses state lines. Unless nurses are licensed in every state in which they practice telenursing, respective regulatory boards are unaware of their presence. The majority of states have laws or regulations that require licensure for telehealth practice (Reed 2005). Pennsylvania's HR549 would permit recognition of RN license among cooperating states, which would facilitate practice across state borders, including telehealth (Piskor 2007).

Authority to practice telenursing across state lines provides the following advantages (National Council of State Boards 1996):

- It establishes the nurse's responsibility and accountability to the board of nursing.
- It establishes legitimacy and availability to practice telenursing.
- It provides jurisdictional authority over the discipline of telenursing in the event that unsafe delivery becomes an issue.

Until this issue has been resolved, nurses must also be cautious when providers from other states give them directions. Several state boards of nursing specifically forbid taking instructions from providers not licensed in the current state. Box 17–4 summarizes barriers to the practice of telehealth.

Licensure Issues

Current licensure issues for telemedicine relate to the state in which healthcare professionals are licensed to practice and the jurisdictional boundaries in which services are delivered. Traditionally telemedicine has required multi-state licensure for healthcare professionals, both for their primary state and for the state in which services are rendered. Application for licensure in additional states can be lengthy and expensive, with the ultimate result of restricting access to services. Telehealth advocates want to remove legal barriers to practice through either nationwide or regional licensing or changes in practice acts that permit practitioners from any state to consult with practitioners from another state without

> **BOX 17–4   Barriers to the Use of Telehealth Applications**
>
> • **Regulatory barriers.** State laws are either unclear or may forbid practice across state lines.
> • **Lack of reimbursement for consultative services.** Most third-party payers do not provide reimbursement unless the client is seen in person.
> • **Costs for equipment, network services, and training time.** Equipment capable of transmitting and receiving diagnostic-grade images is still expensive, although costs are declining.
> • **Fear of healthcare system changes.** Personnel may fear job loss as more clients can be treated at home and hospital units close.
> • **Lack of acceptance by healthcare professionals.** This may stem from liability concerns and discomfort over not seeing a client face-to-face.
> • **Lack of acceptance by users.** This may stem from discomfort with technology, the relationship with the provider, and concerns over security of information and confidentiality.

the need to be licensed in that second state. The Federation of State Medical Boards drafted legislation to address this issue, calling for the establishment of a registry for telehealth physicians, who would enjoy shorter license application periods and lower fees but have some practice restrictions. Some licensing laws pertaining to telehealth have been enacted or are under consideration but no resolution has been achieved as yet. Task forces of the National Council of Nurses suggested multistate licensure as a means to support telenursing. The U.S. Nurse Licensure Compact (NLC) was initiated by the National Council of State Boards of Nursing (NCSBN) during the late 1990s (NCSBN 2007). The resulting mutual recognition model allows a nurse in a state that has adopted the compact to practice in other member states but holds the nurse accountable to the practice laws and regulations in the state where telehealth services are provided. Approximately one-half of the states are compact members at present.

The American Nurses Association (1998) did not support this proposed model, however, citing concerns related to discipline, revenue for individual state boards of licensure, and knowledge issues related to allowable practice in other states. Until additional changes are implemented, delivery of services across some state lines via telehealth may be illegal and practitioners must proceed cautiously. The National Council of State Boards of Nursing (NCSBN) was awarded a grant from the Health Resources and Services Administrations Office for the Advancement of Telehealth to work on licensure portability (NCSBN 2006). The second licensure issue pertains to what jurisdiction the telehealth practitioner is subject to, the physical space of the practitioner, and the jurisdiction of the recipient (Dickens & Cook 2006).

Confidentiality/Privacy

Although telehealth should not create any greater concerns or risks to medical record privacy than any other form of consultation, records that cross state lines are subject to HIPAA regulations and state privacy laws. Security and confidentiality of telehealth services are crucial to acceptance by consumers and professionals (Hildebrand, Pharow, Engelbrecht, Blobel, Savastano, & Hovsto 2006). For this reason experts have called for the creation of standards for e-health, particularly for security and identity management. Nurses need to be mindful of these issues, especially when technicians not bound by professional codes of ethics are present at telehealth sessions.

OTHER TELEHEALTH ISSUES

There are a number of other important issues related to telehealth. They include the following:

- *Lack of standards.* The lack of plug-and-play interoperability among telehealth devices and point-of-care and other clinical information systems is cited as a major obstacle (Craft 2005; Brantley et al. 2004). There is a need for a standard interface specification that allows telehealth data to be merged easily with information from other clinical information systems. Work is in process on the development of these standards using HL7 messages constructed with Extensible Markup Language.
- *National Health Information Infrastructure (NHII).* In succinct terms, the NHII is all about the secure exchange of healthcare information between a requestor and provider. While work is in progress the NHII remains a vision at this time. It requires an identity management system, one trusted on a national scale, that will give information providers a means to validate the electronic identity of a requestor. Similar work is presently under way with the U.S. government. Rules are still needed to create electronic IDs for the NHII. The Department of Health and Human Services, the American Telemedicine Association (ATA), and the Rand Corporation, among other entities, have been discussing the NHII.
- *Homeland security.* The homeland security community has not given significant consideration to telehealth technology when assessing its needs, strategies, and desired outcomes (Brantley et al. 2004). It can make use of various surveillance systems to analyze symptoms on a large scale for possible biological and chemical attacks.
- *Mainstream acceptance.* Despite its advocates, many healthcare professionals have been slow to accept telehealth applications (Williams 2007; Thede 2001). Their reasons include the perception that telehealth applications are not "real" nursing, that telehealth offers few benefits to them, concerns over privacy and legalities, and fears that telehealth applications will reduce the number of healthcare professionals needed.
- *Accreditation and regulatory requirements.* The Joint Commission on Accreditation of Healthcare Organizations first identified medical staff standards for credentialing and privileging for the practice of telemedicine in 2001 and approved revisions in 2003. Practitioners are required to be credentialed and have privileges at the site where the client is located. Credentialing information from the distant site may be used by the originating site to establish privileges if the distant site is accredited by the

Joint Commission. The Food and Drug Administration (FDA) has several guidelines for the use of telehealth-related devices.

- *Patient safety.* The majority of discussions that address patient safety emphasize the potential of telehealth to enhance patient safety through applications such as e-prescribing. Some literature makes mention of threats to patient safety when telehealth applications fail to render the same level of care as hands-on care or when problems occur with the use of electrical devices.

- *Limitations.* Despite its many benefits telehealth suffers some limits as well. One is that the quality of transmitted skin tones is dependent upon room lighting. Another is that the distant provider cannot palpate and is dependent upon the skill of the presenter. A third is the lack of smell. Speed and accessibility to information at any time from any place are essential to quality of service (Babulak 2006). Slowdowns or outages in service are not acceptable.

- *Inadequate funding for technology support.* Descriptions of some telehealth applications describe a lack of monies to establish and maintain the technical infrastructure needed (Bond 2006). In some cases nurses are responsible for the set-up and basic support of telehealth devices. While the wisdom of this approach may be questioned in light of the limited availability of nurses it can be used as an opportunity to establish rapport and comfort with the technology (Starren et al. 2005).

- *Quality of services rendered.* There are two major issues surrounding the quality of telehealth services. One is that services must be at least of the same level of quality as traditional services, particularly for reimbursement services. The second issue is the paradox that geographically isolated populations that stand to derive the largest benefits from telehealth because they have limited access to traditional healthcare services often have the poorest infrastructure, resources, and capability to support telehealth (Liaw and Humphreys 2006). This situation has been exacerbated by a focus on institutional resources rather than rural poor. Telehealth visits can require extra time for equipment management and transmittal of prescriptions (Boodley 2006). There is also a need for extensive research to establish effectiveness and cost and quality relationships (Miller 2007).

ESTABLISHING A TELEHEALTH LINK

Successful establishment and use of a telehealth link require strategic planning as well as consideration of the following factors: necessary infrastructure, costs and reimbursement, human factors, equipment, and technology issues.

Formulating a Telehealth Plan

Any plans for the use of telehealth applications should be in concert with the overall strategic plan of the organization. A telehealth plan minimizes duplicate effort and helps to ensure success. Goals should address the following:

- Current services and deficits
- Telehealth objectives

- Compliance with standards
- Reimbursement policies that favor desired outcomes rather than specific processes
- Periodic review of goals and accomplishments in light of changing technology and needs
- How telecommunication breakdowns will be handled: Will backup be provided? What happens when a power outage in the home severs a link?

The people who will use the system need to be involved in its design from the very beginning. It is wise to start small and expand offerings. Most institutions begin with continuing education and later expand capability. Educational teleconferences require larger rooms that are not suitable for client examinations. Selection of equipment should be based on transmission speed, image resolution, storage capacity, mobility, and ease of use. Higher bandwidth generally improves performance. Equipment should match defined telehealth goals. Box 17–5 lists some strategies to ensure successful teleconferences.

Building the Supporting Framework

Other considerations in telehealth are who will build the infrastructure to support telehealth and what role the federal government should take. Federal and state governments already commit considerable resources to telehealth and related technology. The Department of Commerce, Health Care Financing Administration (HCFA), Office of Rural Health Policy, and Department of Defense are some federal agencies that have conducted telehealth research and demo programs. Most states have projects in process. The National Information Infrastructure Testbed (NIIT) is a consortium of corporations, universities, and government agencies that

---

BOX 17–5   Strategies to Ensure Successful Teleconferences

- Select a videoconferencing system to fit your needs, such as a desktop or mobile system or customized room.
- Locate videoconferencing facilities near where they will be used, yet in a quiet, low-traffic area.
- Schedule sessions in advance to avoid time conflicts. Start on time.
- Establish a working knowledge of interactive conferencing features.
- Provide an agenda to keep the conference on track.
- Introduce all participants.
- Set time limits.
- Send materials needed in advance to maintain focus and involve participants.
- Summarize major points at the conclusion.
- Start by asking all participants if they have a good audio and video feed.
- Participate in a conference call as if it were a face-to-face meeting. Enunciate clearly.
- Minimize background noise or use the mute feature.
- Promote interactivity through questions and answers.
- Have technical support available to resolve any problems that might arise.

views the development of a national information infrastructure as a means to create jobs, promote prosperity, and improve healthcare by reducing redundant procedures and creating an electronic record repository. In their discussion of the infrastructure needed to support telehealth, Nevins and Otley (2002) estimated that an investment of about $20 to $30 billion was needed. In 2005 Kaushal et al. used estimates from experts to project the cost at $156 billion in capital expenditures over five years with another $48 billion in annual operating costs.

Telehealth transmissions can be supported by satellite or microwave, telephone lines, or the Internet. The cost and speed of the service are interrelated. Satellite and microwave transmission is not feasible for most users. **Asynchronous transfer mode (ATM)** service is a high-speed data transmission link that can carry large amounts of data quickly. Speeds range from 0.45 megabits per second (Mbps) to 2.48 gigabits per second (Gbps). ATM works well when large sets of data, such as MRIs, need to be exchanged and discussed. Present ATM use is limited for reasons of cost, availability, and lack of standards. Another option for data transmission is switched multimegabit data service (SMDS), better known as a T1 line. **T1 lines** are high-speed telephone lines that may be used to transmit high-quality, full-motion video at speeds up to 1.544 Mbps. T1 services are leased monthly at a fixed charge independent of use. Next in descending order of speed are DSL (digital subscriber lines) and integrated service digital network (ISDN) lines. DSL uses existing copper telephone wires to transfer high bandwidth data. DSL availability has traditionally been limited by distance from the central telephone office. Variants of DSL technology can rival T1 lines for speed of data transmission. ISDN lines carry 128 kilobits per second (kbps), although lines can be bundled for faster speeds. Each ISDN line costs approximately $30 per month plus costs for calls. ISDN lines support medical imaging, database sharing, desktop videoconferencing, and access to the Internet. Telehealth's identification of 384 kbps as its practical minimum bandwidth renders plain old telephone service (POTS) unsuitable for most applications. Faster access speeds are required for continuing medical education, telemetry, remote consults, and network-based services.

The Internet already carries e-mail for many healthcare professionals and is a powerful tool for obtaining and publishing information. Security and access issues will determine the extent to which client-specific information is interchanged on the Internet. The American Medical Association has published guidelines for e-mail correspondence for clients on its Website.

Cable TV also has the potential to bring high-resolution x-ray images to on-call radiologists at home via its broadband capabilities.

Human Factors

On-site support and commitment from administrators and healthcare professionals are necessary for successful telehealth practice. Acceptance is frequently more difficult to obtain from healthcare providers than it is from clients. Overall, satisfaction is high, particularly when clients perceive that care is easier to obtain or otherwise more convenient (Marcin et al. 2004). Healthcare professionals should provide input about the type of telehealth applications that they would like to see to their professional organizations and healthcare providers. One application, continuing education distance learning programs, is well received and serves to introduce other applications. As a subspecialty area of practice, telehealth has developed its own set of knowledge and skills that must be incorporated into the orientation process for professionals new to the area (Williams 2007). Specific competencies that must be addressed include training time to develop the technical skills needed to set up and use equipment, professional knowledge, interpersonal skills, documentation, professional development, resource management, and practice and administrative issues. Telehealth and all of its applications are new to most people and time is needed to get accustomed to telehealth practices. An example of this may be seen in teleradiology, where radiologists must learn how to interpret images using a monitor. It is possible, however, to enhance images for easier interpretation.

Equipment

Equipment must be reliable, accurate, and flexible enough to meet varying needs. One example of this principle may be seen when equipment purchased for continuing education also supports high-resolution images needed for diagnostic images. However, it is not necessary to have all the latest, most expensive technology to start telehealth. Desktop videoconferencing uses specially adapted personal computers to operate over telephone lines. These PCs may be merged with existing diagnostic imaging systems and other information systems. While it usually lacks broadcast picture quality, desktop teleconferencing provides an opportunity to practice some telehealth applications at a fairly low cost. Consulting parties may be able to see each other and diagnostic images by splitting the PC screen into segments. Box 17–6 lists components needed to support Desktop Video conferencing (DTV).

Telehealth Costs

Estimates for setting up videoconferencing vary greatly, depending on the type of system and applications chosen. Desktop systems are fairly inexpensive. Better resolution increases costs. Costs include equipment purchase, operation,

---

BOX 17–6   Basic DTV Components for Telehealth Applications

- PC
- PC adapter cards
- Camera
- Microphones
- Video overlay cards
- External speakers on existing PCs with broadband switches
- Special adapative tools, such as an electronic stethoscope

and maintenance; network services; and time to learn new skills. Time needed to learn how to use telehealth applications is often underestimated.

Technology Issues

Many of the early technical problems associated with telehealth have been largely resolved. Present issues include resolution, frame rate, standards, and record storage and location. Resolution is the sharpness or clarity of an image. The resolution needed for interpretation of diagnostic images requires a broad bandwidth that is at least 384 kilobits and 30 frames per second (FPS). Video systems work by rapidly displaying a series of still images referred to as *frames.* Frames per second (FPS), or the frame rate, refers to the number of these images that are captured, transmitted, and displayed in one second. The higher the FPS, the smoother the picture. Broadcast quality transmission is 30 FPS. Lower FPS rates produce marginally acceptable video that may be suitable for purposes other than interpretation of diagnostic images. Many DTV systems do not offer broadcast quality at this time. Bandwidth, the efficiency of compression, and hardware and software limitations all determine videoconference frame rates. Another issue related to frame rate is the delay that is noted for one videoconferencing party to respond to another. Although this period is only a few seconds long, it must be factored into teleconferences. Another issue related to resolution is the need to digitize x-rays for transmission and storage. For these reasons, teleradiology applications require more costly equipment and telecommunication services.

Healthcare personnel need to shape the development of technological standards by determining the minimal acceptable standards to ensure quality at the lowest possible costs. Acceptance of international standard H.320 for passing audio and video data streams across networks allowed videoconferencing systems from different manufacturers to communicate. H.320 is a standard for the connection and transfer of multimedia data that allows the transmission and reception of image and sound. It supports a wide range of transmission rates. Prior to the adoption of H.320, only systems produced by the same vendor could communicate. Work continues in this area so that continued improvements can be expected. Other important standards for telehealth include the Digital Image Communication in Medicine (DICOM) standard and the Joint Photographic Experts Group (JPEG) compression standard for digital images. DICOM seeks to promote the communication, storage, and integration of digital image information with other hospital information systems, while JPEG is used to compress images as a means to decrease transmission time and storage requirements. Work is under way for the development of plug-and-play standards to integrate and exchange information captured with telehealth technology with that housed in clinical information systems.

Most discussions of telehealth include the electronic health record (EHR) as a means to make client data readily available and store diagnostic images. **Picture archiving communications systems (PACS)** are storage systems that permit remote access to diagnostic images at a time convenient to the physician. While PACS technology has been available for a number of years, its early history was troubled. Recent technological improvements make PACS feasible.

TELENURSING

At one time the number of references noted in the literature relative to telenursing was limited even though telenursing has been in existence for decades, using available technology to serve its purposes. For example, the telephone has long been used as a communication tool between nurses and healthcare consumers as well as other professionals. As new technology became available, it was also adapted to educate consumers and peers, maintain professional contacts, and provide care to clients at other sites. As a result, nurses currently use telephones, Faxes, computers, smart phones, teleconferences, and the Internet in the practice of telenursing. Potential applications are varied, but common uses are telephone triage, follow-up calls, and checking biometric measurements. Other examples include education, professional consultations, obtaining test results, and taking physician instructions over the phone. Interactive television or teleconferences enable home health nurses to make electronic house calls to clients in their homes; thus nurses can see more clients per day than would be possible via on-site visits. Some advanced practice nurses maintain a primary practice via telehealth (Boodley 2006). Another instance of telenursing is the Telenurse project in Europe, which seeks to standardize the mechanism for describing and communicating nursing care as a means to enable comparisons of nursing practice from one site to another without regard to region or country. In their description of a survey of English-speaking telenurses, Grady and Schlachta-Fairchild (2007) see unlimited opportunities for telenursing, although they note continued issues related to reimbursement, licensure, liability, privacy and confidentiality, quality of care, education, and training for the use of telehealth applications.

The International TeleNurses Association (ITNA) was founded in 1995 to promote and support nursing involvement in telehealth and serve as a resource for nurses. The American Nurses Association (1999) published their Core Principles on Telehealth in 1999. These guidelines are intended to help nurses protect client privacy during the delivery of telehealth services. The American Academy of Ambulatory Care Nursing published its fourth edition of *Telehealth Nursing Practice Standards* in 2007. Other healthcare providers have also developed policy statements or standards of practice, and special interest groups have formed. Telehealth nursing practice is now considered to be a subspecialty of nursing; although Grady and Schlachta-Fairchild (2007) note that the majority of telenurses are not certified in telemedicine, telenursing, or nursing informatics at present, they believe that basic telehealth principles should be integrated into the basic nursing curriculum, which may lead to certification.

A recent study evaluating the feasibility of telenursing in Korea indicated a need to identify telenursing specialties, create a business model, and develop the infrastructure to support practice (Yun & Park 2007).

Despite all of this work a questionnaire administered to Australian nursing students found that the majority of the respondents were largely unaware of what e-health was and how it related to their practice (E-health, what health? 2007).

FUTURE DIRECTIONS

Many providers predict that telehealth will change the way that healthcare is delivered and carve out new roles for healthcare providers. Changes have already started. The way that consumer rights and responsibilites are viewed is changing with the increased use of new technology to deliver care (Finch, Mort, May, & Mair 2005). Telehealth offers new means to locate health information and communicate with practitioners through e-mail and interactive chats or videoconferences. It provides new ways to monitor clients. Smart surveillance cameras and analytic software can be used in the home environment to notify caregivers of changes in acitivity, falls, or lack of movement in the homes of elderly clients. Telehealth cuts down on the need to travel and miss work to seek care. Web-based disease management programs encourage clients to assume greater responsibility for their own care. Applications developed for the military are now available for emergency treatment in some communities. Remote monitoring and use of global positioning systems (GPSs) to direct ambulances to the closest, or best, treatment centers are available now. Mobile technology such as PDAs and point-of-care systems capture data quickly and efficiently facilitate the transmission of data for analysis and use by administrators when they need it, not months or years later. Telehealth services have been slow to take off in the United States primarily due to a lack of reimbursement, but the demand is expected to grow exponentially as Baby Boomers age. Demands for quality, patient safety, and more care options will help change the reimbursement picture, opening the door for more telehealth applications. Brantley et al. (2004) note that better coordination of planning, policy making, and allocation of resources is needed.

Converged devices such as smart phones combine the utility of cell phones and PDAs, allowing users to check e-mail, run applications, and monitor telemetry patients while performing other tasks. These devices provide the potential to increase patient safety, facilitate communication among healthcare professionals, and subsequently reduce liability as orders can be viewed, thus eliminating errors associated with poor handwriting or verbal instructions (Rosenthal 2006).

The Federal Communications Commission (FCC), the National Rural Health Association, the Health Resources and Services Administration (HRSA) Office for the Advancement of Telehealth (OAT), and the Healthcare Information and Management Systems Society have been working to demonstrate how telehealth programs and networks can improve the quality of care in underserved populations and to provide grants (Bazzoli 2004; Federal telepractice grants 2006). The FCC's telemedicine program has not been well utilized. In 2003, new rules were announced that were designed to improve access for rural healthcare programs.

The program enables rural providers to obtain access to modern telecommunication technologies through discounts to telecommunication services charges. These changes are expected to encourage the adoption of more telehealth applications.

Connected health, a new paradigm of care, promises to reduce costs and improve quality by working with clients proactively. People monitor their own health with resulting fewer visits to physicians and inpatient hospital stays (Whitlinger, Ayyagari, McClure, Fisher, & Lopez 2007).

Home-based care will continue its exponential growth as a means to help keep older patients in their own homes and better manage their health (Telemedicine's adolescent angst 2007).

There will be additional work on the national and international telehealth research agenda to supplement that started by Grady and Tschirich (2006) and others that will demonstrate the efficacies of the discipline, standard outcomes, and methodologies. This work will occur in conjunction with various stakeholders. Efforts will entail the education and lobbying of groups with research funds such as the National Institute for Nursing Research (NINR), the Robert Wood Johnson Foundation (RWJ), and the Association of Retired Persons (AARP).

CASE STUDY EXERCISES

17.1   You are the nurse practitioner in St. Theresa's emergency department. A client is brought in with obvious psychiatric problems. You have no psychiatrist available and the nearest psychiatric facility is a one hour drive away. St. Theresa is a Tri-State Health Care Alliance Member. Tri-State has telehealth links with the regional hospital, where a psychiatrist is in the emergency department. What steps would you take to initiate a productive teleconference? Justify your response.

17.2   Erin O'Shell, home health nurse, just set up teleconference equipment for Dr. Bobby to evaluate Mr. Richard Goldstein for possible hospitalization for congestive heart failure. Dr. Bobby and the hospital are a one hour drive away. Just as the teleconference started, but before Dr. Bobby could listen to Mr. Goldstein's lungs or complete other key portions of the examination, a power outage severed the teleconference link. How should Ms. O'Shell handle this situation? Provide your rationale.

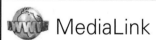 **MediaLink**

Additional resources for this content can be found on the Companion Website at www.prenhall.com/hebda. Click on "Chapter 17" to select the activities for this chapter.

- Glossary
- Multiple Choice
- Discussion Points
- Case Studies
- MediaLink Application
- MediaLink

SUMMARY

- Telehealth is the use of telecommunication technologies and computers to provide healthcare information and services to clients at another location.
- Telehealth is a broad term that encompasses telemedicine but includes the provision of care and the distribution of information to healthcare providers and consumers.
- Efforts to contain costs, improve the delivery of care to all segments of the population, and meet consumer demands make telehealth an attractive tool. Telehealth can help healthcare providers treat clients earlier when they are not as ill and care costs less, provide services in the local community where it is less expensive, improve follow-up care, improve client access to services, and improve the quality of the client's record.
- Telehealth applications vary greatly and include client monitoring, diagnostic evaluation, decision support and expert systems, storage and dissemination of records, and education of healthcare professionals.
- Teleconferencing and videoconferencing are tools that facilitate the delivery of telehealth services.
- Desktop videoconferencing (DTV) is an important development that enables the expansion of telehealth applications into new areas. DTV uses specially adapted personal computers to link persons at two or more sites.
- Telenursing uses telecommunications and computer technology for the delivery of nursing care and services to clients at other sites.
- Neither telemedicine nor telenursing are new. Applications include education of healthcare consumers and professionals as well as the provision of care. In addition to the use of the telephone for triage and information, clients may be monitored at home via telephone or teleconferences. Telehealth is a tool that helps healthcare providers to work more efficiently.
- Major issues associated with the practice of telehealth and telenursing include a lack of reimbursement, infrastructure, plug-and-play standards, licensure and liability issues, and concerns related to client privacy and confidentiality.
- The successful use of telehealth and telenursing is best ensured through the development and implementation of a plan that addresses current services and deficits, goals, technical requirements, compliance with standards and laws, reimbursement, and strategies to handle telecommunication breakdowns.
- Telehealth and telenursing applications are expected to become more commonplace once reimbursement and licensure barriers are removed and technical standards for the exchange of information between telehealth devices and clinical information systems are established.
- Telehealth has the capacity to revolutionize the delivery of healthcare and has already started to do so.

REFERENCES

Agency for Healthcare Research and Quality (AHRQ). (February 2001). *Telemedicine for the Medicare Population. Summary, Evidence Report/Technology Assessment: Number 24*. AHRQ Publication Number 01-E011. Retrieved February 27, 2004, from http://www.ahrq.gov/clinic/epcsums/telemedsum.htm.

American Nurses Association. (October 9, 1996). Telehealth—Issues for nursing. Retrieved February 25, 2004, from http://nursingworld.org/readroom/tele2.htm.

American Nurses Association. (June 24, 1998). Multistate regulation of nurses. Retrieved February 25, 2004, from http://nursingworld.org/gova/multibg.htm.

American Nurses Association. (1999). Core principles on telehealth. Washington, DC: American Nurses Publishing.

ATA adopts telehomecare clinical guidelines. (2007). Retrieved October 4, 2007, from http://www.atmeda.org/news/guidelines.htm.

Bazzoli, F. (January 2004). Telemedicine gets FCC boost. *Healthcare IT News, 1*(1), 11.

Bond, G. E. (2006). Lessons learned from the implementation of a Web-based nursing intervention. *CIN: Computers, Informatics, Nursing. 24*(2), 66–74.

Bonneville, L. & Pare, D. J. (2006). Socioeconomic stakes in the development of telemedicine. *Journal of Telemedicine & Telecare. 12*(5), 217–219.

Boodley, C. (2006). Primary care telehealth practice. *Journal of the American Academy of Nurse Practitioners, 18*(8), 343–345. Retrieved September 29, 2007, from CINAHL with Full Text database.

Brantley, D., Laney-Cummings, K., & Spivack, R. (February 2004). *Innovation, Demand and Investment in Teleheatlh*. A report of the Technology Administration, U.S. Department of Commerce Office of Technology Policy. Retrieved February 28, 2004, from http://www.technology.gov/reports/TechPolicy/Telehealth/2004Report.pdf.

Brennan, P. (October 1996). Nursing informatics: Technology in the service of patient care. Paper presented at the meeting of Alpha Rho Chapter of Sigma Theta Tau, Morgantown, WV.

Brown, N. (2002). Telemedicine coming of age. Retrieved February 29, 2004, from http://trc.telemed.org/telemedicine/primer.asp.

The Centers for Medicare & Medicaid Services (CMS). (2007). Telemedicine overview. Retrieved October 4, 2007, from http://www.cms.hhs.gov/Telemedicine/.

Coen Buckwalter, K., Davis, L. L., Wakefield, B. J., Kienzle, M. G., & Murray, M. A. (2002). Telehealth for elders and their caregivers in rural communities. *Family and Community Health, 25*(3), 31–40.

Coyle, M., Duffy, J., & Martin, E. (2007). Teaching/learning health promoting behaviors through telehealth. *Nursing Education Perspectives, 28*(1), 18–23. Retrieved September 29, 2007, from CINAHL with Full Text database.

Cross, M. A. (2007). Reaching out to rural residents. *Health Data Management, 15*(6), 62–63.

Cudney, S. A., Weinert, C., & Phillips, L. A. (2007). Telephone technical support: An essential adjunct to computer intervention for rural chronically ill women. *CIN: Computers, Informatics Nursing, 25*(4), 221–227.

Cwiek, M. A., Rafiq, A., Qamar, A., Tobey, C., & Merrell, R. C. (2007). Telemedicine licensure in the United States: The need for a cooperative regional approach. *Telemedicine Journal & E-Health, 13*(2), 141–147.

Dannenfeldt, D. (February 2004). Temporary AMA code may increase online consultations. *Healthcare IT News, 1*(2), 23–24.

Department of Veteran Affairs—VistA. (July 2006). Innovations in American Government Award Fact Sheet. Retrieved October 23, 2007, from http://www.innovations.va.gov/innovations/doc/InnovationFactSheet.pdf.

Dickens, B. M. & Cook, R. J. (2006). Legal and ethical issues in telemedicine and robotics. *International Journal of Gynaecology & Obstetrics. 94*(1), 73–78.

Demiris, G., Edison, K., & Vijaykumar, S. (2005). A comparison of communication models of traditional and video-mediated health care delivery. *International Journal of Medical Informatics, 74*(10), 851–856.

Demiris G., Oliver D. P., & Courtney, K. L. (2006). Ethical considerations for the utilization of tele-health technologies in home and hospice care by the nursing profession. *Nursing Administration Quarterly. 30*(1), 56–66.

E-health, what health? (Apr2007). *Australian Nursing Journal.* Retrieved September 29, 2007, from CINAHL with Full Text database.

Ellis, D. G. & Mayrose, J. (2003). The success of emergency telemedicine at the State University of New York at Buffalo. *Telemedicine Journal and e-Health, 9*(1),73–79.

Federal telepractice grants available: funds will assist underserved rural and urban communities. (2006). *ASHA Leader.* Retrieved September 29, 2007, from CINAHL with Full Text database.

Finch, T., Mort, M., May, C., & Mair, F. (2005).Telecare: Perspectives on the changing role of patients and citizens. *Journal of Telemedicine & Telecare. 11*(Supplement 1), 51–53.

Gagnon, M. P., Lamothe, L., Hebert, M., Chanliau, J., & Fortin, J. P. (2006). Telehomecare for vulnerable populations: The evaluation of new models of care. *Telemedicine Journal & E-Health, 12*(3), 324–331.

Garrett, N. & Martini, E. M. (2007). The boomers are coming: A total cost of care model of the impact of population aging on the cost of chronic conditions in the United States. *Disease Management, 10*(2), 51–60.

Goedert, J. (2007). Bringing I.T. into the home. *Health Data Management, 15*(7), 36, 38, 42.

Grady, J. L. & Schlachta-Fairchild, L. (2007). Report of the 2004–2005 International Telenursing Survey. *CIN: Computers, Informatics, Nursing, 25*(5), 266–272.

Grady, J. & Tschirich, P. (October 31, 2006). Creating a national telehealth nursing research agenda. Retreived October 16, 2007, from http://tie.telemed.org/articles/article.asp?path=articles&article=telehealthNursingAgenda_ca_tie06.xml.

Gray, G. A., Stamm, B. H., Toevs, S., Reischl, U., & Yarrington, D. (2006). Study of participating and nonparticipating states' telemedicine Medicaid reimbursement status: Its impact on Idaho's policymaking process. *Telemedicine Journal & E-Health. 12*(6), 681–690.

Hailey D., Foerster, V., Nakagawa, B., Wapshall, T. M., Murtagh, J. A., Smitten, J., et al. (2005). Achievements and challenges on policies for allied health professionals who use telehealth in the Canadian Arctic. *Journal of Telemedicine & Telecare, 11* (Suppl 2), S39–41.

Hildebrand C., Pharow P., Engelbrecht R., Blobel B., Savastano M., & Hovsto A. (2006). Biohealth—the need for security and identity management standards in eHealth. *Studies in Health Technology & Informatics. 121,* 327–336.

Hi-tech home help. (July 2007). *Nursing & Residential Care.* Retrieved September 29, 2007, from CINAHL with Full Text database.

Hogenbirk, J. C., Brockway, P. D., Finley, J., Jennett, P., Yeo, M., Parker-Taillon, D., et al. (2006). Framework for Canadian telehealth guidelines: Summary of the environmental scan. *Journal of Telemedicine & Telecare, 12*(2), 64–70.

Institute of Medicine (IOM). (1996). *Telemedicine: A guide to assess telecommunications in health care.* Retrieved March 2, 2004, from http://books.nap.edu/books/0309055318/html/2.html.

Introducing: Telehealth and telecare. (July 2007). *British Journal of Community Nursing.* Retrieved September 29, 2007, from CINAHL with Full Text database.

Joint Commision for the Accreditation of Healthcare Organizations (JCAHO). (February 2003). Existing requirements for telemedicine practitioners explained. *Joint Commission Perspectives.* Retrieved March 2, 2004, from http://www.atmeda.org/news/JCP-2003-February2.pdf.

Karunanithi, M. (2007). Monitoring technology for the elderly patient. *Expert Review of Medical Devices, 4*(2), 267–277.

Kaushal, R., Blumenthal, B., Poon, E. G., Jha, A. K., Franz, C., Middleton, B., et al. & the Cost of National Health Information Network Working Group (August 2, 2005). The Costs of a National Health Information Network. *Annals of Internal Medicine, 143*(3), 165–173.

Kennedy, C. A. (2005). The challenges of economic evaluations of remote technical health interventions. *Clinical & Investigative Medicine, 28*(2), 71–74.

Kline, S. & Schofield, R. (Spring 2006). Telehealth and care coordination improves outcomes for veterans with heart failure. *Progress in Cardiovascular Nursing, 21*(2), 111–112. Retrieved September 29, 2007, from CINAHL with Full Text database.

Koch, S. (2006). Meeting the challenges—the role of medical informatics in an ageing society. *Studies in Health Technology & Informatics, 124,* 25–31.

Lamprinos, I. E., Prentza, A., & Koutsouris, D. (2006). Communication protocol requirements of patient personal area networks for telemonitoring. *Technology & Health Care, 14*(3), 171–187.

Lehmann, C., Mintz, N., & Giacini, J. (2006). Impact of telehealth on healthcare utilization by congestive heart failure patients. *Disease Management & Health Outcomes, 14*(3), 163–169. Retrieved September 29, 2007, from CINAHL with Full Text database.

Liaw, S. & Humphreys, J. (2006). Rural eHealth paradox: It's not just geography! *Australian Journal of Rural Health, 14*(3), 95–98. Retrieved September 29, 2007, from CINAHL with Full Text database.

The Lewin Group, Inc. (December 2000). *Assessment of approaches to evaluating telemedicine.* Final report prepared for Office of the Assistant Secretary for Planning and Evaluation, Department of Health and Human Services. Retrieved February 27, 2004, from http://www.aspe.hhs.gov/health/reports/AAET/aaet.htm.

Manfredi, L., Shupe, J., & Batki, S. L. (2005). Rural jail telepsychiatry: A pilot feasibility study. *Telemedicine Journal & E-Health, 11*(5), 574–577.

Marcin, J. P., Ellis, J., Mawis, R., Nagrampa, E., Nesbitt, T. S., & Dimand, R. J. (2004). Using telemedicine to provide pediatric subspecialty care to children with special health care needs in an underserved rural community. *Pediatrics, 113* 1 pt. 1, 1–6.

Midwest VA service network deploys $2 million telemedicine network. (September 13, 2007). *Telemedicine and Telehealth News.* Retrieved October 4, 2007, from http:///tie.telemed.org/news/.

Miller, E. A. (July 2007). Solving the disjuncture between research and practice: Telehealth trends in the 21st century. *Health policy, 82*(2), 133–141.

The National Council of State Boards of Nursing (NCSBN). (2007). About. Retrieved January 21, 2008, from https://www.ncsbn.org/156.htm.

The National Council of State Boards of Nursing (NCSBN). (December 14, 2006). NCSBN hosts summit funded by federal grant to promote nurse licensure portability. Retrieved October 23, 2007, from https://www.ncsbn.org/1097.htm.

National Council of State Boards of Nursing, Inc. (1996). Telenursing: The regulatory implications for multistate regulation. *Issues, 17*(3), 1, 8–9.

Nevins, R. & Otley III, V. C. (2002). Demystifying telehealth. *Health Management Technology, 23*(7), 52, 51.

Reed, K. (2005, May). Telemedicine: Benefits to advanced practice nursing and the communities they serve. *Journal of the American Academy of Nurse Practitioners, 17*(5), 176–180. Retrieved September 29, 2007, from Health Source: Nursing/Academic Edition database.

Riverside County Foundation on Aging for the Riverside County Advisory Council on Aging and Riverside County Office on Aging, in partnership with VNA of the Inland Counties and the Riverside Community Health Foundation. (October 2006). Using telehealth and other connective technologies to reach and serve older adults and adults with disabilities.

Rosenberg, H. (2007). Not-for-profit report. Connecting with seniors to reduce hospitalizations. *Nursing Homes: Long Term Care Management, 56*(1), 41–42. Retrieved September 29, 2007, from CINAHL with Full Text database.

Rosenthal, K. (2006). Enjoy "smarter" patient monitoring. *Nursing Management, 37*(5), 52.

Sargeant, J., Allen, M., O'Brien, B., & MacDougall, E. (2003). Videoconferenced grand rounds: Needs assessment for community specialists. *The Journal of Continuing Education in the Health Professions, 23*(2), 116–123.

Schneider, P. (1996). Washington word: Telecom reform. *Healthcare Informatics, 12*(3), 93.

Smith, E. (2004). Telehealth in the Tundra. *Health Management Technology, 25*(3), 24–26.

Starren, J., Tsai, C., Bakken, S., Aidalay, A., Morin, P. C., Hillman, C., et al. & For THE IDEATel Consortium. (2005). The role of nurses in installing telehealth technology in the home. *CIN: Computers, Informatics, Nursing, 23*(4), 181–189.

States require reimbursement for telemedicine. (March 19, 2004). *Psychiatric News, 39*(6), 14.

Stronge, A. J., Rogers, W. A., & Fisk, A. D. (2007). Human factors considerations in implementing telemedicine systems to accomodate older adults. *Journal of Telemedicine & Telecare. 13*(2), 1–3.

Telemedicine's adolescent angst. (2007). *Hospitals & Health Networks, 81*(6), 66, 68, 70.

Thede, L. Q. (2001). Overview and summary: Telehealth: Promise or peril? *Online Journal of Issues in Nursing, 6*(3), Retrieved February 26, 2004, from http://nursingworld.org/ojin/topic16/tpc16top.htm.

Waldo, B. (2003). Telehealth and the electronic medical record. *Nursing Economics, 21*(5), 245.

Wertenberger, S., Yerardi, R., Drake, A. C., & Parlier, R. (2006). Veterans Health Administration Office of Nursing Services exploration of positive patient care synergies fueled by consumer demand: Care coordination, advanced clinic access, and patient self-management. *Nursing Administration Quarterly. 30*(2), 137–146.

Whitlinger, D., Ayyagari, D., McClure, D., Fisher, J., & Lopez, F. (2007). Straight talk. Collaboration fosters connected health: A new paradigm of proactive healthcare. *Modern Healthcare, 37*(21), 4–50.

Williams, C. (2007). Telehealth nursing practice. *AAACN Viewpoint, 29*(1), 12. Retrieved September 29, 2007, from CINAHL with Full Text database.

Yun, E. K. & Park, H. A. (2007). Strategy development for the implementation of telenursing in Korea. *CIN: Computers, Informatics, Nursing, 25*(5), 301–306.

CHAPTER 18

Evidence-Based Practice and Research

After completing this chapter, you should be able to:

1 Describe ways that computers and informatics support evidence-based practice and the research process.

2 Discuss advantages of computerized literature searches over manual methods.

3 Identify selected statistical analysis software programs.

4 Discuss impediments to healthcare research related to health information technology.

5 Examine anticipated impact of increased automation and the electronic health record (EHR) on research efforts and practice change.

6 Examine strategies for best practice to engage healthcare professional students to reap benefits of research tools and technology.

7 Discuss implications and impact of Health Insurance Portability and Accountability Act (HIPAA) legislation on healthcare research.

8 Discuss the role of the healthcare professional in evidence-based practice in a variety of healthcare delivery environments.

THE NEED FOR EVIDENCE-BASED PRACTICE

There is widespread recognition that evidence-based practice is essential to transform healthcare by providing proven effective treatments. At present there is a gap between theory and practice that results in diminished patient care, inefficient practice, and an excessive time lag between the discovery of knowledge and its incorporation into clinical practice (Salmond 2007). The landmark Institute of Medicine (IOM) (2001) report, *Crossing the Quality Chasm*, called for the implementation of evidence-based practice as a means to improve the quality of care. Evidence-based practice is applicable to all healthcare disciplines, and it contributes to the evolution of nursing as a profession (Courey, Benson-Soros, Deemer, & Zeller 2006).

Evidence-based practice (EBP) is an approach to providing care that integrates nursing experience and intuition with valid and current clinical research to achieve best patient outcomes (Dracup & Bryan-Brown 2006; Drenning 2006; Hanberg & Brown 2006; Salmond 2007). Sigma Theta Tau International (STTI), the Honor Society of Nursing, defines evidence-based practice as "an integration of the best evidence available, nursing expertise, and the values and preferences of the individuals, families and communities who are served" (STTI 2005). EBP entails development of best practices based on outcomes and the ability of nurses to access and evaluate current professional literature found both in print and online sources. EBP is a systematic process requiring the following activities (Pipe 2007; Salmon 2007; Zuzelo, McGoldrick, Seminara, & Karbach 2006):

- *Asking a relevant, searchable question.* This determines whether change is needed and helps clarify the problem. An example might include a question asking whether the infection rate associated with central lines is related to the current procedure for central line dressing changes, resulting in policy change based on the findings.
- *Systematically searching for evidence.* This entails a thorough, systematic, exhaustive literature review of studies related to central line dressing change procedures and related infection rates.
- *Critically examining the evidence.* This activity requires practitioners to consider the size and type of studies examined, the quality of research reported, critique of each study examined, results, and recommendations. In the example of the central line dressing change, examining the evidence may lead to recommendations to change the antiseptic agent, the type of dressing material, the frequency at which the dressing is changed, or the dressing change procedure itself; it may also lead to an overall policy review and change.
- *Changing practice as needed.* This requires a re-design of current procedures and workflow as well as timely implementation of needed change. EBP requires sharing results of the examination of evidence and the following up with planned change to educate and acquaint practitioners with the new procedure based on the best evidence.

- *Evaluating the effects of change and maintaining its practice.* This activity involves comparison of pre- and post-change central line infection rates in order to verify the impact or effectiveness of the EBP change. Assuming that problems with the dressing change procedure or wound care material constituted the problem, then one would expect infection rates to continue to decline. One of the greatest challenges with EBP practice change is helping staff break with tradition and integrate the EBP practice change. There is also a need for monitoring the EBP practice change, focusing on outcomes and impact as there is a tendency for staff to resort to previous practices.

EBP provides a better way to treat patients because it replaces tradition with practices supported by research improving outcomes (Dracup & Bryan-Brown 2006; Pipe 2007; Shirey 2006). EBP is exciting to research and implement as it removes reliance on the limited knowledge base of individual practitioners, who may or may not be well-read and skilled in interpretation and application of research findings into clinical practice settings. There is a tremendous knowledge explosion that presents a unique set of challenges for each care provider, making it virtually impossible for any one individual to remain abreast of all the latest technology and developments in one's specialty area at any given time. EBP provides an shared experience for healthcare professions based on systematic and thorough review of scientific data on a given topic. EBP also provides an opportunity to standardize best practice, improve adherence to best practices, and reduce the time an individual provider spends gathering and accessing relevant data, as well as making the EBP data available at the bedside at the time it is most needed (Matter 2006).

EBP advances patient health and safety, providing quality and excellence through systematic examination of the scientific literature. EBP is reported to contribute to increased job satisfaction and vitality because nurses and professionals in other healthcare disciplines feel better about the quality of care they are delivering (Hockenberry, Wilson, & Barrera 2006). Evidence-based practice provides a mechanism for hospitals and other healthcare delivery systems to meet research and excellence requirements inherent in the American Association of Colleges of Nursing (AACN) Magnet designation indicates that a certain level of excellence has been met (Shirey 2006).

THE STATUS OF EVIDENCE-BASED PRACTICE

An extensive body of research knowledge exists now that needs to be incorporated into practice (Drenning 2006). Synder (2007) reports that nurses view evidence-based research favorably. An increasing number of facilities now consider EBP to be part of everyday clinical practice, and evidence-based competencies serve to establish the standards of practice and have built EBP into their clinical ladders (Gardner & Beese-Bjurstrom 2006; Mitchell 2006). Sigma Theta Tau International (2006) completed a landmark EBP study, finding that nurses need information to provide patient care but that many report lacking the comfort, skills, time, or access to appropriate materials needed to personally engage in EBP. This finding of the Sigma Theta Tau (2006) study is particularly true for nurses who entered practice five or more years earlier. Advanced practice nurses indicate higher levels of familiarity with EBP, and it appears that EBP is now integrated into most master's nursing curricula. Nurses entering the profession within the past five years also expressed greater familiarity with EBP from their basic education and report feeling more comfortable with the availability of EBP information.

Shirey (2006) noted that only 15% of the nursing workforce consistently practiced within an EBP framework. Reasons contributing to low utilization of EBP include the following (Chester 2007; Drenning 2006; Hockenberry, Wilson, & Barrera 2006; Mitchell 2006: Pipe 2007; Pravikoff, Tanner, & Pierce 2005; Salmon 2007; Snyder 2007):

- Failure to link theory to practice
- Poor awareness of evidence-based practice
- Lack of literature searching skills
- Lack of confidence with research utilization skills
- Lack of a supportive environment
- Lack of computer access at the bedside
- Lack of effective continuing education to make the transition to evidence-based practice

The National League for Nursing (NLN) recently completed two similar but separate surveys of nurse administrators and faculty in schools of nursing to determine the level of informatics competencies and related requirements. Survey results indicate that computer literacy is reported as a curricular requirement approximately 60% of the time and information literacy approximately 40% of the time (Skiba & Thompson 2007). These preliminary findings are disturbing because professional leaders and the service sector expect nursing graduates to enter the practice setting with computer and information literacy skills. Even when information literacy programs are well established in nursing education, Courey, Benson-Soros, Deemer, and Zeller (2006) noted that it is imperative for nurse educators to determine whether information literacy actually leads to the promotion of evidence-based nursing practice or if there is a missing link between the two skills. For example, just having exposure to computer and information literacy skills does not guarantee competence in these areas.

STRATEGIES TO PROMOTE EVIDENCE-BASED PRACTICE

Evidence-based practice requires a paradigm shift from the traditional model of clinical practice traditionally grounded in intuition, clinical experience, and pathophysiological rationale to a paradigm where there are linkages between clinical expertise and integration of the best scientific evidence, patient values and preferences, and clinical circumstances (Salmond 2007). At the organizational level, EBP must be incorporated into the philosophy and mission of the organization particularly as it relates to the provision of quality patient care provided by expert clinicians. EBP must pervade all levels of the organization, and this can only occur when hospital administration and nurse leaders demonstrate a strong commitment through the creation of an environment that infuses and promotes critical thinking, supports autonomous decision making, and values empowerment processes, including shared governance (Zuzelo et al. 2006). Nurse administrators are obliged to take the initiative in developing EBP models and ensure the availability of information technology supporting EBP models (Matter 2006; Shirey 2006; Simpson 2006). Information technology (IT) tools provide the means to search the literature and apply clinical knowledge, improving practice and safety as well as meeting the standards of excellence required for regulatory and credentialing standards and Magnet status. It is essential that IT tools are accessible at the point of care when needed, providing access to online search engines, journal articles, and databases as well as links through the electronic health record (EHR). Access to essential IT tools requires financial commitment for the technology and subscriptions to database services initially and for upgrades, since there is rapid change in IT. EBP is a shared responsibility among nurses, advanced practice nurses, and nurse researchers (Drenning 2006). The concept of EBP as a basis for nursing practice must be introduced to all nurses during orientation (Dracup & Bryan-Brown 2006; Salmon 2007).

The transition to EBP must be supported through ongoing continuing education initiatives to develop and maintain essential skills; this is particularly relevant for staff accustomed to older, more traditional models of practice. One strategy for success in promoting EBP skills is pairing individuals experienced in EBP with novices. This bringing together of novice and expert provides a fertile area for dialogue and partnership to move EBP forward in the organization, and this model often creates excitement and enthusiasm by taking away perceived barriers as well as IT anxiety. Other strategies for infusion of EBP into the organization include journal clubs that provide a forum for nurses to discuss specific articles and scientific research reviews, as well as the opportunity to invite qualified speakers to address EBP topics.

Database searches of professional journals and credible EBP Websites significantly reduce the time and effort one might expend investigating a clinical question. IT provides access to credible and reliable resources, including secondary sources of reviews of the literature by experts as well as EBP guidelines. These secondary sources of reviews and summaries prepared by experts provide clinical practice guidelines and recommendations (AHRQ 2007). There is broad utility for the implementation of clinical practice guidelines, and these are often available through hospital libraries or via mobile handheld devices such as Personal Digital Assistants (PDAs). PDAs have several attractive features, making them quite portable and allowing the clinician to have access to databases and EBP clinical guidelines at the bedside; there is also increasing evidence that patient safety and nurse satisfaction are increased with PDA use (Thompson 2005; Colevins, Bond, & Clark 2006; Stockwell 2006; Cassey 2007). PDAs are highly regarded by practicing clinicians because they are portable providing current clinical best practice at the bedside. In addition to the PDAs that can be taken to the bedside, other strategies for conducting one's own review of the literature and database searches for EBP include:

- *Record the details of the search.* This includes noting the type and names of search strategies and databases used, whether searches were limited by particular languages (and what those were), the search frame (such as, one year ago, two years ago), key terms used, and the names of Websites explored.
- *Maintain notes on each review.* Notes should include the author name(s), title, study question, type of study, findings, and recommendations for clinical applications. The findings and recommendation are evaluated based on the strength of the evidence. Systematic review or meta-analysis of relevant randomized control trials or practice guidelines based on those reviews are the most highly regarded, followed by evidence obtained from a single well-designed randomized controlled trial (RCT). Other studies, expert opinion, and expert committees are accorded less weight (Hockenberry et al. 2006).
- *Prepare a succinct summary of all the studies reviewed.* The summary should include practice recommendations.

Box 18–1 lists some resources useful to support EBP.

BOX 18–1   Selected Resources Supporting Evidence-Based Practice

Centre for Evidence-Based Nursing

http://www.york.ac.uk/healthsciences/centres/evidence/cebn.htm
Site dedicated to furthering evidence-based nursing practice. This site includes systematic reviews and other resources.

The Cochrane Collaboration of the Cochrane Library

www.cochrane.org
Collection of databases that provides reliable systematic reviews of clinical trials and the efficacy of treatments. Full text retrieval access requires subscription. Databases include the Cochrane Database of Systematic Reviews (CDSR) and the Database of Abstracts of Reviews of Effects.

Database of Abstracts of Reviews of Effectiveness (DARE)

http://www.crd.york.ac.uk/crdweb/
One database in the Cochrane Collaboration. It may also be accessed through the Turning Research into Practice (TRIP) Database.

Evidence-Based Nursing Online

http://ebn.bmjjournals.com/
Provides abstracted, appraised research to subscribers.

Health Information Research Unit (HIRU)

http://hiru.mcmaster.ca
Studies problems of research transfer, develops and tests innovations based on information technology designed to improve the transfer of evidence into practice.

The Joanna Briggs Institute

www.joannabriggs.edu.au/consumer
Australian–based consumer-focused site with links to other countries. Provides access to evidence-based information, publications, online services, education, and training programs.

National Guideline Clearinghouse™ (NGC)

http://www.guideline.gov/
Public resource for evidence-based clinical practice guidelines developed by professional organizations. Available through the U.S. Department of Health and Human Services Agency for Healthcare Research and Quality (AHRQ).

Nursing Best Practice Guidelines

http://www.rnao.org/Page.asp?PageID=861&SiteNodeID=133
Site maintained by the Registered Nurses of Ontario that provides developed guidelines, a toolkit, and guidelines for implementation.

PEDro

http://www.pedro.fhs.usyd.edu.au/
Physiotherapy Evidence Database that offers abstracts of clinical trials, systematic reviews, practice guidelines, and other relevant links.

Sarah Cole Hirsh Institute

http://fpb.case.edu/HirshInstitute/index.shtm
Established by the Frances Payne Bolton School of Nursing, Case Western Reserve University. Provides consulting services, certificates in evidence-based nursing practice, and print and online publications that disseminate evidence-based practice information.

SUMSearch

http://SUMSearch.uthscsa.edu
Uses metasearch techniques to simultaneously search the National Library of Medicine, DARE, and the National Guideline Clearinghouse for medical evidence.

Turning Research Into Practice (TRIP) Database

http://www.tripdatabase.com/index.html
Evidence-based medicine site with access to systematic reviews of medical literature, synopses, guidelines, clinical questions, and other relevant links.

Netting the Evidence

http://www.shef.ac.uk/scharr/ir/netting/
Lists multiple Websites and resources on evidence-based practice. It is organized by 8 categories: library, searching, appraising, implementing, software, journals, databases, and organizations.

Worldviews on Evidence-Based Nursing

A journal published by Sigma Theta Tau International, the Honor Society of Nursing.

Evidence-Based Practice

http://www.biomed.lib.umn.edu/learn/ebp/

(*continued*)

BOX 18–1 (*continued*)

This is a Website that includes an interprofessional tutorial for students in healthcare fields, medicine, faculty, and anyone interested in evidence-based practice.

Medline

http://www.ncbi.nlm.nih.gov/entrez/query.fcgi.
Medline is available through the National Library of Medicine's authoritative and current database of health information for consumers and health professionals and is accessible 24 hours a day.

Agency for Healthcare Quality and Research (AHRQ)

http://ahrq.gov/clinic/epc/
Under the Evidence-based Practice Centers (EPC) Program of the Agency for Healthcare Research and Quality (formerly the Agency for Health Care Policy and Research—AHCPR), 5-year contracts are awarded to institutions in the United States and Canada to serve as EPCs. The EPCs review all relevant scientific literature on clinical, behavioral, and organization and financing topics to produce evidence reports and technology assessments. These reports are used for informing and developing coverage decisions, quality measures, educational materials and tools, guidelines, and research agendas. The EPCs also conduct research on methodology of systematic reviews.

PsychINFO

http://www.ovid.com/site/catalog/DataBase/139.jsp
The American Psychological Association's PsycINFO® database is the comprehensive international bibliographic database of psychology. It contains citations and summaries of peer-reviewed journal articles, book chapters, books, dissertations, and technical reports, all in the field of psychology and the psychological aspects of related disciplines, such as medicine, psychiatry, nursing, sociology, education, pharmacology, physiology, linguistics, anthropology, business, and law. Journal coverage, spanning 1806 to present, includes international material selected from more than 1,900 periodicals written in over 35 languages.

In nursing, there is similarity in many of the techniques, processes, and tools used in both research-based practice and evidence-based practice. The major difference between the two is that research-based practice does not consider clinical expertise or patient preference while EBP uses expertise to translate evidence into an innovative practice change (Drenning 2006). For example, evidence-based practice would involve searching the research to find the best practice based on valid and reliable scientific studies and creating a practice change to implement this best practice—often through developing and implementing a clinical guideline. EBP is also used in policy revision and policy formation. Three of the most frequently cited models for integrating EBP into nursing practice include the Stetler Model, the Iowa Model, and the Rossworm & Larrabee Model (Melnyk & Fineout-Overholt 2005).

USING COMPUTERS TO SUPPORT EVIDENCE-BASED PRACTICE AND RESEARCH

Computers can be used in infinite ways to support the development of evidence-based practice and research, from the earliest stages through the dissemination of findings and the implementation of recommendations and guidelines. While not every student or healthcare professional may conduct research, the current healthcare delivery system calls for practitioners who have skills and competencies in searching literature, demonstrate a basic comprehension of statistics enabling a systematic critique of research studies, and participate in formation and clinical application of evidence-based practice guidelines. It is also relevant that healthcare professionals are called upon to apply fundamental skills in presentation applications. For example, nurses are increasingly expected to share outcomes and impacts of EBP with other units or system-wide in their institutions as part of their clinical ladders and role expectations. Some of the most common computer applications supporting EBP are described in the following paragraphs. Box 18–2 summarizes some ways that computers facilitate evidence-based practice in the research process.

Identification of Searchable Questions and Research Topics

Constant changes in healthcare and the healthcare delivery system create challenges to keep abreast of the latest findings and recommendations for clinical practice, and there is often a time lag between the discovery of knowledge and its application into the clinical setting. Getting the "bench" research translated into "bedside" care has been estimated by some to be as long as 17 years. It is essential that clinicians are more dedicated to narrowing this time to get research from the bench to the bedside in a more expedient manner so there will be much more emphasis on interdisciplinary translational research in the coming decade. While the concept of translational research is new for many nurse clinicians, there are a variety of valid and reliable resources available to promote searchable questions. There are also toolkits to help clinicians locate existing guidelines or clarify searchable questions with the end goal of developing evidence-based practice guidelines. Some of these resources are listed in Box 18–3.

Clinicians interested in and passionate about conducting research frequently have online discussion groups and professional mentors helping them to identify specific areas for EBP or original research. These resources may be specific to a particular subspecialty, including but not limited to critical care nursing, education, and informatics, or to research as an area of concentration. The NURSERES listserv group, at listserv.kent.edu/archives/nurseres.html, is a discussion list for nurse researchers. Additional nursing research opportunities are available online at http://www.nursingsociety.org/Research/ResearchInitatives/Pages/research_finder.aspx. This site provides nurses with names of groups and Web links to various healthcare organizations; it includes a well-defined research section for nurses who have specific

BOX 18–2 Common Computer Applications Supporting Evidenced-Based Practice and Research

- **Topic identification or searchable questions.** Online literature searches, research reports, e-mail, online communities, and discussion groups can be used to identify areas in need of research.
- **Online literature and database searches.** Electronic searches enable the researcher to identify systematic reviews and prior research in an area, as well as articles pertaining to the theoretical framework for proposed studies.
- **Full text retrieval of articles.** This eliminates the need to physically locate journals and photocopy them.
- **Development of resource files.** Computer files replace handwritten reports and may be searched quickly, allowing researchers to spend valuable time performing research and writing reports instead of performing clerical tasks.
- **Selection or development and revision of a data collection tool.** Online literature searches help researchers locate developed data collection tools. If no suitable tool is found, researchers can develop their own tool using a word processing package and then test it by sending it out via e-mail or the Web.
- **Preparation of the grant/study proposal.** Word processing aids the writing process because revisions can be made quickly.
- **Budget preparation and maintenance.** Spreadsheets and financial planning software assist with this process.
- **Determination of appropriate sample size.** The ability to generalize study findings is related to the size of the sample. Power analysis is the process by which an appropriate sample size may be determined. Software is available for this purpose.
- **Data collection.** Computers aid in the collection of data in several ways. Data may be input into a computer through scanned questionnaires, direct entry of field observations, or the use of an online data collection tool. PDAs and notebook computers aid on-site entry of data, eliminating note and paper tools (Hanberg & Brown 2006).
- **Database utilization.** Databases allow organization and manipulation of collected data.
- **Statistical analysis/qualitative text analysis.** Statistical analysis software performs complex computations, while qualitative text analysis allows searches for particular words and phrases in text, noting frequency of appearance and context.
- **Preparation of the research findings for report.** Word processing and graphics programs enable researchers to present their findings without the need for clerical assistance or graphic artists.
- **Bibliographic database managers (BDMs).** This type of software aids the preparation of publications through the importation of references from literature databases without the need to rekey and formats citations and reference lists according to the style selected.
- **Electronic dissemination of findings.** Online journals, Web pages, and e-mail permit researchers to share their findings quickly. This contrasts with the traditional publication of study findings in print media that might take a year or more from the time of submission until distribution.

research interests and lists upcoming conferences where they may submit their research for peer-reviewed presentation.

Timely and ongoing studies allow healthcare educators, providers, agencies, and alliances to explore and examine information trends and react to market changes proactively. For example, an exploration of databases might indicate a new trend in nursing practice based on patient outcomes related to best practice in wound care management. This EBP would serve as an opportunity to examine current policy and would create a clinical guideline to change current policy, resulting in improved patient outcomes, fewer inpatient days, and a reduced cost savings to the unit and institution. Box 18–3 lists examples of selected healthcare informatics topics for research based on readings and discussions with healthcare professionals.

Literature Searches

Systematic literature searches provide an effective means of researching primary research in a logical and systematic manner, providing a more efficient and effective means to find credible scientific information than if one were doing a general

---

BOX 18–3   Suggested Healthcare Informatics Research Topics

The development of informatics competencies

- Nursing education and the development of informatics competencies
- Fostering informatics skills among staff nurses
- Data mining and searching for the best evidence
- Use of informatics in knowledge discovery

Clinical data

- Development and efficacy of acuity and classification systems
- Use of point-of-care devices
- The impact of informatics on clients' families and healthcare providers
- Evidence-based practice guideline development and use, including outcome assessment
- Expert systems, decision trees and support, and artificial intelligence and knowledge engineering
- Client education
- Quality improvement initiatives
- Implementation of ICNP and other standard clinical languages into electronic health records
- Efficacy of telehealth applications
- Tracking resources

Education

- Effectiveness of virtual learning environments
- Models for best practice in unit-based staff development
- Graduate outcome behaviors
- Best pedagogical practice in the nursing classroom
- The impact of mentorship on nurse satisfaction

Web search. This is a relevant concept in the process of locating and examining research because there is opportunity to examine primary data sources in one location (Sigma Theta Tau International 2005). Primary databases for searching nursing literature are the Cumulative Index to Nursing and Allied Health Literature (CINAHL), MEDLINE, and PsychINFO. All three of these primary databases are available for online searches through university and hospital libraries. Students in online educational programs and some of the professional nursing organizations also have free or low-cost access to these online databases to make them readily accessible. For example, MEDLINE is accessed free of charge through the National Library of Medicine's PubMed Web site. CINAHL offers individual subscriptions, although CINAHL does not include medical or basic science journals. MEDLINE incorporates abstracts and references from biomedical journals. PsychINFO is an electronic database produced by the American Psychological Association that includes the behavioral sciences. It is accessed through the American Psychological Association Website. All three of these databases allow users to enter search subjects and then narrow searches by criteria such as language, journal subset, and/or publication year. For example, MEDLINE users can limit a search to nursing journals and/or research reports. CINAHL provides similar capabilities. These features allow potential researchers to quickly determine whether research has been conducted in their area of interest and to peruse the reported findings. The success of search results is directly related to the choice of the terms selected for search. Search terms or key terms act as filters for records stored in the database. Typically authors are asked to supply key terms or concepts for their work. Key terms also vary from database to database. PubMed uses key terms known as Mesh headings. Wong, Wilczynski, and Haynes (2006) noted a 70% overlap in terms between MEDLINE and CINAHL, with CINAHL containing terms unique to nursing. In their analytic study they compared hand searches with CINAHL results to determine the best search strategies to locate research studies and systematic reviews. They used very specific terms such as *exp study design, clinical trial.pt, meta-analysis.mp,* and *meta-analysis.sh.* The use of the "meta-analysis," either in combination with the letters "mp" to refer to multiple posting or "sh" referring to subject heading, represented the best approach to retrieve systematic reviews in CINAHL. Users may view article abstracts and, in some cases, retrieve the full text for articles online through the use of these and other databases. Box 18–4 summarizes a few advantages and disadvantages associated with online literature searches.

Digital Libraries

A **digital library** extends the missions and techniques of physical libraries through information technology (Barroso, Edlin, Sandelowski, & Lambe 2006). Digital libraries are comprised of a set of electronic resources with the related capabilities to create, store, organize, search, and retrieve information to meet the needs of a community of users. While this sounds very much like online access to databases offered by any public or school library, digital libraries extend the capabilities of information retrieval systems to provide open sharing of information to special

BOX 18–4   **Pros and Cons of Online Literature Searches**

Pros

- Searches may be completed quickly.
- Searches may be done without the aid of a librarian.
- Searches may be limited to specific years, languages, or journal subsets.
- Searches may be general or limited to clinical trials and other research reports.
- Online abstracts allow researchers to quickly determine if a particular article suits their purpose.
- When available, full-text retrieval allows the researcher to obtain articles without searching for volumes on a shelf or waiting for copies to arrive from other sites.

Cons

- Searches require a basic level of comfort and skill with online resources and key terms.
- The person conducting the search must be able to narrow the topic area.
- Search results are directly related to the selection of search terms. Poor selection of terms may falsely indicate no or few articles on a given topic or provide a large number of results of limited usefulness.
- Researchers may need the services of a librarian to improve search strategies, selection of search terms, and limiters.
- Online searches may not entirely eliminate the need to locate volumes and photocopy articles or wait for copies to arrive from other libraries unless full-text retrieval is available.
- Online retrieval can be expensive for individuals purchasing articles on a per view basis.

communities of users. For example, the SandBar Digital Library (sonweb.unc.edu/sandbar/index.cfm) is funded by a grant from the National Institute of Nursing Research (NINR) and was built by the University of North Carolina. The purpose of digital libraries is to transform large volumes of data into information and knowledge. SandBar integrates findings from qualitative studies of women with HIV infection. The National Electronic Library for Health (NeLH) was a highly publicized digital library in the United Kingdom, but it has since been replaced by the National Library for Health (http://www.library.nhs.uk/Default.aspx); it provides access to evidence-based reviews, guidelines, various databases, news, and updates. Digital libraries are characterized by open access and sharing and frequently increase access to materials that would otherwise be challenging to access. Digital libraries allow users to search or browse a particular research topic. McCall (2006) noted that clinicians at the bedside need quick access to information with many digital library system searches lasting one minute or less. Digital library access will most likely continue to evolve in the coming decade and beyond as clinicians need scientific data literally at their fingertips.

Data Collection Tools

Data collection tools may be located via online literature searches and discussion lists. Test references provide comprehensive information on published tools that are available for purchase as well as unpublished instruments that appear in journal articles. The use of an existing data collection tool offers the researcher the benefits of established validity and consistency, and the ability to commence research sooner without spending time to devise and test an instrument. A **data collection tool** is a device that has been created for the purpose of accumulating specific details in an organized fashion. Some examples include a physical assessment form, a graphics record, and opinion questionnaires. Once a suitable tool is found, permission for its use often may be obtained more quickly through e-mail than through traditional mail. In the event that a suitable tool is not located, the construction of a data collection tool via word processing software makes revision easy, while online construction yields immediate feedback.

Once the data collection instrument is constructed, discussion lists and chat rooms may be used to test the instrument, solicit study participants, and even collect data. E-mail interviews and Web-based surveys offer alternative methods to collect research data electronically. E-mail allows varying degrees of structure in the interview process, as well as ease of transcription via downloading without interpretation error secondary to pauses and inflection. Data collection via the Internet can offer several advantages. These may include:

- Interactive forms that can be evaluated for completeness and accuracy of data before submission
- Automated data compilation and exportation to other software
- Fast, cost-effective administration of surveys
- Freedom from geographic boundaries
- Ease associated with sending out reminders to complete survey instruments
- Access to previously hidden populations

The Internet population is not representative of the general population. However, because the Internet it is not available to everyone, selection bias is another factor that limits the generalizability of results because the Internet population is nonrepresentative and because open surveys conducted via the Web net volunteer participants. Box 18–5 provides some suggestions for the design and administration of Web-based data collection tools. As with traditional research methods, ethical issues must be considered. These issues include informed consent, protection of privacy, and the avoidance of harm. The ability to use cookies to assign a unique identifier to each person viewing a Web-based questionnaire offers the researcher the ability to determine response and participation rates and to filter out multiple responses. Researchers using cookies should publish a privacy policy, state that cookies will be sent, explain their purpose, and set an expiration date based on the date that data collection will end. Researchers must also recognize that there will be occasional problems with online data collection, including programming errors, usability problems, software incompatibilities, and technical problems (Schleyer & Forrest 2000).

> ### BOX 18–5 Tips for Design and Administration of Web-Based Data Collection Tools
>
> - Determine the objectives for the tool.
> - Write and then edit questions.
> - Include title, introduction, purpose of the tool, and an anonymity statement.
> - Critique the tool for reading level.
> - Ensure that the tool is visually attractive.
> - Limit the amount of information on a page.
> - Ask evaluators to rate the tool for readability and time required for completion and elicit their suggestions.
> - Test the automated data collection process before public posting.
> - Pretest the tool before public posting.
> - Include a few open-ended questions, and provide a wrap-up.

QUANTITATIVE VERSUS QUALITATIVE RESEARCH

Quantitative research uses objective measurements to study structured questions. Typically large numbers of subjects are used to obtain results to be considered statistically valid. A major concern with quantitative research is whether study results can be replicated and the findings subsequently applied to a larger population. This is in contrast to qualitative research where the researcher is examining subjective individual interpretation. Qualitative research examines meanings, concepts, definitions, characteristics, metaphors, symbols, and descriptions of things. Qualitative research uses a variety of methods to collect information, including in-depth interviews and focus groups. Both quantitative and qualitative research methods are supported and facilitated through various information technology applications.

Direct Data Input

Data collection can be expedited through the use of mobile devices such as PDAs and notebook computers at the study site. Data can be transmitted, if needed, to another computer for compilation and analysis. This eliminates transcription errors and lost or illegible paper notes, and speeds the data collection and analysis process. Interactive data collection tools offer the advantages of engaging the participant, eliminating redundant data entry, and decreasing the time and costs needed for cleaning data to ensure its quality.

Data Analysis

Data analysis is the processing of data collected during the course of a study to identify trends and patterns of relationships. This task begins with descriptive statistics in quantitative, and some qualitative, studies. Descriptive statistics permit the researcher to organize the data in meaningful ways that facilitate insight by describing what the data show. Theory development and the generation of hypotheses may emerge from descriptive analysis. In addition to descriptive analysis, there are a number of statistical procedures that a researcher must choose when conducting a study. Until recently, researchers embarking on large studies needed the services of statisticians and large computing centers for data analysis. Many practitioners and students in the healthcare professions thought they were unable to perform meaningful research without these supports. Personal computers now rival larger systems in abilities and can easily link with larger computers, making it easier to conduct research in any setting.

There has been a growing recognition that the huge amounts of data collected within business and healthcare systems might be tapped and used for a variety of purposes. The overwhelming volume of data requires computer processing to turn data into useful information. A variety of terms exist to refer to the use and processing of this data. **Knowledge discovery in databases (KDD)** is a term used in other industries that is now seen in healthcare circles. KDD identifies complex patterns and relationships in collected data. It provides a powerful tool suitable for the analysis of large amounts of data. Commercial packages are available in a range of prices and platforms. KDD may be used to identify risk factors for diseases or efficacy of particular treatment modalities. The confidentiality of individual records may be protected through the use of data perturbation. This is a technique that modifies actual data values to hide confidential information while maintaining the underlying aggregate relationships of the database. Further research is needed on the use of data perturbation and its potential to introduce bias. As healthcare systems continue to expand and explode with large data sets there will be more and more opportunity for KDD to facilitate opportunities to work within these systems and produce population data on a grand scale. **Data mining** is another term for the use of database applications to look for previously hidden patterns. Its use is growing; it has been investigated for marketing purposes, tracking the factors underlying medication errors, and improving financial performance. Data mining supports sifting through large volumes of data at rapid speeds in ways that were not previously possible due to size or speed limitations. Data mining allows real-time access to information for a competitive edge. Data mining in conjunction with electronic records can help physicians quickly determine the number of clients in their practice that need examinations and to generate reminders. Application of mined data is contingent on its quality and on maintaining scientific rigor and scientific processes while gathering it.

Quantitative Analysis The computational abilities of computers readily lend themselves to statistical analysis of qualitative data and render more accurate results than might be available from hand-calculated statistics. Several software packages are available for quantitative analysis; most evolved during the 1960s and 1970s and permit the importation of data from spreadsheet or database software, and sometimes ASCII files. The majority provide versions of their products for a variety of computer platforms. A partial list follows:

- The System for Statistical Analysis (SAS) comprises several products for the management and analysis of data. It is considered an industry standard.
- MINITAB Statistical Software offers an alternative to SAS. Geared to users at every level, it is widely used by high school and college students and incorporates pull-down menus for ease of use.
- BMDP evolved as a biomedical analysis package. It comes in personal and professional editions and offers an easy-to-use interface for data analysis. BMDP also prompts the user until analysis is complete. It offers a comprehensive library of statistical routines.
- SPSS is another well-known software company. SPSS provides products for most computer platforms; it provides statistics, graphics, and data management and reporting capabilities.
- S-Plus is known for its flexibility in allowing users to define and customize functions. It also offers extensive graphics.
- SYSTAT, unlike some of the other packages discussed, was first developed for PC use.
- DataDesk started as a MacIntosh product, but it now is also available for use with Windows.
- JMP started as a MacIntosh product and resembles DataDesk. It is available for use with Windows.

Despite the increased use of statistical analysis packages by nurses, some researchers still argue that nurses should work with the traditional users of supercomputers to develop the skills needed to use these resources and to access large data archives held by government and private agencies. Supercomputers offer the ability to quickly peruse huge databases. This belief gives rise to a new branch of nursing science: nurmetrics. Nurmetrics uses mathematical forms and statistics to test, estimate, and quantify nursing theories and solutions to problems.

Computer Models Computational nursing, a branch of nurmetrics, uses models and simulation for the application of existing theory and numerical methods to new solutions for nursing problems and for the development of new computational methods (Meintz 1994; Van Sell & Kalofissudis 2002). One proposed use of nurmetrics and computational nursing is the formulation and testing of new models for healthcare delivery by using computers. This application is cost effective and can demonstrate how factors such as education may affect health practices and outcomes over time without the need to first implement the program and wait for results. Nursing informatics uses computer science and informatics principles to understand how the structure and function of information may be used to solve problems in nursing administration, nursing education, practice, and research. The College of Nursing at the University of Iowa established the Center for Computational Nursing, which is affiliated with their Institute for Nursing Knowledge.

Qualitative Analysis Computers facilitate organized storage, tabulation, and retrieval of qualitative data. For example, databases can be used like electronic filing cabinets to store data; software can locate key words or phrases in a database, sort data in a prescribed fashion, code observations or comments for later retrieval, support researcher notes, and help create and represent conceptual schemes. As notes, coding, sorting, and pasting are automated, researchers have more time to analyze data. Despite these benefits, critics cite the following challenges:

- Qualitative research may be molded to fit the computer program.
- Computers tempt researchers to use large populations, thus sacrificing in-depth study for breadth.

Software is available to support qualitative research by allowing researchers to automate clerical tasks, merge data, code, and link data. QSR International provides several products that facilitate qualitative research, including NUD*IST and Nvivo. Ethnograph is another product that supports importation of text-based qualitative data into word processing packages. HyperRESEARCH and TAMS Analyzer represent other examples of qualitative software. AQUAD is a specialized program for users with an advanced knowledge of qualitative research. Text must first be entered or scanned into a word processor and converted into ASCII. AQUAD permits coding on the screen, and researchers may define linkages they wish to explore. Words or phrases in text and their frequency may be noted. Listservs that support qualitative research include QUALRS-L, QUALNET-L, and Qual-software.

Data Presentation: Graphics

Once data analysis is complete, graphics presentation software helps the researcher put study findings into a form that is easy for the reader to follow in written study reports and for the listener to follow when findings are presented at professional meetings and conferences. Graphics presentation software allows the researcher to design and make slides for use at presentations without the services of a media department. Harvard Graphics and PowerPoint are two well-known commercial packages. PDAs can now be used to store slide presentations. Figure 18–1 shows a bar graph prepared using a graphics application.

Online Access to Databases

The National Institutes of Health (NIH) offers access to several databases useful to nurses interested in research, health policy, and the identification of funded research projects. One of these databases, the Computer Retrieval of Information on Scientific Projects (CRISP), provides information on research grants supported by the Department of Health and Human Services. CRISP lists the following data for each project: title, grant number, abstract, principal investigator, thesaurus terms, and key words. CRISP is updated weekly and is available at crisp.cit.nih.gov/. Search results may be printed or saved. The

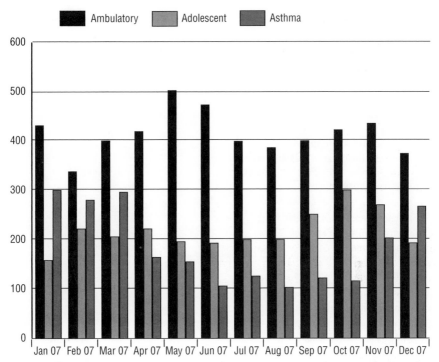

FIGURE 18–1 • Bar graph depicting the number of clinic visits per month for January 2007 through December 2007

Agency for Healthcare Research and Quality (AHRQ) sponsors the National Quality Measures Clearinghouse (NQMC). NQMC is a public repository for evidence-based quality measures and measure sets. NQMC may be accessed through the AHRQ Website at www.ahrq.gov. The intent of this database is to provide detailed information on quality measures and to further their use.

Several other agencies provide access to online databases useful to healthcare researchers, educators, clinicians, and administrators. These include the following:

- The National Library of Medicine (NLM) at www.nlm.nih.gov.
- Sigma Theta Tau's Virginia Henderson International Nursing Library (INL) at www.nursinglibrary.org/portal/main.aspx. The INL provides information on grant opportunities, nurse researchers, meeting proceedings, and access to databases that pertain to nursing research.
- The Cochrane Library at http://www.cochrane.org/reviews/clibintro.htm. The Cochrane Library consists of a regularly updated collection of evidence-based medicine databases, including the Cochrane Database of Systematic Reviews.

There are a number of other sites that contain links to databases and research-related information. These sites are maintained by government agencies, professional organizations, and publishers, among others. Box 18–6 lists some

---

BOX 18–6   Possible Funding Sources for Healthcare

Government Agencies

- National Institutes of Health
- National Institute of Nursing Research
- National Library of Medicine
- Substance Abuse and Mental Health Services Administration
- Centers for Disease Control and Prevention
- Food and Drug Administration
- Agency for Healthcare Research and Quality

Professional Organizations

- Sigma Theta Tau
- American Nurses Association
- Oncology Nursing Foundation
- Specialty Groups

Foundations and Organizations

- Robert Wood Johnson Foundation
- Skin Cancer Foundation
- Epilepsy Foundation
- Myasthenia Gravis Foundation
- American Cancer Society
- March of Dimes
- Arthritis Foundation

---

other sources to consider when seeking research funds. AHRQ is one agency that actively supports research to improve healthcare, particularly studies that can improve patient safety, access to services, and bioterrorism knowledge and preparedness. AHRQ maintains a page for nursing research with links to evidence-based research, funding sources, and news (AHRQ ND).

Collaborative Research

Collaborative computing and research foster productivity by allowing individuals at dispersed sites to share ideas and information in real time. Collaborative computing may use e-mail, desktop videoconferencing, other telecommunication tools, digital libraries, or shared databases to join persons of like interests from locations across the globe.

Collaborative research also offers the potential to help healthcare professionals who lack basic competence and comfort with research methods and skills to develop their skills through mentor relationships. The American Academy of Nursing (AAN) and the AHRQ sponsor the Senior Nurse Scholar in Residence program as a means to encourage a senior nurse researcher to develop areas of investigation that integrate clinical nursing care questions with issues of quality, costs, and access. Information about this program can be found on the AHRQ Website. There are currently initiatives at the NINR to move science forward in more collaborative, synergistic ways than in the past, and the NIH roadmap involves promotion of interdisciplinary teams in addition to clinical and translational research (NINR 2004).

MULTI-INSTITUTIONAL RESEARCH

Automation and uniform languages also aid the simultaneous collection of data from multiple sources. This capability has been limited to healthcare alliances that can, and already do, share data. Predictably there will be even further impetus for the development of national health information networks that can expand linkages to massive databases and solidify those capabilities. The ability to access these large macro databases provides opportunity for multi-institutional research, offering researchers the opportunity to increase the size of their study populations and to eliminate idiosyncrasies associated with a particular place as a contributing factor to the findings. In short, multi-institutional research ensures that findings can be applied to a larger population, increasing the generalizability of one's findings.

RESEARCH IN REAL TIME

The potential of hospital information systems to collect large amounts of data almost instantly allows for research in "real time," or essentially as events occur. This ability helps institutions react quickly to changes noted in client populations. Some systems can perform routine work while automatically channeling study information into an appropriate database according to particular study protocols. This is a desirable feature that would eliminate redundant data entry; however, at the present, few information systems are flexible enough to do this. This lack of flexibility creates the need to collect, gather, and format data separately each time they are needed for a research study.

The Role of Uniform Languages

The lack of a common language to facilitate data collection and decision making was recognized as a problem in healthcare and nursing several years ago. The Unified Medical Language System project represents an attempt to standardize terms used in healthcare delivery in a way that can be understood, measured, and coded across different settings (NLM 2006). The American Nurses Association had a database steering committee working on the Unified Nursing Language System as a means to develop and use other clinical databases to extend nursing knowledge.

A standardized nursing language allows accurate communication among nurses, which aids research and subsequently adds to the body of nursing knowledge. The American Nurses' Association (ANA) (2007) has recognized several standardized languages and terminologies to support nursing practice. These include:

- NANDA for nursing diagnosis.
- The Nursing Interventions Classification (NIC).
- The Nursing Outcomes Classification (NOC).
- The Clinical Care Classification (CCC), which is an interface terminology that contains diagnoses, interventions, and outcomes for use in home care.
- The Home Health Care Classification (HHCC).
- The Omaha System for capturing community health information.
- The Nursing Minimum Data Set (NMDS), which contains clinical data elements.
- Nursing Management Minimum Data Set (NMMDS), which contains nursing administrative data elements.
- The Patient Care Data Set (PCDS), which has since been retired from use.
- The PeriOperative Nursing Data Set (PNDS), a set of diagnoses, interventions, and outcomes for the perioperative area.
- ABC codes (Alternative Billing Concept codes) for use in interventions in nursing and other areas.
- Logical Observation Identifiers Names and Codes (LOINC®) for use of outcome and assessments.
- The Systematic Nomenclature of Medicine Clinical Terms (SNOMED CT®).
- The International Classification for Nursing Practice (ICNP®), which addresses diagnoses, interventions, and outcomes for all of nursing.

SNOMED and ICNP® are the two most widely accepted standards in nursing. At this time standard languages are fodder for research as well as a tool to enhance research through shared meanings. Research has been done to examine mapping between languages. More research will be needed in this area but ICNP® includes all nursing specialties and demonstrates the ability to encompass other standardized nursing languages (ANA 2007; Hyun & Park 2002; Ryan 2006).

In addition to facilitating data collection, uniform languages set the definition of key terms, ensuring that studies can be replicated. Implementation of uniform languages first requires the following:

- Education of staff who are unfamiliar with standardized terms
- Elimination of computer restraints, such as limited characters and lines per field, found with some computer systems
- Database coordination among various clinicians and departments that use terms differently but require access to shared data repositories. This is also known as mapping terms.

IMPEDIMENTS TO HEALTHCARE RESEARCH

From a health information technology perspective, healthcare research has been impeded by slow adoption of data exchange standards and uniform languages, failure to realize a birth-to-death electronic health record, limited interoperability, limited health information exchange, concerns over the confidentiality of private health information, and limited funding. Many technical issues still need to be resolved. From a business perspective competing organizations share the same concerns about sharing information within and between healthcare systems. These concerns present barriers to the creation of large databases required to accurately identify trends related to healthcare problems and to develop successful treatment options, which are so sorely needed. These data from large data sets could certainly hold the key to many of the population-focused challenges confronting healthcare delivery systems, including primary, secondary, and tertiary prevention as well as the shift from inpatient to outpatient care delivery settings. Outcomes and impacts from these data could serve as the basis for policy change at local, state, and federal levels as well.

DISSEMINATION OF RESEARCH FINDINGS

Researchers have a professional obligation to share their research findings. There are multiple opportunities and venues through which one can share and disseminate research findings, such as via traditional paper-based journals, digital libraries, and various online publications. The process of dissemination of research findings can take several weeks from the time a researcher queries a journal to determine if there is interest in publishing his or her study findings until a reply is received. The query and submission process is shortened with electronic publication. Queries, submissions, reviews, and publication can all be done electronically via email. The *Journal of Medical Internet Research* is an example of an online publication with a research focus. Electronic publication has made it possible for more organizations to establish their own journals, and researchers should become familiar with the publication venue that is the best fit for them through conversations with the publisher, mentor, or other colleagues.

Preparing research findings for dissemination through publication is facilitated by using a bibliography database manager (BDM) (Nicoll 2003). This software maintains accuracy of references and properly formats in-text citations as well as the final reference list. BDMs allow the importation of references directly from databases, eliminating the need to rekey and eliminating typographical errors. This process requires an Internet connection to the database, and in some cases a user ID and password to access the database. Selected examples of available BDMs include EndNote, Reference Manager, ProCite, and Biblioscape.

IMPLICATIONS OF HIPAA AND OTHER LEGISLATION FOR HEALTHCARE RESEARCH

The Health Insurance Portability and Accountability Act (HIPAA) originated in 2003 and is now in its 10th year of existence (Shaughnessy, Beidler, Gibbs, & Michael, 2007). The passage of HIPAA brought concerns over its implications for healthcare research, and during the inception of HIPAA, the NIH posted explanatory documents online to clarify information for actual and potential researchers (February 2004; September 2003). Researchers have experienced barriers due to HIPAA, and it seems that clinical researchers now take what has been described as "extra care" while doing clinical research. As of April 2003, HIPAA, also referred to as the Privacy Rule, requires healthcare providers and insurers to obtain additional documentation from researchers related to assurances of patient safety and confidentiality. The key concern is that human subjects, irrespective of age, are protected with a high degree of confidentiality from the person getting access to their personal information. This means there is increased scrutiny and monitoring of requests for access to health information. For example, there may be a need for additional documentation, including written permission from subjects who sign a special authorization form, or a waiver of the authorization requirement from the institutional review board or privacy board. A signed authorization form for research is valid only for a specific research study, not for future projects. Authorization differs from informed consent in that the authorization allows an entity to use or disclose a person's protected health information (PHI) for a specific purpose such as a study, whereas informed consent constitutes permission to participate in the research. The authorization must specify what PHI will be used or disclosed, who can use or disclose it, the purpose of the use or disclosure, and an expiration date. There must also be statements that address the individual's right to revoke the authorization and how that could be accomplished; whether treatment, payment, enrollment, or eligibility of benefits can be based on authorization; and the person's right to know that the Privacy Rule may no longer apply if PHI is redisclosed by the recipient. The authorization form must be signed and dated. Authorization is not required or may be altered when the covered entity obtains appropriate documentation that an institutional review board or a privacy board has granted a waiver or alteration of authorization requirements. Authorization is not required once information has been de-identified according to Privacy Rule standards.

Researchers are not covered entities unless they are also healthcare providers, are employed by a covered entity, or engage in any of the electronic transactions covered under HIPAA. Covered entities include providers that transmit health information electronically for HIPAA transactions, health plans, and clearinghouses. The Privacy Rule allows PHI use or disclosure to researchers to determine if the number and type of study subjects are sufficient to conduct research and if information has been stripped of all or certain identifiers. This second instance is referred to as *limited data*. Covered entities may disclose PHI to researchers to aid in study recruitment. Research started before the enactment of the Privacy Rule may be allowed to continue under a "grandfather" provision. Researchers need to be aware of HIPAA's Privacy Rule because it establishes the conditions under which covered entities can use or disclose PHI. There are implications for the creation and use of databases that contain PHI and that may be used at some future point in time. Researchers may be responsible for drafting the authorization form. Not all researchers must comply with the Privacy Rule.

STUDENTS USING COMPUTERS TO SUPPORT EVIDENCE-BASED PRACTICE AND RESEARCH

Students often believe that research has little significance for them, and few actually carry out the entire research process. This is unfortunate because students need to develop information literacy skills, including the ability to locate and understand research reports as a means to engage in evidence-based practice. A program outcome essential for healthcare students is that they be skilled in applications facilitating electronic literature searches. Despite the availability and merits of this type of search, students fail to find useful information when their choice of search limiters or terms is not appropriate to the database. Online literature searches provide up-to-date information, unlike reference books, which are dated in many areas by the date of publication. Students should also be aware of other resources such as digital libraries that offer systematic reviews of research findings.

A more popular resource is the World Wide Web. It offers a wealth of information for both healthcare professionals and consumers. It is widely accessible at educational institutions for students who have no home Internet access. It even has sites of particular interest to students in the healthcare professions. Students might choose to prepare for a community health teaching project by searching for materials on the Web as long as they are attentive to the quality of sites selected and dates of publication or revision.

Students enrolled in research courses may have occasion to use software for statistical analysis, presentation of graphics, and proposal and report preparation. Many texts include software with study questions for mastery of research content.

Despite the fact that this is considered to be a "digital age" when most students are familiar with a multitude of computer skills, including e-mail, instant messages, Web searches, and file downloads, not all students are equally skilled when it comes to information literacy skills. Reference librarians and faculty are in the ideal position to help foster these skills.

FUTURE DIRECTIONS

Nursing and healthcare both lag behind in the translation of research findings into practice and still need additional information to deliver more effective healthcare at a lower cost. The creation and innovation of new practice models, patient safety outcomes, data driven tests of change, and best practice lie in the ability to work with the resources within our systems. For example, the electronic health record (EHR) provides the database needed to support research and evidence-based practice and has the potential to change and shape care practices. Incorporation of evidence-based guidelines into the EHR and the ability to access data driven information at the bedside puts care and support literally in the hands of clinicians, standardizes evidence-based care, improves quality, and ultimately advances care for patients and satisfaction for providers. The EHR is changing the way in which information is collected and used, ensuring the survival of enterprises that have EHR capability. Eventually one imagines an EHR that contains data from birth to death, making tracking and trending of information across one's life span completely possible with remote access from anywhere in the world. It is hard to imagine these "Star Wars" scenarios, but the technology provides tools and opportunities for system automation unlike ever before. As we move forward in the marriage between clinical practice and technology, there are many considerations that can only be provided by a savvy healthcare provider who is knowledgeable in what the challenges and opportunities are between science and mankind. Above all else, the outcomes and impacts at the bedside are the true gauge of how well we did in the marriage.

CASE STUDY EXERCISES

18.1   You are the staff nurse in a busy medical–surgical department at your community hospital. You and several of your colleagues have an idea that client anxiety is decreased in direct proportion to the amount of teaching that they receive preoperatively. Describe how you might use information technology to look at this issue and prepare a proposal for funding consideration.

18.2   You and your classmates are expected to conduct a health teaching project in a public high school as one of the requirements for your Community Health Nursing course. Identify and discuss resources that you might use to gather material for this project.

18.3   You are working the night shift at your local community hospital. One of your clients was newly diagnosed today with a rare disorder that is unknown to you and your peers. Mrs. Prado is unable to sleep and is asking for more information about her diagnosis. None of the reference books on your unit provide information about her diagnosis. Your unit does, however, have an Internet connection. How might you use resources on hand to meet Mrs. Prado's needs?

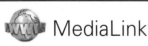 MediaLink

Additional resources for this content can be found on the Companion Website at www.prenhall.com/hebda. Click on "Chapter 18" to select the activities for this chapter.

- Glossary
- Multiple Choice
- Discussion Points
- Case Studies
- MediaLink Application
- MediaLink

SUMMARY

- There is a gap between theory and practice that results in diminished patient care, inefficient practice, and an excessive time lag between the discovery of knowledge and its incorporation into clinical practice. Evidence-based practice represents the attempt to close this gap.
- Evidence-based practice (EBP) is an approach to providing care that integrates nursing experience and intuition with valid and current clinical research to achieve the best patient outcomes.
- Evidence-based practice (EBP) asks a relevant question, searches literature for evidence, critically examines the evidence, changes practice as needed, evaluates the effects of change, and maintains the change that was based upon the integration of best practices.
- Information technology provides the tools to support evidence-based practice and research.
- Research provides the data that allow better allocation of scarce resources and that support the development of knowledge.
- Electronic literature searches, online discussion groups, and digital libraries facilitate both evidence-based practice and research through the identification of questions, location of literature, systematic reviews, and resources.
- Data collection instruments may be located, developed, and even administered online.
- Data analysis is facilitated via the use of software for both qualitative and quantitative analyses.
- Nurmetrics is a branch of nursing science that uses mathematical form and statistics to test solutions to problems. One branch of nurmetrics known as computational nursing uses models and simulations to test solutions and proposed models for care.
- Several organizations maintain databases that contain information useful to nurses conducting research, including CRISP, the National Library of Medicine, the *American Journal of Nursing*, and Sigma Theta Tau.
- The implementation of the electronic health record will provide information required to deliver healthcare more effectively and at lower costs.
- Standardized languages provide a mechanism to ensure common meanings to terms, facilitate data collection, and aid research. The International Classification for Nursing Practice (ICNP®) includes all nursing subspecialties and demonstrates the ability to encompass other standardized nursing languages.
- Automation and the implementation of the electronic health record are expected to increase multi-institutional research efforts as well as research in real time and collaborative research.

- Students in the healthcare professions may reap the benefits of information technology to support evidence-based practice.
- Researchers need to be aware of relevant legislation such as HIPAA and the requirements that such legislation imposes on them in their conduct of research.

REFERENCES

Agency for Healthcare Research and Quality. (ND). NursingResearch. Retrieved January 26, 2008, from http://www.ahrq.gov/about/nursing/.

American Nurses Association. (2004). Nursing Information and Data Set Evaluation Center (NIDSECSM). Retrieved March 10, 2004, from http://www.nursingworld.org/nidsec/.

American Nurses' Association. (June 5, 2007). Relationships among ANA recognized data element sets and terminologies. Retrieved January 14, 2008, from http://nursingworld.org/npii/relationship.htm.

ANCC (2007). *Magnet recognition.* Retrieved February 1, 2008, from http://www.nursecredentialing.org/magnet/.

Barroso, J., Edlin, A., Sandelowski, M., & Lambe, C. (2006). Bridging the gap between research and practice: The development of a digital library of research syntheses. *CIN: Computers, Informatics, Nursing, 24*(2), 85–94.

Cassey, M. Z. (2007, March–April). Keeping up with existing and emerging technologies: An introduction to PDAs. *Nursing Economics, 25*(2), 121–135.

Chester, L. (2007, March). Many critical care nurses are unaware of evidence-based practice…Evidence-based practice is wonderful…sort of (July 2006, 356–358). *American Journal of Critical Care, 16*(2), 106.

Colevins, H., Bond, D., & Clark, K. (2006, April). Refresher students hand from handhelds. *Computers in Libraries, 7–8*, 46–48.

Courey, T., Benson-Soros, J., Deemer, K., & Zeller, R. (2006, November). The missing link: Information literacy and evidence-based practice as a new challenge for nurse educators. *Nursing Education Perspectives, 27*(6), 320–323.

Dracup, K. & Bryan-Brown, C. (2006, July). Evidence-based practice is wonderful… sort of. *American Journal of Critical Care, 15*(4), 356–358.

Drenning, C. (2006, October). Using the best evidence to change practice. Collaboration among to achieve evidence-based practice change. *Journal of Nursing Care Quality, 21*(4), 298–301.

Evidence-based resources for PDAs. *Nursing 2007,* August 2007, 58–61.

Gardner, C. & Beese-Bjurstrom, S. (2006, June). In our unit. RN-driven, evidence-based practice. *Critical Care Nurse, 26*(3), 80.

Hanberg, A. & Brown, S. (2006, November). Bridging the theory—practice gap with evidence-based practice. *Journal of Continuing Education in Nursing, 37*(6), 248–249.

Hardwick, M., Pulido, P., & Adelson, W. (2007, July). The use of handheld technology in nursing research and practice. *Orthopaedic Nursing, 26*(4), 251–255.

Hockenberry, M., Wilson, D., & Barrera, P. (2006, July). Evidence-based practice. Implementing evidence-based nursing practice in a pediatric hospital. *Pediatric Nursing, 32*(4), 371–377.

Hyun, S. & Park, H. A (2002). Cross-mapping the ICNP with NANDA, HHCC, Omaha System and NIC for unified nursing language system development. *International Nursing Review, 49*(2), 99–110.

Institute of Medicine (IOM). (2001). *Crossing the Quality Chasm: A New Health System for the 21st Century.* Washington, DC: National Academy Press.

MacCall, S. L. (2006). Clinical Digital Libraries Project: Design approach and exploratory assessment of timely use in clinical environments. *Journal of the Medical Library Association, 94*(2), 190–197.

Marchioinini, G. & Fox, E. (1999). Progress toward digital libraries: Augmentation through integration. *Information Processing & Management, 35*(3), 219–225.

Matter, S. (2006, December). Empower nurses with evidence-based knowledge. *Nursing Management, 37*(12), 34–37.

Meintz, S. L. (1994). High performance computing for nursing research. In S. J. Grobe and E. S. P. Pluyter-Wenting (Eds.), *Nursing informatics: An international overview for nursing in a technological era. Proceedings of the Fifth IMIA International Conference on Nursing Use of Computers and Information Science* (pp. 448–451). New York: Elsevier.

Melnyk, B. M. & Fineout-Overholt, E. (2005). *Evidence-based practice in nursing & healthcare.* Philadelphia, PA: Lippincott Williams & Wilkins.

Mitchell, P. (2006). Research and development in nursing revisited: Nursing science as the basis for evidence-based practice. *Journal of Advanced Nursing, 54*(5), 528–529.

National Institutes of Health. (September 2003). Privacy boards and the HIPAA privacy rule. Retrieved March 10, 2004, from http://privacyruleandresearch.nih.gov/privacy_boards/hipaa_privacy_rule.asp.

National Institutes of Health. (2004). Clinical Research and the HIPAA Privacy Rule. NIH Publication Number 04–5495. Retrieved March 10, 2004, from http://privacyruleandresearch.nih.gov/clin_research.asp.

National Library of Medicine (NLM). (May 19, 2006). About the UMLS® Resources. Retrieved January 26, 2008, from http://www.nlm.nih.gov/research/umls/about_umls.html.

Nicoll, L. H. (2003). A practical way to create a library in a bibliography database manager: Using electronic sources to make it easy. *CIN: Computers, Informatics, Nursing, Plus, 21*(1), 48–54.

Pipe, T. (2007). Optimizing nursing care by integrating theory-driven evidence-based practice. *Journal of Nursing Care Quality, 22*(3), 234–238.

Pravikoff, D. S., Tanner, A. B. & Pierce, S. T. (2005). Readiness of U.S. nurses for evidence-based practice. *American Journal of Nursing, 105*(9), 40–51.

Proceedings of the National Institute of Nursing Research Integration of NINR Areas of Science with the NIH Roadmap (2004, January 22–23), 1–12.

Ryan, S. (2006). Interview. Multidisciplinary terminology: The International Classification for Nursing Practice (ICNP)…Amy Coenen. *Online Journal of Nursing Informatics, 10*(3), (2p).

Salmond, S. (2007). Advancing evidence-based practice: A primer. *Orthopaedic Nursing, 26*(2), 114–125.

Schleyer, T. K. L. & Forrest, J. L. (2000). Methods for the design and administration of web-based surveys. *Journal of the American Medical Informatics Association,* 416–425.

Shaughnessy, M., Beidler, S. M., Gibbs, K., & Michael, K. (2007). Confidentiality challenges and good clinical practices in human subjects research: Striking a balance. *Topics in Stroke Rehabilitation, 14*(2), 1–4.

Shirey, M. (2006). Evidence-based practice: How nurse leaders can facilitate innovation. *Nursing Administration Quarterly, 30*(3), 252–265.

Sigma Theta Tau International. (2006). 2006 EBP Study summary of findings. Retrieved January 27, 2008, from http://www.nursingknowledge.org/Portal/CMSLite/GetFile.aspx?ContentID=78260.

Sigma Theta Tau International. (2005). Position Statement on Evidence-Based Nursing. Retrieved January 27, 2008, from http://www.nursingsociety.org/aboutus/ PositionPapers/Pages/EBN_positionpaper.aspx.

Simpson, R. (2006). Evidence-based practice: How nursing administration makes it happen. *Nursing Administration Quarterly, 30*(3), 291–294.

Skiba, D. & Thompson, B. (2007). Report of the NLN Survey on Informatics Competencies in the Curriculum, A paper presented at *Evolution or Revolution: Recreating Nursing Education, The National League for Nursing's Annual Education Summit.* Phoenix, AZ.

Snyder, K. (2007). Nurses' thoughts on evidence-based practice. *American Journal of Critical Care, 16*(3), 312–312.

Stockwell, D. C. (2006). Handheld computing in pediatric practice: Is it for you? *Contemporary Pediatrics, 23*(9), 113–120.

Thompson, B. W. (2005). HIPAA guidelines for using PDAs. *Nursing 2005, 35*(11), 24.

Van Sell, S. L. & Kalofissudis, I. (2002). Theory of nursing knowledge and practice. Extracts from their under publication work. The evolving essence of the science of nursing, a complexity integration nursing theory. Retrieved March 9, 2004, from http://www.nursing.gr/theory/Holistic.html.

Wilson, R. L. & Rosen, P. A. (2003). Protecting data through "perturbation" techniques: The impact on knowledge discovery in databases. *Journal of Database Management, 14*(2), 14.

Wong S. S., Wilczynski, N. L., & Haynes, R. B. (2006). Optimal CINAHL search strategies for identifying therapy studies and review articles. *Journal of Nursing Scholarship, 38*(2), 194–199.

Zuzelo, P., McGoldrick, T., Seminara, P., & Karbach, H. (2006). Shared governance and EBP: A logical partnership? *Nursing Management, 37*(6), 45–50.

Appendix A: Internet Primer

This primer is a supplemental reference guide designed to get you up and running on the Internet. The Internet, generally referred to as the "Net," encompasses many different methods of manipulating information and communicating, including the World Wide Web, electronic mail, instant messaging, newsgroups, and file transfer.

TOOLS TO GET ONLINE

If you are not already online through your school or place of work, there are a few things you need to hook up to the Net:

- A computer
- A modem
- A telephone line (if you use your regular telephone line, callers will hear a busy signal when you are online; you can also get a dedicated line) or a cable, dish, Digital Subscriber Line (DSL), or wireless connection
- An Internet service provider (ISP)

Modems

A modem is a piece of equipment that changes computer information to the kind of information that can be passed over telephone or cable lines. It can be an external box or an internal card.

Modems come in different speeds. The speed of a modem determines how quickly you can download or access information from the Internet. Modem speeds keep getting faster, but as of this writing 56K is the fastest available speed available over dial-up connections. Faster connections can be obtained through cable TV companies, satellite connections, or DSL servers, which are available from the telephone company.

Some older computers do not support the fastest speeds for retrieving and displaying content from the Internet and do not provide the same level of service that the newer, faster computers can. Check your computer processor speed, the speed of available connections, and modem types and speeds to determine what is right for you. Your local computer hardware store and Internet service providers can help you with these decisions.

INTERNET SERVICE PROVIDERS

To access the Internet, most users go through an Internet Service Provider (ISP). ISPs are companies that run the computers that enable you to get onto the Net; these computers are called *servers*. When you connect to the Net via dial-up service your modem actually dials the phone number to connect to the ISP's server. DSL subscribers are always connected unless they turn off their computer or disconnect their connection. Some cable and telephone companies provide Internet access, although all levels of services may not be available in all areas.

When choosing an ISP, you should consider:

- *Price.* There are a variety of fee structures for Internet service. It is possible to obtain Internet access at no cost, but these providers generally bombard users with advertisements and may offer little or no technical support. Other providers provide free trial service for a limited time. Some ISPs allow unlimited use for a flat fee, some offer a certain amount of time per month before they begin charging extra, and some charge by the amount of time you are online from the moment you go online. Dial-up service is cheapest but is slow and not satisfactory for applications that require faster speeds or moving large files.
- *Traffic.* For dial-up service find out the "dial up" number (the number your modem calls to link up) of an ISP and call it at different times during the day. Some ISPs get a lot of traffic and it can be difficult to get online; this is particularly true of the larger, national companies.

ELECTRONIC MAIL (E-MAIL)

E-mail is a way of transmitting messages across a telephone line, network, or cable connection to other computers through your ISP. It works like this: You have a program called a mail browser (such as Microsoft Outlook) that enables you to send and read e-mail messages. To send e-mail, first type in the e-mail address. E-mail addresses look like this: user-name@servername.domainname—for example, ClaraBarton@nursingnet.com. Make sure to put what the message is about in the "subject" line. After writing your text in the "body" of the message, you can send it. The message is transmitted across telephone, cable, or network lines to the server, which sorts the mail and sends it to the correct e-mail address.

Whether you use e-mail for work or play, it is generally somewhat informal and not very lengthy. E-mail can be used for sending out memos, writing a note to a friend, and exchanging documents and files. You can even send someone your resume over e-mail (see Appendix B).

Some things to remember when using e-mail:

- Try to check your e-mail every day, especially if you belong to a mailing list (see section on listservs). It is amazing how quickly your mailbox can fill up with messages.
- Do not send lengthy material via e-mail.

- Know your netiquette.
- Do not send anything too confidential or sensitive over e-mail; e-mail is easily accessed by others.
- Try to proofread your e-mail before you send it; it is all too common to see typos in e-mail messages, many of which could be eliminated if the messages were read over just once.
- Do not pass on jokes, stories, and other similar "mass mailings" out to anyone that you do not know well or who prefers to not receive these types of materials.
- Have fun with e-mail! It is a good way to keep in touch, get messages out to a lot of people, and make new friends!

Many people take advantage of free e-mail services offered through Internet access where they work or attend school, or from libraries. In these instances, they use Web-based e-mail accounts that are usually free of charge from Yahoo or other sites.

THE WORLD WIDE WEB (WWW)

The World Wide Web provides a way to access Internet resources by content instead of file names. Since it was launched in 1992, the Web has virtually exploded into mainstream culture.

Browsers

To get to the Web, you must have a computer program called a Web browser. Some of the more popular Web browsers are Netscape Navigator and Microsoft Explorer. Once you are online with your server, you simply open the browser and you are ready to "surf" the Net.

Web Addresses

The Web is made up of millions of Websites (or Web pages). Each Website has an address, which is known as the URL (uniform resource locator). A typical URL looks like this: http://www.prenticehall.com/health; this is the address for the Prentice Hall Website for the health professions. To get to any Website, all you have to do is type the URL in the browser's "go to" box (or something similar, depending on which browser you are using). If you are not certain where this box is, look on the opening page of the browser for a line of characters in print that starts with "http://www."

You can dissect Website addresses and figure out who and what they stand for:

- "http," or HyperText Transport Protocol, appears in every Website address (with a few exceptions). You will always see "://" after "http."
- Generally you will see "www," which tells the server to get the information from the World Wide Web.

- The last two parts of the address are the domain name; in this case, prenticehall.com is the domain name. The domain indicates what kind of site it is. In our case it is ".com" (pronounced "dot-com"), which stands for "commercial." Other domains you will probably come across include: ".edu" = education, ".org" = organization, and ".gov" = government. You get the idea.

Note: Do not get http and HTML confused. HTML stands for HyperText Markup Language, the programming language that enables you to develop a Website. Also, when you read the address for a Website out loud, remember that every "." is pronounced "dot."

Websites

Websites are generally developed around a particular topic, such as nursing or healthcare. The amount of information available on the Web today is staggering and continues to grow. You can use the Web for general research, as an educational tool, as a shopping mall, to find a long lost friend, to get a new job (see Appendix B), or to answer practically any question you might have.

The first page you come to is called the home page, or sometimes the splash page. This page should convey the main ideas behind the entire Website. It generally contains a menu for the entire site.

The home page contains links to other pages. They send you into further detail by a click of the mouse. Links are generally marked by keywords or images. It's like an outline: The home page is your thesis, and each link is a breakdown of main ideas to be covered on that topic. To "follow a link" from the home page, look for highlighted text, buttons, or images and click on them with your mouse. For example, go to http://www.prenticehall.com/health and click on the word "nursing." This is a link to resources for nurses that includes the Prentice Hall book catalog as well as other sites of interest.

Search Engines

Now that you have a basic idea of the workings of the Web, how do you go about finding Websites that may interest you? There are a number of popular directories on the Web called *search engines*. Search engines are Websites that contain Website information (i.e., the URL and a short description) on virtually every topic imaginable.

Some of the larger and more popular search engines are:

- Google at http://www.google.com
- Yahoo! at http://www.yahoo.com

To use a search engine, type in one of the addresses listed above. When the home page for that site comes up, you will notice a search box in which you can type a keyword or phrase. The site will then bring up all the information that it has available on that topic as a list of sites. Sometimes you will need to narrow your search. For example, if you type in "nursing," hundreds of site listings will return. On the other hand, if you are too specific, you may not have any sites returned. You may have to try a few different word combinations to find the sites you are looking for.

Bookmarks

One very useful component of your Web browser is the bookmark tool. Whenever you come to a site that you may want to return to, you can bookmark it. To bookmark a site, go to that site. After it has loaded, choose "bookmark" or a similar command, depending on your browser. Your browser will record the address of that site in your bookmark folder. Anytime you want to return to that site, you simply open the bookmark folder and click on the title of that Website. It is possible to bookmark a Website using special services so you can access your list from anywhere.

Patience

Have patience when using the World Wide Web. Accessing some Websites can take time, depending on how elaborate the site is (e.g., how large it is, how many pictures are on it, and so on), how fast your modem can download the information, and what time of day you are surfing. You can speed things up a bit by turning off the autoload image option in your browser.

Also, you will encounter occasional problems. Sometimes the server of the Website you are trying to reach may be down or there is a lot of activity on that site so it will not be accessible. Try that site later. Dial-up connections are subject to getting disconnected particularly if there is noise on the line. You may notice that your connection is slower on certain days or times of the day depending upon the amount of traffic online at the same time.

Finally, because the Web is so dynamic, sites and links change every day. You might find numerous links on Web pages that go nowhere. There are many reasons for this: People move their pages to new servers, get new Website addresses, or take the pages down. Do not get discouraged; chances are there is another site right around the corner that contains all the information that you need. You can search for a particular site by enclosing the name in quotation marks to find its new location.

MAILING LISTS AND LISTSERVS

Mailing lists are electronic discussion groups that take place through e-mail. They are groups of people who "get together" online to discuss a specific topic. There are numerous mailing lists on nearly every topic imaginable.

A listserv is the software program that is used to run the mailing list. Here is how it works:

- You find out about a mailing list dealing with a subject you are interested in discussing with others (such as culture and nursing).
- To get involved in this discussion group, you have to subscribe to it. This can be done by clicking on a link on an Internet page or sending an e-mail message to that mailing list's listserv.

- Most often, the listserv automatically will subscribe you to the list and send you instructions on how to post to the group. Posting means that you send out a comment to the entire mailing list to which you have subscribed.
- Once you have subscribed, you will begin to receive e-mail messages from the mailing list. Be careful: Some discussion groups have a large following and you may find your mailbox filling up rather quickly.

Newsgroups/Usenet

Newsgroups, like mailing lists, are another popular way of discussing specific topics over the Internet with other people who share the same interest. Unlike a mailing list, however, newsgroups take place on an entirely different network called *Usenet*.

Usenet is composed of thousands of newsgroups. Individual comments that people make to one another on a newsgroup are called *articles*. You post an article when you want to make a comment. The lines of discussion within a newsgroup are called *threads*. To read the discussions on any newsgroup, you must have a software program called a *newsreader*.

Generally, your ISP will provide you with a newsreader program as part of the software package or it may be bundled with your Web browser. When you open the newsreader, it should download any new newsgroups that have been added. You can look through the entire list and choose which newsgroups interest you. When you find one of interest, just open it up and begin reading the articles. Newsgroup addresses are called *hierarchies*. Listed below are some of the standard hierarchies with examples of each. There are many other categories, some of which are from foreign countries.

alt—groups generally alternative in nature (e.g., alt.education.distance, alt.alien.visitors)

bionet—groups discussing biology and biological sciences (e.g., bionet.general, bionet.immunology)

comp—groups discussing computer or computer science issues (e.g., comp.infosystems)

misc—groups that don't fit into other categories (e.g., misc.fitness, misc.jobs)

news—groups about Usenet itself (e.g., news.groups)

rec—groups discussing hobbies, sports, music, and art (e.g., rec.food, rec.humor)

sci—groups discussing subjects related to the science and scientific research (e.g., sci.med.nursing, sci.psychology)

soc—groups discussing social issues, including politics and social programs (e.g., soc.culture, soc.college)

talk—public debating forums on controversial issues (e.g., talk.abortion, talk.religion)

One word of caution: People take newsgroups very seriously. If you want to post an article, be sure you understand the threads (lines of discussions) that have been taking place on the newsgroup. Read a number of articles and understand the threads before putting up your own opinion.

Remember that these discussion groups are frequented by people from all over the world; because of this, newsgroups can offer a wealth of information. Many field experts frequent newsgroups. There may even be groups out there that you can monitor and to which you can provide expert advice.

PORTALS AND VIRTUAL COMMUNITIES

Portals are Websites that offer a personalized view for you based on information provided when you register. Portals organize data into a single, easy-to-use menu providing services such as e-mail, search capability, and online shopping. America Online (AOL) and Yahoo represent general portal sites. There are also special interest or niche portals. Some examples of nursing and healthcare portals include Nursing Net, WebMD, and HealthCentral. Portals continue to evolve. The term *virtual community* refers to a group of people who share common interests, ideas, and feelings online. This may occur through bulletin boards, chat rooms, or user groups. Special interest portals may serve as a tool to create a virtual community that models the features of a neighborhood, complete with shopping and other services.

FTP

FTP stands for file transfer protocol. FTP is a means by which you can send and receive (upload and download) large documents and software over the Internet. FTP sites house these documents and software. Not all sites permit two-way traffic. Look for help with the FTP process under your browser's Help button. FTP is not needed by the majority of users because file compression techniques, faster transfer speeds, and advances in hardware meet the majority of needs.

NETIQUETTE

Netiquette is just like it sounds: etiquette on the Internet. It is just basic, common courtesy to others. Because no single person owns or controls the Internet, it is left to the individual user to be facilitative and kind when participating in discussion groups, authoring Web pages, or sending e-mail messages.

The following list contains general netiquette standards that most people on the Net attempt to abide by:

- Do not make assumptions.
- Do not be judgmental.
- Do not use all capital letters; this is interpreted as SHOUTING.
- Do proofread your messages carefully.

- Do be facilitative.
- Do be honest.
- Do be timely in your replies.
- Do try to make postings brief and to the point.

CONCLUSION

All of this information can be overwhelming at first, but, with time, you can learn to use the many invaluable resources the Internet has to offer. Understanding the many components that make up the Internet and using this knowledge to be discriminatory in the information that you find online will enable you to use the Internet as a research tool, an educational source, a meeting place, and a library. Now that you have this knowledge, you are ready to start surfing the Net.

Appendix B: Career Resources on the Internet

JOB HUNTING IN THE TWENTY-FIRST CENTURY

The advent of computers and the Internet has revolutionized the job search process. If you want to maximize your chances of finding a great job, using the Internet can help. Whether you are a recent nursing school graduate or an experienced nurse, sending out a traditional resume may no longer be enough to land an interview. Furthermore, by the time that a traditional letter and resume reaches a potential employer, the position may have been filled by someone who either sent an inquiry or answered an advertisement via e-mail. The Internet and other computer technologies can help you get the attention of employers, network with colleagues, and research potential new jobs.

JOB SEARCHING ON THE INTERNET

The Internet can help you with your job search in several ways. The first that may come to mind is online job listings. Literally hundreds of sites on the World Wide Web, including local newspaper classified ads, contain help wanted listings. Most have search engines, so you can enter keywords describing the job you are seeking to see whether there are any matches in that database. Looking through all the job listings on the Web can be very time consuming, so you should narrow your search to ads or sites related to healthcare.

Another way to use the Internet in your job search is to post your resume to a database. Again, it is generally best to choose a database that is specific to healthcare or nursing. For guidelines on writing and posting an electronic resume, see the Creating and Posting an Electronic Résumé section of this Appendix.

Some of the most powerful ways to use the Internet to help find a job may be less obvious. The Internet provides a great way to make contacts all over the country. Interested in getting into home healthcare in Florida? Send an e-mail inquiry to some hospitals or ask someone in a chat room or newsgroup, who knows all about it. She or he may even know of a place that is hiring. Many people who spend time online are friendly and willing to help, so post your inquiry anywhere you think you may get a response. As always, be careful about divulging personal information. You can also use e-mail to network with contacts and stay in touch with former classmates, co-workers, and others who may be able to help you find a job.

The World Wide Web can be a great tool for researching careers and potential employers. Many hospitals and other employers have Websites you can peruse. There are also sites for professional organizations, educational institutions, and other groups that may post useful information. Be inquisitive and creative.

HOW RÉSUMÉ DATABASES WORK

More employers are turning to automated applicant-tracking systems to sort and track résumés. These systems are actually databases that allow prospective employers to use keywords to search for applicants who meet certain criteria. For example, say a health maintenance organization is looking for a pediatric acute care nurse. The employer enters words describing her ideal candidate into the automated applicant-tracking system. In this case she may type in "pediatric," "acute care," and "registered nurse" as required keywords that résumés must include to come up in her search results. She may add other keywords if she likes, such as criteria that would be helpful for the job but are not mandatory. The tracking system then searches all the résumés in its system and retrieves those with the keywords the employer specified. Some tracking systems may display a list of résumé "titles" or header lines for each résumé retrieved, such as "LVN/home healthcare/Massachusetts." The employer can then select which résumés she wants to see in full.

How do you find these résumé databases? Some employers have their own in-house automated tracking systems. Employers scan résumés received by mail into the system, and when a position opens up they log onto the database to search for a candidate. Electronic applications and résumés are also stored in the database.

Employers who do not have their own database may use other generic applicant-tracking systems on the Internet. Some of these encompass all job seekers in any field; others are geared to specific areas such as healthcare. With these systems it is up to the job seeker to enter a résumé into the database. The ways to do this vary by systems. One common way to post your résumé online is to type it directly into the database once you have logged onto the site. Many systems allow you to copy your résumé from your word processor and paste it onto the database. You may also be able to send your résumé in via e-mail. Employers search these databases, according to keywords, for your skills, education, experience, or geographic area.

CREATING AND POSTING AN ELECTRONIC RÉSUMÉ

The electronic résumé has many things in common with the traditional résumé. Both prominently display your name, address, and telephone number and list your work experience, education, and special skills. However, there are several differences. An electronic résumé will be seen by prospective employers only if it contains the keywords for which the employers are searching. Many electronic résumés contain a keyword summary section toward the top, listing the standard phrases that describe the applicant's skills, areas of expertise, job titles, and credentials (see Figure B–1). It is a good idea to put the keywords in ascending order of importance. Also use common abbreviations, synonyms, or acronyms for words used in the body of the résumé to increase your odds of matching the employer's keyword specifications. For example, if you list "registered nurse" in the body of your résumé, use "RN" in the keyword summary. To determine what keywords to use, look at the words used in the job listings and use those that describe you. If you have access to electronic résumés, either on your computer or at your library, you can see what keywords others have used as well.

Because your electronic résumé may either be scanned into a computer or sent to a database via e-mail, you will need to ensure that the formatting you use will be readable to any system. Some kinds of formatting and typefaces will

---

Robert William Johnson
1234 Elm Street,
Washington, PA 15301
Home: (724) 229-4321
Cell: (724) 809-1300

Keyword Summary: Nursing, Health Care. RN. BSN. Manager. Home Healthcare. Geriatric. Extended Care. Geriatric Preventive Care. Infection Control. Psychosocial Care. Teaching. Spanish. Relocation.

Current Position

2004–present   Nursing Supervisor, Large Nursing Home, Washington, PA. Coordinated and supervised a nursing team responsible for 24-hour care of geriatric clients at an extended care home. Expanded program of preventive care and reduced hospitalization rate by 20%. Taught in-service programs for floor staff on geriatric care issues. Co-chaired committee on infection control and product evaluation. Effectively represented the unique interests and priorities of the nursing home staff; turnover dropped by 25%.

Previous Positions

1999–2004   Instructor, School of Nursing, Washington Hospital, Washington, PA.

1993–1999   Staff Registered Nurse, Community Teaching Hospital, Washington, PA.

Education

1993   Bachelor of Science, Nursing, Duquesne University, Pittsburgh, PA

Continuing Education Sampling

2007   Seminar: "New Perspectives on Aging"
2007   Workshop: "Care of the Alzheimer's Patient"
2006   Evening course: "The Changing Face of Aging in America"
2005   In-service: "New Studies in Diabetes"

Professional Memberships

1993–present   American Nurses Association
1993–present   Pennsylvania Nurses Association

FIGURE B–1 • Sample electronic resume

turn to gibberish or become unreadable in certain circumstances. To make sure this does not happen, follow these rules of thumb:

- Choose a common typeface, such as Times Roman, Helvetica, or Palatino. Avoid fancy scripts, which are likely to degrade when scanned. Use 12- or 14-point type. Do not use graphics, shading, italics, or underlining; for emphasis, use boldface or capital letters.
- If you are sending your résumé electronically over the Internet, check whether there are formatting specifications you must meet. Some databases require that you meet certain margins or not use tabs. And many require that résumés be sent in plain text or ASCII format.
- If you are sending a hard copy of your résumé, send a copy that is crisp in appearance and easy-to-read, not a photocopy. If you must Fax it, use the fine setting.
- Use plain white $8\frac{1}{2} \times 11$-inch paper with no folds or staples.

ISSUES TO CONSIDER WITH AUTOMATED APPLICANT-TRACKING SYSTEMS

The advantage of getting your résumé into an automated applicant-tracking system is that you will maximize your exposure to employers. There are, however, some disadvantages to consider. It may be difficult for a recent graduate with little experience to shine in a database system, since qualities like independence, perseverance, and reliability are not usually entered as keywords in a search. If you are looking for your first job as a healthcare professional, you may not want to rely solely on an electronic résumé.

There are also confidentiality issues with database résumé systems. While some systems restrict access to subscribers only, others do not. Either way, anyone, including your current boss (who could be a subscriber to the database you are using), can see your résumé posted there. Some services will provide users with a list of subscribers, but this is no guarantee that the information will not get back to your current employer. One way to help protect your privacy is to leave out identifying information about your current employer in your résumé. For example, you could write that you work at "a university medical center" instead of "The University of Texas Medical Center."

Before you post your résumé on any online system, be sure you understand the user guidelines. They will let you know any details about formatting to use or avoid, how long your résumé will remain in the system, how to update it, and whether any fees are charged.

Appendix C: Case Study Exercises—
Suggested Responses

CHAPTER 1

1.1 A client arrives in the emergency department with shortness of breath and complaining of chest pain. Describe how informatics can help nurses and other healthcare providers to more efficiently help the client.

- *Old records (including prior medical history and medications) are available quickly through the use of information systems to all parties involved in the patient's care, no matter what their location.*
- *High-quality care is readily available through telemedicine (electronically submit ECG and chest x-ray to on-call specialists off-site).*
- *The latest research on the patient's drugs and presenting symptoms is available via the Internet.*
- *Expert systems and care maps guide the treatment plan.*

CHAPTER 2

2.1 You are appointed to the hospital's information technology committee as the representative for your nursing unit. The charges of the committee include the following:

- *Identify PC software that is needed to accomplish unit work, such as word processing, spreadsheets, and databases.*
- *Word processing aids the following efforts: committee minutes, writing and revising unit policies and procedures, authoring and revising patient instructions, or developing care maps.*
- *A database can be used to maintain and display personnel information.*
- *The availability of a statistical package fosters unit-based research.*
- *Browser software provides access to materials housed on the intranet such as announcements, policies and procedures, institutional phone numbers, patient education materials, and programs mandated for regulatory bodies. Internet access provides the means to retrieve reference material such as literature search results, drug information, continuing education, and professional groups.*
- *E-mail provides the capability to share information with professional colleagues within the institution and in other facilities.*

- *Determine criteria for the selection and placement of hardware on the units. Discuss these issues and how they affect patient care and workflow.*
- *Avoid high traffic zones—they are subject to multiple interruptions.*
- *Have enough devices for all users.*
- *Provide good lighting and place monitors in areas that avoid screen glare.*
- *Consider ergonomics.*
- *Avoid placing computers in areas subject to liquid or food spills.*
- *Ensure that work surfaces are free from clutter.*

2.2 Your committee is charged with setting up a computer system that will automate transcription of physician orders and reporting of results. Identify the support personnel that you need at this point and write job descriptions for each identified position.

- *Have staff who do the everyday work identify the current workflow.*
- *Have staff and administrators identify information needed by each level of worker.*
- *Meet with staff and information services staff to discuss screen design, information that needs to be exchanged among systems, and desired output.*
- *Get physician and medical record approval for the information displayed in online reports.*
- *Consider whether results will be reported in pending and/or final forms.*
- *Evaluate whether charges for procedures or medications will occur at the time of order, completion, or documentation (or remain a separate process).*
- *Identify a plan for training and implementing the new system.*

2.3 The infection control nurse has traced the spread of a nosocomial infection to a computer keyboard on a hospital unit. It is located in a work area adjacent to four patient rooms. This computer is routinely used by staff for documentation, to check laboratory and radiology results, and to access reference materials. The infection control nurse has asked the unit director and staff to identify strategies to eliminate this problem. Identify measures that can help to eliminate this problem.

- *Identify who is responsible for routine cleaning of computer equipment.*
- *Practice good hand washing techniques.*
- *Have infection control conduct mini programs with interdisciplinary staff.*
- *Replace covers of keyboards as necessary.*
- *Test equipment periodically to identify if one area has specific problems.*

CHAPTER 3

3.1 Agnes Gibbons was admitted through the hospital's emergency department with congestive heart failure. During her admission she was asked to verbally acknowledge whether her demographic data were correct. Ms. Gibbons did so. Extensive diagnostic tests were done, including radiology studies. It was later discovered that all of Ms. Gibbons' information had been entered into another client's file. How would you correct this situation? What departments, or other agencies, would need to be informed of this situation?

- *Contact all clinical parties involved in Ms. Gibbons' care to look at whether she was treated appropriately and review her records in respective ancillary systems. Look at what drugs or blood products she may have been given and potential consequences.*
- *Involve information services, registration, medical records, and the billing department to correct the records.*
- *Determine the length of time it took to discover the error and the manner in which the error was discovered.*
- *Contact legal counsel regarding the situation.*
- *Educate all staff to seek more than one means of validation of patient identity upon admission (health insurance and photo identification in addition to verbal affirmation). Have client view information to validate that it is correct.*
- *Next time, have Ms. Gibbons review the printout of her information and sign it to verify that it is correct. Be prepared to read the information to her.*
- *Delete Ms. Gibbons' information from the other client's record and/or create a new medical record number for the second client.*

3.2   A non-English-speaking Vietnamese man was admitted through the emergency department with suspected tuberculosis (TB). The system carried information under his name. Mr. Nguyen nodded his head when the admitting clerk pointed to the demographic screen. Mr. Nguyen was tested and treated for TB. When the public health nurse went to Mr. Nguyen's address for follow-up, the man was not the Mr. Nguyen who had been treated for TB. How would you address this problem? Explain your rationale.

- *This situation is similar to the one above. A response of "yes" or nodding the head does not ensure that the client has heard or understood what was said.*
- *Validate identity through photo identification plus name and Social Security number.*
- *Obtain a translator as necessary.*
- *Notify all departments involved in the care of this client.*
- *Review client treatment relative to chart information for potentially harmful treatments.*

3.3   You volunteered to serve on a committee to identify information from prior admissions that would be helpful to staff caring for current inpatients. What information, if any, would you select for ready access, and how long would you recommend that it remain active in the system? Remember that your system has limited capacity so that items must be carefully selected and prioritized. Identify the priority assigned to each item and provide your rationale for this priority.

- *Useful information: demographics, medical history, present medications, allergy information, over-the-counter products and herbal or other nontraditional treatments, and advanced directives, in that respective order. Availability of information eliminates repetitious questions and improves care.*

CHAPTER 4

4.1 As the representative for your medical center's Better Care Initiative, a project with the purpose of identifying ways that services can be delivered in a more efficient manner, you have suggested that the Internet be made available to clinicians at the point of care. Develop a report listing both the potential uses as well as potential problems of using the Internet.
   Potential uses

   - *Intranet: to access policies and procedures, telephone numbers, human resources information, and institution-specific references without worry about different versions.*
   - *Internet: to access online databases and research, continuing education and degree programs, full-text retrieval of articles; increased access to experts in the field due to the ease of use of e-mail.*

   Potential problems

   - *Internet: staff may spend more time on the Web than expected, taking them from their other responsibilities and some staff may surf non-work-related sites.*
   - *Personnel may accept information found at face value without evaluating information for quality.*

4.2 One of your clients has a rare genetic defect. The client is requesting additional information about this defect from you, but no reference books on the unit describe this condition. Discuss strategies for how you might obtain quality information using the Internet and electronic communication.

   - *Try a Web search looking for support groups for the client. MEDLINE or one of the other literature databases should have information, possibly in full-text form.*
   - *Use e-mail to write to specialists to request information.*

4.3 The e-health committee at your facility is looking at ways to provide greater client involvement in accessing their own health information. What ramifications must be considered for this to occur in terms of security, interpretation of results, and training?

   - *Do an assessment of users as to their knowledge and understanding of using the Internet.*
   - *Conduct client education and training on the use of the Internet.*
   - *Issue access codes and provide a procedure for changing the codes according to policy.*

- *Review confidential statements frequently.*
- *Have a two-step procedure in place to prevent accessing unauthorized information.*

CHAPTER 5

5.1 You are a nurse participating in the customization and implementation of a barcode medication administration system. Analyze how the process will change from the current manual process. Include potential problem areas and solutions.

- *Provides additional safeguards to ensure that it is the correct patient, correct medication, correct dose and route, and correct time.*
- *Standardizes times for medication administration throughout an organization. Nursing representatives and pharmacists need to discuss these and reach a common agreement.*
- *Clearly displays medications that are due as well as those already given.*
- *Automatically records medications as given once scanned, requiring additional steps if they were not given for some reason.*
- *May create different types of errors. Nursing representatives should evaluate the process to identify potential problem areas as well as a mechanism to identify new types of errors once the system is implemented.*
- *Problematic if system suddenly goes down without warning because there may not be a readily available backup process. Daily or shift worksheets could serve as backup records. Guidelines must be established to determine when "worksheets" might serve as documentation and procedures for late entry once the system is restored.*
- *System requires log-on to review what meds have been given and what still need to be given.*

5.2 You are the physician liaison for the information system department. Recent federal initiatives call for the implementation of CPOE. You have the technology available, but you need to get administrative, nursing, and physician support. How would you go about getting this?

- *Offer several informative meetings.*
- *Post flyer announcements with a catchy phrase that will spark some interest.*
- *Offer demos during physician meetings with food available.*
- *Be available for training at any time that is convenient for the staff.*
- *Conduct progress meetings.*
- *Be flexible and be prepared to answer questions based on individual needs.*
- *Confer with others who have had a successful implementation.*

5.3 You are participating in the customization and implementation of the radiology system. Define the data that must be included in the order entry process. Define the information that the nursing staff would like to view or print from the radiology system.

- *Must include the name of the examination, any modifiers that specify the exact body part to be filmed, date for the examination, and reason for the examination during order entry for treatment and reimbursement purposes.*
- *Output should include the test preparation instructions for staff and the client, notification that the examination has been done, and online results (preliminary and/or final).*

CHAPTER 6

6.1   You are a nurse manager in a hospital that has recently merged with other hospitals, forming a large healthcare enterprise. Each of the hospitals currently uses a different clinical information system. You are a member of the strategic planning committee, which is charged with the task of selecting which of the three systems will be used throughout the enterprise. Describe the process you would use to scan the internal and external environments, as well as the types of data you would collect.

- *Consider the strategic plan for the combined and separate institutions.*
- *Determine current staff satisfaction with each information system.*
- *Look at whether the system is due for major upgrades as well as associated costs. Which one would be easiest to expand? Which one has the most capability for the future? What technology is used?*

6.2   Develop a tool to evaluate each of the three clinical information systems for the scenario described above.

- *Develop a weighted tool that considers ease of use, expandability, compatibility with other systems, ability to customize, ability to generate reports, time needed for training, timeframe for implementation, and overall costs.*

6.3   Your facility belongs to one of three healthcare delivery systems in the city. Competition is fierce. You have been asked to serve on a committee to study and recommend the retention or deletion of certain clinical services. Develop a plan for how you would do that and for how information services might facilitate that task via the use of benchmarking.

- *Compare services delivered to those provided by competitors for total number of cases served, quality of services inclusive of client satisfaction, length of stay as appropriate, cost per case, and profits or loss per cost center. Commercial packages may aid this task.*

6.4   Your facility recently acquired and closed a competing hospital. All paper medical records are stored at a distant site. Records are not readily accessible. Client documentation and results were online but are no longer available after the hospital closure. Some physicians never received test results for clients at the time of shut down. This had a negative impact on client care and satisfaction. How might strategic planning prevent this type of situation from occurring again?

- *Start planning early by sending letters to clients about getting copies of their x-rays, especially mammograms or testing results that will be needed for scheduled surgery.*
- *Notify physician offices and clinics about the impending closure as early as possible.*
- *If results are in the process of being stored at a different site they may not be available for some time. A test might have to be repeated: who will assume the cost?*
- *Set up a hotline that physicians and office staff can call. Have IS personnel available at the old site who are knowledgeable in all system applications, who can answer questions, and who can produce results if necessary.*
- *Consider that the quality and continuity of the clients' care is maintained.*

CHAPTER 7

7.1 You are a member of the committee that will select a clinical documentation system for nurses. Prepare a timeline for the needs assessment and system selection phases. These processes should be accomplished over a 6-month period.

- *Set the target implementation date, then work backward to set other key dates.*
- *Start with a "kickoff" meeting to provide an overview of the process.*
- *Establish an ongoing meeting schedule and develop a project plan.*
- *Anticipate change.*
- *Collect information about workflow processes from end users and administrators.*
- *Identify problems with the current process.*
- *Review the Request for Proposal requirements and compare available products.*
- *Schedule vendor demonstrations and site visits.*
- *Narrow the selection.*

7.2 Develop a list of "musts" and "wants" and assign a weight to each item. Define what your weighting scale will be.

- *Choose a model for the system such as care mapping.*
- *Discuss how the new system will impact other systems.*
- *Develop a numeric scale, say 1–10, with 10 as the most desirable.*
- *Evaluate each of the systems using this scale.*

7.3 Create a list of questions related to the system selection process that you will ask at site visits.

- *Is the system easy to use? What reports and printouts are produced or may be produced? How much time is needed for implementation and training? What roadblocks were encountered? What would you do differently? Can it be adapted easily?*

CHAPTER 8

8.1   You are the project director responsible for creating an implementation time-line that addresses the training and go-live activities for a nursing documentation system, to be implemented on 20 units and involve 350 users. Determine whether the implementation will be staggered or occur simulta-neously on all units, and provide your rationale.

This decision may be influenced by the following:

- *Whether a system is in place now*
- *Administrative support*
- *Staffing and training resource availability*
- *Ability to pull staff from other areas to the pilot unit(s)*
- *The advantages and disadvantages of doing one or all units at a time*

8.2   Create the timeline for the training and go-live schedule for this implementation.

- *Start at least one year in advance, then work backward to make time for all activities.*
- *Plan for 24-hour IS coverage for at least one week (from IS).*
- *Obtain administrative support and a budget.*
- *Plan for the unexpected.*
- *Choose a training system (core trainers, educators versus outside parties).*
- *Determine the number of training hours per staff.*
- *Determine training costs for equipment, trainers, and replacement staffing.*
- *Provide flexibility in the scheduling. Build in extra time before implementation.*
- *Do not start training too early, because people tend to forget.*

8.3   Your present manual medication administration record is being replaced by BCMA, an automated information system. Discuss the specifications you would recommend for reports that the system will generate to notify the nurse when medications are due. Determine how often the reports should print and what information they should contain.

- *Medication administration records need to identify drug name, dose, scheduled time, route, and special instructions. The format for reminders should be determined to be most useful for the staff nurse (that is, shift overview or list by a particular time, patient or group of patients, items not charted or charged). Staff need to determine the most useful frequency for these reports (every 1 or 2 hours or prior to the end of the shift).*

8.4   You have been selected to develop test scripts for interface testing for a new patient care system. Develop a test script with multiple interfaces. Define the output that you should see for each system.

- *An information system would have demographic information, lab results from an outside system, radiology results plus any other diagnostic results, a monitor interface, and possibly a charge interface. Output differs for each interface and function. It must be accurate, and be where it belongs when it is needed. For example, demographic information passes from the registration system and is displayed in the nursing system. Diagnostic results need to pass from other systems into the documentation system. In the case of a charge interface, a message is sent to accounting when a service, supply, or medication is administered.*

8.5 As the manager of the gastrointestinal laboratory in your facility, you are expanding the applications for your information system. At the present, it allows physicians to capture images and produce consults and referral letters in a timely fashion. You have been working with the vendor to expand its features to include the capture of patient history. Consider the pros and cons of interchanging information collected by admitting nurses and physicians.

Pros:

- *Eliminates redundant data entry and preserves data integrity.*
- *It is more convenient because clients do not have to answer the same questions over and over.*
- *Complete history including procedures and reactions that the client encountered would be readily available to all healthcare professionals treating the client.*

Cons:

- *Someone needs to be responsible for verifying that all information is accurate and up to date.*
- *There needs to be agreement between parties as to how information will be communicated.*
- *Uncertainty as to who will have the ability to update the information.*
- *Drug history and reactions to medications must be kept updated.*

CHAPTER 9

9.1 Kevin Gallagher, RN, has access to all client records on his medical-surgical unit. Consider each of the following situations:

- Kevin's mother is admitted to the unit. Is it appropriate for him to view his mother's electronic medical record? Why or why not? *No, unless he is doing so directly on her behalf; otherwise, it is a violation of her privacy.*
- Kevin's unit clerk also has access to Mrs. Gallagher's record. Is it appropriate for her to view Mrs. Gallagher's record? *Only on a need-to-know basis.*
- Kevin's co-worker, Kaneesha, is a client on the unit assigned to another staff nurse's care. Is it appropriate for Kevin to review her chart or laboratory results? *Only on a need-to-know basis and if he is involved in her care.*

9.2 Nancy Whitehorse, RN, routinely accesses client records on her medical unit. Does she violate her confidentiality statement if she performs the following actions?

- She reviews the information and does not discuss it with anyone else. *This is a violation.*
- She discusses information obtained from client records with other healthcare workers on the unit. *This is a violation.*
- She discusses clinical cases, omitting names, in social situations. *This is a violation.*

9.3 Grace Elizaga has been given the charge of training the RNs and unit clerks from the first three client care units slated to start automated order entry at Potter's Medical Center (PMC). The target implementation date is in two months. A total of 93 RNs and 11 unit clerks must receive training before that time. Based on information from other agencies that have the same information system as PMC, eight hours of training time is projected for each individual. As the nurse manager responsible for those units, you have been asked to work with Grace to develop a detailed plan to accomplish this task and submit this plan to your vice president of Client Care Services. Include the following in your plan and provide your rationale:

- Staffing: *Replacement staffing is needed while others train.*
- Costs for your personnel: *Replacement staffing is needed while others train. People also need practice time, and time to apply newly learned skills.*
- Training start and completion dates: *Training must start early and be completed 1–2 weeks before go-live to take care of last-minute stragglers and new hires and to allow practice time.*
- Length and number of training sessions: *Consider the ability of personnel and trainers to get away from the unit, the appropriateness of the training location, and the ability of personnel to learn over a longer session.*

CHAPTER 10

10.1 In the course of conversation, your nurse manager tells you that she loaded a copy of the spreadsheet program she uses on her home office PC onto one of the unit PCs so that she can work on projects at both locations. Your institution has a well-publicized policy against the use of unauthorized, unlicensed software copies. As a staff nurse, what should you do? Explain your response.

- *Talk with your nurse manager, telling her that this is a violation of copyright law and can result in large fines and is probably a violation of institutional policy.*

10.2 You notice several of the new physicians playing computer games on the nursing unit. You had not seen any of these games previously. What, if any, action should you take? Explain your rationale.

- *Remove them. Ask the IS department to "lock" down the machines so that additional software cannot be added without authorization. Approach the residents if necessary and ask them to restrict use on this machine to clinical uses.*

10.3 To remember his computer system password, university nursing instructor Pat Pawakawicz taped his password to the back of his identification badge. When Mr. Pawakawicz lost his identification badge recently, it was turned into hospital security and subsequently the IS department, with his password still attached. When Mr. Pawakawicz picked up his identification badge, he expressed intent to use the same password. Is this an appropriate way to treat a password? Should he use the same password again? Provide your rationale. What, if any, legal ramifications might there be for Mr. Pawakawicz regarding use of his password by unauthorized users?

- *Passwords need to be kept private. When there is any question as to whether they have been compromised, they should be changed immediately. This instructor's behavior may compromise someone's confidentiality. He may face civil or other disciplinary action.*

10.4 The administration at St. John's Hospital takes pride in their strong policies and procedures for the protection of confidential client information. In fact, St. John's serves as a model for other institutions in this area. However, printouts discarded in the restricted access IS department are not shredded. On numerous occasions, personnel working late observed the cleaning staff reading discarded printouts. What action, if any, should these personnel take relative to the actions of the cleaning staff? What action, if any, should be taken by IS administration? Provide your rationale. If current practices are maintained, are there any additional potential risks for unauthorized disclosure of client information? If you answer yes, identify what these risks might be.

- *The IS department needs to practice what it preaches. Printouts should be shredded at the time that they are discarded or, at the very least, the housekeeping personnel should receive inservice training and sign a confidentiality statement.*

10.5 The secretary on 7 Tower Oncology receives a Fax transmission about a client consult. The Fax was intended for a physician's office in the adjacent building. She places the Fax in the out bin of her desk to be delivered later by volunteers. No in-house mailer was used. Is this action appropriate? Explain why or why not.

- *This action is not appropriate. All Faxes should have cover sheets and be placed in a confidential mailer. Staff need inservice training and a reprimand in this case.*

10.6 You notice that the new nurse practitioner for one of your major orthopedic practices has a PDA on which he keeps patient information. Today
he left it in the cafeteria. What should you do?

• *Turn the PDA into the security department or page the nurse practitioner
to tell him that you found his PDA and turned it into security, and that
you are glad you found it instead of someone who might have accessed
information inappropriately.*

CHAPTER 11

11.1 You have been selected as a member of the Integration Project Team, which is
charged with identifying ways that system integration could improve information flow. You work on an inpatient unit that uses a stand-alone nursing
documentation system that is not interfaced or integrated with any other
hospital information system. Identify the implications of this situation, and
suggest integration options that could improve information flow.

• *This situation creates extra work and can compromise data integrity,
leading to several different versions of information for every patient. Data
entry should occur once whenever possible at a point closest to the source.
Substantial cost savings may result for the entire organization by eliminating redundant data entry.*

11.2 You are working to identify elements in your healthcare enterprise that
could be used for a master patient index (MPI). List five basic elements and
describe how each could be used for an MPI.

• *Obvious elements for an MPI include the client's name, medical record,
Social Security number, and date of birth. Name and insurance may change.
Eventually, the universal patient identifier will be a crucial element. Used in
combination, these elements help to ensure access to the correct record.*

CHAPTER 12

12.1 As a new student, identify advantages for when you are gathering information about your assigned patients with an electronic health record.

• *The information can be accessed by more than one person at a time.*
• *It is legible.*
• *It provides a more comprehensive record, incorporating information from
physician offices, ambulatory clinics, and hospital stays.*

12.2 You are a member of the committee charged with designing the EHR
at your facility. Identify which components of nursing documentation
should be retained in the clinical data repository. For example, would
you want to include all client vital signs from the current hospital
admission? Explain why you would include or exclude the various
components.

- *History and assessment, operative notes, allergies and drug reactions, medications, specific lab data such as blood type, and some diagnostic tests need to be retained. Some items, such as all client temperatures, would clutter the record.*

12.3 Identify several external sources of information that would be useful as part of the EHR for access by a home health nurse.

- *Ancillary test results, social history, history and assessment, operative notes, allergies and drug reactions, and medications are useful in every care setting.*

12.4 Discuss the implications of providing nurses in a hospital setting with access to all electronic client information. Identify which types of information are appropriate for access by nurses.

- *Nurses need clinical information but generally do not require billing and payment information. In some cases, it is not necessary for a nurse to know about every aspect of the client's history. For example, the emergency department client who has a laceration from an automobile accident does not need to relate his history of abuse as a child.*

CHAPTER 13

13.1 What benefits do you, as a clinician, perceive associated with HIE?

- *Exchange of information among physicians, clinics, hospitals, pharmacies, and insurance companies will create a more complete, safer record with a more up-to-date list of allergies, treatments, and medications, which will help eliminate redundant tests, treatments, and medications that are contraindicated. It will save time and eliminate the need to ask patients for their health histories over and over again at the risk of missing key information.*

13.2 You work in a prominent surgeon's office. You have noticed that the office manager has accessed the RHIO for information on another employee in the practice who is not currently being treated by the surgeon. How should this situation be handled?

- *Since the office manager is your boss, you may want to initiate a discussion about recent news stories involving inappropriate access of celebrity health records by individuals without a need-to-know, asking your boss if she had heard about what happened to the individuals who committed these acts. If you notice the behavior again you should approach your employing physician, or if you work in a hospital-owned practice, contact the information services department with your concerns.*

13.3 You work in the medical ambulatory clinic. When reviewing your list of patients for the day you notice that one, John Pauvlik, has not had the pneumonia vaccine according to data pulled from the RHIO. What measures should be in place to determine that you have information on the correct patient?

- *Ask the patient to reveal demographic information that you can check against the pulled record for confirmation.*

CHAPTER 14

14.1 You are teaching an undergraduate course titled Nursing Informatics. One class session is scheduled for a discussion on the protection of client record information. How would you summarize the current status of legislative safeguards in the United States? What, if anything, would you suggest that students might personally consider to improve this situation?

- *Traditionally, protection of client information has been patchy from state to state. HIPAA provides protection at a federal level, although many issues remain unclear. Students can uphold standards and serve as advocates for client privacy and write their legislators and senators to view their opinions on the need for additional safeguards or changes to legislation.*

14.2 You have been appointed to the Clinical Information Systems Committee, which is charged with looking at ways that automation can facilitate data collection for the next accreditation visit by the Joint Commission. List examples of how your community hospital demonstrates adherence to Joint Commission information standards, and state your rationale for why you feel these examples display compliance.
Examples include:

- *The existence and use of confidentiality and privacy safeguards, such as individual log-ons, different levels of access based on a need-to-know basis, and user sign-on statements.*
- *Improved access from different locations and by different types of providers at one time for more efficient patient care.*
- *24-hour access with protection against loss via file backup.*
- *More legible and complete documentation of client education than with traditional records.*
- *Improved turnaround time for documentation.*
- *Improved process for the collection of aggregate data to support clinical research and client care.*

14.3 You are the general nursing information systems liaison at Wilson Rehabilitation Institution. CARF accreditation is coming up. What would you do to ensure that your automated documentation is in compliance with CARF standards? Explain your rationale.

- *This preparation should be similar to preparation done with a manual system, although automation can be used to facilitate the process. Reports can be run to show the extent to which required data are collected and in some cases system prompts added to guarantee that those data are provided. Automation also makes it easier to review treatment plans for completeness of documentation and to determine if they are up-to-date. These practices can be used prior to accreditation as a means to pinpoint and correct problem areas.*

14.4 You are instructing new healthcare employees during orientation regarding HIPAA. A question is asked regarding how family members receive information on a delusional client. Discuss how you would deal with the issue and how you would provide additional safeguards over the disclosure of healthcare information.

- *The client should have in his or her file a copy of Durable Power of Attorney and/or Durable Healthcare Power of Attorney and healthcare treatment instructions. The information would be given to healthcare employees to make any necessary decisions. If this is not available, Social Services will get involved and sometimes the court must appoint a guardian to handle these issues.*

14.5 You are part of a research team studying CVA treatments. Discuss how you use client data and how data are de-identified.

- *A Research Consent Form must be reviewed and signed prior to any study. A study number maintained in a filing system separate from the name and address files of the participants identifies all studies. Most researchers have obtained a Certificate of Confidentiality from the Department of Health and Human Services (DHHS). With this certificate, the investigators cannot be forced by court order to disclose research information that may identify a person in any state or local civil, criminal, administrative, legislative, or other proceedings. Disclosures may be necessary, however, upon request of NIH, DHHS, or the IRB for audit or program evaluation purposes. Sometimes studies are requested with a specific area in mind such as by zip codes.*

CHAPTER 15

15.1 As the clinical representative for your unit on the Disaster Planning Committee, you are charged with identifying all forms in your area that require completion of a physical vital records inventory sheet. What forms would you list and why?

- *Look at forms that are frequently consulted, such as staff telephone and pager numbers. Consider whether unavailability to the information creates difficulties. If the answer is yes, then add these forms to the vital records inventory sheet.*

15.2 Work crews at Wilmington Hospital inadvertently cut the cable connecting all terminals at the hospital with the computer center. As the on-duty nursing supervisor, what should you tell your employees, and why? Who would you contact for further information? How do you determine whether to initiate manual alternatives?

- *Tell employees the truth rather than giving the appearance that someone is hiding something. Next try to get an estimate for the expected time-frame that the system will be unavailable. If the downtime is expected to be more than two hours, the institution needs to implement manual alternatives; otherwise, nonemergency procedures may be entered into the system once it is restored, rather than manually.*

15.3 An early-morning train wreck near St. Luke's Hospital derailed seven freight cars carrying chemicals that can emit toxic fumes. The accident took out power lines for the neighborhood and for St. Luke's. Emergency crews evacuated a seven block area, stopping just outside of the hospital's main entrance. Power has already been out for 12 hours and restoration is not expected for at least another 12 to 24 hours. You are on an executive administrative committee charged with determining what information will be brought online first and what will remain in paper form. What would you restore first? What records, if any, would you not restore? Explain your rationale. How would you document, for record-management purposes, that part of the record is automated and part is manual?

- *Demographics and registration information would be restored first because the client must be in the system in order to perform any action.*
- *One of the next features would be the medication administration records (MARs). Not only do MARs have the capability to minimize med errors, but in many settings, charges occur when the medication is charted as given.*
- *Beyond these areas, consideration must be given to treatments and system features that are considered as essential for care. There should be notation in the record of what is in manual form. It may be far too expensive to backload data into the system when a paper record also exists.*

15.4 As the informatics nurse, you are responsible for helping the Renal Department select a new database. One of the top vendors must cancel its Web-based demonstration because its server was stolen. This particular application is designed to run over the Internet with data housed at the vendor site. What questions should this raise for disaster planning with the use of vendor-supported applications?

- *Questions arise relating to the security of client information, because information resides on the vendor's equipment.*

15.5 You recently learned that the information services network engineer responsible for conducting backups on the server for the tumor registry database failed to ensure that regular backups occurred properly. This was discovered when the database was found to be corrupt. Approximately 20,000 entries were lost as a result. As the liaison between the tumor registry and the IS department, how would you ensure that this would not happen again?

- *You must implement a procedure by which backups are accounted for. Make someone in the department accountable to verify that the backups have been completed and document the date this was performed. Perform a periodic checking of the database to verify that all records are available.*

CHAPTER 16

16.1 Locate and evaluate at least one online continuing education offering.

- *There are a number of sites that offer continuing education online. There are several different ways to find sites offering Continuing Education Units, (CEUs). One is to go directly to a professional site, such as the American Nurses Association's NursingWorld.org to look for links to continuing education links. Another way to locate offerings is through a general search engine. Entry of the search terms, "continuing education"+education+nursing returns several sites, some of which are associated with professional organizations or publications. Some have an associated fee while others are free. Users should use discretion at the types of sites that they visit.*

16.2 You are on the education committee at your small community hospital. Your staff development department was eliminated several years ago. You and your colleagues are charged with developing strategies to meet the educational needs of agency registered and licensed practical nurses. Limited capital and the isolated location of your community make this a difficult assignment. Your institution does have Internet and World Wide Web access in the medical library, as well as teleconferencing capability. Develop a proposal to meet your charge using available resources. Be prepared to defend your proposal to an administration loathe to part with monies beyond those already budgeted.

- *Internet access to continuing education eliminates hours of travel and expenses associated with travel.*

16.3 You are the client educator at a medical center in the Pacific Northwest. Your clientele are drawn from a 150-mile radius and beyond. For this reason it is difficult to have clients complete diabetic education or other classes. You have been told to improve client completion of classes or face elimination of your department. The medical center has both teleconferencing capability, presently used for consults, and an established Web page that provides basic information about the institution. How might you use these resources to develop alternative strategies for client education? Address budget considerations, necessary resources, target populations that might be better served, and how you propose to link distant clients with instructional offerings.

- *Submit a proposal to administration to provide education via the Web as well as in the traditional classroom setting. The proposal should address provisions for access for all clients that might include use of computers in local libraries, schools, and senior citizen centers, as well as the possibility of submitting a grant to obtain PCs for clients who do not otherwise have access. Work with the Webmaster for assistance in placing the material on the Web. Consider low-tech options, such as video and the use of the telephone.*

16.4 You recently joined the faculty at a small, private, rural college. Because you express an interest in computers, and are slightly more knowledgeable about computers than your faculty colleagues, you have been asked to establish online sites for all of the traditionally taught courses to post the course syllabi, announcements, handouts, and other relevant course materials as a mechanism to facilitate learning. Your institution already owns a course management system. How would you proceed? What, if any, additional applications might you consider when working on this project?

- *You need to contact the persons responsible for the present course management system to determine whether there are any issues that need to be addressed in terms of number of simultaneous users permitted, whether the current infrastructure can support that number of additional users, and for assistance to get started. You will need to determine whether your facility controls the creation of course or they support faculty in the creation of courses, adding users, and trouble-shooting basic problems. You should determine basic system requirements and current instructional support for yourself as well as for students as you learn how to use this application. You will also need to consult with your peers to determine their plans for the future. For example, do they see the expansion into new markets using online courses? Do they expect to use some of the other course management features such as test administration and electronic gradebooks? And, when do they want to have their training on how to use this application?*

CHAPTER 17

17.1 You are the nurse practitioner in St. Theresa's emergency department. A client is brought in with obvious psychiatric problems. You have no psychiatrist available and the nearest psychiatric facility is a one hour drive away. St. Theresa is a Tri-State Health Care Alliance Member. Tri-State has telehealth links with the regional hospital, where a psychiatrist is in the emergency department. What steps would you take to initiate a productive teleconference? Justify your response.

- *Be prepared to introduce the situation to the psychiatrist as well as to the patient. The patient may or may not be receptive, although the same can be true without a telemedicine link. Ensure that technical support as well as emotional support is available.*

17.2 Erin O'Shell, home health nurse, just set up teleconference equipment for Dr. Bobby to evaluate Mr. Richard Goldstein for possible hospitalization for congestive heart failure. Dr. Bobby and the hospital are a one hour drive away. Just as the teleconference started, but before Dr. Bobby could listen to Mr. Goldstein's lungs or complete other key portions of the examination, a power outage severed the teleconference link. How should Ms. O'Shell handle this situation? Provide your rationale.

- *The backup situation is that the nurse uses the telephone and communicates her findings to the physician. The patient is probably experiencing distress already, which will probably increase without some action. The physician and nurse must work together to determine if this patient needs to go to the hospital or if he should receive further treatment in the home.*

CHAPTER 18

18.1 You are the staff nurse in a busy medical–surgical department at your community hospital. You and several of your colleagues have an idea that client anxiety is decreased in direct proportion to the amount of teaching that they receive preoperatively. Describe how you might use information technology to look at this issue and prepare a proposal for funding consideration.

- *This issue could be addressed in a patient satisfaction survey done during or after the hospitalization. This survey might be completed via telephone or possibly online. An argument for funding this project might be twofold. First, it provides a way to improve patient satisfaction and return visits and is therefore good for business. Second, patient stay may be decreased with cost savings to the institution. The organization may fund the survey or funding may be obtained from a number of different sites that might include professional organizations or various foundations, particularly for a specific population.*

18.2 You and your classmates are expected to conduct a health teaching project in a public high school as one of the requirements for your Community Health Nursing course. Identify and discuss resources that you might use to gather material for this project.

- *There are a huge number of resources that can be tapped for this project. These may include the government, sites such as the National Library of Medicine, as well as information available through other agencies and professional groups, such as the American Academy of Pediatrics. Information from all sites should be evaluated for accuracy, authenticity, and currency before it is shared with others.*

18.3 You are working the night shift at your local community hospital. One of your clients was newly diagnosed today with a rare disorder that is unknown to you and your peers. Mrs. Prado is unable to sleep and is asking for more information about her diagnosis. None of the reference books on your unit provide information about her diagnosis. Your unit does, however, have an Internet connection. How might you use resources on hand to meet Mrs. Prado's needs?

- *Either access your library through your intranet connection to conduct a search and full-text retrieval or access one of the online databases such as MEDLINE through the National Library of Medicine site to do a search and retrieve literature. Consider a Web search as well, although the quality of information obtained will vary greatly and should be reviewed prior to your giving it to Mrs. Prado.*

Glossary

Access code Unique identifier generally provided by a name and password for the specific purpose of restricting computer or information system use to persons who have legitimate authority to view or use information found in the computer or information system.

Administrative information systems Systems that support patient care by managing financial and demographic information and providing reporting capabilities.

Aggregate data Data that are derived from large population groups.

Alphanumeric Numbers and alphabetic characters.

Ambulatory Payment Classification (APC) Describes new reimbursement criteria for ambulatory procedures.

Antivirus software Set of computer programs capable of finding and eliminating viruses and other malicious programs from scanned disks, computers, and networks.

Application security Measures designed to protect a set of computer programs and the information that they create or store, such as timed or automatic sign-off, which prevents unauthorized access by others when users forget to sign off the system.

Application service provider (ASP) Third-party entities that manage and distribute software-based services and solutions to customers across a wide area network from a central data center.

Application software Set of programs designed to accomplish a particular task.

Archetypes Re-usable clinical models of content and processes significant for an initiative to develop a life-long electronic record.

Architecture Structure of the central processing unit and its interrelated elements within an information system.

Arden Syntax Standard language used in the healthcare industry for writing rules.

Arithmetic logic unit (ALU) Component of the central processing unit that executes arithmetic instructions.

Asynchronous Transfer Mode (ATM) High-speed data transmission method suitable for voice, data, image, text, and video information that use fiber or twisted pair. It is faster than ISDN, but less frequently used for reasons of cost, availability, and a lack of standards.

Attachments Files sent with e-mail messages.

Audit trail Electronic tool that can track system access by individual user, by user class, or by all persons who viewed a specific client record.

Authentication Action that verifies the authority of users to receive specified data.

Authoring tools Software programs that allow persons with little or no programming expertise to create instructional computer programs.

Automatic sign-off Mechanism that logs a user off the computer after a specific period of inactivity.

Backloaded Information that is preloaded into the system before the go-live date.

Backup procedure Creation of a second copy of files and information found on a computer, or information system, for the intent of restoring information in the event data are lost or damaged; or an alternative means to accomplish tasks normally done with an information system when that system is not available for some reason.

Backup systems Devices that create copies of system and data files.

Batch processing Manipulation of large amounts of data into meaningful applications at times when computer demands are lowest as a means to maintain system performance during peak utilization hours. Batch processed information is not available before processing and is little used today except to run reports.

Benchmarking Continual process of measuring services and practices against the toughest competitors in the industry.

Bennett Bill Although not passed into law, the Medical Records Confidentiality Act of 1995 was a significant piece of legislation because it attempted to establish the role of healthcare providers in the protection of client information; to fix conditions for the inspection, copying, and disclosure of protected information; and to institute legal protection for health-related information.

Binary code Series of 1s and 0s.

Binary file transfer (BFT) Set of instructions that represents another standard for file transfer.

Biometrics Unique, measurable characteristic or trait of a human being for automatically recognizing or verifying identity.

Bit Smallest unit of data that can be handled by the computer.

Bits per second (bps) Number of bits that can be transferred in 1 second of time.

Bliki A type of Web page that allows collaborative contributions and posts in reverse chronological order.

Blog Abbreviation for Web log.

Blu-ray High density optical disc format rival to HD-DVD.

Body Main portion of an e-mail message.

Browser Retrieval program that allows the user to search and access hypertext and hypermedia documents on the Web by using HTTP.

Bulletin Board Systems (BBS) Originally an online service that offered computerized dial-in meeting and announcements, file sharing, and limited discussions. Now it may refer to a site used to post announcements.

Business continuity planning (BCP) Combines information technology and disaster recovery planning with business functions recovery planning.

Business impact assessment or analysis (BIA) Process of determining the critical functions of the organization and the information vital to maintain operations as well as the applications and databases, hardware, and communications facilities that use, house, or support this information.

Byte Eight bits makes up one byte.

Carpal tunnel syndrome Compression of median nerve as it passes through the wrist along the pathway to the hand resulting in sensory and motor changes to the thumb, index finger, third finger, and radial aspect of the ring finger.

CAPTCHAS Completely automatic public test to tell computers and humans apart.

Central processing unit (CPU) Electronic circuitry that executes computer instructions—reading stored programs one instruction at a time, keeping track of the execution, and directing other computer parts and input and output devices to perform required tasks.

Chief privacy officer (CPO) Individual responsible for the protection of personal health information of patients as required by federal law.

Client/server Distributed approach to computing where different computers work together to carry out a task. The computer that makes requests is known as the client, while the high-performance computer that contains requested files is known as the server.

Clinical data repository Database where information from many different information systems is stored and managed, allowing retrieval of elements without regard to their point of origin.

Clinical decision support Filtered expert information used to guide decisions for clinical care.

Clinical information analyst Person who synthesizes data and interprets its relationship to clinical interventions.

Clinical information systems (CIS) Large computerized database management systems used to access the patient data that are needed to plan, implement, and evaluate care. May also be known as patient care information systems.

Clinical liaisons Clinicians who represent the interests and needs of information system users.

Clinical pathway Suggested blueprint for patient care by diagnosis that includes specific interventions, desired outcomes, and even the projected length of stay of inpatient treatment.

Cold site Company that maintains electronic records and backup media in secure, climate-controlled storage so that information can be used to restore system capability in the event that information and/or system functionality have been lost.

Commission on Accreditation of Rehabilitation Facilities (CARF) Healthcare accrediting body with focus on the improvement of rehabilitative services to people with disabilities and others in need of rehabilitation.

Community Health Information Network (CHIN) Organization that electronically links providers, payers, and purchasers of care for the exchange of financial, clinical, and administrative information via a wide area network in a particular geographic area. Precursor to RHIOs.

Compact discs (CDs) Older form of secondary storage.

Computational nursing Branch of nurmetrics that uses models and simulation to apply existing theory and numerical methods to new solutions for nursing problems.

Computer Electronic device that collects, processes, stores, retrieves, and provides information output under the direction of stored sequences of instructions known as computer programs.

Computer-assisted instruction (CAI) Use of a computer to organize and present instruction primarily for use by an individual learner.

Computer-based patient record (CPR) Automated patient record designed to enhance and support patient care through availability of complete and accurate data as well as bodies of knowledge and other aids to care providers.

Computer-based patient record system (CPRS) People, data, rules and procedures, and computer and communications equipment and support facilities that provide the mechanism by which patient records are created, used, stored, and retrieved.

Computer forensics Collection of electronic evidence for purposes of litigation and internal investigations.

Computer literacy Familiarity with the use of computers, including software tools such as word processing, spreadsheets, databases, presentation graphics, and e-mail.

Computer physician (or provider/prescriber) order entry (CPOE) Process by which the physician or provider directly enters orders for patient care into a hospital information system.

Computer viruses Malicious programs spread via computers that can disrupt or destroy data.

Computer vision syndrome (CVS) Eye and vision problems that result from work done in close proximity such as computer work.

Confidentiality Tacit understanding that private information shared in a situation in which a relationship has been established for the purpose of treatment or delivery of services will remain protected.

Connectivity Process that allows individual users to communicate and share hardware, software, and information using technology such as modems and the Internet.

Consent Process by which an individual authorizes healthcare personnel to process his or her information based on an informed understanding of how this information will be used.

Consumer health informatics Use of electronic information and communication to improve medical outcomes and healthcare decision making from the patient/consumer perspective.

Contingency planning The process of ensuring the continuation of critical business services regardless of any event that may occur.

Continuity planning Essential component of strategic planning designed to maintain business operations.

Control Unit Manages instructions to other parts of the computer, including input and output devices.

Critical Pathway Approach used in automated nursing information systems for designing screens, generating reminders, and providing guideline interventions and documentation.

Current Procedural Terminology (CPT–4) Classification system that lists medical services and procedures performed by physicians and is used for physician billing and payer reimbursement.

Cybercrime Commonly refers to the ability to steal personal information stored on computers such as Social Security numbers.

Data Collection of numbers, characters, or facts that are gathered according to some perceived need for analysis and possibly action at a later point in time.

Database File structure that supports the storage of data in an organized fashion and allows data retrieval as meaningful information.

Database administrator (DBA) Person responsible for overseeing all activities related to maintaining a database and optimizing its use.

Data cleansing Use of software to improve the quality of data to ensure that it is accurate enough for use in data mining and warehousing.

Data collection tool Device created for the purpose of accumulating specific details in an organized fashion.

Data dictionary Tool that defines terms used in a system to ensure consistent understanding and application among all users in the institution. This process may also be achieved through the use of an interface engine.

Data exchange standards Set of agreed-on rules that permit the uniform capture and exchange of data between information systems from different vendors and between different healthcare providers.

Data integrity Ability to collect, store, and retrieve correct, complete, and current data so that the data are available to authorized users when needed.

Data management Process of controlling the storage, retrieval, and use of data to optimize accuracy and utility while safeguarding integrity.

Data mining Technique that looks for hidden patterns and relationships in large groups of data using software.

Data retrieval Process that allows the user to access previously collected and stored data.

Data scrubbing Same as data cleansing.

Data warehouse Provides a powerful method of managing and analyzing data.

Decision-support software Computer programs that organize information to aid choices related to patient care or administrative issues.

Desktop videoconferencing (DTV) Real-time encounter that uses a specially equipped personal computer with an Internet connection to allow face-to-face meetings or simultaneous viewing of the same images.

Digital cameras Means to capture and input still images without film.

Digital Image Communication in Medicine (DICOM) Standard that promotes the communication, storage, and integration of digital images with hospital information systems.

Digital Subscriber Line (DSL) Type of Internet service available over telephone lines that offers greater speed and better connectivity than dial-up service.

Digital Versatile or **Video Discs (DVDs)** Secondary storage device.

Disaster planning Organized approach that anticipates potential problems, maintains security of client information under adverse conditions, and provides an alternative means to support the retrieval and processing of data in the event that the information system fails.

Disease management Multidisciplinary approach to identify patient populations with, or at risk for, specific medical conditions.

Distance learning Use of print, audio, video, computer, or teleconference capability to connect faculty and students who are located at a minimum of two different sites.

Distributed processing Use of a group of independent processors that contain the same information but may be at different sites as a means to maintain information services in the event of a power outage or other disaster.

Document imaging Scanning paper records for conversion to digital files for electronic storage and handling.

Downtime Period of time when an information system is not operational or available for use.

DSL modem Digital Subscriber Line modem.

E-business Refers to services, sales, and business conducted over the Internet.

E-care Broad term used to refer to the automation of all parts of the care delivery process across administrative, clinical, and departmental boundaries.

E-health Wide range of healthcare activities involving the electronic transfer of health-related information on the Internet.

E-learning The delivery of content and stimulation of learning primarily through the use of online telecommunication technologies such as blogs, podcasts, streamed video recorded videos, e-mail, bulletin board systems, electronic whiteboards, inter-relay chat, desktop video conferencing, and the World Wide Web.

Electronic communication Exchange of information through the use of computer equipment and software.

Electronic data interchange (EDI) Communication of data in binary code from one computer to another.

Electronic health record (EHR) Digital version of patient data found in the traditional paper record.

Electronic mail (e-mail) Use of computers to transmit messages to one or more persons. Delivery is almost instant, and attachment files may accompany text messages.

Electronic mail (e-mail) software Computer program that assists the user in sending, receiving, and managing e-mail messages.

Electronic medical record (EMR) Legal record created in hospitals and ambulatory settings of a single encounter or visit that is the source of data for the electronic health record.

Electronic performance support system (EPSS) An application designed to run at the same time as other applications that may supply information, present job aids, or deliver just-in-time training.

Electronic signature Means to authenticate a computer-generated document through a code or digital signature that is unique to each authorized system user.

Encryption Process that uses mathematical formulas to code messages when content needs to be kept secure and confidential.

E-prescribing Electronic transmission of drug prescriptions.

Ergonomics Scientific study of work and space, including details that impact productivity and health.

Error message Computer-generated text that warns the user when entries are missing or improperly constructed for processing. May appear on the monitor screen as data are entered or later via a paper printout.

Evidence-based practice Process by which nurses and other healthcare practitioners use the best available research evidence, clinical expertise, and patient preferences to make clinical decisions.

Expert systems Use of computer artificial intelligence to arrive at a decision that experts in the field would make.

External environment Includes those interested parties and competitors who are outside the healthcare institution.

Extranet Network outside the protected internal network of an organization that uses Internet software and communication protocols for electronic commerce and use by suppliers or customers.

Fax modem Allows computers to transmit images of letters and drawings over telephone lines.

Feature creep Uncontrolled addition of features or functions without regard to timelines or budget.

File Collection of related data stored and handled as a single entity by the computer.

File deletion software Overwrites files with meaningless information so that sensitive information cannot be accessed.

File Transfer Protocol (FTP) Set of instructions that controls both the physical transfer of data across a network and its appearance on the receiving end.

Firewall Type of gateway designed to protect private network resources from outside hackers, network damage, and theft or misuse of information.

Floppy drives Largely obsolete form of a secondary storage device.

Frames per second (FPS) Number of still images captured, transmitted, and displayed in one second of time in a video transmission. The higher the FPS, the smoother the picture. Also referred to as *frame rate*.

Freezing Situation in which a computer will not accept further input and does not process what has already been entered.

Frequently asked questions (FAQ) Document or file, used by many World Wide Web sites, that serves to introduce the group or topic, update new users on recent discussions, and eliminate repetition of questions.

Function Task that may be performed manually or automated.

Gateway Combination of hardware and software used to connect local area networks with larger networks.

Gigahertz Represents 1 billion cycles per second in processor speed.

Goal Open-ended statement that describes what is to be accomplished in general terms, often used in the strategic planning process.

Go-live Date when an information system is first used, or the process of starting to use an information system.

Grand rounds Traditional teaching tool for healthcare professionals in training that involves reviewing a client's case history and present condition inclusive of examination findings before a mutual determination of the best treatment options.

Graphical user interface (GUI) A set of menus, windows, and other standard screen devices that are intended to make using a computer as intuitive as possible.

Hard disk drive Provides storage for digital data.

Hardware Physical components of a computer.

Header Section at the top of an electronic mail message that tells who sent the message, when, to whom and at what location, and the address to which a reply should be directed if different from the sender's address.

Healthcare Information Exchange (HIE) Sharing of patient information such as demographic data, allergies, presenting complaint, diagnostic test values, and other relevant data between providers such as primary physicians, specialists, hospitals, and ambulatory care settings.

Healthcare information system (HIS) Computer hardware and software dedicated to the collection, storage, processing, retrieval, and communication of patient care information in a healthcare organization.

Healthcare information system analyst Person responsible for translating user needs into healthcare information system capability.

Health Insurance Portability and Accountability Act (HIPAA) Also known as the Kennedy–Kassebaum Bill, it is the first federal legislation to protect automatic client records.

Health Level 7 (HL7) Standard for the exchange of clinical data between information systems by means of an extensive set of rules that apply to all data sent.

Help desk First line of user support within an organization. Support service, rather than a specific location, for computer users, often available 24 hours a day by calling a special telephone number. Help desk staff have an information system or computer background and are familiar with all of the software applications and hardware in use.

Helper program Computer application that supports a browser by providing added functionality and performs specific tasks.

High density optical disc format (HD-DVD) Secondary storage device.

Help screens Computer messages displayed on the monitor screen in response to a user's request for assistance by pressing an identified key, or in response to an inappropriate entry by the user. Help screens provide specific directions that the user may follow to reach a desired outcome.

Homegrown software Developed by the consumer to meet specific needs usually because no suitable commercial package is available.

Home page First page seen at a particular Web location.

Hospital information system (HIS) Group of information systems used within a hospital or enterprise that support and enhance patient care. The HIS consists of two major types of information systems: clinical and administrative.

Hot site Facility located at a location separate from that of the healthcare provider and which replicates the provider's information systems for the purpose of quickly restoring information system function in the event of a disaster or disruption to services.

HyperText Markup Language (HTML) Language or set of instructions that is frequently used to write home pages for the Internet, and includes text as well as special instructions known as tags for the display of text and other media. HTML also includes highlighted references to other documents that the user may choose if additional information about that topic is desired.

Hypertext Transfer Protocol (HTTP) Transfer protocol used on Internet pages that establishes a TCP/IP connection between the client and server and sends a request in the form of a command when a link or hypertext is clicked with the mouse.

ID management Administrative area that deals with identifying individuals in a system and controlling their access to resources.

Informatics Science and art of turning data into information.

Informatics Nurse A nurse with advanced preparation in information management.

Informatics Nurse Specialist (INS) A nurse who has educational preparation to conduct informatics research and generate informatics theory.

Information Collection of data that have been interpreted and examined for patterns and structure.

Information literacy Ability to recognize when information is needed as well as the skills to find, evaluate, and use needed information effectively.

Information privacy Right to choose the conditions and the extent to which information and beliefs are shared with others. Informed consent for the release of medical records represents the application of information privacy.

Information security Protection of confidential information against threats to its integrity or inadvertent disclosure.

Information system Computer system that uses hardware and software to process data into information in order to solve a problem.

Information system security Protection of information systems and the information housed on them from unauthorized use or threats to integrity.

Information technology General term that refers to the management and processing of information with the assistance of computers.

Input devices Hardware that allows the user to put data into the computer, such as the keyboard, mouse, track ball, touch screen, light pen, microphone, barcode reader, Fax/modem card, joystick, and scanner.

Instant messaging (IM) Text-based real-time communication characterized by abbreviations that occurs via computers, cell phones, or other mobile devices.

Integrated services digital network (ISDN) High-speed data transmission technology that allows simultaneous, digital transfer of voice, video, and data over telephone lines but at higher speeds than available via dial-up or DSL connections.

Integrated video disk (IVD) Outdated technology that combined the interactivity, information management, and decision-making capability of computers with audiovisual capabilities of videodisk or tape to enhance computer learning.

Integration Process by which different information systems are able to exchange data in a fashion that is seamless to the end user.

Interface Computer program that tells two different systems how to exchange data.

Interface engine Software application that allows different computer systems to access and exchange information.

Internal environment Includes employees of the institution, as well as physicians and members of the board of directors.

International Classification for Nursing Practice (ICNP®) A system that serves to unify various approved nursing languages and classification systems to ensure the acceptance of common meanings across different settings.

International Classification of Disease (ICD–9/ICD–10) System for classification of surgical, diagnostic, and therapeutic procedures.

International standard H.320 Standard for passing audio and video data streams across networks, allowing videoconferencing systems from different manufacturers to communicate.

Internet Worldwide network that connects millions of computers linking governments, university and commercial institutions, and individual users.

Internet relay chat (IRC) Predominantly text-based, interactive form of communication available via the Internet.

Internet service provider (ISP) Company that furnishes Internet access for a fee.

Interoperability The ability of two entities, human or machine, to exchange and predictably use data or information while retaining the original meaning of that data.

Intranet Private computer network that uses Internet protocols and technologies, including Web browsers, servers, and languages, to facilitate collaborative data sharing.

JAVA Programming language that enables the display of moving text, animation, and musical excerpts on Web pages.

Jobs aids Written instructions designed as a reference in training and work settings.

Joint Photographic Experts Group Compression (JPEG) Standard for the compression of digital images for transmission and storage that is also used for diagnostic images.

Joystick Allows the user to control the movement of objects on the screen.

Keyboards Input devices with keys that represent those of a typewriter.

Kilobits (kbps) Data transfer in thousands of bits per second.

Knowledge Synthesis of information derived from several sources to produce a single concept or idea.

Knowledge discovery in databases Extraction of implicit, unknown, and potentially useful information from data.

Knowledge management Structured process for the generation, storage, distribution, and application of both tacit knowledge (personal experience) and explicit knowledge (evidence).

Laboratory Information Systems (LIS) Computer system for use by laboratories that provides many benefits as a result of automated order entry.

Laptop computer Streamlined, portable version of the personal computer.

Learning aids Materials intended to supplement or reinforce lecture or computer-based training. Examples may consist of outlines, diagrams, charts, and maps.

Legacy systems Mainframe vendor-based information systems.

Life cycle Well-defined process that describes the recurring process of developing and maintaining an information system.

Links Also known as hypertext, links are words, phrases, or images used on Internet pages distinguished from the remainder of the document through the use of highlighting or a different screen color that allow users to skip from point to point within or among documents, escaping conventional linear format.

Liquid Crystal Display (LCD) Technology that uses two sheets of polarizing material with a liquid crystal solution between them with each crystal either allowing light to pass through or blocking the light to display text or an image.

Listserv E-mail subscription list program that copies and distributes all e-mail messages to everyone who is a subscriber.

Live data Actual patient and healthcare system.

Local area networks Computers, printers, and other devices linked together to share resources and data within a defined area.

Macintosh computers (Macs) Computers developed by the Apple corporation, said to be very user friendly.

Magnetic tape drive Secondary storage device used primarily with large mainframe computers.

Mainframes Large computers capable of processing large amounts of data quickly.

Main Memory Component of memory that is permanent and remains when power is off. Also known as read only memory (ROM).

Malware Term used to refer to destructive computer programs including viruses, worms, and Trojan Horses.

Mapping Process by which the definition of terms used in one information system are associated with comparable terms in another system, thereby facilitating the exchange of information from one system to another.

Master patient index (MPI) Database that lists all identifiers used in connection with one particular client in a healthcare alliance. Identifiers may include items such as Social Security number, birth date, and name.

Medical informatics Application of informatics to all of the healthcare disciplines as well as the practice of medicine.

Megahertz One megahertz represents 1 million signal voltage cycles per second in processor speed.

Memory Computer storage device in which programs reside during execution. It comprises main memory and random access memory.

Menu List of related commands that can be selected from a computer screen to accomplish a task.

Metadata Set of data that provides information about how, when, and by whom data are collected, formatted, and stored.

Microcomputer Personal computer that is either a stand-alone machine or is networked to other personal computers.

Microprocessor chip Electronic circuits of the CPU etched onto a silicon chip.

Minicomputer Scaled-down version of a mainframe.

Mission Purpose or reason for an organization's existence, representing the fundamental and unique aspirations that differentiate it from others.

m-learning Popular term that denotes the use of mobile technologies, such as the mobile phone, personal digital assistant (PDA), and iPod for learning purposes.

Mobile computing Devices that can be carried or wheeled from one location to another, often with the capability to transmit and receive information.

Modem Communication device that transmits data over telephone lines from one computer to another.

Monitor Screen that displays text and graphic images.

Monitoring systems Devices that automatically monitor biometrics measurements in critical care and specialty areas.

Motherboard Microprocessor chip that contains the electronic circuits of the CPU etched on a silicon chip, mounted on a board.

Mouse Device that can be moved around on the desktop to direct a pointer on the screen.

Multimedia Presentations that combine text, voice, or sound, and still or video images, as well as hardware and software that support the same.

Multiple function devices Combine functions such as printing, scanning, copying, and Fax.

The Net An alternate term to refer to the Internet, a worldwide network that connects millions of computers and serves to link government, university, commercial institutions, and individual users.

Netiquette Set of informal rules for polite communication via electronic means.

Network Combination of hardware and software that allows communication and electronic transfer of information between computers.

Network interface card Provides a physical connection between a computer and network.

News reader software Special browser program needed by individual users to read messages posted on the news group.

Notebook computer Streamlined portable version of the personal computer.

Nurmetrics Branch of nursing science that uses mathematics and statistics to test, estimate, and quantify nursing theories and solutions to problems.

Nursing informatics Use of information and computer technology to support all aspects of nursing practice.

Nursing information system Information system that supports the use and documentation of nursing processes and provides tools for managing the delivery of nursing care.

Nursing Minimum Data Set (NMDS) Consistent collection of data comprising nursing diagnosis, interventions, and outcomes that attempts to collect data that are comparable across different healthcare settings, to project trends, and to stimulate research.

Objective Statement that describes how a goal will be accomplished and the timeframe for this activity.

Offline storage Form of data storage that uses secondary storage devices for data that are needed less frequently, or for long-term data storage.

Off-the-shelf software Commercially available software in which someone else bore the cost for its development and testing.

Online Term indicating a connection to various computer resources, including information systems, the Internet, and the World Wide Web.

Online storage Form of data storage that provides access to current data. An example is a high-speed, hard disk drive.

Online tutorials Detailed instructions available to a user while he or she is using a computer, software application, or information system that show or tell how a particular software application or feature can be implemented.

Open architecture Protocols and technology that follow publicly accepted conventions and are employed by multiple vendors, so that various system components can work together.

Open system See *open architecture.*

Operating system Collection of programs that manage all of the computer's activities.

Optical disk drives They write data to a recording surface media and read it later.

Order entry systems Method by which physician's orders for medications and treatments are entered into the computer and directly transmitted to appropriate areas.

Output devices Hardware that allows the user to see processed data. Terminals or video monitor screens, printers, speakers, and Fax/modem boards are types of output devices.

Outsourcing Process in which an organization contracts with outside agencies for services.

Password Alphanumeric code required for access and use of some computers or information systems as a security measure against unauthorized use. Password does not appear on the monitor display when it is keyed in.

PC specialist Person who provides information and training on computers and software.

Peripheral Any piece of hardware attached to a computer.

Peripheral device interface cards Provide connection between equipment such as printers to the computer for the exchange of information.

Personal computer (PCs) Known as desktop computers. This category provides inexpensive processing power for an individual user.

Personal Computer Memory Card International Association (PCMCIA) card Provide added functionality such as memory to computers.

Personal digital assistants (PDAs) Specialized handheld devices used for calendar and address book functions, access to reference materials, and some input and transmission capabilities.

Personal Health Record (PHR) Lifelong tool for managing health information such as disease conditions, allergies, medications, past surgeries, and other relevant information.

Phishing Ruse to get consumers to divulge personal information through social engineering and technical subterfuge via the use of electronic communication.

Picture archiving communications systems (PACS) Storage systems that permit remote access to diagnostic images at times convenient to the physician.

Plug-in programs Computer applications that have been designed to support browsers by performing specific tasks.

Point-of-care devices Computer access at the actual worksite, which in the delivery of healthcare is at the patient's bedside.

Point-to-point interface Interface that directly connects two information systems.

Portal Websites that may require registration, collect information from the user, and offer personalized features for individual users.

Printer Produces a paper copy of computer generated documents.

Privacy Freedom from intrusion or control over the exposure of self or personal information.

Production environment Point at which a planned information system is actually used to process and retrieve information and support the delivery of services.

Program Set of instructions that tell the computer what to do.

Programmers Persons who write the instructions that tell the computer what to do.

Programming languages Set of rules to create the instructions that direct computers to perform specific functions.

Project scope Defines the size and details of an effort.

Public key infrastructure (PKI) Provides a unique code for each user that is embedded into a storage device.

Qubit Measurement similar to the bit except that it allows for a superposition of both 1 and 0.

Radiology information system (RIS) Provides scheduling of diagnostic tests, communication of patient information, generation of patient instructions and preparation procedures, and file room management.

Random access memory (RAM) Component of memory that can be accessed, used, changed, and rewritten repeatedly while the computer is turned on.

Read-only memory (ROM) Component of memory that contains startup instructions for each time the computer is turned on. ROM is permanent and remains when power is off.

Real-time processing Entry and access to information occurs almost as soon as it is provided.

Redundant array of independent disks (RAID) Duplicate disks with mirror copies of data.

Refresh rate Term used to refer to the speed with which the screen is repainted from top to bottom.

Regional Health Information Organizations (RHIOs) Regional exchange of health and treatment information of patients among healthcare organizations and providers for the collective good.

Relational database Type of database that relies upon the use of tables to represent data.

Remote access Ability to use the resources contained on a network, or an information system, from a location outside of the facility where it is physically located.

Remote backup service (RBS) Company that provides backup services for customers from an off-site location to an on-site location.

Repetitive motion disorders See *repetitive stress injuries (RSIs)*.

Repetitive stress injuries (RSIs) Results from using the same muscle groups over and over again without rest.

Request for Information (RFI) A document sent to vendors that explains the institution's plans for purchasing and installing an information system with the goal of determining which vendors can meet the organization's basic requirements.

Request for Proposal (RFP) Document sent to vendors detailing the requirements of a potential information system with the purpose of soliciting proposals from vendors that describe their capabilities to meet these requirements.

Request for Quote (RFQ) Statement of need that focuses upon pricing, service levels, and contract terms.

Resolution Term used to refer to the sharpness, or clarity, of an image on a computer monitor. Resolution itself is determined by the number of pixels, or tiny dots or squares, displayed per inch on a monitor screen.

Response time Amount of time between a user action and the response from the information system.

Roll out Staggered, or rolling, system implementation, sometimes refers to the preceding marketing campaign as well.

Rule Predefined function that generates a clinical alert or reminder.

Sabotage Intentional destruction of computer equipment or records to disrupt services.

Scan The gathering of information from external and internal environments.

Scanner Input device that converts printed pages or graphic images into a file.

Scope Statement in an organization's mission that defines the type of activities and services that it will perform.

Scope creep Unexpected and uncontrolled growth of user expectations as a project progresses.

Search engines Tool to help users find information on the World Wide Web. Each search engine maintains its own index or list of information on the Web and uses its own method of organizing topics.

Search engine unifier Programs that search servers and databases, such as the World Wide Web, and can shorten search time by looking at several search engines at one time, often yielding more comprehensive data in less time.

Search indexes Automated programs that search the Web when general information is requested.

Secondary storage Form of computer memory that retains data even when the computer is turned off. Examples include hard drives, CDs, DVDs, redundant array of inexpensive disks (RAID), optical disks, and magnetic disks or tape.

Serial Line Internet Protocol (SLIP) Protocol that allows passage of data through communication lines and is used to access the Internet and World Wide Web.

Server Any type of computer that stores files.

Site license Agreement between the computer lab and the software publisher on the terms of use.

Smart card Storage device for patient information that resembles a plastic credit card. The card is kept by the client and presented to healthcare providers when services are rendered, eliminating redundant data entry and the need to store this information on a network.

Software Computer programs, or stored sequences of instructions to the computer.

Software shredder Set of computer programs that prevent recovery of deleted, or discarded, computer files by writing meaningless information over them.

Spam Unwanted or "junk" mail.

SPIM Unsolicited messages often containing a link to a Website that attempts to extract personal information.

Spyware Data collection mechanism that installs itself without the user's permission during Web browsing or downloading software.

Spyware Detection Software Special software that can detect and eliminate spyware.

Standardized Nursing Languages (SNLs) Common set of terms that have been reviewed and accepted by the American Nurses Association.

Strategic planning Development of a comprehensive, long-range plan for guiding the activities and operations of an organization.

Strategy Comprehensive plan used by an organization that states how its mission, goals, and objectives will be achieved.

Structured data Data that follow a prescribed format, often presented as discrete data elements.

Supercomputers Largest, most expensive type of computers. They are complex systems that can perform billions of instructions every second.

Superuser Staff person who has become proficient in the use of the system and mentors others.

Survivability Capability of a system as a whole to fulfill its mission, in a timely manner, in the presence of attacks, failures, or accidents.

Switched multimegabit data service (SMDS) High-speed data transmission service that uses telephone lines, also known as a T1 line. SMDS is faster than ISDN but slower than ATM.

System check Mechanism provided by a computer system to assist users by prompting them to complete a task, verify information, or prevent entry of inappropriate information.

Systemized Nomenclature of Human and Veterinary Medicine (SNOMED) Classification system that includes signs and symptoms of disease, diagnoses, and procedures for the integration of all medical information in an electronic medical record.

T1 lines High-speed telephone lines that may be used to transmit high-quality, full-motion video at speeds up to 1.544 Mbps.

Tablet PC Smaller version of a notebook computer but can be carried like a clipboard that accepts text input via a stylet.

Tape drive Copies files from the computer to magnetic tape for storage or transfer to another machine.

Technical criteria Hardware and software requirements needed to attain a desired level of overall computer or information system performance.

Teleconferencing Use of computers, audio and video equipment, and communication links to provide interaction between two or more persons at two or more sites.

Telehealth Provision of information to healthcare providers and consumers and the delivery of services to clients at remote sites through the use of telecommunication and computer technology.

Telemedicine Use of telecommunication technologies and computers to provide medical information and services to clients at another site.

Telenursing Use of telecommunications and computer technology for the delivery of nursing care to clients at another location.

Terminal Monitor screen and a keyboard once used to input data and receive output from a mainframe computer, now rarely seen.

Test environment Separate software program like that used for the actual application or information system, which permits trial of programming changes prior to their implementation in the actual system, thereby protecting the "real" system from unwanted alterations.

Thin client technology Computing model that allows PCs to connect to a server using a highly efficient network connection.

TIGER Initiative Plan to promote informatics competencies among nurses in order to transform healthcare.

Touchpad Pressure and motion sensitive surface.

Trackball Contains a ball that the user rolls to move the on-screen pointer.

Training Common term used to refer to the introduction of information system skills to workers.

Training environment Separate software application that mirrors the actual information system but permits learners to practice skills without harm to the system or data contained in it. Makes use of fictitious clients and scenarios for instruction and practice.

Training hospital Collection of simulated, or fictitious, client data assembled and stored in a database separate from the actual information system for the purposes of instruction and practice. Incorporates most, if not all, features available on the actual information system.

Training plan Organized approach for the delivery of instruction that should include a philosophy; identification of instructional needs, approaches, and persons responsible for instructional design and delivery; a target date for completion; a budget; and methods for evaluation.

Unified Medical Language System Attempt to standardize terms used in healthcare delivery.

Unified Nursing Language System Attempt to standardize and link nursing databases as a means to extend nursing knowledge.

Uniform Hospital Data Set (UHDS) Most commonly used data set in the United States, even though it does not include data on nursing care and outcomes.

Uniform resource locator (URL) String of characters providing an address that identifies a document's World Wide Web location and the type of server it resides on.

Unique patient identifier Single, universal identifier for client health information that ensures availability of all data associated with a particular client.

Unstructured data Data that do not follow a prescribed format such as that seen in narrative notes.

USB flash drives Small portable storage devices that can be plugged into a computer, and then unplugged and transported.

Usenet news groups Popular Internet feature similar to listservs in content and diversity, with each newsgroup dedicated to a different topic, providing a forum where any user can post messages for discussion and reply.

User class Group of individuals who perform similar functions, and for the purpose of information system training and use, require instruction in how to access and use the same set of system features.

User interface What the user sees when interacting with a computer.

Utility programs Special applications designed to optimize computer operation and control of resident data.

Vendor Company or corporation that designs, develops, sells, and/or supports a product, which in the context of this book is generally a computer, peripheral device, and, more often, an entire information system.

Videoconferencing Face-to-face meeting of persons at separate locations through the use of telecommunications and computer technology.

Virtual Learning Environment (VLE) A system that uses the Internet to assist the educator in developing, managing, and administering educational materials for students.

Virus Malicious program that can disrupt or destroy data.

Web 2.0 An approach to Web design and development that seeks to foster creativity and collaboration through a variety of services such as blogs, wikis, and social networking sites.

Web-based instruction (WBI) Uses the attributes and resources of the World Wide Web, such as hypertext links and multimedia, for educational purposes.

Webcam Small camera used by a computer to send images over the Internet.

Webcast Format that allows multiple learners to access a Website.

Webmaster Person responsible for creating and maintaining a World Wide Web site.

Wide area networks (WANs) Large expansive network systems.

Wiki A type of Web page that allows collaborative contributions such as Wikipedia.

Wireless devices Provide the capability to receive and broadcast signals while in transit, sometimes referred to as *mobile computing*.

Wireless modem Communication device that sends and receives information via access points provided with a subscription to wireless service.

Wisdom Application of knowledge to manage and solve problems.

Work breakdown structure (WBS) Plan to develop the project timelines or schedule a hierarchical arrangement of all specific tasks by using project-planning software.

World Wide Web (WWW) Information service for access to Internet resources by content instead of file names via a graphical user interface (GUI) that supports text, images, sound, and links to documents.

Zip drive Now obsolete form of a high-capacity floppy disk drive.

Index